Rationing and Resource Allocation in Healthcare

Rationing and Resource Allocation in Healthcare

Essential Readings

Edited by

Ezekiel Emanuel, MD, PhD

Andrew Steinmetz, BA

Harald Schmidt, MD, PhD

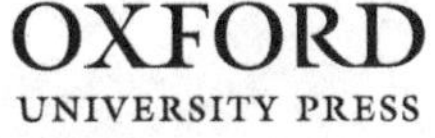

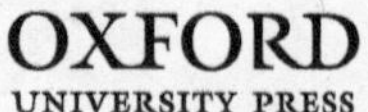

Oxford University Press is a department of the University of Oxford. It furthers the University's objective of excellence in research, scholarship, and education by publishing worldwide. Oxford is a registered trade mark of Oxford University Press in the UK and certain other countries.

Published in the United States of America by Oxford University Press
198 Madison Avenue, New York, NY 10016, United States of America.

Library of Congress Cataloging-in-Publication Data
Names: Emanuel, Ezekiel, 1957– editor.
Title: Rationing and resource allocation in healthcare /
edited by Ezekiel Emanuel, M.D., Ph.D., Andrew Steinmetz, B.A., Harald Schmidt, M.A., Ph.D.
Description: New York : Oxford University Press, 2018. |
Includes bibliographical references and index.
Identifiers: LCCN 2017051754| ISBN 9780190200756 (pbk.) | ISBN 9780190200763 (hardcover)
Subjects: LCSH: Medical ethics. | Health care rationing. | Health facilities—Moral and ethical aspects.
Classification: LCC R724 .R37 2018 | DDC 362.1068/1—dc23
LC record available at https://lccn.loc.gov/2017051754

9 8 7 6 5 4 3 2 1
Paperback printed by Webcom, Inc., Canada
Hardback printed by Bridgeport National Bindery, Inc., United States of America

Contents

1

The Ethics of Rationing, Resource Allocation, and Priority Setting

Introduction

Maria is an attending physician in an intensive care unit (ICU) ward with 12 beds. On an otherwise quiet Sunday afternoon she receives a call from the Emergency Room: Could they send up Patient A, a 29-year-old fireman with a chronic obstructive pulmonary disease (COPD) flare requiring mechanical ventilation? Eleven of the ICU patients urgently require mechanical ventilation and would be certain to die if disconnected. Patient B, in the twelfth bed, is a 54-year-old woman. She is an accomplished single woman, a concert pianist, and a heavy smoker, and she was extubated after a COPD flare 5 hours earlier. She would typically receive 24 hours active follow-up monitoring. As it happens, the fireman is known to Maria personally, and she is aware that he is a caring father of two children aged 3 and 6. Should Maria transfer the smoking single pianist to a non-ICU setting to make place for the fireman with children?

Herman is newly diagnosed with early-stage prostate cancer. Unfortunately, the tumor is somewhat large, about 3 cm, but of a middling Gleason score—a measure of how deranged or malignant the tumor cells appear microscopically—of 5. Fortunately, the cancer has not spread beyond the prostate. Herman's oncologist has delineated his treatment options. These chiefly comprise active surveillance, in which he gets no additional treatment but is carefully followed for possible recurrence; surgical resection of the prostate; and several different kinds of radiation treatments, such as intensity modulated radiotherapy (IMRT) and proton beam therapy. Herman has a friend who had proton beam therapy, and he thinks it is the treatment he wants. However, his insurance company refuses to cover it. Herman is mad. He cannot afford to pay for proton beam out of pocket. On the phone to the insurance company, he screams "You are rationing care! Your rationing decision is going to kill me!"

Is the insurance company rationing Herman's care? Is it acting unethically? On what basis can the insurance company even make this decision not to pay for proton beam therapy? Shouldn't the decision about what treatment to get be made by patients and physicians, instead of insurance companies? These and a vast range of further cases raise a host of complex conceptual, empirical, and terminological issues.

Different words and phrases sometimes mean the same thing. "The evening star" refers to the same object as "the morning star": Venus. This can be confusing: When exactly should you use which term? Moreover, terms are frequently used inaccurately. In this case, Venus is actually a planet, and not a star at all. Mostly, however, different words and phrases mean different things, and the rules that guide their use are such that different expressions illuminate, rather than lead to confusion. One of the central aims of this anthology is to promote clarity and lucid analytic thinking about three fundamental—yet frequently conflated and confused—terms relating to who gets access to what healthcare services. These terms are: *rationing, resource allocation*, and *priority setting*.

The three terms are often used interchangeably, as if they mean the same thing. But it is also common for two people to use the same term but differ in their understanding of it. In part, this lack of clarity has to do with conceptual and ethical difficulties around deciding "who gets what" in healthcare policy and practice. In part it is also to do with the fact these decisions are emotionally and politically charged. Thus, people can use terms in the interest of scoring debating or political points, rather than to be precise and promote rigorous ethical analysis and reasoning. Words can be powerful weapons in shaping the direction of heated debates—often fueled and exacerbated by media coverage that thrives on overdramatized narratives.

Opponents of any form of prioritization typically prefer the term "rationing." Rationing has a negative valence. It has strong connotations of heartless, mechanistic withholding of desirable goods or services by faceless bureaucrats. This effect can prompt the perception that all prioritizations are inherently bad. Consequently, those interested in reasonable discussion about when and under what conditions it might be appropriate to regulate access to healthcare interventions and services often prefer either "resource allocation" or "priority setting." These terms have far fewer negative connotations. In addition to deliberate strategic uses of terminology, there are also various technical characterizations. But none has managed to command universal agreement.

Despite the terminological disagreement, there is, however, agreement that decisions about access to healthcare arise in two distinct types of scarcity: absolute and relative. We seek to clarify the general terminological confusion by using the following definitions that also guide the overall structure of this anthology. *Rationing* should only refer to cases of absolute scarcity. *Resource allocation* should be reserved for situations involving relative scarcity. *Priority setting* is best understood as an overarching umbrella term, denoting the activity of regulating access to beneficial interventions or services in situations of either absolute or relative scarcity.

Rationing is concerned with problems such as how to distribute strictly limited numbers of beds in ICUs, organs for transplantation, or vaccines in a pandemic. Cases of absolute scarcity entail a situation in which demand for resources outstrips supply, and the supply is inherently limited by nature or by the ability to manufacture a product. For instance, there are simply insufficient numbers of livers for transplantation for all the people with chronic liver failure who will die without one. The central ethical issues in situations of absolute scarcity focus on selecting those people in need who will receive medical interventions when not all people who could benefit from an intervention can have access. What criteria should guide choosing the beneficiaries? Which of two desperately ill patients should get the last available ICU bed? Should age matter if we need to choose between 21-year-old Melissa and 62-year-old Felix for the donor liver? Should healthcare workers be prioritized in receiving vaccines during a pandemic? Or should access to vaccines be determined through a lottery, giving everyone—regardless of age, location, occupation, health status, prognosis, or any other characteristic—an equal chance? These are typical questions raised by the tragic but inevitable choices that must be made when there is absolute scarcity of life-saving medical resources.

Resource allocation, by contrast, is concerned with relative scarcity. Choices can be just as challenging. But they differ in nature from choices under absolute scarcity in three important ways.

First, in the case of rationing there is typically no question that what is to be distributed has value in terms of improving health. By contrast, in resource allocation, effectiveness and a clear balance of benefits over risks cannot always be taken for granted. Treatments for specific conditions frequently differ in their benefits and risks. Should payers make available any beneficial medical intervention, regardless of how much additional benefit it offers compared to already existing interventions? Determining effectiveness—and comparative effectiveness—is an inherent part of resource allocation but largely taken for granted in rationing.

Second, the types of choices policy-makers and healthcare workers make differ between rationing and resource allocation. While rationing is chiefly about choosing between people, resource allocation is focused on determining what amount of funds should be given to which patient or disease group, and—directly or indirectly—what the overall healthcare budget should be. Rationing dilemmas typically arise once resource allocation decisions have been made. Often—but not always—rationing choices cannot be eliminated through either immediate or future changes in healthcare budgets. For instance, more money will not solve the problem of too few livers for transplantation. But in resource allocation, budgets are central. For example, how much should a payer of healthcare, whether public or private, spend on neonatal care, and how much on cancer care for people in their 80s? How much for preventive and how much for curative services? How many beds should there be in the ICU and how many in the maternity ward of a hospital? Should patients have to pay for a service, such as deep sedation for a colonoscopy, that is not, strictly speaking, necessary for the procedure, or should insurers or government have to cover it as part of essential healthcare services?

Payers of healthcare are stewards of pooled financial resources—whether these resources come from insurance contributions or taxation. Payers need to ensure that money is well spent: in any case, they ought to. This then raises the question of what methods should be used to assess value within as well as across medical tests and treatments for different conditions. A number of approaches exist to assess the effectiveness, comparative effectiveness, and cost-effectiveness of interventions. But all are controversial and raise deep ethical issues that largely differ from those in rationing. Of course, to avoid these controversies, one response can simply be to provide whatever intervention has been shown to be reasonably safe and effective. But failing to consider the comparative or relative effectiveness and cost is just as much an ethical choice that requires justification. There is no neutral option.

Third, the occurrence of absolute scarcity has clear visibility and high salience. Rationing choices are as inevitable as they are undeniable: no-one disputes that absolute scarcity occurs. Resource allocation decisions are just as inevitable and just as undeniable. Yet the way payers, including governments, decide what services are covered or what cost-sharing patients will experience through copayments, out-of-pocket cost, or variations in insurance premiums, is often far less visible and salient—in fact, frequently the processes are outright opaque.[1] Moreover, the necessity of prioritizing within and across conditions is frequently denied by political leaders, vested interests, or people not inclined to appreciate the inevitable logic of opportunity cost and the fact that healthcare expenditure has an impact on the level of resources devoted to other goods and services, such as education and research. Covering ineffective interventions therefore constitutes unjustifiable waste. And spending

[1] N. Daniels, "Decisions About Access to Health Care and Accountability for Reasonableness," *Journal of Urban Health* 76, no. 2 (1999): pp. 176–191.

on low-value interventions typically affects resources available for higher value services. It is therefore irrational to ignore data on comparative effectiveness and the cost of interventions, to suggest that such considerations have no place in health policy, or to deny that resource allocation requires ethical principles and standards just as rationing does—even if these might be different principles or standards.

Overall, it is fair to say that bioethics has not effectively engaged the questions of rationing and resource allocation. There has been what might be described as mutual avoidance. Health economists and health policy experts who wrestle with rationing and resource allocation issues have often not found the contributions of bioethics particularly helpful. The laying out of the issues without proposing a way forward in terms of policy—a common approach in bioethics—often does not seem particularly insightful to many policy experts. And this can lead to an almost allergic reaction to bioethics and to the framing of rationing and resource allocation issues in ethical terms. Concomitantly, bioethics has not been particularly focused on rationing and resource allocation issues. From whence does this mutual avoidance arise?

At least in bioethics, two reinforcing movements probably account for the avoidance of deeply engaging the issues of rationing and resource allocation. First, the main bioethical principles are of limited utility. Over the past 40 years, particularly through Beauchamp and Childress's influential book, *The Principles of Biomedical Ethics*, now in its seventh edition, four principles have gained prominence as *the* principles of bioethics: autonomy, beneficence, nonmaleficence, and justice.[2] Whether in Beauchamp and Childress's delineation or whether articulated differently by others, these principles have structured bioethical reasoning while other ethical principles, such as priority to the worst-off, have been ignored or minimized. Prominence has been given to autonomy, and attention has focused on elucidating it and on how it could be fully realized in the biomedical and clinical contexts. Conversely, beneficence and nonmaleficence receive less emphasis and decidedly lose out if and when they conflict with autonomy.

Justice, as Beauchamp and Childress acknowledge, has been less well developed in bioethics. One clear emphasis has been on equality, in the sense of treating equals equally, and on nondiscrimination. This basic notion of equality is somewhat helpful—but only somewhat—in dealing with rationing and resource allocation issues. Does treating Melissa and Felix equally mean that we should not take age into account in deciding who gets the liver? Is equality at work when we treat a woman in Botswana with acetic acid and the "see-and-treat" method for cervical cancer screening when her counterpart in Paris would receive Pap cytology and HPV DNA co-testing? There has been comparatively little elucidation of justice in the context of healthcare. This is largely because to do so requires delving into and coming to some settled view on the tensions among utilitarianism, political liberalism, prioritarianism, and other theories of justice.

Second, the substantial emphasis on autonomy within bioethics naturally led to, and was itself reinforced by, the field's focus on clinical and research ethics. Autonomy became the central issue in human subjects research ethics through informed consent and, in clinical ethics, through a patient's rights to consent to treatment and to terminate life-sustaining interventions. Autonomy is an individual-focused principle. Issues of rationing and resource allocation involve populations and society and pose questions of opportunity costs for the community. As bioethics became increasingly focused on autonomy and gave it such prominence, the role and importance of sharing collective resources, fairness, and mutual responsibilities and obligations were necessarily de-emphasized.

Today, bioethics cannot ignore or marginalize rationing and resource allocation issues and

[2] T. L. Beauchamp and J. F. Childress, *Principles of Biomedical Ethics*, Seventh ed. (Oxford University Press, 2012).

still be relevant. It is not that there are no longer important questions in the areas of research or clinical ethics. There are: but the real focus in these areas is on practically implementing the insights of bioethics in the actual care of patients and conducting clinical research studies. Conversely, the challenges in healthcare have moved on to neuroethics, genetics, and priority setting.

In the Fall of 2015, the United Nations adopted the Sustainable Development Goals (SDGs), successors to the Millennium Development Goals (MDGs). A new Goal in the SDGs is dedicated to health and includes as one of its targets achieving universal health coverage (UHC). UHC was first formally endorsed by the World Health Organization in 2005, when countries were called on to provide "access to (necessary) promotive, preventive, curative and rehabilitative health interventions for all at an affordable cost."[3] As such, and as discussed in more detail in Chapters 9 and 10, UHC is generally understood to center around decisions in three key areas: how many people to cover, what services to cover, and what level of cost-sharing, if any, to implement for accessing a given set of health benefits. The SDGs will focus more of the world's attention on UHC. Crucially, decisions about the scope of UHC are not only required of countries making their first steps toward UHC. They are just as relevant for countries that have been engaged in the process for some time and for those that are considered leaders in the field. Both in countries with a long tradition of UHC and new ones, keeping healthcare costs under control is, and inevitably will continue to be, a complex struggle that necessitates addressing coverage, essential services, and cost-sharing decisions.

These are the fundamental questions of the 21st century, and they must be informed by bioethics. Similarly, for bioethics to be relevant to the challenges facing healthcare, it must address, more comprehensively than to date, rationing and resource allocation questions. This will require that bioethicists focus less on autonomy, nonmaleficence, and beneficence and more on the ethical principles related to population health including utility, priority to the worst-off, equality, and the like, and to be much more engaged in balancing or weighing these different principles.

This principal purpose of *Rationing and Resource Allocation in Healthcare* is to provide bioethicists and nonexperts in rationing and resource allocation with easy access to the main issues and arguments in a field that is highly interdisciplinary as well as heterogeneous and wide-ranging in methods and approaches. The anthology is an effort to get people who are engaged in discussions about rationing and resource allocation "up to speed" on the issues and arguments that have been made and the unanswered or poorly answered questions that remain.

The anthology is structured in three parts. Part I concerns overarching conceptual distinctions and broader ethical theory. Part II focuses on issues related to rationing, while Part III focuses on resource allocation. All chapters begin with brief introductions, followed by abridged texts that have either been particularly influential in the debate or are otherwise helpful in view of the purposes of this anthology. Each introduction ends with a set of questions for discussion and a list of additional resources and references, including relevant US and international organizations, films, and other multimedia content that further illuminate the material covered in the chapter.

In Part I, Chapter 2 expands on the proper use of the terms "rationing," "resource allocation," and "priority setting." The introduction reviews common everyday language uses of these terms and uses by organizations active in the field. It then examines alternative and largely mutually exclusive definitions that emphasize different notions as central by highlighting, for example, any activity that determines access to needed or beneficial care, denial of care due to cost reasons, the societal toleration of inequitable access to care, or regulating access through prices in a market situation.

[3] World Health Organization, *57th World Health Assembly: Sustainable Health Financing, Universal Coverage and Social Health Insurance* (Geneva: 2005).

Chapter 3 summarizes major overarching ethical theories that focus on population ethics and underpin principles and policies in both rationing and resource allocation. It begins with two of the historically most influential theories: *utilitarianism*, often understood as requiring the greatest good for the greatest number; and *deontology*, in which respect for persons is central and typically in conflict with both the theoretical foundations of utilitarianism as well as its policy implications. Both utilitarianism and deontology inform much of the current controversies in rationing and resource allocation, as does a theory known as *political liberalism*, which seeks to identify principles of justice to regulate the basic structures of modern pluralistic democratic societies. The introduction and close of the chapter include a set of theories under the umbrella concept of *luck-egalitarianism* that embody a strong principle of treating people as equals but also seek to make rationing and resource allocation decisions sensitive to the choices people make—which can entail penalizing them in different ways for having taken avoidable health risks.

Parts II and III each begin with historical overviews of rationing and resource allocation, respectively. Case studies illustrating paradigmatic issues and challenges in each area help frame the fundamental ethical considerations. In Part II, Chapter 4 explores key historical situations in which individuals and institutions were forced to distribute effective and potentially life-saving medical interventions under conditions of absolute scarcity and had to select which patients would receive them and which ones would not, facing severe illness or death as a consequence. These cases comprise triaging treatment of soldiers in war, regulating diabetes patients' access to insulin, and deciding which people suffering from severe infectious diseases should receive penicillin and which end-stage kidney failure patients should have access to dialysis.

Chapter 5 delineates ethical guidance for rationing decisions. Commentators offer a range of arguments advocating specific principles and criteria that include the likelihood of success of a procedure, prognosis in terms of extending life-expectancy and quality of life, maximizing the numbers of lives saved, personal responsibility for health needs, past or future contributions to society, prioritizing those who are sickest or youngest or oldest, and, finally, just resorting to a lottery.

Chapters 6 and 7 describe the extent to which these ethical principles play out in actual policy. Chapter 6 addresses rationing of organs for transplantation, focusing on livers. It describes how, initially, US policy was driven predominantly by time on the waiting list. This criterion was later replaced by a single measure incorporating three physiological variables that provide a predictor of a patient's risk of death while waiting for a liver transplant. Is waiting time or sickest-first the right criterion? The chapter also considers the ethics of patients being listed at several transplant centers simultaneously, the role of personal responsibility, and questions around multiple transplants that may benefit some of the worst-off patients but could also be used to benefit more than one patient instead.

Chapter 7 concerns access to vaccines in a pandemic. It traces the development of pandemic preparedness policy by the US Department of Health and Human Services that initially began by emphasizing two principles: decreasing health impacts in terms of death or severe morbidity and minimizing societal—including economic—impact. After different types of criticism that suggested moving from focusing on saving most lives to prioritizing younger people over older ones, the Department developed a new scheme.

Part III focuses on resource allocation in the context of relative scarcity and begins, in Chapter 8, with the historical context of chronic dialysis. As set out in Chapter 4, dialysis initially was a rationing problem. However, after a political intervention, the US government decided to cover dialysis for all patients through the Medicare program, generally intended for citizens over 65. Clearly, this was very good news for patients with end-stage renal failure; rationing among people with chronic renal failure was no longer necessary. The conversion of a rationing problem into a resource allocation issue, however, raises a number of questions, such as why single out dialysis?

What about hemophilia? Was the process of deciding what to prioritize fair? Are legislation and political processes appropriate for deciding which diseases to cover? The introduction goes on to trace the background conditions that led to the emergence of health technology assessment (HTA) institutions and other bodies that are concerned with systematically scrutinizing existing and novel interventions to decide whether they should be covered, given the inevitable opportunity cost. Typically, this breaks down to answering three subquestions: Can an intervention work in principle (efficacy), does it work in practice (effectiveness), and does it provide good value for the money spent (efficiency)?

Chapter 9 returns to the foundational ethical principles that are at stake in deciding which interventions to cover in a given benefit package. It focuses on the normative assumptions underlying the method of cost-effectiveness analysis (CEA) and the metric of quality adjusted life years (QALYs) that have major roles in making coverage decisions within and across interventions and disease groups. CEA's utilitarian underpinnings and salient ethical challenges are delineated. These challenges are typically based in alternative ethical theories. How should these competing views be reconciled if we need to have policy that can be acceptable to members of pluralist societies? One option is to settle, once and for all, the question of which is the right normative framework. Alternatively, one could move from striving for agreement on substantive ethical principles to agreement on fair procedures for decision-making. The most influential procedural approach is known as *accountability for reasonableness* and is described along with key criticisms.

Chapter 10 focuses more closely on the current implementation of HTA in a range of countries, including Australia, Germany, the United Kingdom, and the United States. While all face the same basic challenge of ensuring that healthcare budgets obtain value for money, these countries differ considerably in their approaches. All, except for the United Kingdom, began without considering cost—but soon found that the lack of economic assessment severely limited determining value. Countries differ, however, in determining what form of economic assessments they view as reasonable, in whether to use the QALY metric, whether to combine it with more or less fixed cost thresholds, and in whether or not the so-called *rule of rescue* should be adopted, which typically demands genuine commitment of resources in the case of life-threatening conditions for which effective treatments exist.

Chapter 11 provides four cases that illustrate concrete resource allocation dilemmas at the national and global levels. Coverage decisions regarding prostate cancer management options relate to five options that differ considerably in price, somewhat in side effects, and only marginally in terms of survival outcomes: Should all be covered? Chemotherapy for metastatic colon cancer can extend life by several months, but the drugs often differ considerably in their price. A major hospital decided to remove one of two otherwise similar interventions on cost grounds: Does this represent adequate stewardship of resources or unjustifiable interference in patient care? The remaining cases concern the global level. Should Costa Rica cover treatment for an 8-year-old girl suffering from Gaucher's disease, a very rare, but often deadly genetic condition typically requiring lifelong treatment at around $160,000 per year? The final case illustrates a further way in which resource allocation and rationing decisions can be linked. National governments, charitable foundations, nongovernmental organizations (NGOs), and others donate approximately $11 billion per year for HIV/AIDS care and treatment. However, these funds are not sufficient to provide the recommended antiretroviral drug regiment to all in need and some 10–20 million people are untreated. A clear rationing decision arises: Whom should we treat? A broader resource allocation decision is whether efforts are rightly focused on HIV/AIDS, when, for example, almost as many people die of road traffic accidents and diarrhea and far more of pneumonia.

Chapter 12 addresses an issue that is closely related to what criteria and approaches should guide access to a given benefit package: Should it be permissible for the well-off to purchase beneficial interventions or services that are not included in the essential health benefits that are guaranteed to all citizens? Would allowing the rich to pay for specific services or buy supplemental insurance for more services cause the creation of a two-tier system? Would it undermine equality? Does prohibiting a two-tier system undermine individual liberty and the ability of people to spend their own money the way they want to? The requirements to treat people according to need, concerns about the market as a method to distribute health services, and worries that higher tiers have a negative effect on the quality of care provided in the lower tiers all need to be taken into account. The question of tiering is not just a conceptual one but relevant in ethical appraisals of real-world policy. For example, historically, Canada has prohibited insurance companies from selling private coverage for any service provided by the public single-payer system. Patients have sued, arguing that this violates their liberty and timely access to the best care.

While policy-makers and politicians at the higher levels of health systems clearly have major roles in resource allocation, Chapters 13 and 14 concern the role of two other important actors: health professionals and patients themselves. Chapter 13 asks if it might be reasonable to place responsibility for resource allocation decisions on physicians and other frontline healthcare workers. Is it the physician's responsibility to always put his or her patient first? Or should physicians sometimes give priority to the larger population of current and future patients, including people who are not under their care? Might such an active role in resource allocation be an integral part of practicing medicine, as a recently revised Ethics Manual by the American College of Physicians suggests?[4] The chapter provides an overview of the ethical arguments on both sides, provisions in key policy guidance, and empirical findings on physicians' attitudes and practices toward being the allocator of resources.

Chapter 14 begins with the notion that need for healthcare services could be reduced substantially if more attention would be paid to preventing poor health. Many risk factors are modifiable, and the way we behave can have a significant role on our health needs. Correspondingly, there would be reduced need for treatment and funding interventions, thus alleviating resource allocation dilemmas. But how should this situation be addressed in policy? Is it ethical to incentivize health-promoting behaviors through rewards? Is penalizing people for unhealthy behaviors ever ethical? Key policy alternatives are described alongside a number of design features of incentive programs. In addition to the basic ethical questions around personal responsibility touched on in Chapters 3 and 5, the details of incentive policy and practice give rise to a range of nuanced yet important ethical issues.

The final Chapter 15 takes a global perspective, addressing the question of fair distribution of global health assistance. Developed countries have committed to reducing global health inequalities, and major NGOs and private charities have also made significant contributions in efforts to reduce the impact of diseases such as malaria, HIV/AIDS, and tuberculosis. However, in the past few years, overall funding and donations for global health have slowed and continue to be insufficient to ensure access to the most basic interventions for the planet's 7.13 billion people. This dilemma of inadequate health aid raises the question: What should be the priorities for global health assistance? Should HIV/AIDS be the top priority and take the preponderance of resources, or should more money go preferentially to malaria, maternal–child health, family planning, strengthening health systems, or clean water? Approaching this question requires both an understanding of the global burden of disease and an adaptation and expansion of the ethical theories beyond a country's borders to the world.

Flu pandemics entail significant transformations that lead to the emergence of new virus strains for which only very few people have antibodies. Historically, pandemics have

---

[4] L. Snyder, "American College of Physicians Ethics Manual, Sixth Edition," *Annals of Internal Medicine* 156 (2012): pp. 73–104.

occurred about three times a century. The 20th century saw one of the most devastating pandemics in 1918 and two smaller ones some 50 years later. Statistically, the next major pandemic is likely to occur within the lifetime of most people reading this text. Since 1918, the world has become vastly more interconnected. When a pandemic strikes, who should receive priority for vaccines? For respirators? For antiflu drugs? How should countries allocate their health funds in preparing for a pandemic? How much should countries spend stockpiling vaccines, respirators, and antiflu medications?

The SDGs' emphasis on UHC is, without a doubt, to be welcomed unconditionally. But how can we ensure that the pursuit of UHC will complement rather than compete with the other 12 health targets? And how should we strike the balance between clinical curative services, public health services, and action on the social determinants of health—such as education—that may have a greater impact on health than healthcare services?

Far-reaching decisions are not only made by high-level policy-makers. On a daily basis, physicians are confronted with ethical choices. Should they steer patients away from low-value care even if they seem to want it? Should they consider whether patients look after their health or are compliant in treatment in deciding how much time they spend with them?

Rationing and Resource Allocation in Healthcare is an effort to help people understand the ethical issues and analyses underlying common rationing and resource allocation situations. We hope that the cases and readings will facilitate consideration, discussion, and teaching and stimulate the deep reflection and insights needed to address and resolve the underlying issues. Discussions and debates on rationing and resource allocation are as urgent as they are complex. It is our hope that this book will galvanize thinking as well as fair policy and practice.

Part I

Conceptual Distinctions and Ethical Theory

Defining Rationing, Resource Allocation, and Priority Setting

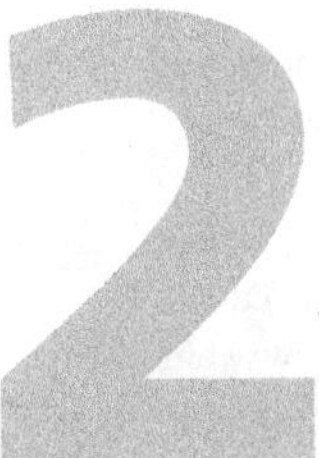

In this chapter, we describe the background to the terms "rationing," "resource allocation," and "priority setting"; introduce five excerpts that provide different characterizations of the concepts; and set out how we will use the concepts in this book.

According to the *Oxford English Dictionary* (OED), *priority setting* is defined as:

> 1. To give priority to; to designate (something) as worthy of special attention; 2. To arrange (items) to be dealt with in order of importance; to establish priorities for (a set of items); to establish priorities for a set of tasks.

As such, the term "priority setting" implies that some kind of criteria are used to determine the worth of an item or sequence of distribution. In general, priority setting has positive connotations, as, for example, evoked in concepts such as "priority boarding" for privileged airline customers. Note that the OED definition does not necessarily entail a situation of scarcity of resources. To return to the example of priority boarding, while everyone with a ticket will be able to board a plane, a prioritization process merely regulates the sequence of entry. In the context of healthcare, priority setting has been defined as "resource distribution among competing needs and demands."[1] It is also in practical use and can be found, for example, in the name of the International Society on Priorities in Health Care (an organization that provides an interdisciplinary forum for exchange between practitioners, policy-makers, academics, and the public). In Sweden, the National Center for Priority Setting in Health Care equally uses the concept in its name, and one of its activities is to develop models that set out which principles and criteria should guide the distribution of medical resources.

Resource allocation, according to the OED, is:

> 1. The action of apportioning or assigning to a special person or purpose;

[1] J. L. Gibson, "Ethics and Priority Setting for HTA: A Decision-Making Framework," April 25, 2005, pp. 1–14.

> apportionment, assignment, allotment; A portion of revenue, etc. assigned to a distinct purpose, constituting a fixed charge upon it; A portion of revenue settled on a particular person; an allowance; The allotment of available materials, provisions, etc., by the government or other authority. 2. The action of allowing or admitting an item in an account; also, the item so allowed. . . .

Compared to priority setting, resource allocation has more neutral, administrative connotations. Resource allocation does not necessarily imply a situation of scarcity. Resource allocation describes a process of distributing goods or services to different people. Thus, resource allocation may not even require explicit criteria—it could be done randomly. The concept is commonly used in the healthcare context, for example, in publications such as: "VA Health Care: Resource Allocation Methodology Has Had Little Impact on Medical Centers' Budgets."[2] In a technical sense, resource allocation has been defined as "earmarking of certain dollars for equipment [or other interventions] to a particular medical use."[3]

Rationing is defined by the OED as follows:

> 1. The regular provision of a fixed amount of supplies to members of the armed services in time of war; an instance of this. Now *rare*; 2. The allocation of a fixed allowance of a specified type of food, clothing, fuel, etc., to each civilian during time of war or shortage; Restriction of the supply of any commodity or service as an economic policy. . . .

Unlike priority setting and resource allocation, rationing relates specifically to a situation of scarcity in which demand may not be met by supply. Imposing limits typically requires specific criteria if rationing is not to be arbitrary. The dictionary definition highlights war as a circumstance in which rationing commonly occurs. Food or fuel are often severely limited in conflict. The need to ration during wartime is embedded in the collective cultural memory of people as symbols of hardship (see also Figure 2.1).

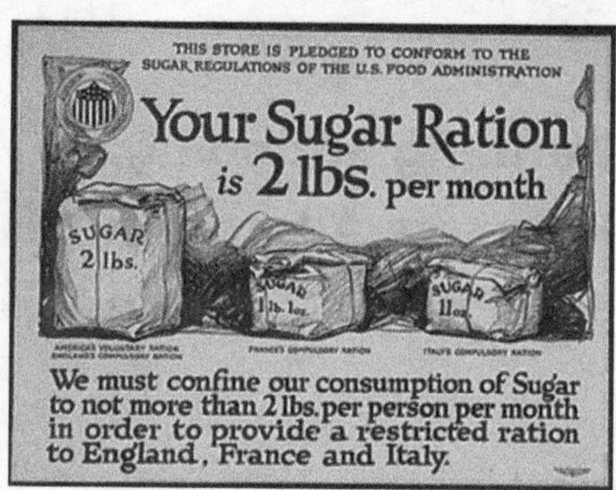

Figure 2.1 Rationing in wartime. This shop window display from 1917 uses the term "ration" to indicate that allowances for US citizens had been capped to ensure that demand in other countries could be met: in order to meet everyone's needs, consumption of some people needed to be limited.

"Your Sugar Ration Is 2 Lbs. Per Month," The Carey Printing Company, 1917, accessed September 5, 2015, http://www.loc.gov/pictures/item/2002707411/.

Rationing is of considerable currency in the health context and is especially frequent in politicians' statements and newspaper headlines. The following examples can be seen as typical in this regard: "Cataracts, Hips, Knees and Tonsils: NHS Begins Rationing Operations,"[4] "Obamacare Rationing Begins, States Cut Prescription Drug Benefits,"[5] "Limited Funds

[2] US General Accounting Office, *VA Health Care: Resource Allocation Methodology Has Had Little Impact on Medical Centers' Budgets: Report to the Committee on Veterans' Affairs, US Senate* (1989).

[3] M. D. Reagan, "Health Care Rationing," *New England Journal of Medicine* 319, no. 17 (1988): p. 1151.

[4] O. Wright, "Cataracts, Hips, Knees and Tonsils: NHS Begins Rationing Operations," *The Independent*, 2011.

[5] S. Ertelt, "Obamacare Rationing Begins, States Cut Prescription Drug Benefits," LifeNews, 2012, accessed July 26, 2015, http://www.lifenews.com/2012/07/31/obamacare-rationing-begins-states-cut-prescription-drug-benefits/.

and Growing Needs Could Require Rationing,"[6] "Seniors Targeted for Rationed Care."[7] The emphasis is usually on denial of goods or services, taking away of benefits, and, frequently, hurting vulnerable people. While priority setting and resource allocations have mostly positive or neutral connotations, these headlines indicate that rationing elicits negative associations. Those who are opposed to any form of limit-setting mostly use the term "rationing," with all its negative connotations, whereas those who see limitations as justified in some cases often seek to avoid it, opting for "resource allocation" or "priority setting" instead.

As the excerpts in this chapter show, there has been little agreement on how the term "rationing" should be used in healthcare. David Hadorn and Robert Brook emphasize that use of the term depends simply on "how the word might be made most useful to the resource allocation debate." In their view, this means that rationing refers to "the societal toleration of inequitable access (e.g., based on ability to pay) to services deemed necessary" (Excerpt 1).[8] The focus here is centrally on the consequences of limit-setting in terms of fairness. Conversely, Robert Brook and Kathleen Lohr emphasize the notions of scarcity and need; accordingly, rationing is "any set of activities that determines who gets needed medical care when resources are insufficient to provide for all" (Excerpt 2).[9]

Some people argue rationing entails the denial of beneficial care because of cost. For instance, Arnold Relman understands the term as: "the deliberate and systematic denial of certain types of services, even when they are known to be beneficial, because they are deemed to be too expensive" (Excerpt 3).[10] Peter Ubel and Susan Goold use the broadest notion of rationing when they argue that it is "any explicit or implicit measure that allows people to go without beneficial health care services" (Excerpt 4).[11] Finally, Uwe Reinardt offers the classic economist perspective arguing that: "free markets . . . [are] one particular form of rationing. Ever since the Fall from Grace, human beings have had to ration everything not available in unlimited quantities, and market forces do most of the rationing" (Excerpt 5).[12]

However, there is full agreement that decisions need to be made along three different dimensions (see also the diagram provided by Ubel and Goold, page 29). First, there can be situations of absolute or relative scarcity. Second, medical interventions or services to which access might be limited can range on a spectrum from being necessary and life-saving to merely beneficial, often offering only marginal benefits. Third, decisions can be made explicitly or implicitly.

In the case of absolute scarcity, natural limitations mean that there are more people requiring a liver, an ICU bed, a vaccine during a pandemic or a drug than are available at a given point in time. However such resources are distributed, some people will inevitably lose out and not get what they need. Tragic choices are therefore inevitable. In the case of relative scarcity, by contrast, the reason that supply cannot meet demand is purely a result of how finances are allocated. Here, tragic choices can often be

---

6 "Willard E. Lund: Limited Funds and Growing Needs Could Require Rationing," Wisconsin State Journal, 2012, accessed July 26, 2015, http://host.madison.com/news/opinion/mailbag/willard-e-lund-limited-funds-and-growing-needs-could-require/article_d15e7ab8-cdc3-11e1-99a0-001a4bcf887a.html.

7 "Seniors Targeted for Rationed Care," AZ Daily Sun, 2012, accessed July 26, 2015, http://azdailysun.com/news/opinion/mailbag/seniors-targeted-for-rationed-care/article_13a0829a-dc33-5cf7-9cc4-30d46f9da600.html.

8 D. C. Hadorn and R. H. Brook, "The Health Care Resource Allocation Debate: Defining Our Terms," *JAMA* 266, no. 23 (1991): pp. 3328–3331.

9 R. H. Brook and K. N. Lohr, *Will We Need to Ration Effective Health Care?* (Santa Monica: Rand, 1991).

10 A. S. Relman, "Is Rationing Inevitable?", *New England Journal of Medicine* 322, no. 25 (1990): pp. 1809–1810.

11 P. A. Ubel and S. Goold, "'Rationing' Health Care: Not All Definitions Are Created Equal," *Archives of Internal Medicine* 158, no. 3 (1998): pp. 209–214.

12 U. E. Reinhardt, "'Rationing' Health Care: What Does It Mean?", *New York Times*, July 3 2009.

Box 2.1 The Concepts of "Rationing," "Resource Allocation," and "Priority Setting" as Used in This Anthology

Rationing:
To regulate, through explicit or implicit means, access to beneficial healthcare under conditions of absolute scarcity

Resource allocation:
To regulate, through explicit or implicit means, access to beneficial healthcare under conditions of relative scarcity

Priority setting:
To regulate, through explicit or implicit means, access to beneficial healthcare under conditions of absolute or relative scarcity

avoided. There can be more flexibility in terms of whose needs are met. For example, HIV drugs were initially not available in South Africa due to high cost. But public pressure led manufacturers to reduce their prices and increased availability.[13] Alternatively, a health plan may decide to no longer fund in vitro fertilization (IVF) on the basis that infertility is not regarded as a medical need and instead cover costly dementia treatments. Put differently, in the case of absolute scarcity, the core of the problem is that there are not enough things, and no further things can be generated in time. Conversely, in the case of relative scarcity, there is not enough money. However, funds might be allocated in different ways, and, moreover, more money can be made available through political or other commitment, as Chapters 8–10 illustrate.

To be clear and precise and to avoid confusion, in this anthology, decisions regarding absolute scarcity should be deemed as cases of *rationing*. Decisions concerned with relative scarcity entail *resource allocation*. The significant difference of the nature of the problem in these two contexts merits emphasis in terminology and reflects most accurately the general characterizations implied by the OED. We see *priority setting* as an overarching concept that relates to decision-making processes in both rationing and resource allocation (Box 2.1).

Deciding not to pay for ineffective interventions constitutes neither rationing nor resource allocation, but rather reduces or prevents waste. Conceptually, such cases are therefore easily excluded from the debates that are at the center of the discussion here. However, it is not always straightforward to determine when something is completely ineffective. Similarly, there is no clear-cut division between the concepts of necessary and beneficial treatments. What is necessary to one group of people may merely be useful to another and vice versa.[14] Whereas in cases of rationing, effectiveness of interventions is largely taken for granted, determining the scope of benefit is an inherent part of resource allocation. Overall, both rationing and resource allocation decisions are centered on interventions that have some benefit.

Rationing and resource allocation decisions do not need to be explicit decision processes only, embodied in laws, guidelines, coverage policies of health plans, or other binding codes. Decisions about changes to coverage and benefit design may be made on an informal ad hoc basis, with very direct implications on patients' access to healthcare. Rationing and resource allocation can therefore be both explicit and implicit.

Finally, rationing and resource allocation decisions can occur at three different levels of the healthcare system: micro, meso, and macro. The micro level commonly refers to the interaction of patients and healthcare workers at the bedside or in an office visit. For example, a physician may advise a patient during a consultation against an imaging study because the

[13] D. G. McNeil, "Companies to Cut Cost of Aids Drugs for Poor Nations," *New York Times*, May 12, 2000.

[14] As perhaps illustrated by the example of IVF: an infertile couple may argue that access is absolutely necessary for their livelihood and should be provided by their health plan, whereas the health plans' manager, or certain population groups, may find that infertility should be accepted as part of life, and that healthcare resources should be used for issues where need is far less controversial, such as in the treatment of neurocognitive diseases.

benefits are likely to be only very marginal. At the meso level, a hospital may decide to include some medications in its drug formulary, but not others, even though the excluded ones are known to be effective. Health plans often make similar inclusion and exclusion decisions in the design of their benefit packages. At the macro level, governments decide what funding will be made available to publicly funded healthcare as opposed to other areas such as education. Chapter 8 describes how the US government decided to pay for all patients with chronic renal failure though federally collected funds. Macro-level decisions can have very direct effects on the question of who gets what. The following chapters will show that, moreover, rationing and resource allocation at all three levels engage some kind of criteria and entail medical, scientific, and economic as well as value judgments.

Questions for Discussion

1. What are the principal similarities and differences between the OED dictionary definitions of rationing, resource allocation, and priority setting?
2. Which of the following do you think is the best definition of rationing?
   A. "The societal toleration of inequitable access to [necessary] health services"
   B. "Any set of activities that determines who gets needed medical care when resources are insufficient to provide for all"
   C. "The deliberate and systematic denial of certain types of services, even when they are known to be beneficial because they are deemed to be too expensive"
   D. "Any explicit or implicit measures that allow people to go without beneficial healthcare services"
   E. "To regulate, through explicit or implicit means, access to beneficial healthcare under conditions of absolute scarcity"
3. Hadorn and Brook have some sympathy for the view that rationing might be avoided if "useless or marginal care" would be eliminated (Excerpt 1). Suppose you are a consultant advising a policy-maker. The policy-maker is interested in reducing care with marginal benefits. Practically, how should a health system go about this? Which stakeholders are most likely to resist the approach?
4. In Excerpt 3, Relman notes that Joseph A. Califano, a lawyer and former secretary of the US Department of Health, Education, and Welfare, argued that physicians can play a major role in improving efficiency, thereby obviating the need for rationing. State on what grounds you agree or disagree.
5. Consider the illustration by Ubel and Goold on page 29 in Excerpt 4, and give examples of cases in each of the eight quadrants. What do you notice in the process?

EXCERPTS

NOTE: The following excerpts have generally been edited for length, and omissions are indicated with ellipses. Editing includes footnotes and endnotes, which have also been renumbered. For citation and related purposes, the full original source texts should be used.

EXCERPT 1

Abridged text from:

D. C. Hadorn and R. H. Brook, "The Health Care Resource Allocation Debate: Defining Our Terms," *JAMA* 266, no. 23 (1991): pp. 3328–3331.

The Health Care Resource Allocation Debate: Defining Our Terms

David C. Hadorn, MD, MA, and Robert H. Brook, MD, ScD

. . .

Th[e] broader usage generally follows Aaron and Schwartz's widely quoted definition that rationing occurs when "not all care expected to be beneficial is provided to all patients[1] . . .

Other recent definitions of rationing move even farther from the word's original roots in scarcity and fairness. In an article entitled "Health care rationing through inconvenience,"[2] Grumet in effect equated rationing with "cost-containment"; indeed, the word rationing did not appear anywhere in the article except in the title. Callahan has advocated the "rationing of medical progress,"[3] meaning the deliberate curtailment of certain forms of applied medical research (eg, artificial hearts). Aaron and Schwartz have recently redescribed rationing as "the denial of commodities to those who have the money to buy them."[4] . . .

How should the word rationing be used? The answer, we believe, lies in considering how the word might be made most useful to the resource allocation debate. . . .

We believe that the best solution is to restrict the use of rationing to something close to Relman's definition: the withholding of services acknowledged to be beneficial, based on ability to pay. Such withholding is potentially far more common and problematic than are the isolated areas of medicine (eg, organ transplants) to which the traditional meaning of rationing can be legitimately applied.

We do not, however, believe that the withholding of care must be "deliberate and systematic," as Relman would have it. Simple toleration by society of inequitable barriers to effective care should also qualify as rationing; otherwise, it would be too easy for society to say that it simply cannot produce an equitable situation, and that the situation is, therefore, not deliberately brought about. ("Inequitable barriers" here refers primarily to restrictions on access due to wealth or insurance status, but could be extended to race and other sociodemographic factors. Geographic distance ordinarily would not count as an inequitable barrier, any more than the reduced availability of police and fire protection in rural areas is today considered unfair to the people who choose to live in the country.) Another important consideration with respect to defining rationing is that withholding care acknowledged to be beneficial is potentially avoidable through the identification and elimination of useless or marginal care. Brook and Lohr have estimated that 30% or more of the health care services currently rendered in this country might safely be forgone, and that elimination of this subset of care could permit society to save enough money to avoid the

[1] M. D. Reagan, "Health Care Rationing," *New England Journal of Medicine* 319, no. 17 (1988): pp. 1149–1151.

[2] G. W. Grumet, "Health Care Rationing Through Inconvenience," *New England Journal of Medicine* 321, no. 9 (1989): pp. 607–611.

[3] D. Callahan, "Rationing Medical Progress," *New England Journal of Medicine* 322, no. 25 (1990): pp. 1810–1813.

[4] H. Aaron and W. Schwartz, "Rationing Health Care: The Choice before Us," *Science* 247, no. 4941 (1990): pp. 418–422.

need to ration effective health care.[5] While good evidence on this subject is relatively meager, subsequent studies and a recent review of available literature have tended to confirm Brook and Lohr's views in this area.[6,7,8,9,10] Nevertheless, whether or not the elimination of unnecessary services would save enough money to provide all deemed-necessary services must be considered an unresolved issue at this time. . . .

If, in fact, sufficient savings can be realized from the curtailment of payment for unnecessary care, American society might avoid rationing (in Relman's sense of the word) by identifying sufficiently beneficial or effective services and providing coverage for these services under all basic-level plans. Thus, a further advantage to the recommended, restricted use of the word rationing is that society remains able to distinguish between the withholding of truly effective care (rationing) from the curtailment of services of dubious or unproven benefit (not rationing). The distinction is vital and should be clearly maintained both conceptually and in our language.

Schwartz and Aaron have observed that the elimination of marginal or useless care would result in only a onetime savings, because new essential services are created continuously through research. This is the primary reason that Callahan has suggested that certain types of medical progress be rationed, as noted above.[11] While limits on (tax supported) medical innovation may be necessary someday, we believe that by subjecting new technology to strict evaluations of expected benefit before extending coverage under insurance plans, the heretofore unbridled tide of progress can be reined in to a significant extent. . . .

Health Care Needs

So far, we have defined rationing as the toleration of inequitable access to beneficial services. An important modification is required in this definition before we are finished. A clear and important connotation found in the original scarcity and fairness usage of rationing (and in the dictionary definition cited earlier) is that rationed goods and services are necessary or basic to a continued decent existence. Food and water—two basic necessities—are rationed around the world today, but automobiles and television sets are not rationed anywhere because these latter commodities are not considered necessary to a minimally decent life. . . .

The notion of necessity as it pertains to health care rationing is not completely captured by commonly used words like "beneficial," "effective," or "appropriate." Indeed, it is clearly possible for a medical service to be beneficial or appropriate without being truly necessary. . . .

We conclude that the definition of rationing should be modified to mean the withholding of care duly deemed necessary—as opposed to effective, appropriate, or beneficial.

---

[5] R. H. Brook and K. N. Lohr, *Will We Need to Ration Effective Health Care?* (Rand, 1986).

[6] M. R. Chassin, et al., "Does Inappropriate Use Explain Geographic Variations in the Use of Health Care Services?: A Study of Three Procedures," *JAMA* 258, no. 18 (1987): pp. 2533–2537.

[7] C. Winslow, et al., "The Appropriateness of Performing Coronary Artery Bypass Surgery," *Journal of the American Medical Association* 260, no. 4 (1988): pp. 505–509.

[8] R. H. Brook, et al., "Predicting the Appropriate Use of Carotid Endarterectomy, Upper Gastrointestinal Endoscopy, and Coronary Angiography," *New England Journal of Medicine* 323, no. 17 (1990): pp. 1173–1177.

[9] M. R. Chassin, et al., *The Appropriateness of Use of Selected Medical and Surgical Procedures and Its Relationship to Geographic Variations in Their Use* (Ann Arbor, MI: Association for Health Services Research and Health Administration Press, 1989).

[10] R. H. Brook, et al., "Appropriateness of Acute Medical Care for the Elderly: An Analysis of the Literature," *Health Policy* 14, no. 3 (1990): pp. 225–242.

[11] Callahan, "Rationing Medical Progress."

. . .

The connection between medical needs and rationing is fundamental to a clear understanding of the current policy debate. If we can identify "really necessary" health care interventions and ensure that all patients have equitable access to these interventions, rationing can be avoided. The main difficulty with this plan, of course, lies in the ambiguity inherent in the concept of health care needs. . . .

We believe it is possible to narrowly define need so as to permit the salutary application of this critical concept to the health care resource allocations debate. To do so, it will be necessary to develop objective criteria by means of which health care needs can be distinguished from "mere desires." Indeed, some form of objective criteria is always required to evaluate claims of need against others or against society.[12]

In the case of health care, suitable objective criteria might coherently take the form of a special type of clinical guideline—necessary-care guidelines—that would depict the indications (namely, "types of patients") for which specified services are considered necessary.[13] These guidelines would be developed by duly constituted and representative bodies or panels, based on available outcome data, public testimony, and expert consensus. Necessary-care guidelines would specify the clinical indications for which various interventions (eg, carotid endarterectomy, radiation therapy for cancer, magnetic resonance imaging) have been "clearly demonstrated ('or reasonably well demonstrated') to provide significant net health benefit over no or alternative treatment."[14] Net benefit would be defined in terms of longevity plus quality of life. Services judged to provide only insignificant net health benefits would be deemed unnecessary, and desires for such services would not be considered needs. Necessary-care guidelines would be updated regularly and appeals mechanisms would be available to accommodate atypical patient cases. . . .

Conclusion

The current debate over possible solutions to the health care cost and access problem is too important, too complex, and too sensitive to be burdened with imprecise usage of critical terms. All who are working in this area should speak a common language in order to facilitate progress toward reasonable solutions.

In this article we have suggested how certain fundamental terms might best be conceptualized and defined. The term rationing, we believe, should be used to mean societal toleration of inequitable access (eg, based on ability to pay) to services deemed necessary, as defined by reference to appropriate clinical guidelines. . . .

---

[12] T. M. Scanlon, "Preference and Urgency," *Journal of Philosophy* 72, no. 19 (1975): pp. 655–669.

[13] D. C. Hadorn, "Necessary-Care Guidelines: Defining Health Care Needs Using an Explicit Standard of Proof," April 24, 1991.

[14] D. C. Hadorn, "Setting Health Care Priorities in Oregon: Cost-Effectiveness Meets the Rule of Rescue," *Journal of the American Medical Association* 265, no. 17 (1991): pp. 2218–2225.

EXCERPT 2

Abridged text from:
R. H. Brook and K. N. Lohr, *Will We Need to Ration Effective Health Care?* (Santa Monica: Rand, 1991).

Will We Need to Ration Effective Health Care?

Robert Henry Brook and Kathleen N. Lohr

The central health policy issue for the remainder of the decade, if not the century, is whether the nation will accept and act on the premise that it must ration effective medical services. Rationing can be simply defined as any set of activities that determines who gets needed medical care when resources are insufficient to provide for all. Put another way, it is the provision of some service to one patient at the risk of denying it to an equally deserving patient. At the most basic level, it is the problem clinicians face in deciding who to treat when not all can be treated.[1]

The rhetoric of the times conveys the impression that only the rationing of care—either by direct means (for example, by denying the patient access to a certain procedure) or by some general economic mechanism (such as increasing deductibles in health insurance policies or reducing income eligibility levels for Medicaid)—will halt the persistent escalation in health care costs and expenditures, which now constitute more than 10% of the nation's gross national product.

Most of the health debate today focuses on how best to implement rationing and which mechanisms to use, not on whether rationing is necessary. We believe that the correct question is whether deliberate rationing of services by nonmedical or nonclinical means is needed. The answer, we contend, is "no."

. . .

The rationing issue is not an idle or merely intellectual one, because the social costs of rationing can be high. If the country decides to ration effective services, no matter how well it does so, it will have a greater impact on the elderly, the poor, and the chronically ill than on the rich, the middle class, or the healthy. With explicit, stringent rationing, people with resources will find ways to obtain needed medical services; those lacking such resources will do without, at least temporarily. . . .

Along with numerous colleagues we have just completed a major social experiment on the effects of differing levels of cost sharing on health. About 2,000 families in six sites in the United States were given health insurance that differed only in the amount of money the family members were required to pay out of pocket. All of the insurance plans were representative of the US population, except the elderly were excluded. They chose their own physicians and paid on a fee-for-service basis. Expenditures were 40% higher on the plan in which services were free than on the plans that required patient cost sharing.[2]

These large differences in expenditures had negligible, if any, effects on the health of the average adult or child.[3] However, at the end of the experiment, low-income children with anemia may have been worse off with cost sharing. And low-income adults who were sick, especially with hypertension, were also worse off on the cost-sharing plans. Because of higher resulting higher blood pressure, these adults on the cost-sharing plan had an estimated 15% greater chance of dying within five years than

---

[1] W. A. Knaus, "Rationing, Justice, and the American Physician," *Journal of the American Medical Association* 255 (1986): pp. 1176–1177.

[2] J. P. Newhouse, et al., "Some Interim Results from a Controlled Trial of Cost Sharing in Health Insurance," *New England Journal of Medicine* 305, no. 25 (1981): pp. 1501–1507.

[3] R. H. Brook, et al., "Does Free Care Improve Adults' Health?", *New England Journal of Medicine* 309, no. 23 (1983): pp. 1426–1434.

those on the freecare plan. These outcomes can be attributed to the lower physician contract resulting from cost sharing.[4]

. . .

Evidence that rationing effective services in the United States may be unnecessary comes from three areas: the wide variation in per-person rates of use of all forms of medical care, the unproven effectiveness of many procedures used to diagnose and treat illness, and the unquestioned assumption among both medical practitioners and the public that doing more at least doing something is preferable to doing nothing.

First, the per-person rates of use of certain services vary widely in this country among people who appear to be similar in all the characteristics that usually predict use.[5] These characteristics include basic health status, age, sex, and other demographic, social, and economic factors.

Examples are numerous and telling:

- Per-person medical expenditure for elderly residents of Miami, Florida are more than twice as high as those for seniors in Rochester, New York.
- Hospital use is 60% higher in the North Central regions of the country than the West.
- The rates of use of computerized tomography (CAT) scans to diagnose problems affecting the brain per patient discharged from acute care hospitals were seven times higher in the West North Central states (Iowa, Kansas, Minnesota, Missouri, Nebraska, North Dakota, and South Dakota) than in the Mountain states (Arizona, Colorado, Idaho, Montana, Nevada, New Mexico, Utah, Wyoming).

. . .

If the figures at the lower end of these ranges represent appropriate and adequate care, then 30% to 50% of the nation's health bill might be said to consist of expenditures on care that produces little or no demonstrable health benefits. If these ineffective services were selectively eliminated, the pressure to ration effective services would be markedly relieved. However, if the figures at the upper end of these ranges represent adequate care, then expenditures on health care do not appear so out of line. The question is, what is appropriate?

Unfortunately, the medical or clinical data with which to determine whether procedures are generally overused or underused are sparse. Some information, however, can be marshaled. Consider, for instance, the appropriateness of hospital use. A hospital day, which is an expensive commodity is termed appropriate if the services provided can be done only while the patient is hospitalized and if these services are medically effective; that is, they will do more good than harm. Recent studies indicate that about 25% of all hospital days are inappropriate because the services performed did not require hospitalization. For example, the only care the patient received may have been oral medication, which could Just as easily have been taken at home.[6]

Having an unnecessary operation or diagnostic test also represents inappropriate care. If such services are provided in the hospital setting, and if they are the only reason for that hospitalization, then the percentage of hospital days that are inappropriate rises dramatically. Preliminary work in a few hospitals suggest that one-third or more of the coronary angiographies and coronary artery bypass surgeries may be medically inappropriate; that is, the risk to the patient is,

[4] E. B. Keeler, et al., "How Free Care Reduced Hypertension in the Health Insurance Experiment," *Journal of the American Medical Association* 254, no. 14 (1985): pp. 1926–1931.

[5] R. H. Brook, et al., "Geographic Variations in the Use of Services: Do They Have Any Clinical Significance?", *Health Affairs* 3, no. 2 (1984): pp. 63–73; K. Lohr, W. Lohr and R. H. Brook, *Geographic Variations in the Use of Medical Services and Surgical Procedures: A Chartbook* (Washington, DC: National Health Policy Forum, George Washington University, 1985); M. R. Chassin, et al., "Variations in the Use of Medical and Surgical Services by the Medicare Population," *New England Journal of Medicine* 314, no. 5 (1986): pp. 285–290.

[6] J. D. Restuccia, et al., "A Comparative Analysis of Appropriateness of Hospital Use," *Health Affairs* 3, no. 2 (1984): pp. 130–138.

on average, as great as the procedure's benefit.[7] Similar results have been found for carotid endarterectomies (a procedure to remove clots in arteries leading to the brain) performed in selected Veterans Administration hospitals.[8] If these results, which have not been obtained from hospitals selected for poor performance or questionable practices, are representative of all hospitals, then the 30% to 50% figures cited earlier may not appear farfetched. They may even be an underestimate.

Some of the nation's health care dollars go to services and technologies whose efficacy (performance under ideal circumstances, for example by the best physicians in the best hospitals) and effectiveness (performance under ordinary circumstances such as in the common private practice setting) have never been satisfactorily examined.[9] Even when the efficacy of a surgical procedure or new drug has been demonstrated, it is not clear that results achieved under these ideal conditions will also be achieved by the average practitioner. More studies are needed that describe the risks and benefits of procedures when performed by the average practitioner. Carotid endarterectomy, for example, may be an appropriate procedure for some patients, but only when the surgeon's postoperative complication rate is very low. If the average surgeon who performs the procedure has a higher complication rate, then the risk to the patient may outweigh the benefit.

. . .

Another problem relates to the "do something" mentality. One manifestation of this problem is that physicians have not been taught how to an accurate value on additional diagnostic information. The urge to obtain yet more (relatively uninformative) data pervades the diagnostic process, and the consequences of this attitude are subtle, costly, and sometimes harmful. It may, for instance, obscure the diagnosis of something as simple as appendicitis in patients coming to an emergency room with belly pain.

An example from a recent book by David Sackett and his colleagues in illustrative.[10] A 35-year-old man goes to a physicians with nonexertional chest pain that occurs after a heavy meal. No other cardiovascular risk factor is present. After taking a personal history and doing a physical examination, the physician concludes that the patient has about a 5% chance of having coronary artery disease. The question, then, is whether he should order an exercise stress test to determine more conclusively whether the patient has heart disease, even though the odds are about 19 to 1 that the patient does not.

Many physicians would automatically order the stress test. If the test were positive, as dye study of circulation of the heart (coronary angiography) would be ordered. If a blockage of the left main coronary artery were eventually found (an unlikely event in this example), then coronary artery bypass surgery would be performed. If no untoward events occurred during the test or operation, the diagnostic and therapeutic process would be declared a success.

If, however, 1,000 such patients were put through this process, more harm than good would probably be done, and at great cost. The stress test is not totally accurate in ruling illness in or out (respectively, "sensitive" or "specific" in technical terms). Thus, some patients will suffer from being falsely labeled as ill or having heart disease; others who truly have heart disease may be incorrectly reassured about their state of health. An occasional patient, who may or may not have heart disease, could suffer a serious complication of the test or even die. Because all these problems can and do occur with this test, the net gain (in either accurate information or

---

[7] C. Winslow et al., "The Appropriateness of Use of Coronary Angiography and Coronary Artery Bypass Surgery," *Clinical Research* 34 (1986): p. 635A.

[8] N. J. Merrick and R. H. Brook, "Estimates of the Influence of Comorbidity on the Appropriateness of Carotid Endarterectomy," 1985.

[9] R. H. Brook and K. N. Lohr, "Efficacy, Effectiveness, Variations, and Quality. Boundary-Crossing Research," *Med Care* 23, no. 5 (1985): pp. 710–722

[10] D. L. Sackett, R. B. Haynes and P. Tugwell, *Clinical Epidemiology: A Basic Science for Clinical Medicine* (Little, Brown, 1985).

improved health status) from administering it to 1,000 men, each of whom has only a 5% chance of having coronary disease in the first place, is less than its associated risks.

The point can be generalized. Deciding to use a diagnostic technology, even a relatively inexpensive one, can be both harmful and costly. Greater knowledge about the sensitivity and specificity of diagnostic tests, better appreciation of the strengths and limitations of such tests in specific clinical situations, and wider application of formal decision analysis skills (skills that physicians typically do not learn or apply in daily practice) would go far to rationalize medical practice and reduce costs. Moreover, patients appear willing to give up the "more is better" philosophy for tests or procedures when their physicians explain why the test or procedure is not needed.[11]

From these bits of evidence, we can speculate that perhaps one-third of the financial resources devoted to health care today are being spent on ineffective or unproductive care. If these expenditures could be identified and reduced, explicit rationing or stringent economic measures would not be necessary. Even if the above calculations are slightly off and the nation's total health bill increased slightly as a proportion of gross national product, these changes would nonetheless help produce a health care system that is based on demonstrably effective services and is more responsive to the needs of all citizens.

Eliminating inefficiency in the medical system, however, will not be easy. It will require changes in federal policies, funding decisions, and medical education, and it will necessitate an extensive research effort to assess the quality of care. In addition, some of the necessary steps will challenge traditional practices and ingrained habits of both the medical profession and the public Because such changes are difficult and time-consuming to implement, it is important to begin the discussion now.

. . .

[11] J. H. C. Sox, I. Margulies and C. H. Sox, "Psychologically Mediated Effects of Diagnostic Tests," *Annals of Internal Medicine* 95, no. 6 (1981): pp. 680–685.

EXCERPT 3

Abridged text from:

A. S. Relman, "Is Rationing Inevitable?", *New England Journal of Medicine* 322, no. 25 (1990): pp. 1809–1810.

Is Rationing Inevitable?

Arnold S. Relman

. . . Payers—government, business, and the health insurance companies—are at the end of their economic rope. Unable to support the continued escalation of medical costs, they are determined to use whatever means they can to control expenditures. Two consequences, are a growing morass of regulations and bureaucracy and an increasing surveillance of physicians' decisions—particularly those involving the use of hospitals.

. . .

Few observers expect present cost-containment efforts to be successful. Conventional wisdom holds that unrestrained consumer demand coupled with the relentless development of increasingly sophisticated new technology will keep driving costs up until some major new approach is adopted. The most likely next step, many now believe, will be some form of systematic rationing.

Limited access to medical care has always been with us. Over five years ago Fuchs pointed out in the *Journal* that patients' income and the geographic location of physicians and facilities have historically restricted the availability of medical services to many Americans.[1] And Grumet has also reminded us that reimbursement regulations imposed by third-party payers (a part of what is euphemistically called "managed care") can similarly result in a kind of rationing. But what is now being contemplated is something quite different: the deliberate and systematic denial of certain types of services, even when they are known to be beneficial, because they are deemed too expensive. This kind of rationing is different from global governmental budgetary restraints on facilities and personnel, such as occurs in centrally planned health economies like those of Great Britain or Sweden. Instead, it would be achieved through decisions not to pay doctors and hospitals for the delivery of particular services to particular groups of patients under defined circumstances.

Two articles deal with this kind of rationing. One is by Daniel Callahan, director of the Hastings Center for Bioethics, who has recently written two thoughtful books about the role of medical care in our society.[2,3] In the present essay, he criticizes what he calls our national addiction to new medical technology and our expectations of unlimited medical progress. He argues that to afford decent health care for all, as well as the other social goods with which our medical care budget presumably competes, we shall have to set some limits on the use of new technology and accept that "some, perhaps many, beneficial applications will have to be passed over on grounds of cost and other, more pressing social priorities."[4] In his earlier writings Callahan suggested that we ration high-technology care for the aged and the terminally ill. The other article, by Norman Levinsky,[5] rejects that view and argues strongly against age as a criterion for rationing. Although Levinsky takes no stand on rationing in general, he maintains that the elderly should not be the exclusive targets if a decision is made to ration health care.

The first proposal for explicit, systematic, and publicly accountable rationing of health

---

[1] V. R. Fuchs, "The Rationing of Medical Care," *New England Journal of Medicine* 311, no. 24 (1984): pp. 1572–1573.

[2] D. Callahan, *Setting Limits: Medical Goals in an Aging Society* (Georgetown University Press, 1995).

[3] D. Callahan, *What Kind of Life?: The Limits of Medical Progress* (Georgetown University Press, 1995).

[4] D. Callahan, "Rationing Medical Progress," *New England Journal of Medicine* 322, no. 25 (1990): pp. 1810–1813.

[5] N. G. Levinsky, "Age as a Criterion for Rationing Health Care," *New England Journal of Medicine* 322, no. 25 (1990): pp. 1813–1816.

care services at the state level has recently been made by the Oregon legislature, and it is attracting much comment, pro and con.[6] The idea is to use federal and state Medicaid funds to provide basic health services to all Oregonians below the poverty line, not just the fraction who qualify under the usual Medicaid rules. To provide such universal access, the state has enlisted physicians and other citizens to join in constructing a comprehensive list of medical services, in order of priority based on clinical effectiveness and social value. State payment will extend as far down the list of services as available funds allow. In this way, Oregon hopes to ration health services to the poor in a manner that ensures public participation in the difficult task of establishing funding priorities.

At the recent annual meeting of the Massachusetts Medical Society, these issues were the subject of a lively debate by a panel that included Daniel Callahan, and Joseph A. Califano (a lawyer and former secretary of the US Department of Health, Education, and Welfare). . . . Callahan defended rationing as a reasonable, equitable, and inevitable policy for the allocation of limited health care resources. He was supportive of the Oregon initiative. Califano, on the other hand, was not convinced. He urged instead that physicians join in an effort to make our health care system more efficient and affordable, thereby obviating the need for rationing. He objected to the Oregon plan because it would limit services to the poor and would not address the more fundamental problems in the health care system that have caused the present economic crisis. His list of needed reforms included the following: greater emphasis on preventive medicine and more healthful lifestyles; changes in payment mechanisms to eliminate perverse incentives for oversupply and duplication of high-technology services; reforms in health manpower to put more emphasis on primary care; and a comprehensive solution to the malpractice-liability problem. Although agreeing that these reforms are needed, Callahan doubted that the system could be improved enough to avoid rationing.

This, in essence, is the health policy debate of the 1990s. Can we improve our health care system sufficiently, and soon enough, to avoid either systematic rationing or more restriction of access through pricing? Like Califano, I am convinced that we can. In a country that spends as much as we do on health care, there should be no need to deny medically necessary services (including the best of modern technology) to anyone. We need not become the helpless economic victims of technology unless we lack the will to evaluate it critically and employ it only when medically indicated.[7] All the evidence suggests that there are vast savings to be made through the elimination of unnecessary services and facilities.

The quality and efficiency of medical care depend primarily on the behavior of physicians, although government must also do its part. If physicians work in good faith with government to devise better ways to deliver health services, there is realistic hope for an affordable system that will guarantee access to an acceptable standard of care for all Americans, without resorting to rationing of any kind. In any case, this decade should tell the story. By the turn of the century we shall either have helped the United States to improve its health care system substantially or we shall find our services to patients externally regulated and rationed as never before.

---

[6] "The Oregon Rationing Plan: Inspired or Misguided?", *Healthweek* (1990): p. 18.

[7] M. Angell, "Cost Containment and the Physician," *Journal of the American Medical Association* 254, no. 9 (1985): pp. 1203–1207.

EXCERPT 4

Abridged text from:

P. A. Ubel and S. Goold, "'Rationing' Health Care: Not All Definitions Are Created Equal," *Archives of Internal Medicine* 158, no. 3 (1998): pp. 209–214.

Rationing & Health Care: Not All Definitions Are Created Equal

P. A. Ubel and S. Goold

Despite consensus among most experts that health care costs need to be contained, there is great controversy about whether it is ever acceptable to ration health care. Part of this controversy results from disagreement about whether health care costs can be adequately contained by eliminating waste, rather than by rationing health care. Another part of this controversy, however, may arise from disagreement about what it means to ration health care. . . .

Rationing has taken on such negative connotations that few people think that the word can apply to justifiable actions. Many people think health care rationing, by definition, is unacceptable, raising questions about the usefulness of debating whether we ever need to ration health care. At the same time, a number of people argue that health care rationing is either inevitable or justifiable. Do people disagree on whether it is ever justifiable to withhold beneficial health care services from patients? Or do they simply disagree on whether withholding those services qualifies as health care rationing? In a highly controversial and important area such as health care rationing, it is crucial to be clear about what we mean by rationing.

In this article, we explore various definitions of health care rationing and provide a simple schematic to understand and categorize these definitions. We argue that not all these definitions are equally acceptable. Instead, we favor a broad interpretation of health care rationing, whereby rationing encompasses any explicit or implicit measures that allow people to go without beneficial health care services. We argue that this broad view of health care rationing has several advantages, most important being that it highlights the frequency with which we allow patients to go without beneficial health care services because of their cost.

Definitions of Rationing

The medical literature is filled with numerous casual and formal definitions of health care rationing. A sample will suffice to show the range of meanings people place on these words. Some state that health care rationing involves inequitable distribution of resources based on inability to pay.[1] Others define rationing as "the equitable distribution of scarce resources,"[2] as the "denial of commodities to those who have the money to buy them,"[3] as "the deliberate and systematic denial of certain types of services, even when they are known to be beneficial, because they are deemed too expensive,"[4] and as "any set of activities that determines who gets needed medical care when resources are insufficient to provide for all."[5]

This confusing array of definitions reflects different notions of what constitutes health care rationing. Rationing definitions differ in

---

[1] *The American Heritage Illustrated Encyclopedic Dictionary* (Boston, MA: Houghton Mifflin Co, 1987).

[2] D. C. Hadorn and R. H. Brook, "The Health Care Resource Allocation Debate: Defining Our Terms," *Journal of the American Medical Association* 266, no. 23 (1991): p. 3331.

[3] L. R. Churchill, *Rationing Health Care in America: Perceptions and Principles of Justice* (University of Notre Dame Press, 1987).

[4] H. Aaron and W. Schwartz, "Rationing Health Care: The Choice Before Us," *Science* 247, no. 4941 (1990): pp. 418–422.

[5] A. S. Relman, "Is Rationing Inevitable?", *New England Journal of Medicine* 322, no. 25 (1990): pp. 1809–1810.

several ways. First, they differ according to whether something has to be explicit to qualify as rationing. . . .

Second, they differ according to whether a resource must be absolutely scarce before its distribution qualifies as rationing. . . .

Third, they differ according to whether rationing only involves limits on necessary services, or whether limits on any beneficial services qualify as health care rationing. . . .

Figure [2.2] captures these 3 distinctions among rationing definitions. In Figure [2.2], the vertical line separates medical services that are being limited explicitly vs those that are being limited nonexplicitly. This line is to the left of the midpoint to suggest that more services are withheld nonexplicitly than explicitly, although the exact ratio of explicit-to-nonexplicit limitations is not represented. The horizontal line separates absolutely scarce resources from those that are not absolutely scarce. The horizontal line is above the midpoint of the diagram to suggest that few resources are absolutely scarce, although the exact ratio of scarce-to-nonscarce resources is not represented. Finally, within Figure [2.2] is a circle. Inside the circle are those health care services believed to be necessary; outside the circle are those health care services that are believed to be beneficial but not necessary.

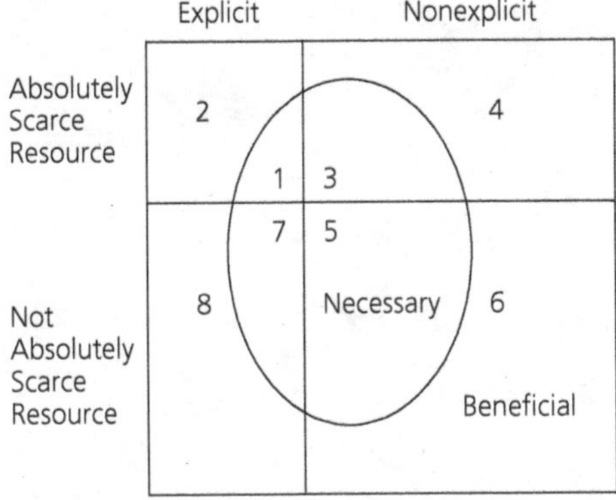

Figure [2.2] Distinctions among rationing definitions. The vertical line separates medical services that are being limited explicitly versus those limited nonexplicitly. The horizontal line separates absolutely scarce resources from those not absolutely scarce. For a more complete description, see the "Definitions of Rationing" section of the text.

Figure [2.2] is helpful in illustrating differences among various definitions of health care rationing. For example, the view that rationing only includes the explicit distribution of absolutely scarce and necessary resources, such as life-saving transplantations, is represented by section 1 of Figure [2.2]. The slightly less restrictive view, that rationing includes explicit distribution of absolutely scarce resources that are either necessary or beneficial, is represented by sections 1 and 2. And our view, that rationing includes any mechanism that allows people to go without beneficial health care services, is represented by sections 1 through 8. Nevertheless, as we discuss later, the 8 areas delineated by Figure [2.2] are not always distinct from each other. Instead, the lines between absolutely scarce and not absolutely scarce, between explicit and nonexplicit, and between necessary and beneficial are often fuzzy.

. . .

Choosing a Broad Definition of Health Care Rationing

We contend that health care rationing is best defined as implicitly or explicitly allowing people to go without beneficial health care services. By arguing for this broad definition of health care rationing, we do not suggest that there is only 1 meaning of the term *health care rationing*. Instead, we argue that a broad definition of health care rationing is a more useful starting point for debates about health care policy and health care priority setting.

We have primarily argued for this broad definition of rationing by pointing out problems with more restricted definitions that seek to limit rationing to explicit mechanisms, absolutely scarce resources, or necessary health care services.

But another type of argument leads us to the same broad definition of health care rationing. As mentioned earlier, the dividing lines illustrated in Figure [2.2], between absolutely scarce and nonscarce resources, between explicitly and implicitly withheld resources, and between necessary and beneficial resources, are not nearly as sharp as Figure [2.2] suggests. Where, for example, is the line between beneficial and necessary health care services? Given the fuzziness of these distinctions, it seems arbitrary to limit rationing to any of the narrow definitions that rely on maintaining these distinctions. Instead, a broad definition of rationing, by acknowledging the arbitrariness of these distinctions, focuses our attention less on distinctions and more on whether particular health care services are appropriate to withhold from patients. While we could debate whether cosmetic surgery is necessary or beneficial, it is much more important to decide whether all patients who want a specific type of cosmetic surgery should receive it.

Our broad definition of rationing will include many occurrences that do not strike most people as morally problematic and will include others where it is clearly wrong to withhold services from patients. It will force people to deal with the gray areas in moral debates about what patients ought to receive and what they should be allowed to live without. This broad definition of rationing forces us to deal with the moral issues in their full and troubling complexity.

By choosing this broad definition of health care rationing, we create room for many types of rationing, a number of which are suggested by the distinctions discussed earlier. For example, there is explicit rationing and implicit rationing, rationing of absolutely scarce resources and of fiscally scarce resources, and rationing of necessary resources and of beneficial but unnecessary resources. Similarly, it is highly likely that there are more and less justifiable types of rationing. By this broad definition of health care rationing, rationing is not defined as de facto inappropriate. Indeed, a major advantage of this broad view of rationing is that it forces us to decide when it is acceptable to allow particular patients to go without beneficial health care services.

. . .

EXCERPT 5

Full text from:

U. E. Reinhardt, "'Rationing' Health Care: What Does It Mean?", *New York Times*, July 3, 2009.

"Rationing" Health Care: What Does It Mean?

Uwe E. Reinhardt

As the dreaded R-word—rationing—once again worms its way into our debate on health care reform, it may be helpful to relearn what is taught about rationing in freshman economics.

In their well-known textbook Microeconomics, the Harvard professor Michael L. Katz and the Princeton professor Harvey S. Rosen, for example, put it thusly:

> Prices ration scarce resources. If bread were free, a huge quantity of it would be demanded. Because the resources used to produce bread are scarce, the actual amount of bread has to be rationed among its potential users. Not everyone can have all the bread that they could possibly want. The bread must be rationed somehow; the price system accomplishes this in the following way: Everyone who is willing to pay the equilibrium price gets the good, and everyone who does not, does not. [Italics added.]

In short, free markets are not an alternative to rationing. They are just one particular form of rationing. Ever since the Fall from Grace, human beings have had to ration everything not available in unlimited quantities, and market forces do most of the rationing.

Many critics of the current health reform efforts would have us believe that only governments ration things.

When a government insurance program refuses to pay for procedures that the managers of those insurance pools do not consider worth the taxpayer's money, these critics immediately trot out the R-word. It is the core of their argument against cost-effectiveness analysis and a public health plan for the nonelderly.

On the other hand, these same people believe that when, for similar reasons, a private health insurer refuses to pay for a particular procedure or has a price-tiered formulary for drugs—e.g., asking the insured to pay a 35% coinsurance rate on highly expensive biologic specialty drugs that effectively put that drug out of the patient's reach—the insurer is not rationing health care. Instead, the insurer is merely allowing "consumers" (formerly "patients") to use their discretion on how to use their own money. The insurers are said to be managing prudently and efficiently, forcing patients to trade off the benefits of health care against their other budget priorities.

These thoughts popped into my head as I sat as a guest in the White House East Room during last week's ABC News town hall meeting. There a neurologist suggested in his question that the president and his policy-making team seek to impose rationing of health care so that more lower-income Americans can receive it, all the while refusing to countenance that rationing for their own families.

One must wonder where people worried about "rationing" health care have been in the last 20 years. Could they possibly be unaware that the United States health system has rationed health care in spades for many years, on the economist's definition of rationing, and that President Obama and Congress are now desperately seeking to reduce or eliminate that form of rationing?

Let me remind rationing-phobes what they would find in the huge body of research literature and media reports on our health system, should they ever trouble themselves to read it:

- Many Americans without health insurance or very high deductibles routinely forgo prescribed medicine or follow-up visits with a doctor because they cannot afford it, risking more serious illness later on.
- A 2008 peer-reviewed study by researchers at the Urban Institute found that health spending for uninsured nonelderly

Americans is only about 43% of health spending for similar, privately insured Americans. Unless one argues that the extra 57% received by insured Americans is all waste, these data imply rationing by price and ability to pay.

- A few years ago, The Wall Street Journal featured a series of articles reporting how often uninsured middle-class Americans are charged the highest prices at pharmacies and in hospitals, and how sometimes they are hounded over medical bills to the point of being jailed for failed court appearances.
- Studies have shown that solid middle-class American families—even ostensibly insured families—can lose all of their savings and sometimes their homes over mounting medical bills in the case of severe illness.
- In its report Hidden Cost, Value Lost: The Uninsured in America, the prestigious Institute of Medicine a few years ago estimated that some 18,000 Americans yearly die prematurely for want of the timely health care that health insurance makes possible and that can prevent catastrophic illness.
- A recent study by an M.I.T. professor found that uninsured victims of severe traffic accidents receive 20% less health care than equivalent, insured victims and are 37% more likely to die from their injuries.

Need I go on?

As I read it, the main thrust of the health care reforms espoused by President Obama and his allies in Congress is first of all to reduce rationing on the basis of price and ability to pay in our health system.

An important allied goal is to seek greater value for the dollar in health care, through comparative effectiveness analysis and payment reform. As I reported in an earlier post on this blog, even the Business Roundtable, once a staunch defender of the American health system, now laments that relative to citizens in other developed countries, Americans receive an estimated 23% less value than they should, given our high health care spending.

To suggest that the main goal of the health reform efforts is to cram rationing down the throat of hapless, non-elite Americans reflects either woeful ignorance or of utter cynicism. Take your pick.

Wittgenstein, Ludwig. *Philosophical Investigations*. Ed. G. E. M. Anscombe. 3rd ed. (New York: Pearson), 1973.

Further Resources

Literature

Bruce, Andrea. "Drug Shortages Forcing Hard Decisions on Rationing Treatments," *New York Times*, January 29, 2016.

Pipes, C. Sally. "Obama Will Ration Your Health Care," *The Wall Street Journal*, December 30, 2008.

Singer, Peter. "Why We Must Ration Health Care," *New York Times*, July 25, 2009.

Other Media

Anne Curzan. "What makes a word 'real'?" TED video, 17:09, March, 2014. https://www.ted.com/talks/anne_curzan_what_makes_a_word_real?language=en: The speakers discusses that although we heavily rely on dictionaries, we rarely consider who the authority figures making these books are.

3 General Ethical Theory

Imagine you are walking in a forest. On your way back to the parking lot, you approach some railroad tracks that you crossed heading out. As you near, you notice that a runaway trolley with an unconscious driver is headed down a hill toward five railroad employees wearing earmuffs, engrossed in their work on the tracks with heavy machinery. Right where you cross the tracks there happens to be a switch. Instantly, you reach for it, to divert the train away from the workers onto another track. However, just as you are about to move the lever, you notice with horror that that there is a sixth worker on this track, equally equipped and absorbed in his work. Should you throw the switch and divert the trolley so that instead of killing five workers, only one is killed?[1]

While this scenario might be viewed merely as a philosopher's abstract thought experiment, it also has very clear analogies to many rationing and resource allocation decisions. For example, if it is permissible to throw the switch, should it also be permissible to turn off the power of a patients' life support in the ICU to use her liver, heart, kidneys, and pancreas to save the lives of five other dying patients?

Cases such as these raise the question of which fundamental ethical principles should guide individual actions or broader policies when we have to make rationing or resource allocation decisions. Among philosophers, there is no agreement on how to answer this question. Over time, there have been two dominant—and largely opposing—theories: deontology and utilitarianism. As comprehensive ethical theories, they are systematic attempts to address ethical choices based on fundamental conceptions of what is valuable in human life. Although they have not been set out with the aim of addressing rationing or resource allocation decisions, they had much influence in shaping underlying value frameworks. In addition, there have been other influential alternative theories that have been set out largely in response to deontology and utilitarianism and that seek to sidestep some of the central problems that they face. The most influential

[1] J. J. Thomson, "The Trolley Problem," *The Yale Law Journal* 94, no. 6 (1985): pp. 1395–1415.

of the alternative approaches described here is known as *political liberalism*. This theory aims to offer a response to the fact that pluralist democracies will typically include a wide range of fundamental normative positions—including those sympathetic to either deontological and utilitarian approaches—while still needing to make policy that is supported as reasonable by as many people as possible. The chapter also includes excerpts setting out different understandings of *egalitarianism*, a group of theories in political philosophy that posit as a primary objective to treat people equally, with central implications for allocation decisions and particularly also the role that personal responsibility should play.

To return to the trolley dilemma, a line of reasoning that is based on the thinking of the British philosophers Jeremy Bentham (1748–1832) and John Stuart Mill (1806–1873) can lend support to positions inclined to save the most lives. Bentham and Mill observe that people typically seek pleasure and avoid pain. Mill, further developing Bentham's work, set out some of utilitarianism's key tenets in an essay originally published in a popular magazine article in 1861 under the title of *Utilitarianism* (Excerpt 1).[2] He defines what came to be known as the Greatest Happiness Principle, according to which

> actions are right in proportion as they tend to promote happiness, wrong as they tend to produce the reverse of happiness. By happiness is intended pleasure, and the absence of pain; by unhappiness, pain, and the privation of pleasure.

Bentham and Mill argue that utility obtains insofar as actions maximize pleasure and minimize pain, leading them to call their approach "Utilitarianism." Importantly, the level at which the balance of pleasure over pain is assessed is not merely that of the individual concerned, but of all beings capable of pleasure and pain. This type of assessment requires an impartial perspective: "As between his own happiness and that of others, utilitarianism requires [an agent] to be as strictly impartial as a disinterested and benevolent spectator."[3] The supreme principle of Utilitarianism is therefore maximizing happiness from a universal and impartial viewpoint. Accordingly, the Greatest Happiness Principle is typically understood as requiring the realization of the greatest good for the greatest number.

Utilitarianism thus focuses centrally on the consequences of actions. In later developments, this gave rise to a formal distinction between *act utilitarianism* and *rule utilitarianism*. Act utilitarianism aims to maximize utility in each individual action. Rule utilitarianism recognizes that an individual act may increase utility temporarily, but also takes a broader perspective. It additionally recognizes the possibility that the routine adoption of some actions that temporarily increase utility could eventually lower overall utility. For instance, sacrificing a person on life support to use her organs to extend the lives of five others would be an act that, in the short term, increases overall utility. But doing so routinely could have other unintended consequences. Many people might become reluctant to go to the hospital for fear of becoming an organ "donor," thereby lowering overall utility of the practice in the longer term. When utility maximizing acts would lead to such consequences, rule utilitarians try to find rules that can avoid the unintended consequences. John Smart's discussion of the rightness and wrongness of actions discusses the distinction between act and rule utilitarianism in abstract terms in more detail and illustrates it further through two concrete examples (Excerpt 2).[4]

Utilitarianism seems to lead to repugnant conclusions when it comes to rationing decisions. It would seem to be acceptable to divert the trolley to kill one person rather than five and acceptable to take one person off life support and harvest her organs to save five other patients. Yet, as Chapters 9 and 10 show, its

[2] J. S. Mill, *Utilitarianism, Liberty & Representative Government* (J. M. Dent, 1910), pp. 5–24.

[3] Ibid.

[4] J. J. Smart and B. Williams, *Utilitarianism: For and Against* (New York: Cambridge University Press, 1973), pp. 97–100.

focus on maximizing overall welfare or utility from an impartial point of view is at the core of the dominant paradigm of cost-effectiveness analysis (CEA) that underlies resource allocation. CEA aims to assess from an objective perspective the relative effectiveness of healthcare interventions to maximize health gains—utility. Unqualified, CEA focuses on the total sum and not on the distribution of benefits: it is intentionally blind to who or which groups of patients benefit and centers on maximizing overall health gains per unit of cost.

A fundamentally different ethical theory is that of *deontology*. The name is derived from the Greek terms *logos* and *to deon*, referring to the teaching or science of what is proper, required, or a duty. This theory focuses on what constitutes an ethical duty. The rightness or wrongness of actions or rules is decidedly not dependent on their outcomes. And the focus is not on saving the most lives but on acting from duty. The German Enlightenment philosopher Immanuel Kant (1724–1804) set out a systematic account with far-reaching influence in his *Groundwork of the Metaphysic of Morals* (Excerpt 3).[5] The work opens with a broadside against utilitarianism:

> There is nothing it is possible to think of anywhere in the world, or indeed anything at all outside it, that can be held to be good without limitation, excepting only a good will. [. . .] The good will is good not through what it effects or accomplishes, not through its efficacy for attaining any intended end, but only through its willing, i.e., good in itself, and considered for itself, without comparison, it is to be estimated far higher than anything that could be brought about by it in favor of any inclination, or indeed, if you prefer, of the sum of all inclinations.

Kant observes that humans can act in two distinct ways. Acting in an instrumental or practical way, we can find means to accomplish certain ends. For example, when we are hungry, we can find food and stop being hungry. But what matters ethically is that we are also able to reflect on our actions and act in ways in which the reason for action is not satisfaction of some physical desire or primal need, but to act in accordance with principles that fulfill moral standards. On Kant's view, it is only when we act on the basis of ethical principles—with a good will—that we are acting freely and thus morally.

In the case of seeking food because of hunger, the will only executes because it is determined by need. But imagine a situation in which we could lie to someone in a way that would confer a disadvantage on him but an advantage on ourselves. For example, there might be an opportunity to cheat someone out of money. If we refrain from doing so because we view the action as wrong, the will is determined from within us and aligned with a fundamental moral principle. Kant argues that what matters is that we act in ways that are universalizable: if there was no trust that people would hold explicit and implicit promises, moral agents would be constantly frustrated and fundamental institutions of society—such as promise-keeping—would collapse. As a guide for moral action, Kant therefore set out a test for actions in the form of what he calls the *categorical imperative*: "I ought never to conduct myself except so that I could also will that my maxim become a universal law."[6] As long as we act in accordance with this imperative, Kant argues, our actions are principled, free, and ethical.

Kant discusses several different formulations of the categorical imperative. The second version applies the imperative to how we should treat other people. This version came to be known as the *formula of humanity*, and it emphasizes that all persons have equal moral worth and are equally deserving of respect: "Act so that you use humanity, as much in your own person as in the person of every other, always at the same time as an end and never merely as means."[7] What this means in the case of harvesting one person's organs to save the lives of

---

[5] I. Kant, *Groundwork for the Metaphysics of Morals* (New Haven: Yale University Press, 2002).

[6] Ibid.

[7] Ibid.

five people is that the act is impermissible, as the one person is treated merely as a means. Pure instrumentalization is prohibited by the formula of humanity. Many would argue that denying cancer patients costly treatment that extends their lives by a few months also violates the formula. The way such arguments feature in actual policy will be considered later in Chapters 9 and 10 in relation to what has been termed the "rule of rescue."

The tension between deontology and utilitarianism can be summarized in the following way: utilitarianism determines whether an action or rule is ethical by assessing its consequences. That action or rule that produces the most benefit—which can be assessed as a balance of pleasure over pain, happiness, or, more commonly, utility—is the ethical thing to do. Deontology determines whether an action is ethical by assessing whether the person doing it is acting from duty. Acting from duty entails following a rule or imperative that can be universalizable. Regarding the treatment of people, this means that we should never treat people merely as means, but also always as ends in themselves.

In the 20th century, utilitarianism seemed dominant in many areas and influenced much of public policy. John Rawls (1921–2002), an American political philosopher, was dissatisfied by utilitarianism and its implications (Excerpt 4).[8] In particular, utilitarianism insufficiently valued individual rights. Rights were only honored when they increased utility or happiness and could be overridden when more utility or happiness could result. Furthermore, Rawls was concerned that utilitarians centered on maximizing utility or happiness, and then seemed to ignore how that utility or happiness was distributed among people. Ironically, despite utilitarianism's emphasis on being impartial in distributing benefits, its conception of neutrality would permit that a small number of people receive all the benefits—as long as that is how most overall benefits are produced. Rawls thought such distributions should not be acceptable and that there should be principles that could ensure a more fair distribution.

Rawls's goal was to find ethical principles not for personal action but to guide political or public policy decisions. He was also acutely aware that, in the public sphere, people have different values. What one person considers beneficial another person may not. Some might be utilitarians, others deontologists. His challenge was to find a set of ethical principles that reasonable people with different values and views of what is good in life could agree to. To find the answer, he developed a hypothetical or imaginary scenario: the *original position*.

Imagine we bring together all people living in a society with as yet to be determined structures and institutions. These people do not know anything about the specifics of their future lives. They do not know if they are a man or woman, Catholic, Muslim, Buddhist, Protestant, Jewish, Hindu, or have no religion at all. They do not know if they will be rich or poor, or what job, if any, they have. They do not know what they value, which talents, abilities, or possible disabilities they have. This constrained view about the specific position in society that the people in the original position have Rawls calls the "veil of ignorance."[9] What these hypothetical people do know is that they will have different values and ideas about what makes a good life. That is, they will have what Rawls calls different comprehensive doctrines or systems of religious and moral beliefs. The original position is intended to neutralize personal knowledge about natural talents and social circumstances, and then asks people to imagine what principles they would want to govern their society, what principles of justice they would think would be fair. Rawls argues that by neutralizing natural endowment and social circumstance, the principles agreed to in the original position under a veil of ignorance would be fair and ethical ones to govern public policy decisions.

So what kind of principles would reasonable people choose? Rawls identifies three principles (although he expresses them as two,

[8] J. Rawls, *A Theory of Justice, Revised Edition* (Cambridge: Harvard University Press, 1999).

[9] Ibid., p. 160.

see Excerpt 9).[10] First, and most fundamentally, people would grant each other basic political rights and liberties, such as freedom of speech, assembly, and religion, one-person-one vote, and due process of law. This has been termed the Liberty Principle. Second, Rawls asserts, there would be consensus on what he calls the Fair Equality of Opportunity Principle. Powerful offices and careers should not be available only to the rich and powerful, but open to all, based on their capabilities. This principle means that offices, jobs, and other positions should be open to everyone to compete for. No governmental position or other job should be reserved only for men, or Protestants, or, perhaps, children of certain aristocratic families. This second principle seeks to ensure that there is fair opportunity for people who start out poor and disadvantaged to develop their talents, work hard, and move up in society. Correspondingly, it calls for societal structures that enable such movement.

Third, Rawls argues that people would agree that it is permissible to distribute basic (or primary) social and economic goods such as income and wealth in an unequal way—but only in so far as the inequality is to the greatest benefit of the least-advantaged members of society. This is called the Difference Principle. It means that it is ethical to allow people with superior talents and skills to have far higher incomes than others, as long as that inequality also improves the situation of those who are the worst-off in society. Consider the following options of distributing lifetime-average levels of income, shown in Table 3.1 compared to a hypothetical benchmark A that embodies strict equality:[11]

Table 3.1
Income Distribution Scenarios

Economic Scenarios	Worst-Off Group	Middle Group	Best-Off Group	Total Aggregate Income
A	10,000	10,000	10,000	30,000
B	12,000	15,000	20,000	40,000
C	20,000	30,000	50,000	110,000
D	17,000	50,000	100,000	167,000

Utilitarianism would favor scenario D because it generates the highest overall utility. But the difference principle would support option C only: although both of the better-off groups are worse-off than in scenario D, and although the total aggregate income is lower, the worst-off group fares the best compared to scenario A. For Rawls, injustice results from "inequalities that are not to the benefit of all."[12]

In Excerpt 5, Will Kymlicka outlines important internal tensions arising from Rawls's work that have influenced much subsequent thinking in political philosophy.[13] Kymlicka focuses centrally on issues around compensating for natural inequalities and subsidizing people's choices. He asserts that Rawls "leaves too much room for the influence of natural inequalities, and at the same time leaves too little room for the influence of our choices."[14] These issues are highly relevant for discussions in rationing and resource allocation.

First, Kymlicka emphasizes that Rawls's approach views two people as equally well-off as long as they have the same bundle of social primary goods—even if one of them may have higher resource needs because of poor health or physical or mental disability. But this seems implausible. In the same way, Kymlicka finds unpersuasive that a person should be viewed

[10] R. J. Arneson, "Luck, Egalitarianism and Prioritarianism," *Ethics* 110, no. 2 (2000): pp. 339–349.

[11] L. Wenar, "John Rawls," Stanford Encyclopedia of Philosophy, 2012, accessed July 26, 2015, http://plato.stanford.edu/entries/rawls/.

[12] Rawls, *A Theory of Justice*, p. 54.

[13] W. Kymlicka, *Contemporary Political Philosophy* (Oxford: Clarendon Press, 1990), pp. 70–76.

[14] Ibid., p. 70.

as better-off simply because she has more primary goods than another. Having nominally more may still result in challenges for the person concerned, for it can be the case that "the extra income is not enough to pay for extra costs she faces due to some natural disadvantage—e.g. the costs of medication for an illness, or of special equipment for some handicap."[15]

Second, Kymlicka argues that when "inequalities in income are the result of choices not circumstances, the difference principle creates, rather than removes, unfairness."[16] He illustrates this with the case of two people who are identical in natural endowment and primary goods. One of them uses his resources to purchase land for a garden to grow vegetables for his own consumption and to sell the remainder to make a living. The other purchases land to build a tennis court to play all day long, working just enough on a nearby farm to sustain basic needs such as housing, food, and clothing. Soon, the gardener is better off than the tennis player in terms of available primary goods. The difference principle would require redistributing some of the gains of the gardener to the tennis player—but this, Kymlicka says, would be "peculiar," as treating "people with equal concern requires that people pay for the costs of their own choices."[17]

The latter tension is not unique to Rawls, but also arises in many egalitarian theories that comprise a wide variety of approaches unified in the basic tenet that all human persons are equal in some fundamental way, echoing Kant's universalist conception.[18] When it comes to tennis players and gardeners, what does respecting people as equals mean? And what are the implications for the context of this anthology: Should rationing and resource allocation decisions be sensitive to the choices we make? Or should policy and practice be dependent or independent of whether, for example, people live healthily, or, perhaps, smoke, or eat and drink excessively?

An influential variety of theories that came to be termed "luck-egalitarian" address this issue directly. As Richard Arneson[19] notes in Excerpt 6, in luck-egalitarianism,

> the aim of justice as equality is to eliminate so far as is possible the impact on people's lives of bad luck that falls on them through no fault or choice of their own. In the ideal luck egalitarian society, there are no inequalities in people's life prospects except those that arise through processes of voluntary choice or faulty conduct, for which the agents involved can reasonably be held responsible.

The approach has attracted strong criticism on the grounds that it can be overly harsh and abandon people to their dire fates.[20] Arneson seeks to avoid key elements of such criticism by defending what he terms *responsibility-catering prioritarianism*, the view that

> justice requires us to maximize a function of human well-being that gives priority to improving the well-being of those who are badly off and of those who, if badly off, are not substantially responsible for their condition in virtue of their prior conduct.

Arneson emphasizes that "priority is assigned to aiding an individual in virtue of how badly his life is going, as measured by an objective scale," and therefore tilts distributing benefits in favor of those who are badly off—while still, of course, requiring, "misfortune due to bad luck" as a condition for entitlement to assistance.[21] In Excerpt 7, Shlomi Segall also seeks to defend a version of luck-egalitarianism, but goes further than Arneson in being inclusive toward people

---

15 Ibid., p. 71.

16 Ibid., p. 73.

17 Ibid., p. 74.

18 R. Arneson, "Egalitarianism," Stanford Encyclopedia of Philosophy, 2013, http://plato.stanford.edu/entries/egalitarianism/.

19 R. J. Arneson, "Luck, Egalitarianism and Prioritarianism," *Ethics* 110, no. 2 (2000): pp. 339–349.

20 E. S. Anderson, "What Is the Point of Equality?", *Ethics* 109, no. 2 (1999): pp. 287–337.

21 Arneson, "Luck, Egalitarianism and Prioritarianism."

who have made bad choices.[22] After a review of five strategies that seek to avoid the objection that luck-egalitarianians are unduly harsh on people who are responsible for needs, he proposes to supplement the theory with a value outside of it: autonomy. The core of his argument is that since luck-egalitarian justice requires compensation of losses that people are not responsible for, the underlying requirement is that people

> need to be held responsible for their actions. To meet that purpose individuals must be autonomous, for surely people cannot be held responsible when lacking the autonomy to do otherwise. And, in order to safeguard such autonomy, certain threshold requirements must be satisfied (minimal healthy functioning, adequate nutrition, the social basis of minimal self-respect, etc.). Indeed, it is essential for a luck egalitarian regime to observe these threshold requirements, for, once victims of bad option luck are allowed to slip below the material prerequisites of autonomy, their subsequent choices and actions invariably fall under the brute luck category, as the agents cannot be held responsible for the resulting disadvantages.[23]

So what role would this characterization leave for the choices people made in policy and practice? Segall is willing to accept personal responsibility as a tie-breaker in situations where two patients are in equal need of treatment, but in one case the need arose because of avoidable risk taking, and in the other case because of faulty judgment. That is, in the case of a car crash, where we are forced to choose between treating a reckless driver and his equally needy innocent passenger, "we would then need a justification for not using considerations of self-responsibility as tie-breakers"—and Segall emphasizes that this need of justification equally applies to other normative theories, and is not confined to luck-egalitarianism.[24]

In Excerpt 8, Scheffler examines two questions:[25] to what extent luck-egalitarians, as often claimed, can draw support from Rawls, and whether luck-egalitarianism itself is a plausible form of egalitarianism. On both counts his answer is negative. While some commentators suggest that Rawls simply failed to appreciate that his approach would commit him to adjusting for peoples' choices in what goods they are entitled to, Scheffler reviews Rawls' project to underline that it was about determining

> which principles of distributive justice are most appropriate for a modern democratic society. . . . In other words, the question is which principles of justice are most consistent, in modern conditions, with the freedom and equality of persons. Equality is understood as a social and political ideal that governs the relations in which people stand to one another. The core of the value of equality does not, according to this understanding, consist in the idea that there is something that must be distributed or allocated equally"

Scheffler therefore argues that instead of providing foundations for luck-egalitarianism, Rawls's conception of free and equal people favors a more general conception of equality as a social and political ideal.

He objects to luck-egalitarianism as a plausible form of egalitarianism because he finds that the degree of weight that the position "places on the distinction between choices and circumstances [is] both philosophically dubious and morally implausible."[26] He is concerned that it is not clear at all how to determine when exactly an action can be seen as truly voluntary given that specific behaviors are often based on a complex entanglement that includes unchosen personality traits and social circumstance

[22] S. Segall, *Health, Luck, and Justice* (Princeton University Press, 2009).

[23] Ibid., p. 63.

[24] Ibid., p. 70.

[25] S. Scheffler, "What Is Egalitarianism?", *Philosophy & Public Affairs* 31, no. 1 (2003): pp. 5–39.

[26] Ibid.

along with what seems to stand out as a person's deliberate choice. He reviews several attempts at defending the luck-egalitarian position against these and further charges but finds them all falling short of being satisfactory.

Rationing and resource allocation decisions always have ethical foundations, whether they are stated explicitly—by referring in transparent ways to broader theories—or can be reconstructed more implicitly by analyzing the underlying principles of specific policies. One attraction of, for example, CEA, is that is can be based explicitly on utilitarian principles. Transparency and accountability can help people affected by decisions to know what drives policy, and possible criticism can be directed at concrete elements of policy or the underlying theory. However, a major problem with a monolithic theoretical framework as a basis for rationing and resource allocation is found in Rawls's point that people typically have different comprehensive doctrines, worldviews, or value systems—not everyone affected by CEA used in resource allocation agrees with utilitarianism. Clearly, all types of egalitarians, as well as proponents of other theories, are aware of the fact of pluralism. Yet, for better or worse, Rawls can be credited with pushing hard to abandon seemingly irresolvable arguments about the rightness and wrongness of ethical standards (including those governing rationing and resource allocation decisions). In Excerpt 9, Ezekiel Emanuel emphasizes that the focus on neutrality by attempting to accommodate the range of holders of different comprehensive doctrines is understandable but ultimately has a major drawback in that it risks undecideability—a problem to which we return in Chapters 5, 9, and 10.[27]

Suppose that you have the following situation: a ward holds 15 patients and all face certain death. Ten patients can be cured with one pill, 5 each require two. All 15 patients are similar in other respects, although 3 have contributed to their disease by heavy drinking. You only have 10 pills. How would you distribute the pills? What should be the hospital's policy?[28] Should you give the pills to patients who just need 1 pill and save 10 lives? Should you give them to the patients who need 2 pills and save 5 lives? Should you choose a lottery and give everyone a chance, most likely saving fewer than 10 lives? Should you exclude those who drank themselves to ill health and then use a lottery? A utilitarian would typically favor the first option. A deontologist would feel more pressure toward the lottery, and a Rawlsian framework might also support this policy. Some versions of Prioritarianism and most—though not all—luck-egalitarians would accept depri-oritizing those among the patients requiring 2 pills who have contributed to their condition through excessive use of alcohol. The following excerpts and subsequent chapters will illuminate in more detail the reach and relevance of normative theories in shaping principles and policies for making rationing and resource allocation decisions.

---

[27] E. Emanuel, *The Ends of Human Life: Medical Ethics in a Liberal Polity* (Cambridge: Harvard University Press, 1991), pp. 35–37.

[28] D. W. Brock and D. Wikler, "Ethical Issues in Resource Allocation, Research, and New Product Development," in *Disease Control Priorities in Developing Countries, 2nd Edition*, edited by D. Jamison, et al. (Washington, DC: Oxford University Press and The World Bank, 2006), p. 264.

Questions for Discussion

1. A runaway trolley is headed toward five railroad workers. You stand at a switch. You can divert the trolley towards a track with one worker. Should you divert the trolley?
2. You're a gifted transplant surgeon. Five patients need five different organs. UNOS is on strike. There's a hospitalized motorcyclist with compatible organs for each of the five patients. She's an organ donor—and she has no family or friends. She is recovering, but she is on life support. Should you take her off life support?
3. The Golden Rule is often stated as "Do unto others as you would have them do unto you." Is this the same as, or something different from, Kant's categorical imperative?
4. Kymlicka criticizes Rawls by arguing that when "inequalities in income are the result of choices not circumstances, the difference principle creates, rather than removes, unfairness." Restate Rawls's difference principle and set out whether you agree or disagree with Kymlicka's charge (you may wish to draw on his discussion of the tennis player and the gardener in Excerpt 5).
5. In Excerpt 6, Arneson notes that "In the ideal luck egalitarian society, there are no inequalities in people's life prospects except those that arise through processes of voluntary choice or faulty conduct, for which the agents involved can reasonably be held responsible." Assume that you are a country's most senior health official. After a recent election, the new government tasks you with organizing health policy according to the luck-egalitarian ideal. In which area of health policy do you expect the greatest challenges?

EXCERPTS

Note: The following excerpts have generally been edited for length, and omissions are indicated with ellipses. Editing includes footnotes and endnotes, which have also been renumbered. For citation and related purposes, the full original source texts should be used.

EXCERPT 1

Abridged text from:

J. S. Mill, *Utilitarianism, Liberty & Representative Government* (J. M. Dent, 1910), pp. 5–24.

Chapter 11 What Utilitarianism Is

John Stuart Mill

. . .

The creed which accepts as the foundation of morals, Utility, or the Greatest Happiness Principle, holds that actions are right in proportion as they tend to promote happiness, wrong as they tend to produce the reverse of happiness. By happiness is intended pleasure, and the absence of pain; by unhappiness, pain, and the privation of pleasure. To give a clear view of the moral standard set up by the theory, much more requires to be said; in particular, what things it includes in the ideas of pain and pleasure; and to what extent this is left an open question. But these supplementary explanations do not affect the theory of life on which this theory of morality is grounded—namely, that pleasure, and freedom from pain, are the only things desirable as ends; and that all desirable things (which are as numerous in the utilitarian as in any other scheme) are desirable either for the pleasure inherent in themselves, or as means to the promotion of pleasure and the prevention of pain.

. . .

According to the Greatest Happiness Principle . . . the ultimate end, with reference to and for the sake of which all other things are desirable (whether we are considering our own good or that of other people), is an existence exempt as far as possible from pain, and as rich as possible in enjoyments, both in point of quantity and quality; the test of quality, and the rule for measuring it against quantity, being the preference felt by those who, in their opportunities of experience, to which must be added their habits of self-consciousness and self-observation, are best furnished with the means of comparison. This, being, according to the utilitarian opinion, the end of human action, is necessarily also the standard of morality; which may accordingly be defined, the rules and precepts for human conduct, by the observance of which an existence such as has been described might be, to the greatest extent possible, secured to all mankind; and not to them only, but, so far as the nature of things admits, to the whole sentient creation.

. . .

The utilitarian morality does recognise in human beings the power of sacrificing their own greatest good for the good of others. It only refuses to admit that the sacrifice is itself a good. A sacrifice which does not increase, or tend to increase, the sum total of happiness, it considers as wasted. The only self-renunciation which it applauds, is devotion to the happiness, or to some of the means of happiness, of others; either of mankind collectively, or of individuals within the limits imposed by the collective interests of mankind. I must again repeat, what the assailants of utilitarianism seldom have the justice to acknowledge, that the happiness which forms the utilitarian standard of what is right in conduct, is not the agent's own happiness, but that of all concerned. As between his own happiness and that of others, utilitarianism requires him to be as strictly impartial as a disinterested and benevolent spectator. In the golden rule of Jesus of Nazareth, we read the complete spirit of the ethics of utility. To do as one would be done by, and to love one's neighbour as oneself, constitute the ideal perfection of utilitarian morality. As the means of making the nearest approach to this ideal, utility would enjoin, first, that laws and social arrangements should place the happiness, or (as speaking practically it may be called) the interest, of every individual, as nearly as possible in harmony with the interest of the whole; and secondly, that education and opinion, which have so vast a power over human character, should so use that power as to establish in the mind of every individual an indissoluble association between his own happiness and the good of the whole; especially between his own happiness and the practice of such modes of conduct, negative and positive, as regard for the universal happiness prescribes: so that not only he may be unable to conceive the possibility of happiness to himself, consistently with conduct opposed to the general good, but also that a direct impulse to promote the general good may be in every individual one of the habitual motives of action, and the sentiments connected therewith may fill a large and prominent place in every human being's sentient existence. If the impugners of the utilitarian morality represented it to their own minds in this its true character, I know not what recommendation possessed by any other morality they could possibly affirm to be wanting to it: what more beautiful or more exalted developments of human nature any other ethical system can be supposed to foster, or what springs of action, not accessible to the utilitarian, such systems rely on for giving effect to their mandates.

The objectors to utilitarianism cannot always be charged with representing it in a discreditable light. On the contrary, those among them who entertain anything like a just idea of its disinterested character, sometimes find fault with its standard as being too high for humanity. They say it is exacting too much to require that people shall always act from the inducement of promoting the general interests of society. But this is to mistake the very meaning of a standard of morals, and to confound the rule of action with the motive of it. It is the business of ethics to tell us what are our duties, or by what test we may know them; but no system of ethics requires that the sole motive of all we do shall be a feeling of duty; on the contrary, ninety-nine hundredths of all our actions are done from other motives, and rightly so done, if the rule of duty does not condemn them. It is the more unjust to utilitarianism that this particular misapprehension should be made a ground of objection to it, inasmuch as utilitarian moralists have gone beyond almost all others in affirming that the motive has nothing to do with the morality of the action, though much with the worth of the agent. He who saves a fellow creature from drowning does what is morally right, whether his motive be duty, or the hope of being paid for his trouble: he who betrays the friend that trusts him, is guilty of a crime, even if his object be to serve another friend to whom he is under greater obligations. [B]ut to speak only of actions done from the motive of duty, and in direct obedience to principle: it is a misapprehension of the utilitarian mode of thought, to conceive it as implying that people should fix their minds upon so wide a generality as the world, or society at large. The great majority of good actions are intended, not for the benefit of the world, but for that of individuals, of which the good of the world is made up; and the thoughts of the most virtuous man need not on these occasions travel beyond the particular persons concerned, except so far as is necessary to assure himself that in benefiting them he is not violating the rights—that is, the legitimate and authorized expectations—of any one else. The multiplication of happiness is, according to the utilitarian ethics, the object of virtue: the occasions on which any person (except one in a thousand) has it in his power to do this on an extended scale, in other words, to be a public benefactor, are but exceptional; and on these occasions alone is he called on to consider public utility; in every other case, private utility, the interest or happiness of some few persons, is all he has to attend to. Those alone the influence of whose actions extends to society in general, need concern themselves habitually about so large an object. In the case of abstinences indeed—of things which people forbear to do, from moral considerations, though the consequences in the particular case might be beneficial—it would be unworthy of an intelligent agent not to be consciously aware that the action is of a class which, if practised generally, would be generally injurious, and that this is the ground of the obligation to abstain from it. The amount of regard for the public interest implied in this recognition, is no greater than is demanded by every system of morals;

for they all enjoin to abstain from whatever is manifestly pernicious to society. The same considerations dispose of another reproach against the doctrine of utility, founded on a still grosser misconception of the purpose of a standard of morality, and of the very meaning of the words right and wrong. It is often affirmed that utilitarianism renders men cold and unsympathizing; that it chills their moral feelings towards individuals; that it makes them regard only the dry and hard consideration of the consequences of actions, not taking into their moral estimate the qualities from which those actions emanate. If the assertion means that they do not allow their judgment respecting the rightness or wrongness of an action to be influenced by their opinion of the qualities of the person who does it, this is a complaint not against utilitarianism, but against having any standard of morality at all; for certainly no known ethical standard decides an action to be good or bad because it is done by a good or a bad man, still less because done by an amiable, a brave, or a benevolent man or the contrary. These considerations are relevant, not to the estimation of actions, but of persons; and there is nothing in the utilitarian theory inconsistent with the fact that there are other things which interest us in persons besides the rightness and wrongness of their actions. The Stoics, indeed, with the paradoxical misuse of language which was part of their system, and by which they strove to raise themselves above all concern about anything but virtue, were fond of saying that he who has that has everything; that he, and only he, is rich, is beautiful, is a king. But no claim of this description is made for the virtuous man by the utilitarian doctrine. Utilitarians are quite aware that there are other desirable possessions and qualities besides virtue, and are perfectly willing to allow to all of them their full worth. They are also aware that a right action does not necessarily indicate a virtuous character, and that actions which are blameable often proceed from qualities entitled to praise. When this is apparent in any particular case, it modifies their estimation, not certainly of the act, but of the agent. I grant that they are, notwithstanding, of opinion, that in the long run the best proof of a good character is good actions; and resolutely refuse to consider any mental disposition as good, of which the predominant tendency is to produce bad conduct. This makes them unpopular with many people; but it is an unpopularity which they must share with every one who regards the distinction between right and wrong in a serious light; and the reproach is not one which a conscientious utilitarian need be anxious to repel.

EXCERPT 2

Abridged text from:
J. J. Smart and B. Williams, *Utilitarianism: For and Against* (New York: Cambridge University Press, 1973), pp. 30–57, 97–100.

Utilitarianism: For and Against

J. J. Smart and B. Williams

6. Rightness and Wrongness of Actions

I shall now state the act-utilitarian doctrine. Purely for simplicity of exposition I shall put it forward in a broadly hedonistic form. If anyone values states of mind such as knowledge independently of their' pleasurableness he can make appropriate verbal alterations to convert it from hedonistic to ideal' utilitarianism. And I shall not here take sides on the issue between hedonistic and quasi-ideal utilitarianism. I shall concern myself with the evaluation signified by "ought" in "one ought to do that which will produce the best consequences," and leave to one side the evaluation signified by the word "best."

Let us say, then, that the only reason for performing an action *A* rather than an alternative action *B* is that doing *A* will make mankind (or, perhaps, all sentient beings) happier than will doing *B*. (Here I put aside the consideration that in fact we can have only probable belief about the effects" of our actions, and so our reason should be more precisely stated as that doing *A* will produce more probable benefit than will doing B. For convenience of exposition I shelve this question of probability for a page or two.) This is so simple and natural a doctrine that we can surely expect that many of my readers will have at least some propensity to agree. For I am talking, as I said earlier, to sympathetic and benevolent men, that is, to men who desire the happiness of mankind. Since they have a favourable attitude to the general happiness, surely they will have a tendency to submit to an ultimate moral principle which does no more than express this attitude. It is true that these men, being human, will also have purely selfish attitudes. Either these attitudes will be in harmony with the general happiness (in cases where everyone's looking after his own interests promotes the maximum general happiness) or they will not be in harmony with the general happiness, in which case they will largely cancel one another out, and so could not be made the basis of an interpersonal discussion anyway. It is possible, then, that many sympathetic and benevolent people depart from or fail to attain a utilitarian ethical principle only under the stress of tradition, of superstition, or of unsound philosophical reasoning. If this hypothesis should turn out to be correct, at least as far as these readers are concerned, then the utilitarian may contend that there is no need for him to defend his position directly, save by stating it in a consistent manner, and by showing that common objections to it are unsound. After all, it expresses an ultimate attitude, not a liking for something merely as a means to something else. Save for attempting to remove confusions and discredit superstitions which may get in the way of clear moral thinking, he cannot, of course, appeal to argument and must rest his hopes on the good feeling of his readers. If any reader is not a sympathetic and benevolent man, then of course it cannot be expected that he will have an ultimate pro-attitude to human happiness in general. . . .

The utilitarian's ultimate moral principle, let it be remembered, expresses the sentiment not of altruism but of benevolence, the agent counting himself neither more nor less than any other person. Pure altruism cannot be made the basis of a universal moral discussion because it might lead different people to different and perhaps incompatible courses of action, even though the circumstances were identical. When two men each try to let the other through a door first a deadlock results.

Altruism could hardly commend itself to those of a scientific, and hence universalistic, frame of mind. If you count in my calculations why should I not count in your calculations? And why should I pay more attention to my calculations than to yours? Of course we often tend to praise and honour altruism even more than generalized benevolence. This is because people too often err on the side of selfishness, and so altruism is a fault on the right side. If we can make a man try to be an altruist he may succeed as far as acquiring a generalized benevolence.

Suppose we could predict the future consequences of actions with certainty. Then it would be possible to say that the total future consequences of action *A* are such-and-such and that the total future consequences of action *B* are so-and-so. In order to help someone to decide whether to do *A* or to do *B* we could say to him: "Envisage the total consequences of *A*, and think them over carefully and imaginatively. Now envisage the total consequences of B, and think them over carefully. As a benevolent and humane man, and thinking of yourself just as one man among others, would you prefer the consequences of *A* or those of B?" That is, we are asking for a comparison of one (present and future) *total* situation with another (present and future) *total* situation. So far we are not asking for a *summation* or *calculation* of pleasures or happiness. We are asking only for a comparison of total situations. And it seems clear that we can frequently make such a comparison and say that one total situation is better than another. For example few people would not prefer a total situation in which a million people are well-fed, well-clothed, free of pain, doing interesting and enjoyable work, and enjoying the pleasures of conversation, study, business, art, humour, and so on, to a total situation where there are ten thousand such people only, or perhaps 999,999 such people plus one man with toothache, or neurotic, or shivering with cold. In general, we can sum things up by saying that if we are humane, kindly, benevolent people, we want as many people as possible now and in the future to be as happy as possible. . . .

Sometimes, of course, more needs to be said. For example one course of action may make some people very happy and leave the rest as they are or perhaps slightly less happy. Another course of action may make all men rather more happy than before but no one very happy. Which course of action makes mankind happier on the whole? Again, one course of action may make it highly probable that everyone will be made a little happier whereas another course of action may give us a much smaller probability that everyone will be made very much happier. In the third place, one course of action may make everyone happy in a pig-like way, whereas another course of action may make a few people happy in a highly complex and intellectual way.

It seems therefore that we have to weigh the maximizing of happiness against equitable distribution, to weigh probabilities with happiness, and to weigh the intellectual and other qualities of states of mind with their pleasurableness. Are we not therefore driven back to the necessity of some calculus of happiness? Can we just say: "envisage two total situations and tell me which you prefer"? If this were possible, of course there would be no need to talk of summing happiness or of a calculus. All we should have to do would be to put total situations in an order of preference. . . .

Let us now consider the question of equity. Suppose that we have the choice of sending four equally worthy and intelligent boys to a medium-grade public school or of leaving three in an adequate but uninspiring grammar school and sending one to Eton. (For sake of the example I am making the almost certainly incorrect assumption that Etonians are happier than other public-school boys and that these other public-school boys are happier than grammar-school boys.) Which course of action makes the most for the happiness of the four boys? Let us suppose that we can neglect complicating factors, such as that the superior Etonian education might lead one boy to develop his talents so much that he will have an extraordinary influence on the well-being of mankind, or that the unequal treatment of the boys might cause jealousy and rift in the family. Let us suppose that the Etonian will be as happy as (we may hope) Etonians usually are, and similarly for the other boys, and let us suppose that remote effects can be neglected. Should we prefer the greater happiness of one boy to the moderate happiness of all four? Clearly one parent may prefer one total situation (one boy at Eton and three at the grammar school) while another may prefer the other total situation (all four at, the medium-grade public school). Surely both parents have an equal claim to being sympathetic and benevolent, and yet their difference of opinion here is not founded on an empirical disagreement about facts. I suggest, however, that there are not in fact many cases in which such a disagreement could arise. Probably the parent who wished to send one son to Eton would draw the line at sending one son to Eton plus giving him expensive private tuition during the holidays plus giving his other sons no secondary education at all. It is only within rather small limits that this sort of disagreement about equity can arise. Furthermore the cases in which we can make one person *very* much happier without increasing *general* happiness are rare ones. The law of diminishing returns comes in here. So, in most practical cases, a disagreement about what should be done will be an empirical disagreement about what total situation is likely to be brought about by an action, and will not be a disagreement about which total situation is preferable. For example the inequalitarian parent might get the other to agree with him if he could convince him that there was a much higher probability of an Etonian benefiting the human race, such as by inventing a valuable drug or opening up the mineral riches of Antarctica, than there is of a non-Etonian doing so. (Once more I should like to say that I do not myself take such a possibility very seriously!) I must again stress that since disagreement about what causes produce what effects is in practice so much the most important sort of disagreement, to have intelligent moral discussion with a person we do not in fact need complete agreement with him about ultimate ends: an approximate agreement is sufficient.

7. The place of rules in act-utilitarianism

According to the act-utilitarian, then, the rational way to decide what to do is to decide to perform that one of those alternative actions open to us (including the null-action, the doing of nothing) which is likely to maximize the probable happiness or well-being of humanity as a whole, or more accurately, of all sentient beings. The utilitarian position is here put forward as a criterion of rational choice. It is true that we may choose to habituate ourselves to behave in accordance with certain rules, such as to keep promises, in the belief that behaving in accordance with these rules is generally optimistic, and in the knowledge that we most often just do not have time to work out individual pros and cons. When we act in such an habitual fashion we do not of course deliberate or make a choice. The act-utilitarian will, however, regard these rules as mere rules of thumb, and will use them only as rough guides. Normally he will act in accordance with them when he has no time for considering probable consequences or when the advantages of such a consideration of consequences are likely to be outweighed by the disadvantage, of the waste of time involved. He acts in accordance with rules, in short, when there is no time to think, and since he does not think, the actions which he does habitually are not the outcome of moral thinking. When he has to think what to do, then there is a question of deliberation or choice, and it is precisely for such situations that the utilitarian criterion is intended.

It is, moreover, important to realize that there is no inconsistency whatever in an act-utilitarian's schooling himself to act, in normal circumstances, habitually and in accordance with stereotyped rules. He knows that a man about to save a drowning person has no time to consider various possibilities, such as that the drowning person is a dangerous criminal who will cause death and destruction, or that he is suffering from a painful and incapacitating disease from which death would be a merciful release, or that various timid people, watching from the bank, will suffer a heart attack if they see anyone else in the water. No, he knows that it is almost always right to save a drowning man, and in he goes. Again, he knows that we would go mad if we went in detail into the probable consequences of keeping or not-keeping every trivial promise: we will do most good and reserve our mental energies for more important matters if we simply habituate ourselves to keep promises in all normal situations. Moreover he may suspect that on some occasions personal bias may prevent him from reasoning in a correct utilitarian fashion. Suppose he is trying to decide between two jobs, one of which is more highly paid than the other, though he has given an informal promise that he will take the lesser paid one. He may well deceive himself by underestimating the effects of breaking the promise (in causing loss of confidence) and by overestimating the good he can do in the highly paid job. He may well feel that if he trusts to the accepted rules he is more likely to act in the way that an unbiased act-utilitarian would recommend than he would be if he tried to evaluate the consequences of his possible actions himself.

. . .

(1) George, who has just taken his Ph.D. in chemistry, finds it extremely difficult to get a job. He is not very robust in health, which cuts down the number of jobs he might be able to do satisfactorily. His wife has to go out to work to keep them, which itself causes a great deal of strain, since they have small children and there are severe problems about looking after them. The results of all this, especially on the children, are damaging. An older chemist, who knows about this situation, says that he can get George a "decently paid" job in a certain laboratory, which pursues research into chemical and biological warfare. George says that he cannot accept this, since he is opposed to chemical and biological warfare. The older man replies that he is not too keen on it himself, come to that, but after all George's refusal is not going to make the job or the laboratory go away; what is more, he happens to know that if George refuses the job, it will certainly go to a contemporary of George's who is not inhibited by any such scruples and is likely if appointed to push along the research with greater zeal than George would. Indeed, it is not merely concern for George and his family, but (to speak frankly and in confidence) some alarm about this other man's excess of zeal, which has led the older man to offer to use his influence to get George the job . . . George's wife, to whom he is deeply attached, has views (the details of which need not concern us) from which it follows that at least there is nothing particularly wrong with research into CBW. What should he do?

(2) Jim finds himself in the central square of a small South American town. Tied up against the wall are a row of twenty Indians, most terrified, a few defiant, in front of them several armed men in uniform. A heavy man in a sweat-stained khaki shirt turns out to be the captain in charge and, after a good deal of questioning of Jim which establishes that he got there by accident while on a botanical expedition, explains that the Indians are a random group of the inhabitants who, after recent acts of protest against the government, are just about to be killed to remind other possible protestors of the advantages of not protesting. However, since Jim is an honoured visitor from another land, the captain is happy to offer him a guest's privilege of killing one of the Indians himself. If Jim accepts, then as a special mark of the occasion, the other Indians will be let off. Of course, if Jim refuses, then there is no special occasion, and Pedro here will do, what he was about to do when Jim arrived, and kill them all. Jim, with some desperate recollection of schoolboy fiction, wonders whether if he got hold of a gun, he could hold the captain, Pedro and the rest of the soldiers to threat, but it is quite clear from the set-up that nothing of that kind is going to work: any attempt at that sort of thing will mean that all the Indians will be killed, and himself. The men against the wall, and the other villagers, understand the situation, and are obviously begging him to accept. What should he do?

To these dilemmas, it seems to me that utilitarianism replies, in the first case, that George should accept the job, and in the second, that Jim should kill the Indian. Not only does utilitarianism give these answers but, if the situations are essentially as described and there are no further special factors, it regards them, it seems to me, as *obviously* the right answers. But many of us would certainly wonder whether, in (I) could possibly be the right answer at all; and in the case of (2), even one who came to think that perhaps that was the answer, might well wonder whether it was obviously the answer. Nor is it just a question of the rightness or obviousness of these answers. It is also a question of what sort of considerations come into finding the answer. A feature of utilitarianism is that it cuts out a kind of consideration which for some others makes a difference to what they feel about such cases: a consideration involving the idea, as we might first and very simply put it, that each of us is specially responsible for what *he* does; rather than for what other people do. This is an idea closely connected with the value of integrity. It is often suspected that utilitarianism, at least in its direct forms, makes integrity as a value more or less unintelligible. I shall try to show that this suspicion is correct. Of course, even if that is correct, it would not necessarily follow that we should reject utilitarianism; perhaps, as utilitarians sometimes suggest, we should just forget about integrity, in favour of such things as a concern for the general good. However, if I am right, we cannot merely do that, since the reason why utilitarianism cannot understand integrity is that it cannot coherently describe the relations between a man's projects and his actions.

EXCERPT 3

Abridged text from:

I. Kant, *Groundwork for the Metaphysics of Morals* (New Haven: Yale University Press, 2002), Section 1.

First Section: Transition from the Common Rational Knowledge of Morals to the Philosophical

Immanuel Kant

There is nothing it is possible to think of anywhere in the world, or indeed anything at all outside it, that can be held to be good without limitation, excepting only a good will. Understanding, wit, the power of judgment,[1] and like talents of the mind,[2] whatever they might be called, or courage, resoluteness, persistence in an intention, as qualities of temperament, are without doubt in some respects good and to be wished for; but they can also become extremely evil and harmful, if the will that is to make use of these gifts of nature, and whose peculiar constitution is therefore called character,[3] is not good. It is the same with gifts of fortune. Power, wealth, honor,[4] even health and that entire well-being and contentment with one's condition, under the name of happiness, make for courage and thereby often also for arrogance,[5] where there is not a good will to correct their influence on the mind,[6] and thereby on the entire principle of action, and make them universally purposive; not to mention that a rational impartial spectator can never take satisfaction even in the sight of the uninterrupted welfare of a being, if it is adorned with no trait of a pure and good will; and so the good will appears to constitute the indispensable condition even of the worthiness to be happy.

. . .

The good will is good not through what it effects or accomplishes, not through its efficacy for attaining any intended end, but only through its willing, i.e., good in itself, and considered for itself, without comparison, it is to be estimated far higher than anything that could be brought about by it in favor of any inclination, or indeed, if you prefer, of the sum of all inclinations. Even if through the peculiar disfavor of fate, or through the meager endowment of a step-motherly nature, this will were entirely lacking in the resources to carry out its aim, if with its greatest effort nothing of it were accomplished, and only the good will were left over (to be sure, not a mere wish, but as the summoning up of all the means insofar as they are in our control): then it would shine like a jewel for itself, as something that has its full worth in itself. Utility or fruitlessness can neither add to nor subtract anything from this worth. It would be only the setting, as it were, to make it easier to handle in common traffic, or to draw the attention of those who are still not sufficiently connoisseurs, but not to recommend it to connoisseurs and determine its worth.

. . .

But now in order to develop the concept of a good will, to be esteemed in itself and without any further aim, just as it dwells already[7] in the naturally healthy understanding, which does not need to be taught but rather only to be enlightened, this concept always standing over the estimation of the entire worth of our actions and constituting the condition for everything else: we will put before ourselves the concept of duty, which contains that of a good will, though under certain subjective limitations

---

[1] R. B. Louden and K. Manfred, eds., *Kant: Anthropology from a Pragmatic Point of View* (Cambridge University Press, 2006), Ak 7.

[2] *Geist.*

[3] For Kant's distinction between "temperament" and "character," see *Anthropology from a Pragmatic Point of View*, Ak 7; see also Ak 4.

[4] Power, wealth, and honor are for Kant the three objects of the principal social passions. See *Anthropology from a Pragmatic Point of View*, Ak 7:271–274.

[5] *Mut und hierdurch öfters auch Übermut.*

[6] *Gemüt.*

[7] This word added in 1786.

and hindrances, which, however, far from concealing it and making it unrecognizable, rather elevate it by contrast and let it shine forth all the more brightly.

I pass over all actions that are already recognized as contrary to duty, even though they might be useful for this or that aim; for with them the question cannot arise at all whether they might be done from duty, since they even conflict with it. I also set aside the actions which are actually in conformity with duty, for which, however, human beings have immediately no inclination, but nevertheless perform them because they are driven to it through another inclination. For there it is easy to distinguish whether the action in conformity with duty is done from duty or from a self-seeking aim. It is much harder to notice this difference where the action is in conformity with duty and the subject yet has besides this an immediate inclination to it. E.g., it is indeed in conformity with duty that the merchant should not overcharge his inexperienced customers, and where there is much commercial traffic, the prudent merchant also does not do this, but rather holds a firm general price for everyone, so that a child buys just as cheaply from him as anyone else. Thus one is honestly served; yet that is by no means sufficient for us to believe that the merchant has proceeded thus from duty and from principles of honesty; his advantage required it; but here it is not to be assumed that besides this, he was also supposed to have an immediate inclination toward the customers, so that out of love, as it were, he gave no one an advantage over another in his prices. Thus the action was done neither from duty nor from immediate inclination, but merely from a self-serving aim.

By contrast, to preserve one's life is a duty, and besides this everyone has an immediate inclination to it. But the often anxious care that the greatest part of humankind takes for its sake still has no inner worth, and its maxim has no moral content. They protect their life, to be sure, in conformity with duty, but not from duty. If, by contrast, adversities and hopeless grief have entirely taken away the taste for life, if the unhappy one, strong of soul, more indignant than pusillanimous or dejected over his fate, wishes for death and yet preserves his life without loving it, not from inclination or fear, but from duty: then his maxim has a moral content.

. . .

The second proposition[8] is: an action from duty has its moral worth not in the aim that is supposed to be attained by it, but rather in the maxim in accordance with which it is resolved upon; thus[9] that worth depends not on the actuality of the object of the action, but merely on the principle of the volition, in accordance with which the action is done, without regard to any object of the faculty of desire. It is clear from the preceding that the aims we may have in actions, and their effects, as ends and incentives of the will, can impart to the actions no unconditioned and moral worth. In what, then, can this worth lie, if it is not supposed to exist in the will, in the relation of the actions to the effect hoped for? It can lie nowhere else than in the principle of the will, without regard to the ends that can be effected through such action; for the will is at a crossroads, as it were, between its principle a priori, which is formal, and its incentive a posteriori, which is material, and since it must somehow be determined by something, it must be determined through the formal principle in general of the volition if it does an action from duty, since every material principle has been withdrawn from it.

The third proposition, as a consequence of the first two, I would express thus: Duty is the necessity of an action from respect for the law. For the object, as an effect of my proposed action, I can of course have an inclination, but never respect, just because it[10] is merely an effect and not the activity of a will.[11] Just as little can I have respect for inclination in general, whether my own or another's; I can at most approve it in the first case, in the second I can sometimes even love it, i.e., regard it as favorable to my

[8] Kant does not say explicitly what the "first proposition" was, but presumably it is that an action has moral worth only if it is done from duty.

[9] This word added in 1786.

[10] Kant's pronoun here is in the feminine, which could refer to "effect" but not to "object," which seems to be the intended referent. Editors therefore often emend the pronoun to the neuter.

[11] 1785: "an effect of my will."

own advantage. Only that which is connected with my will merely as a ground, never as an effect, only what does not serve my inclination but outweighs it, or at least wholly excludes it from the reckoning in a choice, hence only the mere law for itself, can be an object of respect and hence a command. Now an action from duty is supposed entirely to abstract from[12] the influence of inclination, and with it every object of the will, so nothing is left over for the will that can determine it except the law as what is objective and subjectively pure respect for this practical law, hence the maxim[13] of complying with such a law, even when it infringes all my inclinations.

The moral worth of the action thus lies not in the effect to be expected from it; thus also not in any principle of action which needs to get its motive from this expected effect. For all these effects (agreeableness of one's condition, indeed even the furthering of the happiness of others) could be brought about through other causes, and for them the will of a rational being is therefore not needed; but in it alone the highest and unconditioned good can nevertheless be encountered. Nothing other than the representation of the law in itself, which obviously occurs only in the rational being insofar as it, and not the hoped-for effect, is the determining ground of the will, therefore[14] constitutes that so pre-eminent good which we call "moral," which is already present in the person himself who acts in accordance with it, but must not first of all be expected from the effect.[15]

But what kind of law can it be, whose representation, without even taking account of the effect expected from it, must determine the will, so that it can be called good absolutely and without limitation? Since I have robbed the will of every impulse that could have arisen from the obedience to any law, there is nothing left over except the universal lawfulness of the action in general which alone is to serve the will as its principle, i.e., I ought never to conduct myself except so that I could also will that my maxim become a universal law. Here it is mere lawfulness in general (without grounding it on any law determining certain actions) that serves the will as its principle,

[12] *Absondern.*

[13] A maxim is the subjective principle of the volition; the objective principle (i.e., that which would serve all rational beings also subjectively as a practical principle if reason had full control over the faculty of desire) is the practical law.

[14] 1785: "thus."

[15] One could accuse me of merely taking refuge behind the word respect in an obscure feeling instead of giving a distinct reply to the question through a concept of reason. Yet even if respect is a feeling, it is not one received through influence but a feeling self-effected through a concept of reason and hence specifically distinguished from all feelings of the first kind, which may be reduced to inclination or fear. What I immediately recognize as a law for me, I recognize with respect, which signifies merely the consciousness of the subjection of my will to a law without any mediation of other influences on my sense. The immediate determination of the will through the law and the consciousness of it is called respect, so that the latter is to be regarded as the effect of the law on the subject and not as its cause. Authentically, respect is the representation of a worth that infringes on my self-love. Thus it is something that is considered as an object neither of inclination nor of fear, even though it has something analogical to both at the same time. The object of respect is thus solely the law, and specifically that law that we lay upon ourselves and yet also as in itself necessary. As a law we are subject to it without asking permission of self-love; as laid upon us by ourselves, it is a consequence of our will, and has from the first point of view an analogy with fear, and from the second with inclination. All respect for a person is properly only respect for the law (of uprightness, etc.) of which the person gives us the example. Because we regard the expansion of our talents also as a duty, we represent to ourselves a person with talents also as an example of a law, as it were (to become similar to the person in this) and that constitutes our respect. All so-called moral interest consists solely in respect for the law. [The parenthetical material in the penultimate sentence was added in 1786. Cf. *Critique of Practical Reason*, Ak 5:71–89. In the *Metaphysics of Morals*, Kant lists four feelings that are produced directly by reason and can serve as moral motivation. These are "moral feeling," "conscience," "love of human beings," and "respect" (*Metaphysics of Morals*, Ak 6:399–403).]

and also must so serve it, if duty is not to be everywhere an empty delusion and a chimerical concept; common human reason,[16] indeed, agrees perfectly with this in its practical judgment, and has the principle just cited always before its eyes.

Let the question be, e.g.: When I am in a tight spot, may I not make a promise with the intention of not keeping it? Here I easily make a distinction in the signification the question can have, whether it is prudent, or whether it is in conformity with duty, to make a false promise. The first can without doubt often occur. I do see very well that it is not sufficient to get myself out of a present embarrassment by means of this subterfuge, but rather it must be reflected upon whether from this lie there could later arise much greater inconvenience than that from which I am now freeing myself, and, since the consequences of my supposed cunning are not so easy to foresee, and a trust once lost to me might become much more disadvantageous than any ill I think I am avoiding, whether it might not be more prudent to conduct myself in accordance with a universal maxim and make it into a habit not to promise anything except with the intention of keeping it. Yet it soon occurs to me here that such a maxim has as its ground only the worrisome consequences. Now to be truthful from duty is something entirely different from being truthful out of worry over disadvantageous consequences; in the first case, the concept of the action in itself already contains a law for me, whereas in the second I must look around elsewhere to see which effects might be bound up with it for me. For if I deviate from the principle of duty, then this is quite certainly evil; but if I desert my maxim of prudence, then that can sometimes be very advantageous to me, even though it is safer to remain with it. Meanwhile, to inform myself in the shortest and least deceptive way in regard to my answer to this problem, whether a lying promise is in conformity with duty, I ask myself: Would I be content with it if my maxim (of getting myself out of embarrassment through an untruthful promise) should be valid as a universal law (for myself as well as for others), and would I be able to say to myself that anyone may make an untruthful promise when he finds himself in embarrassment which he cannot get out of in any other way? Then I soon become aware that I can will the lie but not at all a universal law to lie; for in accordance with such a law there would properly be no promises, because it would be pointless to avow my will in regard to my future actions to those who would not believe this avowal, or, if they rashly did so, who would pay me back in the same coin; hence my maxim, as soon as it were made into a universal law, would destroy itself.

Thus I need no well-informed shrewdness to know what I have to do in order to make my volition morally good. Inexperienced in regard to the course of the world, incapable of being prepared for all the occurrences that might eventuate in it, I ask myself only: Can you will also that your maxim should become a universal law? If not, then it is reprehensible, and this not for the sake of any disadvantage impending for you or someone else, but because it cannot fit as a principle into a possible universal legislation; but for this legislation reason extorts immediate respect from me, from which, to be sure, I still do not have insight into that on which it is grounded (which the philosopher may investigate), but I at least understand this much, that it is an estimation of a worth which far outweighs everything whose worth is commended by inclination, and that the necessity of my actions from pure respect for the practical law is what constitutes duty, before which every other motive must give way because it is the condition of a will that is good in itself, whose worth surpasses everything.

. . .

If, then, there is supposed to be a supreme practical principle, and in regard to the human will a categorical imperative, then it must be such from the representation of that which, being necessarily an end for everyone, because it is an end in itself, constitutes an *objective* principle of the will, hence can serve as a universal practical law. The ground of this principle is: *Rational nature exists as end in itself.* The human being necessarily represents his

[16] 1785: "but common human reason."

own existence in this way;[17] thus to that extent it is a *subjective* principle of human actions. But every other rational being also represents his existence in this way as consequent on the same rational ground as is valid for me; thus it is at the same time an *objective* principle, from which, as a supreme practical ground, all laws of the will must be able to be derived. The practical imperative will thus be the following: *Act so that you use humanity,*[18] *as much in your own person as in the person of every other, always at the same time as end and never merely as means.* We will see whether this can be accomplished.

In order to remain with the previous examples,

First, in accordance with the concept of the necessary duty toward oneself, the one who has suicide in mind will ask himself whether his action could subsist together with the idea of humanity *as an end in itself.* If he destroys himself in order to flee from a burdensome condition, then he makes use of a person merely *as a means,* for the preservation of a bearable condition up to the end of life. The human being, however, is not a thing, hence not something that can be used *merely* as a means, but must in all his actions always be considered as an end in itself. Thus I cannot dispose of the human being in my own person, so as to maim, corrupt, or kill him.[19] (The nearer determination of this principle, so as to avoid all misunderstanding, e.g., the amputation of limbs in order to preserve myself, or the risk at which I put my life in order to preserve my life, etc., I must here pass over; they belong to morals proper.)[20]

Second, as to the necessary or owed duty toward others, the one who has it in mind to make a lying promise to another will see[21] right away that he wills to make use of another human being *merely as means,* without the end also being contained in this other. For the one I want to use for my aims through such a promise cannot possibly be in harmony with my way of conducting myself toward him and thus contain in himself the end of this action.[22] Even more distinctly does this conflict with the principle of other human beings meet the eye if one approaches it through examples of attacks on the freedom and property of others. For then it is clearly evident that the one who transgresses the rights of human beings is disposed to make use of the person of others merely as a means, without taking into consideration that as rational beings, these persons ought always to be esteemed at the same time as ends, i.e., only as beings who have to be able to contain in themselves the end of precisely the same action.*

Third, in regard to the contingent (meritorious) duty toward oneself, it is not enough that the action does not conflict with humanity in our person as end in itself; it must also *harmonize with it.* Now in humanity there are predispositions

---

[17] See *Conjectural Beginning of Human History,* Ak 8:114; *Anthropology in a Pragmatic Respect,* Ak 7:127, 130.

[18] *Menschlichkeit*; this term refers to one of our three fundamental predispositions: (1) animality (through which we have instincts for survival, procreation, and sociability); (2) humanity, through which we have the rational capacities to set ends, use means to them, and organize them into a whole (happiness); and (3) personality, through which we have the capacity to give ourselves moral laws and are accountable for following them (see *Religion within the Boundaries of Mere Reason,* Ak 6:26–28; *Anthropology in a Pragmatic Respect,* Ak 7:322–325). "Humanity" thus means the same as "rational nature," and Kant's use of it involves no retraction of the claim that moral commands must be valid for all rational beings, not only for members of the human species.

[19] In the *Metaphysics of Morals,* Kant discusses the duty not to maim oneself in connection with the duty forbidding suicide (Ak 6:422–23). *Verderben* ("corrupt") therefore probably carries with it the broad sense of ruining or destroying (sc. one's body or parts of it) rather than the narrower sense of moral corruption. Duties to oneself as a moral being, which Kant classifies as duties against lying, avarice, false humility (or servility), and duties as moral judge of oneself, are dealt with separately, 6:428–442.

[20] *Zur eigentlichen Moral.*

[21] *Einsehen.*

[22] It is essential to Kant's conception of a promise that it involves a "united will" of the promisor and the promisee (*Metaphysics of Morals,* Ak 6: 272).

to greater perfection, which belong to ends of nature in regard to the humanity in our subject; to neglect these would at most be able to subsist with the *preservation* of humanity as end in itself, but not with the *furthering* of this end.

Fourth, as to the meritorious duty toward others, the natural end that all human beings have is their own happiness. Now humanity would be able to subsist if no one contributed to the happiness of others yet did not intentionally remove anything from it; only this is only a negative and not a positive agreement with *humanity as end in itself*, if everyone does not aspire, as much as he can, to further the ends of others. For regarding the subject which is an end in itself: if that representation is to have its *total* effect on me, then its ends must as far as possible also be *my* ends.

EXCERPT 4

Abridged text from:

J. Rawls, *A Theory of Justice, Revised Edition* (Cambridge: Harvard University Press, 1999), pp. 10–19, 52–55.

A Theory of Justice: Revised Edition

John Rawls

3. The Main Idea of the Theory of Justice

My aim is to present a conception of justice which generalizes and carries to a higher level of abstraction the familiar theory of the social contract as found, say, in Locke, Rousseau, and Kant.[1] In order to do this we are not to think of the original contract as one to enter a particular society or to set up a particular form of government. Rather, the guiding idea is that the principles of justice for the basic structure of society are the object of the original agreement. They are the principles that free and rational persons concerned to further their own interests would accept in an initial position of equality as defining the fundamental terms of their association. These principles are to regulate all further agreements; they specify the kinds of social cooperation that can be entered into and the forms of government that can be established. This way of regarding the principles of justice I shall call justice as fairness.

Thus we are to imagine that those who engage in social cooperation choose together, in one joint act, the principles which are to assign basic rights and duties and to determine the division of social benefits. Men are to decide in advance how they are to regulate their claims against one another and what is to be the foundation charter of their society. Just as each person must decide by rational reflection what constitutes his good, that is, the system of ends which it is rational for him to pursue, so a group of persons must decide once and for all what is to count among them as just and unjust. The choice which rational men would make in this hypothetical situation of equal liberty, assuming for the present that this choice problem has a solution, determines the principles of justice.

In justice as fairness the original position of equality corresponds to the state of nature in the traditional theory of the social contract. This original position is not, of course, thought of as an actual historical state of affairs, much less as a primitive condition of culture. It is understood as a purely hypothetical situation characterized so as to lead to a certain conception of justice.[2] Among the essential features of this situation is that no one knows his place in society, his class position or social status, nor does any one

---

[1] As the text suggests, I shall regard Locke's Second Treatise of Government, Rousseau's The Social Contract, and Kant's ethical works beginning with The Foundations of the Metaphysics of Morals as definitive of the contract tradition. For all of its greatness, Hobbes's Leviathan raises special problems. A general historical survey is provided by J. W. Gough, *The Social Contract*, 2nded. (Oxford: Clarendon Press, 1957), and O. Gierke, *Natural Law and the Theory of Society, trans.* with an introduction by Ernest Barker (Cambridge: Cambridge University Press, 1934). A presentation of the contract view as primarily an ethical theory is to be found in G. R. Grice, *The Grounds of Moral Judgment* (Cambridge: Cambridge University Press, 1967).

[2] Kant is clear that the original agreement is hypothetical. See *The Metaphysics of Morals*, pt. I (Rechtslehre), especially §§47, 52; and pt. II of the essay "Concerning the Common Saying: This May Be True in Theory but It Does Not Apply in Practice," in Kant's Political Writings, ed. Hans Reiss and trans. by H. B. Nisbet (Cambridge: Cambridge University Press, 1970), pp. 73–87. See Georges Vlachos, *La Pensée politique de Kant* (Paris: Presses

know his fortune in the distribution of natural assets and abilities, his intelligence, strength, and the like. I shall even assume that the parties do not know their conceptions of the good or their special psychological propensities. The principles of justice are chosen behind a veil of ignorance. This ensures that no one is advantaged or disadvantaged in the choice of principles by the outcome of natural chance or the contingency of social circumstances. Since all are similarly situated and no one is able to design principles to favor his particular condition, the principles of justice are the result of a fair agreement or bargain. For given the circumstances of the original position, the symmetry of everyone's relations to each other, this initial situation is fair between individuals as moral persons, that is, as rational beings with their own ends and capable, I shall assume, of a sense of justice. The original position is, one might say, the appropriate initial status quo, and thus the fundamental agreements reached in it are fair. This explains the propriety of the name "justice as fairness": it conveys the idea that the principles of justice are agreed to in an initial situation that is fair. The name does not mean that the concepts of justice and fairness are the same, any more than the phrase "poetry as metaphor" means that the concepts of poetry and metaphor are the same.

Justice as fairness begins, as I have said, with one of the most general of all choices which persons might make together, namely, with the choice of the first principles of a conception of justice which is to regulate all subsequent criticism and reform of institutions. Then, having chosen a conception of justice, we can suppose that they are to choose a constitution and a legislature to enact laws, and so on, all in accordance with the principles of justice initially agreed upon. Our social situation is just if it is such that by this sequence of hypothetical agreements we would have contracted into the general system of rules which defines it. Moreover, assuming that the original position does determine a set of principles (that is, that a particular conception of justice would be chosen), it will then be true that whenever social institutions satisfy these principles those engaged in them can say to one another that they are cooperating on terms to which they would agree if they were free and equal persons whose relations with respect to one another were fair. They could all view their arrangements as meeting the stipulations which they would acknowledge in an initial situation that embodies widely accepted and reasonable constraints on the choice of principles. The general recognition of this fact would provide the basis for a public acceptance of the corresponding principles of justice. No society can, of course, be a scheme of cooperation which men enter voluntarily in a literal sense; each person finds himself placed at birth in some particular position in some particular society, and the nature of this position materially affects his life prospects. Yet a society satisfying the principles of justice as fairness comes as close as a society can to being a voluntary scheme, for it meets the principles which free and equal persons would assent to under circumstances that are fair. In this sense its members are autonomous and the obligations they recognize self-imposed.

One feature of justice as fairness is to think of the parties in the initial situation as rational and mutually disinterested. This does not mean that the parties are egoists, that is, individuals with only certain kinds of interests, say in wealth, prestige, and domination. But they are conceived as not taking an interest in one another's interests. They are to presume that even their spiritual aims may be opposed, in the way that the aims of those of different religions may be opposed. Moreover, the concept of rationality must be interpreted as far as possible in the narrow sense, standard in economic theory, of taking the most effective means to given ends. I shall modify this concept to some extent, as explained later (§25), but one must try to avoid introducing into it any controversial ethical elements. The initial

Universitaires de France, 1962), pp. 326–335; and J. G. Murphy, *Kant: The Philosophy of Right* (London: Macmillan, 1970), pp. 109–112, 133–136, for a further discussion.

situation must be characterized by stipulations that are widely accepted.

In working out the conception of justice as fairness one main task clearly is to determine which principles of justice would be chosen in the original position. To do this we must describe this situation in some detail and formulate with care the problem of choice which it presents. These matters I shall take up in the immediately succeeding chapters. It may be observed, however, that once the principles of justice are thought of as arising from an original agreement in a situation of equality, it is an open question whether the principle of utility would be acknowledged. Offhand it hardly seems likely that persons who view themselves as equals, entitled to press their claims upon one another, would agree to a principle which may require lesser life prospects for some simply for the sake of a greater sum of advantages enjoyed by others. Since each desires to protect his interests, his capacity to advance his conception of the good, no one has a reason to acquiesce in an enduring loss for himself in order to bring about a greater net balance of satisfaction. In the absence of strong and lasting benevolent impulses, a rational man would not accept a basic structure merely because it maximized the algebraic sum of advantages irrespective of its permanent effects on his own basic rights and interests. Thus it seems that the principle of utility is incompatible with the conception of social cooperation among equals for mutual advantage. It appears to be inconsistent with the idea of reciprocity implicit in the notion of a well-ordered society. Or, at any rate, so I shall argue.

I shall maintain instead that the persons in the initial situation would choose two rather different principles: the first requires equality in the assignment of basic rights and duties, while the second holds that social and economic inequalities, for example inequalities of wealth and authority, are just only if they result in compensating benefits for everyone, and in particular for the least advantaged members of society. These principles rule out justifying institutions on the grounds that the hardships of some are offset by a greater good in the aggregate. It may be expedient but it is not just that some should have less in order that others may prosper. But there is no injustice in the greater benefits earned by a few provided that the situation of persons not so fortunate is thereby improved. The intuitive idea is that since everyone's well-being depends upon a scheme of cooperation without which no one could have a satisfactory life, the division of advantages should be such as to draw forth the willing cooperation of everyone taking part in it, including those less well situated. The two principles mentioned seem to be a fair basis on which those better endowed, or more fortunate in their social position, neither of which we can be said to deserve, could expect the willing cooperation of others when some workable scheme is a necessary condition of the welfare of all.[3] Once we decide to look for a conception of justice that prevents the use of the accidents of natural endowment and the contingencies of social circumstance as counters in a quest for political and economic advantage, we are led to these principles. They express the result of leaving aside those aspects of the social world that seem arbitrary from a moral point of view.

The problem of the choice of principles, however, is extremely difficult. I do not expect the answer I shall suggest to be convincing to everyone. It is, therefore, worth noting from the outset that justice as fairness, like other contract views, consists of two parts: (1) an interpretation of the initial situation and of the problem of choice posed there, and (2) a set of principles which, it is argued, would be agreed to. One may accept the first part of the theory (or some variant thereof), but not the other, and conversely. The concept of the initial contractual situation may seem reasonable although the particular principles proposed are rejected. To be sure, I want to maintain that the most appropriate conception of this situation does lead to principles of justice contrary to utilitarianism and perfectionism, and therefore that the contract doctrine provides an alternative to these views. Still, one may dispute this contention even though one grants that the

[3] For the formulation of this intuitive idea I am indebted to Allan Gibbard.

contractarian method is a useful way of studying ethical theories and of setting forth their underlying assumptions.

. . .

4. The Original Position and Justification

I have said that the original position is the appropriate initial status quo which insures that the fundamental agreements reached in it are fair. This fact yields the name "justice as fairness." It is clear, then, that I want to say that one conception of justice is more reasonable than another, or justifiable with respect to it, if rational persons in the initial situation would choose its principles over those of the other for the role of justice. Conceptions of justice are to be ranked by their acceptability to persons so circumstanced. Understood in this way the question of justification is settled by working out a problem of deliberation: we have to ascertain which principles it would be rational to adopt given the contractual situation. This connects the theory of justice with the theory of rational choice.

If this view of the problem of justification is to succeed, we must, of course, describe in some detail the nature of this choice problem. A problem of rational decision has a definite answer only if we know the beliefs and interests of the parties, their relations with respect to one another, the alternatives between which they are to choose, the procedure whereby they make up their minds, and so on. As the circumstances are presented in different ways, correspondingly different principles are accepted. The concept of the original position, as I shall refer to it, is that of the most philosophically favored interpretation of this initial choice situation for the purposes of a theory of justice.

But how are we to decide what is the most favored interpretation? I assume, for one thing, that there is a broad measure of agreement that principles of justice should be chosen under certain conditions. To justify a particular description of the initial situation one shows that it incorporates these commonly shared presumptions. One argues from widely accepted but weak premises to more specific conclusions. Each of the presumptions should by itself be natural and plausible; some of them may seem innocuous or even trivial. The aim of the contract approach is to establish that taken together they impose significant bounds on acceptable principles of justice. The ideal outcome would be that these conditions determine a unique set of principles; but I shall be satisfied if they suffice to rank the main traditional conceptions of social justice.

One should not be misled, then, by the somewhat unusual conditions which characterize the original position. The idea here is simply to make vivid to ourselves the restrictions that it seems reasonable to impose on arguments for principles of justice, and therefore on these principles themselves. Thus it seems reasonable and generally acceptable that no one should be advantaged or disadvantaged by natural fortune or social circumstances in the choice of principles. It also seems widely agreed that it should be impossible to tailor principles to the circumstances of one's own case. We should insure further that particular inclinations and aspirations, and persons' conceptions of their good do not affect the principles adopted. The aim is to rule out those principles that it would be rational to propose for acceptance, however little the chance of success, only if one knew certain things that are irrelevant from the standpoint of justice. For example, if a man knew that he was wealthy, he might find it rational to advance the principle that various taxes for welfare measures be counted unjust; if he knew that he was poor, he would most likely propose the contrary principle. To represent the desired restrictions one imagines a situation in which everyone is deprived of this sort of information. One excludes the knowledge of those contingencies which sets men at odds and allows them to be guided by their prejudices. In this manner the veil of ignorance is arrived at in a natural way. This concept should cause no difficulty if we keep in mind the constraints on arguments that it is meant to express. At any time we can enter the original position, so to speak, simply by following a certain procedure, namely, by arguing for principles of justice in accordance with these restrictions.

It seems reasonable to suppose that the parties in the original position are equal. That is, all have the same rights in the procedure for choosing principles; each can make proposals, submit reasons for their acceptance, and so on. Obviously the purpose of these conditions is to represent equality between human beings as moral persons, as creatures having a conception of their good and capable of a sense of justice. The basis of equality is taken to be similarity in these two respects. Systems of ends are not ranked in value; and each man is presumed to have the requisite ability to understand and to act upon whatever principles are adopted. Together with the veil of ignorance, these conditions define the principles of justice as those which rational persons concerned to advance their interests would consent to as equals when none are known to be advantaged or disadvantaged by social and natural contingencies.

There is, however, another side to justifying a particular description of the original position. This is to see if the principles which would be chosen match our considered convictions of justice or extend them in an acceptable way. We can note whether applying these principles would lead us to make the same judgments about the basic structure of society which we now make intuitively and in which we have the greatest confidence; or whether, in cases where our present judgments are in doubt and given with hesitation, these principles offer a resolution which we can affirm on reflection. There are questions which we feel sure must be answered in a certain way. For example, we are confident that religious intolerance and racial discrimination are unjust. We think that we have examined these things with care and have reached what we believe is an impartial judgment not likely to be distorted by an excessive attention to our own interests. These convictions are provisional fixed points which we presume any conception of justice must fit. But we have much less assurance as to what is the correct distribution of wealth and authority. Here we may be looking for a way to remove our doubts. We can check an interpretation of the initial situation, then, by the capacity of its principles to accommodate our firmest convictions and to provide guidance where guidance is needed.

In searching for the most favored description of this situation we work from both ends. We begin by describing it so that it represents generally shared and preferably weak conditions. We then see if these conditions are strong enough to yield a significant set of principles. If not, we look for further premises equally reasonable. But if so, and these principles match our considered convictions of justice, then so far well and good. But presumably there will be discrepancies. In this case we have a choice. We can either modify the account of the initial situation or we can revise our existing judgments, for even the judgments we take provisionally as fixed points are liable to revision. By going back and forth, sometimes altering the conditions of the contractual circumstances, at others withdrawing our judgments and conforming them to principle, I assume that eventually we shall find a description of the initial situation that both expresses reasonable conditions and yields principles which match our considered judgments duly pruned and adjusted. This state of affairs I refer to as reflective equilibrium.[4] It is an equilibrium because at last our principles and judgments coincide; and it is reflective since we know to what principles our judgments conform and the premises of their derivation. At the moment everything is in order. But this equilibrium is not necessarily stable. It is liable to be upset by further examination of the conditions which should be imposed on the contractual situation and by particular cases

[4] The process of mutual adjustment of principles and considered judgments is not peculiar to moral philosophy. See N. Goodman, *Fact, Fiction, and Forecast* (Cambridge, MA.: Harvard University Press, 1955), pp. 65–68, for parallel remarks concerning the justification of the principles of deductive and inductive inference.

which may lead us to revise our judgments. Yet for the time being we have done what we can to render coherent and to justify our convictions of social justice. We have reached a conception of the original position.

. . .

11. Two Principles of Justice

I shall now state in a provisional form the two principles of justice that I believe would be agreed to in the original position. The first formulation of these principles is tentative. As we go on I shall consider several formulations and approximate step by step the final statement to be given much later. I believe that doing this allows the exposition to proceed in a natural way.

The first statement of the two principles reads as follows.

> First: each person is to have an equal right to the most extensive scheme of equal basic liberties compatible with a similar scheme of liberties for others.
>
> Second: social and economic inequalities are to be arranged so that they are both (a) reasonably expected to be to everyone's advantage, and (b) attached to positions and offices open to all.

There are two ambiguous phrases in the second principle, namely "everyone's advantage" and "open to all." Determining their sense more exactly will lead to a second formulation of the principle in §13. The final version of the two principles is given in §46; §39 considers the rendering of the first principle.

These principles primarily apply, as I have said, to the basic structure of society and govern the assignment of rights and duties and regulate the distribution of social and economic advantages. Their formulation presupposes that, for the purposes of a theory of justice, the social structure may be viewed as having two more or less distinct parts, the first principle applying to the one, the second principle to the other. Thus we distinguish between the aspects of the social system that define and secure the equal basic liberties and the aspects that specify and establish social and economic inequalities. Now it is essential to observe that the basic liberties are given by a list of such liberties. Important among these are political liberty (the right to vote and to hold public office) and freedom of speech and assembly; liberty of conscience and freedom of thought; freedom of the person, which includes freedom from psychological oppression and physical assault and dismemberment (integrity of the person); the right to hold personal property and freedom from arbitrary arrest and seizure as defined by the concept of the rule of law. These liberties are to be equal by the first principle.

The second principle applies, in the first approximation, to the distribution of income and wealth and to the design of organizations that make use of differences in authority and responsibility. While the distribution of wealth and income need not be equal, it must be to everyone's advantage, and at the same time, positions of authority and responsibility must be accessible to all. One applies the second principle by holding positions open, and then, subject to this constraint, arranges social and economic inequalities so that everyone benefits.

These principles are to be arranged in a serial order with the first principle prior to the second. This ordering means that infringements of the basic equal liberties protected by the first principle cannot be justified, or compensated for, by greater social and economic advantages. These liberties have a central range of application within which they can be limited and compromised only when they conflict with other basic liberties. Since they may be limited when they clash with one another, none of these liberties is absolute; but however they are adjusted to form one system, this system is to be the same for all. It is difficult, and perhaps impossible, to give a complete specification of these liberties independently from the particular circumstances—social, economic, and technological—of a given society. The hypothesis is that the general form of such a list could be devised with sufficient exactness to sustain this conception of justice. Of course, liberties not on the list, for example, the right to own certain kinds of property (e.g., means of production) and freedom of contract as understood by the doctrine of laissez-faire are not basic; and so they are not protected by the priority of the first principle. Finally, in regard to the second principle, the distribution of wealth and income, and positions of authority and responsibility, are to be consistent with both the basic liberties and equality of opportunity.

The two principles are rather specific in their content, and their acceptance rests on certain assumptions that I must eventually try to explain and justify. For the present, it should be observed that these principles are a special case of a more general conception of justice that can be expressed as follows.

> All social values—liberty and opportunity, income and wealth, and the social bases of self-respect—are to be distributed equally unless an unequal distribution of any, or all, of these values is to everyone's advantage.

Injustice, then, is simply inequalities that are not to the benefit of all. Of course, this conception is extremely vague and requires interpretation.

As a first step, suppose that the basic structure of society distributes certain primary goods, that is, things that every rational man is presumed to want. These goods normally have a use whatever a person's rational plan of life. For simplicity, assume that the chief primary goods at the disposition of society are rights, liberties, and opportunities, and income and wealth. (Later on in Part Three the primary good of self-respect has a central place.) These are the social primary goods. Other primary goods such as health and vigor, intelligence and imagination, are natural goods; although their possession is influenced by the basic structure, they are not so directly under its control. Imagine, then, a hypothetical initial arrangement in which all the social primary goods are equally distributed: everyone has similar rights and duties, and income and wealth are evenly shared. This state of affairs provides a benchmark for judging improvements. If certain inequalities of wealth and differences in authority would make everyone better off than in this hypothetical starting situation, then they accord with the general conception.

Now it is possible, at least theoretically, that by giving up some of their fundamental liberties men are sufficiently compensated by the resulting social and economic gains. The general conception of justice imposes no restrictions on what sort of inequalities are permissible; it only requires that everyone's position be improved. We need not suppose anything so drastic as consenting to a condition of slavery. Imagine instead that people seem willing to forego certain political rights when the economic returns are significant. It is this kind of exchange which the two principles rule out; being arranged in serial order they do not permit exchanges between basic liberties and economic and social gains except under extenuating circumstances (§§26, 39).

EXCERPT 5

Abridged text from:
W. Kymlicka, *Contemporary Political Philosophy* (Oxford: Clarendon Press, 1990), pp. 70–76.

Contemporary Political Philosophy

W. Kymlicka

Chapter 3 Liberal Equality

. . .

3. The Social Contract Argument

. . .

(a) The Convergence of the Two Arguments

. . .

A really successful criticism of Rawls must either challenge his fundamental intuitions, or show why the difference principle is not the best spelling out of these intuitions (and hence why a different description of the original position should be part of our reflective equilibrium). [. . .] Can we find any problems internal to Rawls's theory, criticisms not of his intuitions, but of the way he develops them?

(b) Internal problems

One of Rawls's central intuitions, . . . concerns the distinction between choices and circumstances. His argument against the prevailing view of equality of opportunity depends heavily on the claim that it gives too much room for the influence of our undeserved natural endowments. [. . .] But Rawls himself leaves too much room for the influence of natural inequalities, and at the same time leaves too little room for the influence of our choices.

(i) Compensating for natural inequalities

I will look at the question of natural talents first. Rawls says that people's claim to social goods should not be dependent on their natural endowments. The talented do not deserve any greater income, and they should only receive more income if it benefits the less well off. So, according to Rawls, the difference principle is the best principle for ensuring that natural assets do not have an unfair influence.

But Rawls's suggestion still allows too much room for people's fate to be influenced by arbitrary factors. This is because Rawls defines the worst off position entirely in terms of people's possession of social primary goods—i.e. rights, opportunities, wealth, etc. He does not look at people's possession of natural primary goods in determining who is worst off. Two people are equally well off for Rawls (in this context) if they have the same bundle of social primary goods, even though one person may be untalented, physically handicapped, mentally disabled, or suffering from poor health. Likewise, if someone has even a small advantage in social goods over others, then she is better off on Rawls's scale, even if the extra income is not enough to pay for extra costs she faces due to some natural disadvantage—e.g. the costs of medication for an illness, or of special equipment for some handicap.

But why should the benchmark for assessing the justice of social institutions be the prospects of the least well off in terms of social goods? This stipulation conflicts with both the intuitive and contract arguments. In the contract argument, the stipulation is unmotivated in terms of the rationality of the parties in the original position. If, as Rawls says, health is as important as money in being able to lead a successful life, and if the parties seek to find a social arrangement that guarantees them the greatest amount of primary goods in the worst possible outcome (the maximin reasoning) then why would they not treat lack of health and lack of money as equally cases of being less well off for the purposes of social distribution? Every person recognizes that she would be less well off if she suddenly became disabled, even if her bundle of social goods remained the same. Why would she not want society also to recognize her disadvantage?

The intuitive argument points in the same direction. Not only are natural primary goods as necessary as social goods for leading a good life, but people do not deserve their place in the distribution of natural assets, and so it is wrong for people to be privileged or disadvantaged because of that place. . . . Rawls thinks this intuition leads to the difference principle, under which people only receive extra rewards for their talents if doing so is to the benefit of the less well off: "we are led to the difference principle if we wish to set up the social system so that no one gains or loses from his arbitrary place in the distribution of natural assets or his initial position in society without giving or receiving compensating advantages in return."[1] But that is wrong, or at least misleading. We are only led to the difference principle if by "gains or loses" we mean gains or loses in terms of social goods. The difference principle ensures that the well endowed do not get more social goods just because of their arbitrary place in the distribution of natural assets, and that the handicapped are not deprived of social goods just because of their place. But this does not entirely "mitigate the effects of natural accident and social circumstance."[2] For the well endowed still get the natural good of their endowment, which the handicapped undeservedly lack. The difference principle may ensure that I have the same bundle of social goods as a handicapped person. But the handicapped person faces extra medical and transportation costs. She faces an undeserved burden in her ability to lead a satisfactory life, a burden caused by her circumstances, not her choices. The difference principle allows, rather than removes, that burden.[3]

[1] J. Rawls, *A Theory of Justice* (Cambridge, MA: Harvard University Press, 1971), p. 102.

[2] Ibid., p. 101.

[3] This objection is raised by Barry and Sen, although they mistakenly blame the problem on Rawls's commitment to using primary goods to define the least well-off position in B. M. Barry, *The Liberal Theory of Justice: A Critical Examination of the Principal Doctrines in A Theory of Justice by John Rawls* (Oxford: Clarendon Press, 1973) and A. Sen, "Equality of What?", in *The Tanner Lecture on Human Values*, edited (Cambridge University Press, 1980). The problem actually lies in Rawls's incomplete use of primary goods—i.e. his arbitrary exclusion of natural primary goods from the index. Rawls does discuss the idea of compensating natural disadvantages, but only in terms of a "principle of redress" under which compensation is made in order to remove the direct effects of the handicap and thereby create equality of opportunity in *A Theory of Justice*. Rawls rightly rejects this view as both impossible and undesirable. But why not view compensation as a way of eliminating an undeserved inequality in overall primary goods? Compensating people for the unchosen costs of their natural disadvantages should be done, not so that they can compete with others on an equal footing, but so they can have the same ability to lead a satisfying life. For more on this, compare F. Michelman, "Constitutional Welfare Rights and A Theory of Justice," in *Reading Rawls: Critical Studies on Rawls' A Theory of Justice*, edited by N. Daniels (Stanford University Press, 1975), pp. 330–339, A. Gutmann, *Liberal Equality* (Cambridge University Press, 1980), pp. 126–127, and N. Daniels, *Just Health Care* (Cambridge University Press, 1985), ch. 3 with T. W. M. Pogge, *Realizing Rawls* (Cornell University Press, 1989), pp. 183–188 and D. Mapel, *Social Justice Reconsidered: The Problem of Appropriate Precision in a Theory of Justice* (University of Illinois Press, 1989), pp. 101–106.

Some commentators argue that Rawls does support compensating natural disadvantages, but not as a matter of justice. Instead he views our obligations to the naturally disadvantaged as "duties

Rawls seems not to have realized the full implications of his own argument against the prevailing view of equality of opportunity. The position he was criticizing is this: (1) Social inequalities are undeserved, and should be rectified or compensated, but natural inequalities can influence distribution in accordance with equality of opportunity. Rawls claims that natural and social inequalities are equally undeserved, so (1) is "unstable." Instead, he endorses: (2) Social inequalities should be compensated, and natural inequalities should not influence distribution. But if natural and social inequalities really are equally undeserved, then (2) is also unstable. We should instead endorse: (3) Natural and social inequalities should be compensated. According to Rawls, people born into a disadvantaged class or race not only should not be denied social benefits, but also have a claim to compensation because of that disadvantage. Why treat people born with natural handicaps any differently? Why should they not also have a claim to compensation for their disadvantage (e.g. subsidized medicine, transportation, job training, etc.), in addition to their claim to non-discrimination?

So there are both intuitive and contract reasons for recognizing natural handicaps as grounds for compensation, and for including natural primary goods in the index which determines who is in the least well-off position. There are difficulties, in trying to compensate for natural inequalities. . . . It may be impossible to do what our intuitions tell us is most fair. But Rawls does not even recognize the desirability of trying to compensate such inequalities.

(ii) Subsidizing people's choices

The second problem concerns the flip side of that intuition. People do not deserve to bear the burden of unchosen costs, but how should we respond to people who choose to do costly things? We normally feel that unchosen costs have a greater claim on us than voluntarily chosen costs. We feel differently about someone who spends $100 a week on expensive medicine to control an unchosen illness, compared with someone who spends $100 a week on expensive wine because they enjoy its taste. Rawls appeals to this intuition when criticizing the prevailing view for being insensitive to the unchosen nature of natural inequalities. But how should we be sensitive to people's choices?

Imagine that we have succeeded in equalizing people's social and natural circumstances. To take the simplest case, imagine two people of equal natural talent who share the same social background. One wants to play tennis all day, and so only works long enough at a nearby farm to earn enough money to buy land for a tennis-court, and to sustain his desired lifestyle (i.e. food, clothing, equipment). The other person wants a similar amount of land to plant a garden, in order to produce and sell vegetables for herself and others. Furthermore, let us imagine, with Rawls, that we have started with an equal distribution of resources, which is enough for each person to get their desired land, and start their tennis and gardening. The gardener will

---

of public benevolence," R. Martin, *Rawls and Rights* (University Press of Kansas, 1985), pp. 189–191, or "claims of morality," Pogge, *Realizing Rawls*, 186–191, 275. These obligations to the disadvantaged are not matters of mere charity, for they should be compulsorily enforced through the state, but nor are they claims of justice. According to Pogge and Martin, Rawls's theory of justice is about "fundamental justice," whereas compensation for the naturally disadvantaged is about "the overall fairness of the universe," Martin, *Rawls and Rights*, 180; Pogge, *Realizing Rawls*, 189. Unfortunately, neither author explains this contrast, nor how it is consistent with Rawls's emphasis on "mitigating the effects of natural accident and social fortune" Rawls, *A Theory of Justice*, 585. Martin, for example, seems to say that mitigating the effects of differential natural *assets* is a matter of fundamental justice, whereas mitigating the effects of differential natural *handicaps* is a matter of benevolence Martin, *Rawls and Rights*, 178. It is hard to see what, within a Rawlsian approach, justifies this distinction. (Brian Barry argues that this restriction is only legitimate if Rawls is abandoning the whole idea of justice as equal consideration and adopting instead the Hobbesian idea of justice as mutual advantage—B. M. Barry, *The Liberal Theory of Justice*, 243–246).

quickly come to have more resources than the tennis-player, if we allow the market to work freely. While they began with equal shares of resources, he will rapidly use up his initial share, and his occasional farm work only brings in enough to sustain his tennis-playing. The gardener, however, uses her initial share in such a way as to generate a steadier and larger stream of income through larger amounts of work. Rawls would only allow this inequality if it benefits the least well off—i.e. if it benefits the tennis-player who now lacks much of an income. If the tennis-player does not benefit from the inequality, then the government should transfer some of her income to him in order to equalize income.

But there is something peculiar about saying that such a tax is needed to enforce equality, where that is understood to mean treating both people as equals. Remember that the tennis-player has the same talents as the gardener, the same social background, and started with an equal allotment of resources. As a result, he could have chosen income-producing gardening if he wished, just as she could have chosen non-income-producing tennis. They both faced a range of options which offered varying amounts and kinds of work, leisure, and income. Both chose that option which they preferred. The reason he did not choose gardening, therefore, is that he preferred playing tennis to earning money by gardening. People have different preferences about when it is worth giving up potential leisure to earn more income, and he preferred leisure while she preferred income.

Given that these differences in lifestyle are freely chosen, how is he treated unequally by allowing her to have the income and lifestyle that he did not want? Rawls defends the difference principle by saying that it counteracts the inequalities of natural and social contingencies. But these are not relevant here. Rather than removing a disadvantage, the difference principle simply makes her subsidize his expensive desire for leisure. She has to pay for the costs of her choice—i.e. she forgoes leisure in order to get more income. But he does not have to pay for the costs of his choice—i.e. he does not forgo income in order to get more leisure. He expects and Rawls requires that she pay for the costs of her own choices, and also subsidize his choice. That does not promote equality, it undermines it. He gets his preferred lifestyle (leisureful tennis), plus some income from her taxes, while she gets her preferred lifestyle (income-producing gardening) minus some income that is taxed from her. She has to give up part of what makes her life valuable in order that he can have more of what he finds valuable. They are treated unequally in this sense, for no legitimate reason.

When inequalities in income are the result of choices; not circumstances, the difference principle creates, rather than removes, unfairness. Treating people with equal concern requires that people pay for the costs of their own choices. Paying for choices is the flip side of our intuition about not paying for unequal circumstances. It is unjust if people are disadvantaged by inequalities in their circumstances, but it is equally unjust for me to demand that someone else pay for the costs of my choices. In more technical language, a distributive scheme should be "endowment-insensitive" and "ambition-sensitive."[4] People's fate should depend on their ambitions (in the broad sense of goals and projects about life), but should not depend on their natural and social endowments (the circumstances in which they pursue their ambitions).

Rawls himself emphasizes that we are responsible for the costs of our choices. This in fact is why his account of justice measures people's share of primary goods, not their level of welfare. Those who have expensive desires will get less welfare from an equal bundle of primary goods than those with more modest tastes. But, Rawls says, it does not follow that those with modest tastes should subsidize the extravagant, for we have "a capacity to assume responsibility for our ends." Hence "those with less expensive tastes have presumably adjusted their likes and dislikes over the course of their lives to the income and wealth they could

---

[4] R. Dworkin, "What Is Equality? Part 2: Equality of Resources," *Philosophy and Public Affairs* 10, no. 4 (1981): p. 311.

reasonably expect; and it is regarded as unfair that they now should have less in order to spare others from the consequences" of their extravagance.[5,6,7,8,9,10] So Rawls does not wish to make the gardener subsidize the tennis-player. Indeed he often says that his conception of justice is concerned with regulating inequalities that affect people's life-chances, not the inequalities that arise from people's life-choices, which are the individual's own responsibility.[11,12,13,14] Unfortunately, the difference principle does not make any such distinction between chosen and unchosen inequalities. Hence one possible result of the difference principle is to make some people pay for others' choices, should it be the case that those with the least income are, like the tennis-player, in that position by choice. Rawls wants the difference principle to mitigate the unjust effects of natural and social disadvantage, but it also mitigates the legitimate effects of personal choice and effort.

So while Rawls appeals to this choices-circumstances distinction, his difference principle violates it in two important ways. It is supposed to mitigate the effect of one's place in the distribution of natural assets. But because Rawls excludes natural primary goods from the index which determines who is least well off, there is in fact no compensation for those who suffer undeserved natural disadvantages. Conversely, people are supposed to be responsible for the costs of their choices. But the difference principle requires that some people subsidize the costs of other people's choices. Can we do a better job of being "ambition-sensitive" and "endowment-insensitive"? This is the goal of [the legal philosopher Ronald] Dworkin's theory.

[5] J. Rawls, "Social Unity and Primary Goods," in *Utilitarianism and Beyond*, edited by A. Sen and B. Williams (Cambridge University Press, 1982), pp. 168–169.

[6] J. Rawls, "Fairness to Goodness," *The Philosophical Review* (1975): p. 553.

[7] J. Rawls, "Kantian Constructivism in Moral Theory," *The Journal of Philosophy* 77, no. 9 (1980): p. 545.

[8] J. Rawls, "Reply to Alexander and Musgrave," *The Quarterly Journal of Economics* (1974): p. 643.

[9] J. Rawls, "The Basic Structures as Subject," in *Values and Morals*, edited by A. Goldman and J. Kim (Dordrecht: Reidel, 1978), p. 63.

[10] J. Rawls, "Justice as Fairness: Political Not Metaphysical," *Philosophy and Public Affairs* 14, no. 3 (1985): pp. 243–244.

[11] Rawls, *A Theory of Justice*, pp. 7, 96.

[12] Rawls, "The Basic Structures as Subject," p. 56.

[13] J. Rawls, "A Well-Ordered Society," in *Philosophy, Politics, and Society*, edited by P. Laslett and J. S. Fishkin (New Haven: Yale University Press, 1979), pp. 14–15.

[14] Rawls, "Social Unity and Primary Goods," p. 170.

EXCERPT 6

Abridged text from:

R. J. Arneson, "Luck, Egalitarianism, and Prioritarianism," *Ethics* 110, no. 2 (2000): pp. 339–349.

Luck, Egalitarianism, and Prioritarianism

Richard J. Arneson

In her recent, provocative essay "What Is the Point of Equality?", Elizabeth Anderson argues against a common ideal of egalitarian justice that she calls "luck egalitarianism" and in favor of an approach she calls "democratic equality."[1] According to the luck egalitarian, the aim of justice as equality is to eliminate so far as is possible the impact on people's lives of bad luck that falls on them through no fault or choice of their own. In the ideal luck egalitarian society, there are no inequalities in people's life prospects except those that arise through processes of voluntary choice or faulty conduct, for which the agents involved can reasonably be held responsible. Anderson asserts that the adherents of luck egalitarianism, which can be elaborated in many different ways, include John Roemer, Erik Rakowski, Thomas Nagel, Ronald Dworkin, Gerald Cohen, Richard Arneson, and (with a qualification) Philippe Van Parijs.[2] In contrast, according to the democratic equality conception, justice as equality requires an end to oppressive social relationships. In the ideal society of democratic equality, the social conditions of everyone's freedom are secured, each stands to every other in a relationship of fundamental equality, including equal respect, and all have real freedom to participate in democratic self-government.

Anderson's criticisms of luck egalitarianism score good points against a variety of views, including views I have defended.[3] In this comment I do not aim to defend luck egalitarianism across the board, but rather to identify one (outlier) member of the luck egalitarian family that is not vulnerable to Anderson's criticisms, is plausible in its own right, and in particular emerges as superior to the "democratic equality" conception of egalitarian justice. The version of egalitarian justice that I endorse I call responsibility-catering prioritarianism.[4] Roughly stated, the idea is that justice requires us to maximize a function of human well-being that gives priority to improving the well-being of those who are badly off and of those who, if badly off, are not substantially responsible for their condition in virtue of their prior conduct. Further elaboration is given below.

As characterized by Anderson, luck egalitarianism amounts to the following combination of claims: (1) it is morally bad if some are badly off through no fault or choice of their own, (2) it is morally bad if some are worse off than others through no fault or choice of their own, and (3) social justice requires us to eliminate, so far as is possible, the moral bads described in (1) and (2). To capture the luck

---

[1] E. S. Anderson, "What Is the Point of Equality?", *Ethics* 109, no. 2 (1999): pp. 287–337.

[2] J. E. Roemer, *Theories of Distributive Justice* (Harvard University Press, 1998); E. Rakowski, *Equal Justice* (Clarendon Press, 1991); T. Nagel, *Equality and Partiality* (Oxford University Press, 1991); R. Dworkin, "What Is Equality? Part 2: Equality of Resources," *Philosophy and Public Affairs* 10, no. 4 (1981): pp. 283–345; G. A. Cohen, "On the Currency of Egalitarian Justice," *Ethics* 99, no. 4 (1989): pp. 906–944; R. J. Arneson, "Equality and Equal Opportunity for Welfare," *Philosophical Studies* 56, no. 1 (1989): pp. 77–93; P. Van Parijs, *Real Freedom for All: What (If Anything) Can Justify Capitalism?* (Clarendon Press, 1997).

[3] See also R. J. Arneson, "Rawls, Responsibility, and Distributive Justice," in *Justice, Political Liberalism, and Utilitarianism: Themes from Harsanyi and Rawls*, edited by M. Salles and J. A. Weymark (Cambridge: Cambridge University Press, 2010).

[4] On prioritarianism, see D. Parfit, *Equality or Priority?* (University of Kansas, 1995); also D. Mckerlie, "Equality and Priority," *Utilitas* 6, no. 01 (1994): pp. 25–42; also P. Weirich, "Utility Tempered with Equality," *Nous* 17, no. 3 (1983): pp. 423–439. On the variant responsibility-catering prioritarianism, see R. J. Arneson, "Equality of Opportunity for Welfare Defended and Recanted," *Journal of Political Philosophy* 7, no. 4 (1999): pp. 488–497.

egalitarian ideal, both claims (1) and (2) are necessary.[5] By itself, (2) would not support the judgment that it is morally unfortunate if disastrous bad luck brings it about that everyone is made far worse off so long as everyone ends up equally badly off.

Luck egalitarianism seems to involve a conditional affirmation of equality—it is morally desirable that everyone's condition should be the same unless differential merit or differences in people's voluntary choices give rise to inequality. The prioritarianism I defend is committed to claim (1) but not claim (2), and involves no commitment whatsoever to the idea that it is morally desirable, from the standpoint of distributive justice, that everyone's condition be equal. So there may seem to be a mismatch, in that what I defend is not quite what Anderson attacks. However, Anderson explicitly mentions the leximin version of priority to the worse off as a variant of luck egalitarianism that falls within the intended scope of her criticisms.[6] It should be of some interest to explore whether or not any of her criticisms inflicts damage on what I regard as a plausible close cousin of luck egalitarianism. Moreover, what I say in defense of prioritarianism casts doubt on Anderson's democratic equality conception of social justice.

. . .

Second criticism: Luck egalitarianism misconceives the role of individual responsibility in distributive justice. Anderson holds that luck egalitarianism builds consideration for individual responsibility into the theory of justice in the wrong way, with disastrous results. The luck egalitarian identifies justice with minimizing and equalizing the effects of bad brute luck on people, luck that falls on people in ways that are beyond their power to control, but this involves a harsh toleration of misfortune that falls on people through their fault or choice. In a society that is just by luck egalitarian standards, some members of society must be allowed to fall into utter destitution that is deemed to arise through their fault or choice. The luck egalitarian imperative of making social decisions to help or decline to help needy individuals on the basis of the degree to which they have exercised or failed to exercise responsibility in socially approved ways is unfair to the needy who are labelled faulty and left to languish. But the social process of distinguishing responsible from irresponsible, deserving from nondeserving citizens is inherently disrespectful and unfair to all members of society. Those who receive aid are stigmatized as incompetent failures. Those who are deemed unworthy of aid are stigmatized as morally irresponsible and undeserving. In a luck egalitarian society all members will find their privacy violated by intrusive and offensive

[5] A further complication should be noted. Claims (1) and (2) are compatible with (3): It is morally bad if some are as well off as others through no merit of their own. Moreover, (1) through (3) are compatible with the denial of a straight assertion of equality, (4): It is morally bad if some are worse off than others. What Anderson calls "luck egalitarianism" might then be interpreted as a principle of moral meritocracy along the lines of (5): It is morally desirable that each person be exactly as well off or badly off as she deserves on the basis of her moral merit. So far as I can see, my responses to Anderson's criticisms of luck egalitarianism and to her grounds for endorsing the rival "democratic equality" view are not affected by ambiguity in her characterization of luck egalitarianism.

[6] Anderson, p. 291. (Leximin holds that we ought, as a first priority, maximally to improve the condition of the worst-off individual, then as a second priority, maximally to improve the condition of the second-worst-off, and so on up to the best-off. Prioritarianism holds that we ought to maximize a weighted sum of benefit that gives extra weight to obtaining a benefit for a person, the worse off she is prior to receipt of the benefit. This will imply giving priority to helping the worse off. Since prioritarianism welcomes chance events that increase people's well-being, it is not, strictly speaking, a member of the luck egalitarian family of views, just a close cousin. Prioritarianism prefers the outcome in which a random meteor shower confers benefits costlessly on some already advantaged people to the status quo ante in which well-being is less for some people and better for none, but more equally divided. Leximin, an extreme version of prioritarianism, dictates the same preference ordering over these two alternatives.

investigative procedures that aim to classify them according to the level of badness of their lives and the degree of irresponsibility of their life choices. These invasions of privacy signal that taking the imperative of justice to be undoing the effects of all brute bad luck inherently erases the line between what is the legitimate concern of society and what should be left to individual discretion.

Some versions of luck egalitarianism attempt to mitigate harsh treatment of those deemed irresponsible and undeserving by recommendations of paternalistic restriction of freedom designed to protect these putatively irresponsible and undeserving individuals from self-harming conduct. Here the thought is that some people may be incapable of prudent and responsible conduct, so we must restrict their liberty in self-regarding matters to give them a fair opportunity for a decent life. Anderson finds paternalism so motivated to be unacceptable because it inherently expresses adverse judgments on citizens' lives which no society should make.

In response: I agree for the most part with Anderson's characterization of the luck egalitarian line on individual responsibility, which the version of prioritarianism I embrace also follows. I argue below that Anderson is wrong to reject individual responsibility so construed. Before developing this response, I place Anderson's third criticism of luck egalitarianism on the table and describe a doctrine of responsibility-catering prioritarianism (RCP) that can withstand both criticisms.

Third criticism: Luck egalitarianism violates the norm that we should respect persons. According to Anderson, luck egalitarianism is defective in a deeper way than has been noted to this point. This theory fails to express equal concern and respect for all persons. The considerations that are the basis for adopting luck egalitarian principles essentially involve appeal to a contemptuous pity of the unfortunate on the part of the fortunate and in return envy of the haves that gnaws at the have-nots. Neither the attitude of pity for those viewed as worse off nor envy of those deemed to be better off is compatible with a proper egalitarian regard for persons. Luck egalitarian principles embody the idea that what fundamentally matters morally is how well off one person is as compared to others. At the root of this conception is a morally incorrect perspective that leads to distorted notions of what we owe to one another.

This last objection misfires if it is aimed at the prioritarian branch of the family of egalitarian principles. Prioritarianism holds that institutions and practices should be set and actions chosen to maximize moral value, with the stipulation that the moral value of obtaining a benefit (avoiding a loss) for a person is greater, the greater the well-being gain that the person would get from it (the smaller the loss in well-being), and greater, the lower the person's lifetime expectation of well-being prior to receipt of the benefit (loss). Prioritarianism is egalitarian in tilting in favor of those who are badly off. But priority is assigned to aiding an individual in virtue of how badly his life is going, as measured by an objective scale of well-being, not intrinsically by any comparison between his life and that of others. If the attitude that a theory expresses is given by the reasons that warrant its adoption, then I see no basis for associating with prioritarianism with a psychology of pity and envy. The root idea of prioritarianism is that one ought as a matter of justice to aid the unfortunate, and the more badly off someone is, the more urgent is the moral imperative to aid. The moral ground for helping someone is the badness of their situation, not any determination of how one person's situation compares with another's. So envy is not in play. Moreover, the misfortune that is supposed to trigger the obligation to aid according to prioritarianism is misfortune due to bad luck, so there is no basis here for holding oneself superior if one happens to have experienced good luck rather than bad, and to be in the position of helper rather than beneficiary.

Prioritarianism aside, Anderson's association of luck egalitarianism with unseemly emotions of rancorous envy and contemptuous pity is off the mark. Claims (1) and (2) as stated above express the root idea of luck egalitarianism, so the invocation of emotions that feed on social status is otiose. More generally, I doubt that invocation of an ideal of respect for persons can do any work in selecting principles of justice or in determining that some candidate principles are driven by unseemly motives. If one wants to be fair and do what is just, and after full reflection one is convinced that some version of luck egalitarianism is the correct theory of justice, then one's adoption of luck egalitarianism reflects one's belief that this doctrine picks out what justice requires coupled with one's desire to conform to the requirements of justice. One expresses due respect for persons and treats them respectfully by acting toward persons in accordance with the moral principles that are best supported by reasons. In this sense respect for persons looks to be an unobjectionable but purely formal idea, neither a clue to what principles are best supported by moral reasons nor a constraint on what principles might be chosen.

Prioritarianism as stated does not attribute moral value per se to channeling benefits toward the more deserving and responsible, though such considerations would no doubt play an instrumental role in a fully articulated prioritarian theory. I myself am inclined to think that if two persons voluntarily engage in high stakes gambling, from which the loser emerges with unfavorable future life prospects, it is intrinsically, not merely instrumentally more valuable to provide the means to a one-unit gain of well-being to someone who is just as badly off as the unlucky gambler but arrives at this condition through bad luck that is beyond his power to control than to the unlucky gambler. Hence it is better to amend prioritarianism to responsibility-catering prioritarianism. According to the latter doctrine, the moral value of altering a state of affairs in a way that makes someone better off or worse off depends, other things being equal, on the degree of responsibility the person bears for her present condition. It is morally more valuable to provide a gain in well-being of a given size for a person with a given well-being prospect if she is less rather than more responsible for her present condition (if it is bad). In a similar way, less moral disvalue is produced by bringing about a loss in well-being of a given size to a person with a given well-being prospect if the person is less rather than more responsible for her present condition (if it is good). To have a theory, rather than a quick sketch of a theory, one would have to provide an account of responsibility and attach weights to the three elements of well-being, priority for the badly off, and responsibility in responsibility-catering prioritarianism (RCP).

RCP even if fully articulated would be an abstract moral theory, a set of principles of justice, not a specification of just institutions or just practices. These latter would vary with circumstances, which determine what institutions and practices and actions would best achieve the RCP moral goals. On any remotely plausible theory of human well-being, even if in principle interpersonal cardinal well-being and responsibility judgments can be made, in practice individuals and institutions would not have access to such information, so in practice we would be designing the most relevant and appropriate proxies we can find for the values that really matter to us. Anderson's attractive ideals of democratic equality are pitched at a somewhat lower level of abstraction than RCP, and might for all I know be a reasonably good set of means for implementing prioritarian values under favorable modern circumstances. Indeed, some of her criticisms of luck egalitarianism might be interpreted as criticisms of inept strategies for implementing RCP values.

Real disagreement arises when allegedly wrongful policies that invade privacy, restrict people's liberty for their own good, and restrict rights to equal participation in democratic politics would improve the quality of people's lives and distribute these improvements fairly according to the weighted well-being standard. One aspect of the disagreement is that Anderson accords priority to freedom on her favored interpretation of it (see below). According to RCP, having real freedom to achieve basic human goods is valuable both instrumentally and for its own sake, insofar as having wide freedom is itself a constituent of a good human life. But freedoms according to RCP are important as constituents of well-being, and the ultimate moral standard is the extent of (appropriately weighted) well-being that we achieve. To enhance weighted well-being, this or that freedom must sometimes give way. Freedom, even freedom on its morally most adequate interpretation, is not an absolute moral value that trumps all others. For example, perhaps all paternalism inevitably carries some cost of insult and stigma imposed on those whose freedom is restricted for their own good. But when paternalistic policy satisfies RCP, the insult and stigma cost is outweighed by genuine well-being gains, and is not then inherently disrespectful.

. . .

Democratic equality characterized and criticized. Anderson's arguments against luck egalitarianism pave the way for the democratic equality conception that she proposes to replace it. The latter is complex; this discussion just highlights some main features. The democratic equality ideal requires that all members of society should have a fundamental equal status, constituted by the real freedom possessed by all over the entire course of their lives to function as humans, to participate in civil society, and to participate in democratic political decision making. In other words, all persons are equally guaranteed the capacity to achieve a threshold acceptable level in these three domains, the generic human, the sphere of association, and the political. The maintenance of these equal freedoms is to be guaranteed over the course of people's entire adult lives, come what may. This guarantee is asserted to contrast favorably with luck egalitarianism, which countenances allowing people to languish in bondage or squalor if they are deemed to have had a fair opportunity and squandered their opportunities through their own fault or choice. Democratic equality guarantees only freedom at an acceptable threshold level. Inequalities above the threshold are not deemed per se morally undesirable. This limited guarantee imposes on individuals the responsibility to order their lives as they choose above the threshold and eschews the politics of envy that Anderson associates with luck egalitarianism. Personal responsibility also receives its due in the democratic equality norm in another significant way: The guarantees that democratic equality enforces are guarantees of access to functionings (real freedom to achieve a set level of functioning), not a guarantee of any achieved level of functioning.

This democratic equality ideal is intended to be a sketch of a theory that needs further refinement, so criticism may be premature. But as presented so far, the implications of democratic equality are implausible where they disagree with those of RCP. Democratic equality holds that once someone is above the basic capability threshold, justice is unconcerned with whether or not his life goes better or worse. Why not? Suppose that society faces an issue, say a choice of tax policy, where the interests of those who are far above the basic capability threshold (and thus on the average high in well-being) are starkly opposed to the interests of those who are just above the threshold (and thus on average significantly lower in well-being). Unfortunately someone's ox must be gored. Whose? RCP says that on the facts as described, other things equal we should favor the worse off in order to fulfill the requirements of justice. Democratic equality says that the issue is a "don't care" from the standpoint of justice. I disagree.

The force of this criticism could be blunted to some extent if the threshold of basic capability is set at a very high level. But only to an extent. Moreover, this move brings another difficulty into view. Democratic equality extends an unconditional guarantee that each member of society shall have access to the basic functioning level. But this priority ranking is too stringent. When misfortune strikes, it is a regrettable fact that some people cannot be sustained at the threshold level no matter what resources are poured into the coffers earmarked for their aid. In other cases, sustaining an individual at the threshold level is possible only at too great a cost. Morally sensitive cost and benefit calculation must be carried out to determine whether maintaining an individual at the guaranteed level (or at some specified distance from the level) is morally worthwhile all things considered, but democratic equality is inhospitable to the needed tradeoffs. The higher the threshold level of basic capability is set, the more glaring this problem becomes.

Democratic equality eschews moralizing judgments about the quality of individual lives and hectoring assessments of the degree to which individuals have behaved responsibly.

Is this avoidance an advantage? To focus on the relevant issues, ignore questions concerning the availability of the information needed for making these judgments and assessments and concerning the moral cost of discovering this information if it is available. RCP affirms that what is morally right to do depends on this information. But in circumstances in which the information is unavailable or costly to obtain, RCP affirms whatever norms and policies will most efficiently advance the RCP goals. Consider then simple examples in which the relevant information is readily available. Suppose that a national park service rescue team can choose between one of three lifesaving missions. Each involves significant risk of severe harm to rescue workers, but promises a significant net saving of lives. Suppose these risks and benefits are the same for each of the three rival missions. The park rescue team must choose either to assist (a) a party of stranded schoolchildren caught in an unanticipated blizzard while on a school outing, (b) a party of experienced climbers who carefully chose to pursue a difficult route under hazardous conditions which then suddenly turned desperate, or (c) a party of tourists who ignored warning signs and the stern advice of park rangers to venture on a foolhardy hike across a treacherous steep slope, rendered more treacherous by their mid-hike alcohol consumption. One might suppose that the rescue team's policy should be set in part by consideration of its incentive effects on the behavior of future park visitors, but suppose the park is about to be shut down and there are no such incentive effects to consider. I take it to be a datum in this case that the fully voluntary choice of the climbers to shoulder the risk they take and the grossly reckless conduct of the hikers reduce their moral claims to be aided by comparison with the claim of the stranded school children. This is the basic idea of the responsibility-catering element in responsibility-catering prioritarianism. A proposed theory of justice that excludes it excludes a factor that is intrinsically morally important.

Anderson's democratic equality attempts to balance concern for the well-being of the badly off and concern for individual responsibility by guaranteeing each individual a level of material provision that secures the status of equal democratic citizen for all, and above this line, by allowing individuals to obtain whatever outcomes result from the ensemble of individual voluntary choices. But this way of splitting the difference between social guarantees and individual responsibility does not fully take the measure of the problem of accommodating individual responsibility within egalitarian distributive norms. In the Andersonian democratic equality society with guarantees of a threshold of guaranteed functionings for all, some individuals might behave culpably irresponsibly, again and again, so that the cost of maintaining them at the guaranteed threshold level becomes prohibitive, or swallows up all social resources. In this situation the guaranteed social minimum would be unfairly draining resources that should go to other members of society/ RCP would deny that such a guaranteed social minimum not qualified by the reciprocal requirement of a threshold level of responsible conduct by citizens could be just. At the level of practical policy, a guaranteed minimum of some sort might be the best we can do to balance conflicting considerations, but at the level of principle, the democratic equality synthesis cannot be upheld as morally fair and just.

RCP also incorporates the belief that what we should do depends both on how much good we can do for people and how badly off they will be absent our intervention. In the example, policy should respond to the consideration that it is objectively worse to have one's life cut short as a child, other things being equal, than to have one's life abruptly ended after one has lived longer and had ample opportunity to sample the goods basic to a normal human life. No doubt measurements of well-being and well-being prospects are beset by conceptual difficulties such that commensurability is only partial even in principle, quite aside from the practical difficulties of acquiring the information that in theory is needed for assessment. But I have never seen a good argument for maintaining an asymmetry between the good and the right in this regard: If one supposes no rational agreement on the good is possible, one's skepticism will by parity of reasoning lead one to conclude that no rational agreement on the right is possible, and one should abandon moral theory as a lost cause.

If one rejects wholesale moral skepticism, then liberal egalitarian teleology remains a viable contender for our reflective allegiance, and responsibility-catering prioritarianism stands as one interpretation of its fundamental principle. The point of equality I would say is to improve people's life prospects, tilting in favor of those who are worse off, and in favor of those who have done as well as could reasonably be expected with the cards that fate has dealt them.

EXCERPT 7

Abridged text from:
S. Segall, *Health, Luck, and Justice* (Princeton University Press, 2009), ch. 4.

Chapter 4

Tough Luck?: Why Luck Egalitarians Need Not Abandon Reckless Patients

S. Segall

Introduction

I [began] by presenting the abandonment dilemma, namely, how to sustain a responsibility-sensitive account of egalitarian justice that is yet able to justify universal and unconditional (i.e., one that does not deny it from imprudent patients) medical care. . . . I argue that luck egalitarianism can escape the abandonment objection if, when applied to health care policy (and social policy more generally), it is complemented with other moral considerations (including other considerations of justice), such as those of meeting basic needs.

The . . . abandonment objection is largely credited to Elizabeth Anderson.[1] Anderson claims that luck egalitarians are harsh on victims of option luck (such as those taking risks with their health), for they abandon such victims to their dire fates.[2] In response to Anderson, I claim that luck egalitarians can escape this objection unscathed. . . . In order to do so I first look at recent luck egalitarian responses to the abandonment objection. I examine five such responses. . . . [I then] suggest that the concern for meeting basic needs . . . could complement luck egalitarianism and, as such, potentially lay to rest the abandonment objection.

I. Luck Egalitarian Attempts to Deflect the Abandonment Objection

How might luck egalitarians respond to the abandonment objection? Here are five such attempts.

The first luck egalitarian response I want to look at here has some affinity with the all-luck egalitarian position surveyed in the previous chapter. It is similar in the sense that it also questions the distinction between brute and option luck. This response therefore similarly questions the alleged luck egalitarian commitment to abandoning those who suffer bad option luck (e.g., unlucky smokers). However, it is somewhat less radical and so,

[1] E. S. Anderson, "What Is the Point of Equality?", *Ethics* 109, no. 2 (1999): pp. 287–337. For criticism of Anderson, see R. J. Arneson, "Luck, Egalitarianism and Prioritarianism," *Ethics* 110, no. 2 (2000): pp. 339–349; T. Christiano, 'Comment on Elizabeth Anderson's "What Is the Point of Equality,"' http://www.brown.edu/Departments/Philosophy/bears/9904chri.html; D. Sobel, 'Comment on Elizabeth Anderson's "What Is the Point of Equality,"' http://www.brown.edu/Departments/Philosophy/bears/9904sobe.html. For sympathetic reviews, see S. Scheffler, "What Is Egalitarianism?", *Philosophy & Public Affairs* 31, no. 1 (2003): pp. 5–39; D. Wikler, "Personal and Social Responsibility for Health," in *Public Health, Ethics and Equity*, edited by S. Anand, F. Peter, and A. K. Sen (Oxford University Press, 2004), pp. 109–134.

[2] "[J]ustice does not permit the exploitation or abandonment of anyone, even the imprudent." Anderson, "What Is the Point of Equality?" p. 298 (see also pp. 295–296). See also Scheffler: "[T]he fact that a person's urgent medical needs can be traced to his own negligence or foolishness or high-risk behavior is not normally seen as making it legitimate to deny him the care he needs" ("What Is Egalitarianism?" pp. 18–19); and S. Scheffler, "Choice, Circumstance, and the Value of Equality," *Politics, Philosophy & Economics* 4, no. 1 (2005): pp. 5–28.

consequently, is its conclusion. The response, as offered by Peter Vallentyne, says that in some cases, the rational thing to do, that is, the course of action that yields the highest expected utility, does involve taking some risk. To flatly deny compensation in all cases of bad option luck, regardless of the "quality" of the risk, is to discourage individuals from taking calculated risks, and is therefore inefficient and wasteful. Efficient, and thereby just (pace Vallentyne), institutions would therefore compensate for bad option luck (in cases where taking a gamble is the rational course of action).[3]

Vallentyne's argument cannot, however, meet the abandonment objection fully. As Vallentyne himself points out, his argument does not "eliminate" the abandonment objection, it only "softens" it, for it does not recommend compensating all cases of bad option luck. Specifically, he acknowledges that we should not compensate for bad option luck when taking the risk in question was irrational (that is, not the course of action yielding the highest expected utility).[4] Note also that Vallentyne's contribution is in demonstrating that it is efficient (and thereby, arguably, just) to provide incentives for risk-taking when doing so is the prudent course of action. Vallentyne does not argue, then, that luck egalitarians are committed to compensating risk-taking when to do so would be imprudent. It therefore seems that Vallentyne's proposal cannot be used for meeting the abandonment of the imprudent objection. It rather redefines (correctly, I think) what counts as imprudence (where some risk-taking is prudent, and therefore should be compensated).[5] In effect, then, Vallentyne's proposal is consistent with the criticism that depicts luck egalitarianism as abandoning the imprudent (rather than abandoning all victims of bad option luck), and thus cannot serve as a response to it.

Here is a second luck egalitarian response to the abandonment objection. As a response to that objection, Ronald Dworkin advocates adding a residual layer of mandatory social insurance to his famous (voluntary) hypothetical insurance, so as to cover incidents of bad option luck that lead to destitution and loss of basic capabilities. This mandatory scheme insures individuals against ending up lacking the most basic of capabilities needed to lead a decent life, regardless of the personal history that led them to require such assistance.[6] Critics such as Anderson, however, dismiss Dworkin's solution by arguing that it is paternalistic, and as such, disrespectful of those it aids.[7] Dworkin (in later writings) deflects that accusation by saying that his proposed health insurance, although compulsory, compensates incidents of bad option luck that

[3] Peter Vallentyne, "Brute Luck, Option Luck, and Equality of Initial Opportunities," *Ethics* 112, no. 3 (2002): pp. 529–557. See also M. Fleurbaey, "Egalitarian Opportunities," *Law and Philosophy* 20, no. 5 (2001): pp. 499–530, esp. pp. 513–522. As mentioned in the previous chapter, Kasper Lippert-Rasmussen offers a somewhat similar argument for compensating bad option luck, but one that combines the current response with the one surveyed in the previous chapter. (See his L. R. by Kasper, "Egalitarianism, Option Luck, and Responsibility," *Ethics* 111, no. 3 (2001): pp. 548–579). In a recent unpublished manuscript, Richard Arneson has identified this group of philosophers as "desert luck egalitarians," for they hold that prudent risks (as well as altruistic conduct) convert a case of bad option luck into one deserving compensation. See his "Luck Egalitarianism Interpreted and Defended," *Philosophical Topics* (2004): pp. 1–20.

[4] Vallentyne, "Brute Luck, Option Luck, and Equality of Initial Opportunities," p. 556.

[5] On the claim that what counts as a responsible action would depend on what risks it is conventionally reasonable to undertake, see A. Ripstein, "Equality, Luck, and Responsibility," *Philosophy & Public Affairs* 23, no. 1 (1994): pp. 3–23.

[6] R. Dworkin, *Sovereign Virtue: The Theory and Practice of Equality* (Harvard University Press, 2002), chs. 2, 9. See also R. Dworkin, *Foundations of Liberal Equality* (University of Utah Press, 1990), p. 85; R. Dworkin, "Sovereign Virtue Revisited," *Ethics* 113, no. 1 (2002): p. 11; R. Dworkin, "Equality, Luck and Hierarchy," *Philosophy & Public Affairs* 31, no. 2 (2003): p. 192.

[7] Anderson, "What is the Point of Equality?" p. 301.

individuals behind a veil of ignorance would most likely choose to insure against and is therefore not clearly paternalistic or badly so. Since everyone wants to avoid leading a "horribly grim" life, it follows that individuals are not averse to an insurance scheme that guarantees them basic resources such as adequate unemployment benefits and basic health care.[8] [. . .]

A third luck egalitarian suggestion for meeting the abandonment objection relies on pointing out that it is unfair to hold individuals responsible for the degree to which they are responsible agents to begin with. In a postscript to his canonical 1989 article, Richard Arneson suggested that people's capacity for prudence varies along with natural talent and upbringing, and therefore a modified version of luck egalitarianism should take account also of the degree to which people's imprudence is itself a matter of bad luck.[9] A somewhat similar solution is offered also by John Roemer in his famous "pragmatic theory of responsibility." Roemer proposes to identify "types" of individuals clustered around their ability to act prudently (schoolteachers are generally more prudent than steelworkers, say), identify a mean rate of prudent behavior within those types, and treat conduct that is less prudent than that mean as imprudent behavior for the purposes of distributive justice.[10] If imprudence is, to an extent, itself a matter of bad brute luck, it would follow that the imprudent should be compensated, thus avoiding the abandonment objection.

Meeting the abandonment objection, it is important to note, is perhaps not Arneson's and Roemer's main motivation in advancing the above argument. My evaluation of that particular argument's ability to meet the abandonment objection is therefore not intended as a criticism of that argument itself. What I do want to say about Arneson's and Roemer's proposal is that even though this type of modification brings luck egalitarianism closer to meeting the abandonment objection, it is unable to do so fully: Arneson and Roemer only relocate the boundary between prudence and imprudence (and hence between option luck and brute luck), rather than show that imprudence is impossible (and that all luck is brute). Had they shown that, perhaps they would have answered the problem of imprudent agents pointed out by Anderson. Arneson's and Roemer's reinterpretation still leaves a spectrum of cases of genuine option luck, and therefore does not entitle its victims to luck egalitarian compensation. Thus, the abandonment objection still stands.

A fourth potential response to the abandonment objection relies on the plausible premise that, in reality, option luck almost never occurs. Option luck understood as "a deliberate and calculated risk,"[11] taken with full information, hardly ever occurs in real life. Rather, almost all disadvantages suffered in contemporary market societies have an element of bad brute luck about them.[12] Being unemployed, for example, almost always entails a structural element that is beyond one's control. It would follow that in contemporary societies, the abandonment objection does not arise, simply because there are no pure cases of bad option luck that would be ignored by luck egalitarians. If anything, the abandonment objection is worth worrying about once we have reached an egalitarian utopia.

Let us suppose then that the abandonment objection arises only in fully egalitarian societies. Notice that even then, the objection still represents an embarrassment to luck egalitarians, whose theory is an attempt to say something of universal truth with regard to the

[8] See "Sovereign Virtue Revisited," p. 114.

[9] R. J. Arneson, "Equality and Equal Opportunity for Welfare," in *Equality: Selected Readings*, edited by L. P. Pojmanand and R. Westmoreland (New York: Oxford University Press, 1997), p. 239. See also Anderson, "What Is the Point of Equality?" p. 300; S. L. Hurley, *Justice, Luck, and Knowledge* (Harvard University Press, 2005).

[10] J. E. Roemer, "A Pragmatic Theory of Responsibility for the Egalitarian Planner," *Philosophy & Public Affairs* (1993): pp. 146–166.

[11] Dworkin, *Sovereign Virtue,* p. 73.

[12] D. Miller, "What Kind of Equality Should the Left," in *Equality* (London: Institute for Public Policy Research, 1997): p. 91.

requirements of egalitarian justice. But even setting that thought aside, it is still doubtful that this fourth response can go all the way in rescuing luck egalitarianism from the abandonment objection. Consider this. The response only concerns the moral arbitrariness of luck, and thus of the need to compensate risk takers. But the abandonment objection refers not only to cases of reckless risk-taking, but also to cases of deliberate waste and self-harm. That is to say, the broad category of option luck includes not only risk takers but also individuals who deliberately inflict disadvantages, including illnesses, upon themselves. They do so not as a result of a risk badly taken but out of a conscious decision to bear the costs of a certain course of action in order to enjoy some other advantage that that course of action may bring. Smokers, for example, are not all necessarily risk takers, as they may simply be willing to sacrifice the later years of their lives for the pleasure of smoking throughout their (shorter) lives. Here again luck appears to be irrelevant. Daniels's fair opportunity approach and Anderson's democratic equality approach would support treating patients with that kind of history, while luck egalitarians arguably are committed to abandoning them. It appears, therefore, that this luck egalitarian response does not cope well with such self-inflicted harm cases.[13] The claim that option luck hardly ever occurs cannot, then, help luck egalitarians to meet fully Anderson's abandonment objection.

The final luck egalitarian response to the abandonment objection that I shall look at invokes the requirements of autonomy. Since it holds that individuals should be compensated for losses that they are not responsible for, luck egalitarian justice must demand, to be consistent, that individuals be held responsible for their actions. To meet that purpose individuals must be autonomous, for surely people cannot be held responsible when lacking the autonomy to do otherwise. And, in order to safeguard such autonomy, certain threshold requirements must be satisfied (minimal healthy functioning, adequate nutrition, the social basis of minimal self-respect, etc.). Indeed, it is essential for a luck egalitarian regime to observe these threshold requirements, for, once victims of bad option luck are allowed to slip below the material prerequisites of autonomy, their subsequent choices and actions invariably fall under the brute luck category, as the agents cannot be held responsible for the resulting disadvantages. Thus, a luck egalitarian regime would have to compensate these individuals continuously, which is surely wasteful. For that reason, it is imperative that those who suffer bad option luck do not fall below the subsistence level required for autonomous conduct.

This purported luck egalitarian response to the abandonment objection is attractive. However, upon reflection this autonomy response turns out to be a nonegalitarian consideration (and therefore it cannot constitute a luck egalitarian response). To explain: it is not a requirement of luck egalitarian justice that victims of option luck be raised to the level of autonomy. For it is not unfair to abandon them, according to this reading; it is only inefficient.[14] Since it offers a potential solution to the abandonment objection nevertheless (only not an egalitarian one), I will return to consider this response [below]

It may be the case that the five responses examined here do not exhaust the array of potential luck egalitarian replies to the abandonment objection. However, if they do, and if, as I have argued, these luck egalitarian responses cannot meet the abandonment objection fully, then any attempt to rescue luck egalitarianism from that objection

[13] This response's only means of sidestepping such cases would be to assert that all cases of self-inflicted harm result, at bottom, from lack of true agency, and thus still fall under brute luck. But it is difficult to respond to such an assertion short of immersing ourselves "up to our necks in the free will problem," as Cohen as noted. G. A. Cohen, "On the Currency of Egalitarian Justice," *Ethics* 99, no. 4 (1989): p. 934.

[14] N. Barry, "Defending Luck Egalitarianism," *Journal of Applied Philosophy* 23, no. 1 (2006): p. 99.

would have to be an external one (i.e., a non-justice-based reason). I turn to examine that suggestion now.

IV. A Potential Solution?

One potential nonegalitarian response to the abandonment objection is the autonomy argument [i.e.:] that it is mandatory to treat the imprudent, for it would be wasteful to allow individuals to fall below the level of subsistence needed for autonomous agency. Another, perhaps even stronger reason to treat the imprudent is that we must not allow basic needs, including medical needs, to go unmet. The obligation to meet basic needs is a well-entrenched moral requirement in ethics and political philosophy.[15] It is based on the recognition that individuals have a deep interest in having their needs met. The more basic the need is, the deeper the interest of the individual is in having it met. We commonly think that there is some urgency about meeting needs, urgency that is not necessarily there when we consider meeting people's mere preferences.[16] We consequently think that individuals would be harmed if their basic needs are not met.[17] Since it is plausible to think that we owe each other equal protection from harm, this is often seen as capable of grounding a universal entitlement to health care.[18] Health care, on this account, is simply part of the social minimum that society ought to guarantee to its citizens.[19] . . . [C]oupling the moral requirement to meet basic needs, including basic medical needs, with luck egalitarian distributive justice allows for a comprehensive ethical guide to health care, and one that escapes the abandonment objection.

The requirement to meet basic needs whomever they belong to can be seen as following from individuals' equal moral worth, and the equal respect society ought to show toward them. . . . This is a moral requirement that is external, and prior (in the sense of being more fundamental), to the one of egalitarian distributive justice. The moral requirement to meet basic needs coupled with luck egalitarian distributive justice thus requires us to treat imprudent patients who are needy. In this way, luck egalitarian health care avoids the abandonment objection. It is relatively easy, notice, for the sort of luck egalitarianism I defend here to allow the concern for basic needs to complement the requirements of egalitarian distributive justice. For, . . . my version of luck egalitarianism is distinct from the ideal of desert. It does not insist on punishing individuals or on matching the level of their well-being to the level of their deservingness (prudence-wise). It is therefore not a requirement of justice, on my account, that the imprudent be left to suffer. The account thus lends itself to being coupled with the rather straightforward concern for meeting basic needs.

Notice that by supplementing the requirements of egalitarian distributive justice with those of meeting basic needs we are thereby adding a layer of sufficientarian distribution to the egalitarian one required by luck egalitarianism. . . . I suggest that that sufficientarian

[15] Norman Daniels himself recognizes that "we have a widely recognized moral obligation to meet people's medical needs." N. Daniels, *Just Health: Meeting Health Needs Fairly* (Cambridge University Press, 2007), p. 111.

[16] T. M. Scanlon, "Preference and Urgency," *Journal of Philosophy* 72, no. 19 (1975): pp. 655–669.

[17] D. Wiggins, *Needs, Values, Truth: Essays in the Philosophy of Value* (Clarendon Press, 1998).

[18] A. E. Buchanan, "The Right to a Decent Minimum of Health Care," *Philosophy & Public Affairs* (1984): pp. 55–78.

[19] This has been recognized also by Rawls in his most recent writing. Rawls writes of the social minimum: "the expectation of an assured provision of health care at a certain level (calculated by estimated cost) is included as part of that minimum." J. Rawls, *Justice as Fairness: A Restatement* (Harvard University Press, 2001), p. 173. On the concept of social minimum more generally, see S. White, "Social Minimum," *Stanford Encyclopedia of Philosophy* (2010).

distribution is justified on grounds of the moral requirement to meet basic needs. . . .

How, then, does the requirement of meeting basic needs combine with the luck egalitarian conception of fairness to form a coherent ethical guide to policy? [Fairness can] sometimes be indeterminate. More specifically, . . . treating the imprudent is, under the luck egalitarian conception of fairness, neither fair nor unfair. The requirement of meeting basic needs, in turn, tells us to meet all members' basic needs irrespective of how (im) prudent their antecedent conduct was. Thus, the combination of indeterminate luck egalitarian fairness with the concern for basic needs yields a coherent guide to policy that avoids the abandonment objection.

Now notice that even when luck egalitarian distributive justice is supplemented with a sufficientarian concern for meeting basic needs, it does not escape the following dilemma. Often, given the scarcity of resources, we must give priority to treating one patient rather than another. Suppose two patients are in equal need but one of them is so out of her own fault while the other is not. Suppose the situation is one of a car crash, where one of the injured individuals is the reckless driver and the other, equally needy, is her innocent passenger. Though both are equally needy, considerations of luck egalitarian justice would determine that the innocent passenger should be assigned priority and get treated first. Now, some may be troubled by that conclusion, for it implies, at least in the example as I construed it, that a small measure of recklessness may lead to what amounts to a death sentence (when resources are scarce). This may again seem harsh toward the reckless driver. To quote Arneson again: "His "punishment"—the quality of life he gets after the accident—does not fit his "crime"—the brief lapses of judgment."[20] It seems then that even coupled with the concern for meeting basic needs, luck egalitarianism is unable to escape being harsh.

Let me make two points in response. The first point is that this objection is not peculiar to luck egalitarianism (although luck egalitarianism might, admittedly, exacerbate the problem here). Second, I would like to suggest a possible way out of this dilemma for luck egalitarians. Here is the first point. Suppose we supplemented luck egalitarianism with the considerations of autonomy. . . . In the example above, autonomy will be harmed if we leave either patient untreated. Considerations of autonomy therefore do not forbid assigning priority to the innocent driver. In fact, even responsibility-insensitive accounts of justice in health care . . . are not immune from the need to justify not giving priority to the innocent passenger. It would [for example,] represent an equal loss of democratic capabilities, or an equal loss of opportunity to pursue one's life plan, to leave either injured motorist untreated. Assuming that we are forced to choose between the two, we would then need a justification for not using considerations of self-responsibility as tie-breakers here.

The dilemma of whether or not to assign lower priority in treatment to those who have brought the medical condition upon themselves is therefore not peculiar to luck egalitarians. Whatever justification one has for providing health care, one would still have to decide whether or not to allow considerations of personal responsibility to affect the way in which medical resources, which are inevitably scarce, are distributed. For example, the dilemma of whether or not to assign priority in anti-retroviral therapies to AIDS patients who have been infected by contaminated blood (as the Chinese government has recently decided) is one that all theories of justice, and not just a luck egalitarian one, have to address.[21] It does not matter, for that purpose, whether one justifies health care on grounds of providing opportunities for life plans or safeguarding basic

[20] R. J. Arneson, "Luck Egalitarianism Interpreted and Defended," *Philosophical Topics* (2004): pp. 1–20. See also M. Fleurbaey, "Equal Opportunity or Equal Social Outcome?", *Economics and Philosophy* 11, no. 01 (1995): pp. 25–55; R. E. Goodin, "Negating Positive Desert Claims," *Political Theory* (1985): pp. 575–598.

[21] See for example, Daniels, *Just Health*, p. 298.

democratic capabilities. In the absence of reasons to the contrary, health care systems would be justified in assigning priority to a patient who has been harmed by the health care system itself.[22] It is plausible to think that we have reasons to prefer a patient who is needy out of other people's fault over one whose need is no one's fault (not to mention the one whose need is her own fault). In short, the need to justify neutrality (with regard to considerations of personal responsibility) in medical care is a challenge facing all theories of justice in health care, and not just luck egalitarianism.

. . .

Still, assigning absolute priority to the innocent passenger over the reckless driver in the case of only one available rescue might seem harsh on the reckless driver. Although she is at fault for the accident, and certainly more so compared to her passenger, we still feel uneasy about allowing this difference to result in something that may well amount to an automatic death sentence. There is indeed a simple and obvious way around this problem (and that is the second point I promised to make) and that is to apply, at least in principle, a mechanism of weighted lottery. Suppose we agree that the reckless driver is more at fault compared to her innocent passenger. And suppose we also agree that she does not deserve an automatic death sentence for what could be a rather small amount of imprudence (not stopping at a stop sign, say). We could then accordingly toss an imaginary coin between the two patients, one that is slightly weighted in favor of the innocent passenger. Thus, we are able to have a responsibility-sensitive account that is not unduly harsh (in circumstances of scarce resources).

. . .

[22] If our obligation toward the AIDS patient who contracted the disease while receiving transfusion is strong, our obligation toward the patient who has contract it while *donating* blood (say, from an infected needle) is even stronger. Of course, things get a little complicated if we determine that the blood donation was a matter of option luck (the person chose to give blood) whereas the blood transfusion was one of brute luck (the patient had to have a blood transfusion). Yet, if giving blood is something that it would be unreasonable to expect people not to do, then we may cast the case of AIDS following a donation as one constituting a brute luck disadvantage. I am grateful to Kristin Voigt for helping me clarify this point.

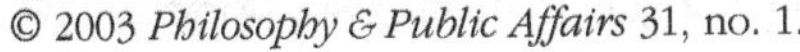

EXCERPT 8

Abridged text from:

S. Scheffler, "What Is Egalitarianism?", *Philosophy & Public Affairs* 31, no. 1 (2003): pp. 5–39.

What Is Egalitarianism?

Samuel Scheffler

One of the most significant theories of distributive justice to have emerged since the publication of *A Theory of Justice* is the form of distributive egalitarianism that Elizabeth Anderson has dubbed "luck egalitarianism."[1] This theory has different variants, but the central idea is common to all of these variants. The core idea is that inequalities in the advantages that people enjoy are acceptable if they derive from the choices that people have voluntarily made, but that inequalities deriving from unchosen features of people's circumstances are unjust. Unchosen circumstances are taken to include social factors like the class and wealth of the family into which one is born. They are also deemed to include natural factors like one's native abilities and intelligence.

Luck egalitarianism overlaps with but also diverges from the prevailing political morality in most liberal societies, both with respect to the unacceptability of inequalities deriving from people's circumstances and with respect to the acceptability of inequalities deriving from their choices. Consider first the unacceptability of inequalities deriving from people's circumstances. The prevailing political morality holds that intentional discrimination based on largely unchosen factors such as race, religion, sex, and ethnicity is unjust, and that distributive inequalities resulting from such discrimination are unjust as well. It also holds that people of equal talent from different social classes should have equal access to the social positions for which their talents qualify them, and that it is unjust if inequalities result from a society's failure to provide this kind of equal opportunity. Thus, the prevailing morality agrees with luck egalitarianism in rejecting certain kinds of inequalities deriving from unchosen features of people's circumstances. However, in rejecting all inequalities of advantage resulting from differing circumstances, luck egalitarianism goes far beyond the prevailing political morality, which, against a background of nondiscrimination and equal opportunity, is prepared to tolerate significant distributive inequalities deriving from differences of talent and ability. By contrast, luck egalitarianism denies that a person's natural talent, creativity, intelligence, innovative skill, or entrepreneurial ability can be the basis for legitimate inequalities.

Consider next the acceptability of inequalities deriving from people's choices. If some people make more money than others because they choose to work longer hours, then the prevailing morality certainly agrees with luck egalitarianism that that is not in itself objectionable. Unlike luck egalitarianism, however, the prevailing political morality does not go so far as to say that any extra income deriving from people's choices should, in principle, be exempt from redistributive taxation. In determining one's tax burden, the prevailing morality makes no attempt to identify, let alone to shield from taxation, the portion of one's income that is traceable specifically to one's choices as opposed to one's natural abilities.

The upshot is that although there are substantial areas of overlap between luck egalitarianism and the prevailing political morality, luck egalitarianism is in one way much more willing than the prevailing morality to engage in redistributive taxation, but also in one way much less willing. In this sense at least, luck egalitarianism is both more and less egalitarian than the prevailing political morality.[2]

---

[1] E. S. Anderson, "What Is the Point of Equality?", *Ethics* 109, no. 2 (1999): pp. 287–337.

[2] I do not mean to imply that these two factors cancel each out so that there is no net difference in the redistributive implications of the two positions. Luck egalitarians differ among themselves about the how much redistribution is justified, in part because they disagree about the extent to which actual inequalities are the result of differences in people's circumstances as opposed

Unlike Rawls's theory, which became the focus of intense critical scrutiny as soon as *A Theory of Justice* appeared in print, luck egalitarianism has been relatively slow to attract critical attention, despite the impressive level of influence it has attained and the lively debates that have taken place among proponents of its different variants. This state of affairs has begun to change, however, and in this article I wish to make a modest contribution to the project of critical examination that Anderson and others have initiated.[3] I am indebted to Anderson's discussion in many ways, some of which I will acknowledge more specifically as I proceed. But my primary emphases will be different from hers, and I hope that my main points are sufficiently independent as to be of interest in their own right.

Luck egalitarianism is often presented as an extension and generalization of some Rawlsian arguments whose substantive implications Rawls himself failed fully to appreciate. Thus, luck egalitarianism is often said by its advocates to be truer than Rawls's own conception of justice to some of his fundamental insights. In part because of its putative Rawlsian pedigree, perhaps, luck egalitarianism's supporters have done less than one might expect to provide an independent defense of the position at the fundamental level. In this article, however, I argue that luck egalitarianism can draw little support from Rawls. In addition, I present reasons for doubting whether it is either a plausible position in its own right or a compelling interpretation of egalitarianism.

II.

[M]any discussions of luck egalitarianism are addressed primarily to other egalitarians. They simply assume that an ideal of distributive equality has an important role to play in our thinking about distributive justice, and they ask how that ideal is best to be understood. Arneson makes the point explicitly. His arguments, he writes, are "addressed to egalitarians, not their opponents."[4] As with Arneson's own essay, most of the luck-egalitarian literature is devoted to considering two closely related questions. The first question is what exactly egalitarians wish to equalize.[5] This question is often formulated as a question about the correct "metric" of equality. The candidates for equalization that have been debated include

to differences in their choices. The "prevailing political morality" also encompasses a range of positions on the extent of legitimate redistribution, for although, as I have said, adherents of the prevailing morality have no principled objection to taxing income that derives from people's choices, they disagree among themselves about how much taxation is justified and why. In general, however, most luck egalitarians think that the economic regimes of contemporary liberal societies should be significantly more redistributive than those regimes have usually been in practice, and more redistributive than the prevailing political morality would allow. As I note in Section II, it is therefore striking that the rise of luck egalitarianism occurred during a period in which liberal societies were in fact becoming much less redistributive.

[3] See, in addition to the paper of Anderson's cited above, J. Wolff, "Fairness, Respect, and the Egalitarian Ethos," *Philosophy & Public Affairs* 27, no. 2 (1998): pp. 97–122; S. V. Shiffrin, "Paternalism, Unconscionability Doctrine, and Accommodation," *Philosophy & Public Affairs* 29, no. 3 (2000): pp. 205–250; T. Hinton, "Must Egalitarians Choose Between Fairness and Respect?", *Philosophy & Public Affairs* 30, no. 1 (2001): pp. 72–87. Debra Satz has also pursued related themes in her as yet unpublished work.

[4] R. J. Arneson, "Equality and Equal Opportunity for Welfare," *Philosophical Studies* 56, no. 1 (1989): pp. 77–93.

[5] Indeed, in some luck-egalitarian writings, this is not only the first question but also the first sentence. John Roemer, for example, begins his essay "Equality of Talent" by asking: "If one is an egalitarian, what should one want to equalize?" And Roemer's essay "A Pragmatic Theory of Responsibility for the Egalitarian Planner" begins: "What should an egalitarian seek to equalize?" Both essays are included in *J. E. Roemer, Egalitarian Perspectives: Essays in Philosophical Economics* (Cambridge University Press, 1996).

welfare, resources, opportunity for welfare, and access to advantage, among others. The second question is which forms of disadvantage should receive compensation in the name of equality. Here there has been discussion of physical handicaps, medical needs, limited talents, unfavorable social positions, unsuccessful gambles, expensive tastes, expensive religious commitments, undesirable aspects of temperament, and so on.

The rise of luck egalitarianism as an important position within political philosophy, which took place during roughly the last two decades of the twentieth century, coincided with a marked increase in inequalities of income and wealth in the United States and other liberal societies.[6] Those decades were characterized by a strong trend, intensified by the collapse of the Soviet Union, toward increased privatization and reliance on the market, and a steady erosion in political support for distributive egalitarianism of any kind. Thus there was a sharp disparity between the luck egalitarianism that was becoming increasingly influential in philosophical discussions of distributive justice, and the actual distributive practices of the societies in which those discussions took place—and this despite the fact that one of the aims of luck-egalitarian theorists is to demonstrate that egalitarians need not, in general, be hostile to markets, and must indeed rely upon them in important ways. Of course, the existence of a disparity between luck-egalitarian theory and actual political practice does not by itself tell against the luck-egalitarian position. Justice is a normative notion, and so no proposed principle of justice can be falsified simply by pointing out that actual practice does not, in fact, to conform to it. Yet the starkness of the contrast between luck-egalitarian theory and contemporary political practice makes it especially important to address fundamental questions about the moral defensibility of the core luck-egalitarian idea. What needs to be considered is whether luck egalitarians have latched on to an idea of equality that has real appeal as a social and political value.

. . .

In my view, the luck-egalitarian position is open to doubt on a number of grounds. Perhaps the most obvious difficulty is that the degree of weight that the luck egalitarian places on the distinction between choices and circumstances seems, on its face, to be both philosophically dubious and morally implausible. Philosophically, the question is whether the distinction is deep enough to bear the kind of weight that luck egalitarians place on it. Some luck-egalitarian writings seem implicitly to suggest that whatever is assigned to the category of unchosen circumstance is a contingent feature of the causal order, which is not under the individual's control and does not implicate his or her personhood, whereas voluntary choices are fully under the control of individuals and constitute pure expressions of their agency. But this contrast is, of course, untenable. In any sense of identity that actually matters to people, unchosen personal traits and the social circumstances into which one is born are importantly, albeit not exclusively, constitutive of one's distinctive identity.[7] And, in any ordinary sense of "voluntary," people's voluntary choices are routinely influenced by unchosen features of their personalities, temperaments, and the social contexts in which they find themselves. In his defense of a version of luck egalitarianism,[8] G. A. Cohen concedes that reliance on the distinction between choices and circumstances may leave luck egalitarians "up to our necks in the free will problem," but he says—perhaps with some irony?—that "that is just tough luck."[9] Cohen points out that one of the achievements of luck egalitarianism is to demonstrate that

[6] For some of the relevant US data, see US Census Bureau, *Income Inequality (1967–1998)*, at www.census.gov/hhes/income/incineq/p60204/. For data on other liberal democracies, see T. M. Smeeding and A. Grodner, *Changing Income Inequality in OECD Countries: Updated Results from the Luxembourg Income Study (Lis)* (Springer, 2000).

[7] This is a theme of several of the essays included in my *Boundaries and Allegiances* (New York: Oxford University Press, 2001).

[8] G. A. Cohen, "On the Currency of Egalitarian Justice," *Ethics* 99, no. 4 (1989): pp. 906–944.

[9] Ibid., p. 934.

egalitarians can incorporate "the most powerful idea in the arsenal of the anti-egalitarian right: the idea of choice and responsibility."[10] Yet, in so doing, luck egalitarianism invites the objection that, like the political philosophies of the anti-egalitarian right, it tacitly derives much of its appeal from an implausible understanding of the metaphysical status of the category of choice.

This objection would be easier to dismiss if the luck-egalitarian account of the significance of choice were morally compelling. But in fact that account seems on its face to be morally implausible. It is morally implausible, for example, that justice requires individuals to be fully compensated for disadvantages that derive from unchosen features of their circumstances but not to be compensated at all for disadvantages that result from their voluntary choices. As Anderson has argued, it is morally implausible that choice should have that kind of significance or make that degree of difference. On the one hand, there are many unchosen personal attributes that may be disadvantageous but for which we do not, in fact, demand compensation from others. On the other hand, the fact that a person's urgent medical needs can be traced to his own negligence or foolishness or high-risk behavior is not normally seen as making it legitimate to deny him the care he needs. Still less do people automatically forfeit any claim to assistance if it turns out that their urgent needs are the result of prudent or well-considered choices that simply turned out badly.[11] We are neither so systematically alienated from the unchosen aspects of our own identities nor so uniformly confident of and identified with our role as choosers as to regard the presence or absence of choice as having this kind of make-or-break significance. This helps explain why the appeal of luck egalitarianism may seem tacitly to depend on a form of metaphysical libertarianism, for libertarianism may appear to promise a basis in metaphysics for a dichotomy that would otherwise seem so stark as to be morally untenable.[12]

Some luck-egalitarian writers have sought to address these difficulties by qualifying the luck-egalitarian principle or limiting its application in various ways. And some writers have suggested that certain of the difficulties can be avoided by drawing the line between choices and circumstances differently. Dworkin, for example, in explaining the differences between his view and Cohen's, argues that the line should be rooted in "ordinary people's ethical experience."[13] If the distinction is drawn

[10] Ibid., p. 933.

[11] See Anderson, "What is the Point of Equality," pp. 296–300.

[12] In S. Scheffler, "Responsibility, Reactive Attitudes, and Liberalism in Philosophy and Politics," *Philosophy & Public Affairs* (1992): pp. 299–323, I argued that contemporary liberalism has been exposed to conservative attack because of a perceived tendency among many liberals, both in politics and in philosophy, to rely on a reduced conception of individual agency and responsibility. The points made in the last two paragraphs might be taken to suggest that what luck egalitarianism has done, in effect, is to overcompensate for that perceived tendency.

[13] Dworkin's reply to Cohen takes up sections II through IV of chap. 7 of *Sovereign Virtue*. The quoted phrase occurs on pp. 289–290. There is additional discussion of the ethical interpretation of the distinction between choices and circumstances on pp. 322–325. It is worth noting that in his original formulations of his equality of resources scheme, Dworkin did not characterize the relevant distinction as a distinction between choices and circumstances at all. He tended to speak instead of a distinction between the person and his circumstances. See, for example, *Sovereign Virtue*, pp. 81 and 140. He was criticized for this by Cohen (in Section IV of "On the Currency of Egalitarian Justice"), who argued that the relevant notion is choice rather than personality. In more recent discussions, such as those cited at the beginning of this note, Dworkin does indeed characterize the distinction as a distinction between choices and circumstances (or choice and chance), but he preserves a link with his earlier characterization by asserting that people's "choices reflect their personalities" (*Sovereign Virtue*, p. 322). My argument in the text is that this does not yield a distinction between choices and circumstances that is helpful to Dworkin's position.

in this way, he says, then various aspects of one's personality that are not in straightforward sense chosen—including one's ambitions, tastes, preferences, convictions, and traits of character—will nevertheless fall on the choice side of the line. The reasons are twofold. First, all of these features of personality are relevant to the choices that one makes, either because they supply motives for one's actions or because they "affect [one's] pursuit of" one's ends.[14] Second, people normally identify with these aspects of their personalities and see themselves as having to take "consequential responsibility" for them, in the sense that they expect to have to bear the costs of possessing them.[15] One conclusion Dworkin draws from this is that people cannot normally demand compensation for expensive values or tastes. Even though such tastes are not actually chosen, they nevertheless fall on the choice side of the line by his standards, at least when people identify with them. Eric Rakowski, who takes a similar position, says that people's values and beliefs are "constitutive elements of themselves for which they must assume responsibility,"[16] and that even though one does not choose one's preferences, one can nevertheless choose to strengthen or weaken them, so that they too are appropriately situated on the choice side of the line.[17]

However, this way of drawing the line between choices and circumstances leads to further difficulties. By the criteria that Dworkin and Rakowski suggest, people's talents and abilities, no less than their ambitions and preferences, may also deserve to be situated on the choice side of the line. After all, people's talents and abilities are often relevant to their choices, either because they shape people's motives or because they affect people's pursuit of their ends. In addition, people frequently view their talents, no less than their values and preferences, as importantly constitutive of their identities. And even if talents are themselves unchosen, people can nevertheless choose whether to develop them. Furthermore, many people also expect to take "consequential responsibility" for their talents, in the sense that they believe they are entitled to the differential rewards that such talents may enable them to secure. If this is correct, then the effect of broadening the category of choice to include not only the actions one actually chooses but also the various constitutive features of oneself that underlie one's choices, is to cast doubt on the capacity of the distinction between choices and circumstances to support the substantive positions that luck egalitarians favor.[18]

There is a further point that a number of critics have made. Luck egalitarianism, as it is often presented, appears to treat equality as being an essentially distributive ideal whose fundamental aim is to eliminate the effects on distribution of "brute luck." Because of this concern to neutralize brute luck, the luck egalitarian arrives at allocative decisions on the basis of judgments that are strongly "inward looking." That is, an individual's claim to be compensated in the name of equality for some disadvantage always depends on a judgment about the source of the disadvantage in different aspects of the self. We cannot know whether an individual's disadvantage entitles her to egalitarian compensation without disentangling the respective contributions made by her will, on the one hand, and by unchosen features of her talents and personal circumstances,

[14] R. Dworkin, *Sovereign Virtue: The Theory and Practice of Equality* (Harvard University Press, 2002), p. 322.

[15] Ibid., p. 290.

[16] E. Rakowski, Equal Justice (Clarendon Press, 1991), p. 63.

[17] Ibid., pp. 57–72.

[18] At one point (*Sovereign Virtue*, pp. 260–263), Dworkin himself insists on the importance, for ethical purposes, of identification with aspects of one's unchosen circumstances. These "parameters," which help define what counts as a good life for an individual, are distinguished from those circumstances that count instead as "limitations" on one's ability to lead a good life. However, as Anthony Appiah suggests in his review of *Sovereign Virtue*, it is very unclear how a recognition of the ethical role of parameters is to be reconciled with the assignment of fundamental significance to the distinction between choices and circumstances. (See A. Appiah, "Equality of What?", *The New York Review of Books* [2001]: pp. 63–68.)

on the other hand, to the processes that put her at that disadvantage. For this reason, luck egalitarianism encourages her to look inward in deciding whether she has a legitimate claim on fellow citizens, and, as Anderson and Wolff have emphasized,[19] it encourages those fellow citizens both to scrutinize the deepest aspects of her self and to arrive at heavily moralized judgments about the degree of responsibility she bears for her own misfortune.

In all of the respects I have mentioned, the luck-egalitarian conception of equality diverges from a more familiar way of understanding that value. Equality, as it is more commonly understood, is not, in the first instance, a distributive ideal, and its aim is not to compensate for misfortune. It is, instead, a moral ideal governing the relations in which people stand to one another. Instead of focusing attention on the differing contingencies of each person's traits, abilities, and other circumstances, this ideal abstracts from the undeniable differences among people. It claims that human relations must be conducted on the basis of an assumption that everyone's life is equally important, and that all members of a society have equal standing. As Anderson insists, in defending a version of this ideal, equality so understood is opposed not to luck but to oppression, to heritable hierarchies of social status, to ideas of caste, to class privilege and the rigid stratification of classes, and to the undemocratic distribution of power. In contrast to the inward-looking focus of luck egalitarianism, it emphasizes the irrelevance of individual differences for fundamental social and political purposes. As a moral ideal, it asserts that all people are of equal worth and that there are some claims that people are entitled to make on one another simply by virtue of their status as persons. As a social ideal, it holds that a human society must be conceived of as a cooperative arrangement among equals, each of whom enjoys the same social standing. As a political ideal, it highlights the claims that citizens are entitled to make on one another by virtue of their status *as* citizens, without any need for a moralized accounting of the details of their particular circumstances. Indeed, it insists on the very great importance of the right to be viewed simply as a citizen, and to have one's fundamental rights and privileges determined on that basis, without reference to one's talents, intelligence, wisdom, decision-making skill, temperament, social class, religious or ethnic affiliation, or ascribed identity.

Of course, things are not quite so simple. The *social and political ideal* of equality, as I will call it, itself has distributive implications. Furthermore, even if that ideal emphasizes the importance, for certain purposes, of abstracting from the differing contingencies of individuals' situations, it must also concede the necessity of attending to such differences for other purposes. People may claim equal rights as citizens, but the interpretation and application of those rights will often depend on features of their individual circumstances. And special circumstances may at times give rise to special rights. Still, one will think about the distributional implications of equality very differently than luck egalitarianism tempts us to do if one insists that, in the end, the relevant question is about the bearing on distribution of a morally-based ideal of human social and political relations—and not about the optimal way of reflecting in our economy a metaphysical distinction between individuals' choices and their unchosen circumstances. Granted, the social and political ideal of equality may itself be understood in different ways.[20] But unless distributive egalitarianism is anchored in some version of that ideal, or in some other comparably general understanding of equality as a moral value or normative ideal, it will be arbitrary, pointless, fetishistic: no more

[19] Anderson, "What Is the Point of Equality?" (at, for example, p. 310); Wolff, "Fairness, Respect, and the Egalitarian Ethos" (especially pp. 113–118).

[20] One important interpretative issue, about which there is no general consensus, is what the ideal implies about the relations among people who are not citizens of the same country or members of the same political society. Debra Satz discusses this issue in her unpublished paper, "Inequality of What and Between Whom? When and Where Does Inequality Matter? The Case of Inequality Between Nations."

compelling than a preference for any other distributive pattern.

If one keeps firmly in mind the fact that questions about egalitarian distributive norms must be controlled by some broader understanding of equality, then the appeal of luck egalitarianism seems to me limited. As I have already suggested, many people accept what I have called the social and political ideal of equality. That ideal does not support the ambition of purging the influence of brute luck from human relations, which is just as well since one has only to describe that ambition for its folly to be evident. As Anderson argues, questions of distribution are important, for people who are committed to the social and political value of equality, not because a properly designed set of distributive institutions can help to minimize the influence of luck, but rather because certain kinds of distributive arrangements are incongruous with that social and political value. Clearly, for example, people whose basic needs have not been met—people who lack adequate food, clothing, shelter, education, or medical care—cannot participate in political life or civil society on a footing of equality with others, or can do so only with great difficulty. Even if basic needs have been met, a society cannot be considered a society of equals if the resources that individuals have available to pursue their most cherished ends is left entirely at the mercy of market forces. Moreover, significant distributive inequalities can all too easily generate inequalities of power and status that are incompatible with relations among equals. Thus, those who accept the social and political ideal of equality will have compelling reasons to avoid excessive variations in people's shares of income and wealth, and this will mean, among other things, that they have reason to oppose institutions that allow too much scope for differences in people's natural and social circumstances to translate into economic inequalities. But, on the one hand, this is very different from having the general ambition of eradicating the distributive effects of brute luck, and, on the other hand, it does not assume that inequalities arising from people's choices are always acceptable.

From this perspective, the most important questions concern not the neutralization of luck but rather, for example, the nature of people's "basic needs," the proper criteria for political institutions to use in distinguishing between genuine needs and what are merely very strong preferences, the appropriate measure for the social and political institutions of a complex modern society to employ when assessing the well-being of individual citizens, and, especially, the degree of material inequality that is compatible with a conception of society as a fair system of cooperation among equals. Depending on how these questions are answered, people who are committed to the social and political ideal of equality may end up supporting a system that tolerates either more or less inequality of income and wealth than luck egalitarianism does. In either case, however, the motivation for their position will be different from the motivation for a luck-egalitarian outlook. Since the position that adherents of the ideal favor will have been developed in response to questions that differ, at least in part, from the ones that luck egalitarians ask, the basis for their position will lie in considerations that differ from the ones that luck egalitarians cite.[21]

III.

[I]t is misleading to treat Rawls's theory of justice as representing a kind of incipient luck egalitarianism. Notwithstanding his remarks about the moral arbitrariness of people's natural attributes and of the social positions into which they are born, his failure to claim that justice

[21] In "Equality and Justice," in *Ideals of Equality*, ed. Andrew Mason (Oxford: Blackwell, 1998), pp. 21–36, David Miller draws a distinction between distributive equality and social equality that is similar to the distinction I have drawn in this section, although Miller takes a different view of the relations between the two notions than I would. In the same volume, Richard Norman ("The Social Basis of Equality," pp. 37–51) invokes Miller's chapter in defending what he calls "socially-located egalitarianism."

requires people to be compensated for all disadvantages resulting from unchosen features of their circumstances is no mere oversight. Despite occasional remarks to the effect that his conception of justice "nullifies the accidents of natural endowment and the contingencies of social circumstance as counters in [a] quest for political and economic advantage,"[22] it is quite clear from his discussion as a whole that the underlying motivation for Rawls's theory of justice is not the general elimination of the influence of brute luck on distribution. Indeed, Rawls explicitly emphasizes the differences between his own theory and what he calls "the principle of redress." This is "the principle that undeserved inequalities call for redress; and since inequalities of birth and natural endowment are undeserved, these inequalities are somehow to be compensated for."[23] Rawls says that the principle of redress is plausible "only as a prima facie principle, one that is to be weighed in the balance with others."[24] His own theory, accordingly, "gives some weight to the considerations singled out by the principle of redress,"[25] but it is clearly "not the same as"[26] that principle.

Rather than trying to devise a conception of justice that will minimize the effects of brute luck, Rawls aims to identify the most reasonable conception of justice to regulate the basic structure of a modern democratic society. For the purposes of this enterprise, a society is conceived of as a fair system of cooperation among free and equal people, each of whom is taken to have the capacity for a sense of justice and the capacity to develop and pursue a rational plan of life which is constitutive of his or her good. Different plans are rational for different people, and the human good is irreducibly heterogeneous. Rawls cites the "moral arbitrariness" of natural attributes and social contingencies, not because his ultimate aim is to extinguish the influence of all arbitrary factors but rather because he thinks the arbitrariness of the factors he cites serves to undermine both an important objection and an influential alternative to his view. The objection is that those people who are more talented or intelligent or hard-working than others deserve greater economic rewards than his theory would permit them to secure. And the alternative that many of those who press this objection favor is "the system of natural liberty," which, as we have seen, allows people to compete in a largely unregulated free market, constrained only by the need to respect one another's basic liberties and by a requirement of formal equality of opportunity.

Rawls believes that the appeal of the system of natural liberty is morally spurious. The extent to which the system allows people's material prospects to be influenced by their natural assets and the social circumstances into which they are born is indefensible. It is indefensible because it is incongruous with people's status as equals and because the distribution of those contingencies does not itself have any moral basis. If we take seriously the idea that all citizens have equal standing in society, and the idea that each has an equally important interest in developing and pursuing a rational plan of life within a fair cooperative framework, then it is inappropriate to set up an institutional scheme that makes people's chances of carrying out their plans depend so heavily on natural and social contingencies that in themselves have no moral authority. Rawls's emphasis on the moral arbitrariness of people's natural attributes and social starting points is meant to undercut our tendency to treat those factors as morally authoritative, especially when doing so would compromise something morally fundamental.

What is relevant for Rawls, in other words, is the conjunction of two points. The first point is that the distribution of natural and social contingencies lacks any moral basis. The second point is that a system that allows the economic distribution to track the distribution of those contingencies too closely will compromise the status of some citizens as equals,

---

22 Rawls, *A Theory of Justice*, p. 15.

23 Ibid., p. 100.

24 Ibid., p. 101.

25 Ibid., p. 100.

26 Ibid., p. 101. Rakowski believes (mistakenly, in my view) that Rawls relies on the principle of redress as a premise of his argument. See *Equal Justice*, pp. 112–114.

for it will undermine their ability to satisfy the equally legitimate interest that each citizen has in developing and pursuing a rational plan of life that is constitutive of his or her good. If Rawls is right, the conjunction of these two points gives us reason to reject the system of natural liberty, once we conceive of society as a fair system of cooperation among free and equal people. But the importance of these points neither derives from nor commits Rawls to the general ambition of neutralizing all of the distributive effects of bad brute luck. For Rawls, what is fundamental is the status of citizens as equals, and the moral arbitrariness of people's natural and social starting points is important because it helps to clarify the distributive implications of taking equal citizenship seriously.

Rawls's defense of his reliance on primary goods as the basis for interpersonal comparisons of well-being also looks very different when it is not seen through the lens of luck-egalitarian concerns. In saying that citizens in a well-ordered society are expected to take responsibility for their ends, in the sense that they are expected to "regulate and revise their ends and preferences in the light of their expectations of primary goods,"[27] Rawls is certainly not making a claim about the moral significance of a putative metaphysical distinction between voluntary choices and unchosen circumstances. Instead, he is making an observation about how his principles of justice serve, in effect, to allocate responsibility between society and the individual. He writes:

> This conception [of justice] includes what we may call a social division of responsibility: society, the citizens as a collective body, accepts the responsibility for maintaining the equal basic liberties and fair equality of opportunity, and for providing a fair share of the other primary goods for everyone within this framework, while citizens (as individuals) and associations accept the responsibility for revising and adjusting their ends and aspirations in view of the all-purpose means they can expect, given their present and foreseeable situation.[28]

As Rawls notes, this allocation of responsibility would make no sense if, in general, people were unable "to moderate the claims they make on social institutions"[29] because they lacked the capacity to adjust their plans in light of the resources they could expect to have at their disposal under the terms of a fair distribution.

By the same token, the allocation of responsibility would make no sense if society as a whole lacked the capacity to establish institutions capable of guaranteeing the basic liberties and fair equality of opportunity. In fact, as Rawls suggests, it does not seem unreasonable to suppose that people normally do have the capacity to adjust their plans in light of their fair expectations. What is more important for the purposes of our discussion, however, is that the suggestion that they have such a capacity is not a metaphysical thesis about the relation of causation and the will, nor, in any case, does it provide the *motivation* for the allocation of responsibility. People are asked to accept responsibility for their ends, in Rawls's sense, not because the metaphysics of the will makes it fitting that people should bear the costs of their choices, but rather because it is reasonable to expect people to make do with their fair shares. And what makes shares fair, according to Rawls, is not that they compensate people for all unchosen disadvantages while leaving them to bear the costs (or reap the rewards) of their voluntary choices. Shares are fair when they are part of a distributive scheme that makes it possible for free and equal citizens to pursue their diverse conceptions of the good within a framework that embodies an ideal of reciprocity and mutual respect.[30]

In addition, Rawls emphasizes that his reliance on primary goods as the basis for

---

27 J. Rawls, *Collected Papers*, ed. Samuel Freeman (Harvard University Press, 1999), p. 370.

28 Ibid., p. 371.

29 Ibid.

30 For a related discussion of the passage from Rawls discussed in this paragraph, see T. M. Scanlon, "The Significance of Choice," in *Tanner Lectures on Human Values*, edited by S. McMurrin

interpersonal comparisons is limited to the special case of social justice. As he says, "Primary goods are not . . . to be used in making comparisons in all situations but only in questions which arise in regard to the basic structure. It is another matter entirely whether primary goods are an appropriate basis in other kinds of cases."[31] What is distinctive about the case of social justice is that interpersonal comparisons must be capable of providing grounds for adjudicating among conflicting claims in a way that all citizens can recognize as fair. It follows, Rawls believes, that we need a practical basis for making these comparisons and that this basis must lie in features of people's situations that are publicly accessible and can be appraised without violating people's liberties or subjecting them to unduly intrusive examination. As he says, "the idea is to find a practicable basis of interpersonal comparisons in terms of objective features of citizens' social circumstances open to view."[32] This is in striking contrast to the inward-looking focus of luck egalitarianism. Whereas the aim of neutralizing the distributive effects of brute luck requires intrusive and conceptually problematic judgments about the inner sources of people's disadvantages, the aim of adjudicating fairly among the claims of free and equal citizens requires judgments that rest on a practicable and public basis.

None of this is to suggest that Rawls's views are beyond criticism. It is perfectly possible to argue, for example, that the difference principle inappropriately rewards those who are among the worst-off, as measured in terms of primary goods, only because they prefer greater leisure to greater income and so choose to work at less demanding jobs or not to work at all. It is also perfectly possible to argue that Rawls's reliance on primary social goods as the measure of well-being renders him incapable of taking adequate account, as an acceptable theory of justice surely must, of those who have special medical conditions that are unusually costly to treat.

Indeed, Rawls himself concedes the force of both of these criticisms. In response to the first, he indicates that despite some reservations, he is prepared to contemplate an expansion of the list of primary goods to include leisure time.[33] In response to the second, he acknowledges the importance of making provision for those with special medical needs but treats this as a "problem of extension"[34] which is to be deferred until after "the first problem of justice"[35] has been addressed. This problem concerns the relations among "citizens who are normally active and fully cooperating members of society over a complete life."[36] Accordingly, for the purpose of addressing this problem, Rawls makes the frankly idealized assumption that all citizens have, "at least to the essential minimum degree, the moral, intellectual, and physical capacities that enable them to be fully cooperating members of society over a complete life."[37] Elsewhere he describes himself as assuming "that all citizens have physical and psychological capacities within a certain normal range."[38] He speculates that the problem of special medical needs can be dealt with "at the legislative stage when the prevalence and kinds of these misfortunes are known and the costs of treating them can be ascertained and balanced along with total government expenditure."[39]

These tentative lines of response may or may not prove adequate. Perhaps they are too

(Salt Like City: University of Utah Press, 1988), pp. 151–216, at 197–201. I have also discussed Rawls's doctrine of "responsibility for ends" in section IV of "Responsibility, Reactive Attitudes, and Liberalism in Philosophy and Politics" (see *Boundaries and Allegiances*, pp. 29–30).

[31] Rawls, *Collected Papers*, 364.

[32] Rawls, "The Priority of Right and Ideas of the Good," in *Collected Papers*, pp. 449–472 at pp. 454–455.

[33] See Rawls, *Collected Papers*, pp. 252–253 and 455.

[34] See J. Rawls, *Political Liberalism* (Columbia University Press, 2005), pp. 21–22, and *Collected Papers*, p. 531.

[35] See Rawls, Collected Papers, pp. 259 and 368.

[36] Ibid., p. 368.

[37] Rawls, *Political Liberalism*, p. 183.

[38] Rawls, *Collected Papers*, p. 368.

[39] Rawls, *Political Liberalism*, p. 184.

ad hoc or require intuitionistic balancing of a kind that Rawls had hoped to avoid. But it is a mistake to regard the criticisms to which he is responding as the thin end of a wedge: that is, as leading inexorably to luck egalitarianism. The aim that informs Rawls's response to the problem of special medical needs, and that would also have to inform any better response, is the aim of "restor[ing] people by health care so that once again they are fully cooperating members of society."[40] This, once again, is entirely independent from and does not commit Rawls to the aim of compensating people for all disadvantages resulting from unchosen circumstances. Instead, the aim of enabling people to be fully cooperating members of society provides an independent standard for judging which disadvantages should be compensated. By this standard, some disadvantages should be compensated even if they result from bad "option luck," whereas others should not be compensated even if they result from bad "brute luck." For example, the standard may require that people be provided with medical care even if their need for care results from choices that they made voluntarily but that turned out badly. On the other hand, it does not require that people be compensated for expensive tastes simply because those tastes result from unchosen features of their upbringing, for such compensation is not normally necessary to enable people to be cooperating members of society. As Rawls says, "We don't say that because the preferences arose from upbringing and not choice that society owes us compensation. Rather, it is a normal part of being human to cope with the preferences our upbringing leaves us with."[41]

In discussing the relation between Rawls's view and the luck-egalitarian position, my primary concern has not been interpretative. By emphasizing the differences between the two positions I have hoped instead to accomplish two things. The first is to make clear that the philosophical underpinnings of luck egalitarianism are not to be found in Rawls's work. Thus, if luck egalitarianism is to be supplied with a compelling motivation, that motivation will need to come from somewhere else; it cannot simply ride piggy-back on Rawls's remarks about the arbitrariness of the natural lottery or about the need for citizens to take responsibility for their ends.

My second aim has been to illustrate how a plausible form of distributive egalitarianism can be anchored in a more general conception of equality as a social and political ideal. Rawls's theory shows how this can be done. For Rawls, people are conceived of as free and equal citizens, and the aim is to determine which principles of distributive justice are most appropriate for a modern democratic society whose members are so understood. In other words, the question is which principles of justice are most consistent, in modern conditions, with the freedom and equality of persons. Equality is understood as a social and political ideal that governs the relations in which people stand to one another. The core of the value of equality does not, according to this understanding, consist in the idea that there is something that must be distributed or allocated equally, and so the interpretation of the value does not consist primarily in seeking to ascertain what that *something* is. Instead, the core of the value is a normative conception of human relations, and the relevant question, when interpreting the value, is what social, political, and economic arrangements are compatible with that conception.

---

[40] Ibid.

[41] Ibid., p. 185n. Of course, luck egalitarians disagree among themselves as to whether people should receive compensation for expensive unchosen tastes, for they disagree about whether such tastes are properly subsumed under the heading of "choice" or of "circumstance." Dworkin, as we have seen, assimilates most preferences to the "choice" side of the luck-egalitarian divide, despite the fact that they are not themselves chosen, and he concludes that in general no compensation is called for. For Rawls, however, the question is not whether preferences are properly subsumed within the category of "choices." The question, instead, is whether compensation for expensive tastes is necessary to enable people to participate in the scheme of social cooperation.

EXCERPT 9

Full text from:

E. Emanuel, *The Ends of Human Life: Medical Ethics in a Liberal Polity* (Cambridge: Harvard University Press, 1991), pp. 35–37.

2 The Nature of Liberal Political Philosophy: Two Forms of Liberalism

Ezekiel Emanuel

I have claimed that political philosophy provides the framework for addressing medical ethical questions and that the persistent irresolution of these questions in American society derives from its liberal political philosophy. What is the nature of this liberal political philosophy?

One of the "constitutive principles of liberalism"[1] is the ideal of neutrality. In modern societies, individuals typically espouse a plurality of conceptions of the meaning, purpose, and value of life, that is, conceptions of the good life. According to the ideal of neutrality, the state should tolerate these different conceptions of the good life and not try to impose a particular view of what is worthy or good. The state is neutral when it does not base its laws on any particular conception of the good life, and thereby permits people to affirm and pursue their own ideas of what is worthy. This liberal ideal of neutrality does not claim that state policies will not have a differential effect on the pursuits of citizens; clearly different policies will generally help some rather than others. Neutrality of effect is impossible, an absurd ideal. Instead, the ideal is for neutrality in justification.[2] "The basic [political] institutions and public policy are [neither] to be designed to favor any particular" conception of the good life nor to be justified by appeal to any particular conception of the good life.[3] On liberal grounds, the state's institutions and policies should create a political framework within which individuals who hold different views can pursue their own conception of the good life. Dworkin succinctly summarizes the ideal of neutrality: "[Liberalism] supposes [as its constitutive political morality] that political decisions must be, so far as possible, independent of any particular conception of the good life, or of what gives value to life. Since the citizens of a society differ in their conceptions, the government does not treat them as equals if it prefers one conception to another."[4]

There are different ways of understanding and justifying this neutrality, and therefore different forms of liberalism. One of the dominant forms is *moral liberalism,* which justifies neutrality by appeal to individual autonomy.[5] The highest human good, according to moral liberalism, is for individuals to fashion their own lives by their own lights. An individual can be autonomous only when he actually exercises his own capacities of choice, judgment, and the like. Autonomy, and the full flourishing of the individual, require that the state let individuals exercise these capacities themselves,

---

[1] R. Dworkin, *A Matter of Principle* (Harvard University Press, 1985), p. 4.

[2] C. E. Larmore, *Patterns of Moral Complexity* (Cambridge University Press, 1987), pp. 42–50.

[3] J. Rawls, "The Priority of the Right and the Ideas of the Good" (unpublished manuscript, August 24, 1987), p.14.

[4] Dworkin, *A Matter of Principle*, 191. This is one of those places in which we can see Dworkin adopting a liberalism which is hostile to the moral liberalism he seemed to adopt in arguing for state support of the arts. But the view expressed here seems more naturally congenial to his true position, although given the apparent conflicts among his positions one can never be sure what his true position really is.

[5] This dichotomy is borrowed from John Rawls, "Justice as Fairness: Political not Metaphysical," *Philosophy and Public Affairs* 14 (1985): pp. 223–251. I use slight different terms from his, but the grounds of the distinctions are the same.

without interference. The limits on government action and the content of government policies—an extensive set of individual rights and opportunities—are necessary to ensure that individuals realize the ideal of autonomy. Where government policies are necessary, the justification should be to enhance each individual's ability to choose and create her own life. In education policy, for instance, the objective should be to ensure that children have sufficient knowledge and exposure to choose and create their own lives. The moral liberal believes:

> The content of children's right to education will depend upon what is adequate for living a full life within their society-for being capable of choosing among available conceptions of the good and of participating intelligently in democratic politics if they so choose . . . [Consequently moral liberals] rank children's rights to education above their rights to religious freedom since [moral liberals] believe that this restriction of their present liberty is necessary to create the conditions for future enjoyment of religious and other freedoms. Without education, liberal freedoms lose a great deal, even if not all, of their value.[6]

Similarly, the moral liberal endorses state support of art because it will enhance the opportunity of individuals to create their own lives.[7]

Historically, moral liberalism has been a dominant strand both in philosophy, including Kant and Mill, and in American culture.[8] However, it has been attacked as being not really, or not sufficiently, liberal. Moral liberalism guarantees governmental neutrality and extensive individual freedom from state interference, but it does so to promote a single conception of the good life. Since the principle of individual autonomy is used to justify state laws and policies, moral liberalism permits the state to promote a single conception of the good life to all citizens, regardless of their individual values. In moral liberalism, therefore, there is no neutrality of justification because governmental neutrality is justified by appeal to a view of the highest human good: autonomy.

An alternative has been proposed: *political liberalism*.[9] Articulated by Rawls, Dworkin, and others, this liberalism informs contemporary American political and legal thought. And the fundamental conceptions of political liberalism—its notions of pluralism, autonomy, equality, and its framework for relating these ethical conceptions have implicitly and explicitly influenced medical ethics.[10] My purpose is not to provide a detailed interpretation of political liberalism; but neither is it sufficient simply to review Rawls's two principles of justice to reveal

[6] A. Gutmann, "Children, Paternalism, and Education: A Liberal Argument," *Philosophy & Public Affairs* 9, no. 4 (1980): pp. 338–358. Subsequently in *Democratic Education* (Princeton, N.J.: Princeton University Press, 1987) Gutmann shifts away from this position, but the justification quoted here is a typical moral liberal view.

[7] See Dworkin, *A Matter of Principle*, ch. 11, in which he argues that state subsidy of art is justified when it enhances "a rich cultural structure, one that multiplies distinct possibilities or opportunities of value" (229).

[8] G. Kateb, "Democratic Individuality and the Claims of Politics," *Political Theory* 12, no. 3 (1984): pp. 331–360.

[9] This term was initially used in J. Rawls, "The Idea of an Overlapping Consensus," *Political Theory* 23 (1984): pp. 1–25.

[10] The influence of political liberalism is fairly clear. Explicitly, Rawls's theory of justice has had a profound effect on how justice in medical ethics is approached. Similarly, the notion of autonomy and neutrality has dominated thinking about medical ethics. See, for example, President's Commission for the Study of Ethical Problems in Medicine and Biomedical and Behavioral Research, *Making Health Care Decisions* (Washington, DC: US Government Printing Office, 1982), chap. 2; and President's Commission for the Study of Ethical Problems in Medicine and Biomedical and Behavioral Research, *Deciding to Forego Life-Sustaining Treatment* (Washington, DC: US Government Printing Office, 1983), chap 2.

the importance of political liberalism for medical ethics.[11] To understand how such principles are to be interpreted, to what social goods they apply, requires some appreciation for the complexity of the theory. Indeed, it is only through understanding the basic conceptions of political liberalism and the framework they create that their effect on medical ethics can be illustrated.

The Tenets of Political Liberalism

Political liberalism can be understood as being constructed from seven tenets. The first three define the practical and philosophical back ground for political liberalism, indeed for any political philosophy; the remaining four are the constitutive tenets characteristic of political liberalism.[12]

1. The Circumstances of justice. Two facts of social life form the *practical* background to considerations of justice: scarcity of resources and pluralism of beliefs. Scarcity means that there will always be more demand than supply of resources, which requires a theory delineating social cooperation and the distribution of resources. Pluralism is the historical fact that in modern society people "hold opposing religious and philosophical beliefs, and affirm not only diverse moral and political doctrines, but also conflicting ways of evaluating arguments and evidence when they try to reconcile these oppositions."[13] In modern society there is no agreed-upon view of the good life to guide enactment of laws and policies.

2. The Justification of justice. Because of pluralism, political philosophy cannot be justified by appeal to any transcendental religion or philosophy. Instead, political philosophy is the articulation, elaboration, and formulation of ethical ideals implicit or latent in existing institutions, traditions, and practices. This theory is then revised by comparison with shared ethical judgments—for instance, that racial and religious discrimination is wrong—and traditional theories. The ultimate aim is to achieve both a coherence between the theory and individual ethical judgments and generalized agreement on the particular philosophy. On this view, the justification of a political philosophy rests on all things—ethical convictions, traditions, practices, and the philosophy—"fitting together" into a consistent whole.[14] Thus, political philosophy is a structure without foundations that is justified by a dynamic "reflective equilibrium" in which there is mutual support—and potential for revision—between particular ethical judgments, ethical ideals, and general principles. This implies that we cannot simply apply principles to cases; "the study of our substantive moral" judgments informs general principles, indeed may lead to their revision or rejection. It also means that political philosophy "starts from within a certain political tradition" and is informed by the values of that tradition.[15]

3. The Objectives of justice. The purpose of political philosophy is practical; it provides

[11] Frequently medical ethicists erroneously believe that a mechanical application of Rawls's two principles of justice to the distribution of health care resources is possible. The consequences are usually at odds with the theory more fully understood. See S. Gorovitz, *Doctors' Dilemmas: Moral Conflict and Medical Care* (Macmillan, 1982) and R. M. Veatch, *A Theory of Medical Ethics* (Basic Books, 1981) for this error, and see N. Daniels, *Just Health Care* (Cambridge University Press, 1985) for the more comprehensive approach to political liberalism and just health care.

[12] The seven tenets outlined here are merely an adaptation of Rawls's own outline of his philosophy as being "built up from six fundamental intuitive ideas." However, as anyone familiar with Rawls's work will recognize, my outline leaves out two ideas commonly thought to be critical to understanding Rawls, the original position and the veil of ignorance. Not only do I believe these ideas are completely dispensable to understanding political liberalism, I think they have lead to more confusion than elucidation and should be passed over.

[13] J. Rawls, "Kantian Constructivism in Moral Theory," *The Journal of Philosophy* 77, no. 9 (1980): pp. 515–572.

[14] J. Rawls, *A Theory of Justice* (Cambridge, Mass.: Harvard University Press, 1971), p. 579.

[15] J. Rawls, "Justice as Fairness," p. 225.

a shared ethical "framework for deliberation" that citizens appeal to in assessing the justice of social institutions, laws, and policies.[16] Most important, a political philosophy's frame work serves to guide the assessment and restructuring of the "basic structure" of society, that is, "the way in which the major social institutions distribute fundamental rights and duties and determine the division of advantages from social cooperation."[17] These institutions—including the constitution, the legal system, property, economic institutions, educational institutions, and the like—receive primary attention because they define the background into which we are born and in which we create and pursue our lives; this background has a pervasive effect on our lives and their possibilities from birth.

I now move from the general tenets that apply to all political philosophies to the specific claims distinctive of political liberalism.

4. The Ideal of Neutrality. According to political liberalism, the only way to accept pluralism while avoiding "the autocratic use of state power" is to espouse neutrality. Excluding from politics the diverse conceptions of a good life found in a modern, pluralistic society is the only way to secure political agreement and resolve social problems. But while pluralism precludes agreement on a detailed conception of the good life, it does not preclude the sharing of some values and principles by people with diverse conceptions of the good. Thus we can all agree that religious or racial discrimination is wrong. These shared values can provide the "kernel of an overlapping consensus" from which the basic framework of political philosophy is elaborated. Neutrality is preserved because the political philosophy is justified by appeal to values shared by different conceptions of the good life and not by appeal to any particular detailed conception of the good life.

5. The Conception of the Person. The entire framework and particular principles of political liberalism depend upon its conception of a person.[18] A person has two moral powers or capacities: "A sense of justice is the capacity to understand, to apply, and to act from the public conception of justice which characterizes the fair terms of social co operation. The capacity for a conception of the good is the capacity to form, to revise, and rationally to pursue a conception of one's rational advantage or good."[19] By possessing these two moral powers, citizens are *equal* and entitled to the benefits of social cooperation. Citizens are *free* in the sense that they can choose their own good and take responsibility for it, but the particular ends they choose do not affect their political standing, rights, opportunities, or privileges. In other words, our political freedom inheres in the ability to stand apart from our conception of the good. Our political rights do not depend upon our choice of final ends; we are free from politically punitive actions resulting from our choice of religion, political views, careers, or spouses, and from any changes, minor or radical, that we make in these choices during our lives.

6. The Conception of justice. The principles of justice indicate how to distribute goods. To clarify Rawls's now famous two principles of justice, I shall restate them as three principles:

a. Each person has an equal right to the most extensive scheme of equal basic liberties compatible with a similar scheme for all.
b. Offices and positions must be open to all under conditions of fair equality of opportunity.
c. Inequalities of wealth and income must be to the greatest advantage of the least advantaged members of society.

In essence, the first principle is one of strict equality—all citizens get the same rights; the second is one of fair equality of opportunity, ensuring that those who possess the same talents, abilities, and drive should have the same

[16] See Rawls, "Kantian Constructivism in Moral Theory," 560–564; "Justice as Fairness"; and "The idea of an Overlapping Consensus."

[17] Rawls, *A Theory of Justice*, p. 7.

[18] In "Kantian Constructivism in Moral Theory" Rawls claims that both the principles of justice and the notion of primary goods "rest upon a particular conception of that person."

[19] Rawls, "Justice as Fairness," p. 233.

prospects of success regardless of their starting point in the social hierarchy or their family's income;"'[20] and the third is Rawls's well-known difference principle requiring the distribution of incomes to ensure that the worst-off people are maximally benefited. These principles are "lexically ordered" so that the first one must be fully satisfied before the succeeding ones are applied.

7. The Conception of the Good. The primary goods are the things to be distributed by the three principles of justice. Each person, regard less of his particular conception of the good life, affirms the liberal conception of a person. Therefore, each person recognizes that people should exercise their two moral powers as well as have a chance to pursue their own particular conception of the good life. The primary goods are those things "generally necessary as social conditions and all-purpose means to enable human beings to realize and exercise their moral powers and to pursue their final ends."[21] These primary goods, then, are deemed good by every person and define a common standard of what each citizen needs that is derived from the conception of a person but independent of any particular conception of the good life. The five primary goods are as follows:

a. First, the basic liberties as given by a list, for example: freedom of thought and liberty of conscience, freedom of association, and the freedom defined by the liberty and integrity of the person, as well as the rule of law, and finally the political liberties;
b. Second, freedom of movement and choice of occupations against a background of diverse opportunities;
c. Third, powers and prerogatives of offices and positions of responsibility, particularly those in the main political and economic institutions;
d. Fourth, income and wealth; and
e. Finally, the social bases of self-respect.[22]

Once the conception of a person, the principles of justice, and the primary goods have been defined, their integral relationship to each other, their mutual dependence, should be clear.[23]

This summary of the seven tenets of political liberalism will help to clarify why liberal political philosophy produces the persistent irresolution surrounding medical ethical issues in contemporary America. Simultaneously, this examination will provide a test of the *philosophical* plausibility of political liberalism. The study of the issues of terminating care and allocating medical resources will show how the liberal ideal of neutrality, the prohibition against justifying state laws and policies by appeal to a conception of the good life, precludes, even in theory, any resolution to these medical ethical issues.

[20] Fair equality of opportunity is stronger than simple equality of opportunity because it requires not just elimination of overt discrimination but programs to ensure that social disadvantages are compensated for, permitting children with the same talents and motivation the same chance of success. Practically, this may require heavy investment in education and other programs to support poorer children.

[21] Rawls, "Kantian Constructivism in Moral Theory," p. 526.

[22] J. Rawls, "Social Unity and Primary Goods," in *John Rawls: Collected Papers*, edited by S. Freeman (Cambridge: Harvard University Press, 1999), pp. 359–397.

[23] This presentation should make clear that political liberalism recognizes "spheres of justice." (See M. Walzer, *Spheres of Justice: A Defense of Pluralism and Equality* (Basic Books, 2008)). There are three different principles of distribution in the public sphere related to different goods. The principles are different in part because the goods—rights, opportunities, and income—have different social significance because of how they are related to a conception of the person. Furthermore, completely excluded from this scheme are the distributions made in the private sphere. The social distributions of "private" goods will have their own principles of distribution which need not bear any relationship to the political principles. Thus scientific associations might distribute honors and awards which might be based not on equality or the difference principle but on merit or contribution. Hence political liberalism has a complex view of distributions which includes at least four different "spheres" of justice.

Further Resources

Relevant Organizations

Governmental

The NIH Department of Bioethics: A US center for bioethics scholarship and training. Additional information can be found at www.bioethics.nih.gov/

Presidential Commission for the Study of Bioethical Issues: Advises the President of the United States on bioethical issues. Additional information can be found at www.bioethics.gov

Nongovernmental

International Bioethics Committee (IBC): Part of UNESCO, an agency of the United Nations, the IBC is a global forum for reflection in bioethics. Additional information can be found at http://www.unesco.org/new/en/social-and-human-sciences/themes/bioethics/international-bioethics-committee**The Hastings Center:** A US-based bioethics research institute. Additional information can be found at www.thehastingscenter.org

World Medical Association (WMA): Aims to set standards in Medical Education, Medical Science, Medical Art, Medical Ethics, and Health Care. Additional information can be found at www.wma.net

Nuffield Council on Bioethics: A UK-based organization that examines and reports on ethical issues in biology and medicine. Additional information can be found at www.nuffieldbioethics.org

American Medical Association (AMA): Produces an ethics code for all physicians and medical students. Additional information can be found at http://www.ama-assn.org/ama/pub/physician-resources/medical-ethics/code-medical-ethics.page

American College of Physicians: An organization of internal medicine physicians that produces an ethics code. Additional information can be found at https://www.acponline.org/clinical-information/ethics-and-professionalism/acp-ethics-manual-sixth-edition-a-comprehensive-medical-ethics-resource

Literature

Bentham, Jeremy, *An Introduction to the Principles of Morals and Legislation*. Ed. J. H. Burns and H. L. A. Hart. (Oxford: Clarendon, 1996).

Bok, Hilary, *Freedom and Responsibility* (Princeton, NJ: Princeton University Press, 1998).

Locke, John, *Two Treatises of Government*. Ed. Peter Laslett. 3rd ed. (Cambridge: Cambridge University Press, 1988).

Pauly, Bernadette M., Colleen Varcoe, and Jan Storch. "Framing the Issues: Moral Distress in Health Care." *Hec Forum* 24, no. 1 (03/25 2012): 1–11.

Rohlf, Michael, "Immanuel Kant," The Stanford Encyclopedia of Philosophy (Spring 2016 Edition), Edward N. Zalta (ed.), http://plato.stanford.edu/archives/spr2016/entries/kant/.

Rousseau, Jean-Jacques, *The Social Contract* (Harmondsworth: Penguin, 1968).

Scheunemann, Leslie P., and Douglas B. White. "The Ethics and Reality of Rationing in Medicine." *Chest* 140, no. 6: 1625–1632.

Wenar, Leif, "John Rawls," The Stanford Encyclopedia of Philosophy (Winter 2013 Edition), Edward N. Zalta (ed.), http://plato.stanford.edu/archives/win2013/entries/rawls/.

Wilson, Fred, "John Stuart Mill," The Stanford Encyclopedia of Philosophy (Spring 2016 Edition), Edward N. Zalta (ed.), http://plato.stanford.edu/archives/spr2016/entries/mill/.

Other Media

Arkin, Alan. *Catch-22*. DVD. Directed by Mike Nichols. Hollywood: Paramount Pictures: A bomber waits as long as possible to drop bombs to save as many lives as possible.

Bale, Christian. *The Dark Knight*. DVD. Directed by Christopher Nolan. Burbank: Warner Home Video, 2008: Batman must make a decision on who to save—a childhood friend or the District Attorney.

Bale, Christian. *The Dark Knight Rises*. DVD. Directed by Christopher Nolan. Burbank: Warner Bros. Entertainment Inc.: Batman must decide if he should sacrifice himself to save a city from a nuclear bomb.

Connery, Sean. *The Rock*. DVD. Directed by John Schwartzman and Michael Bay. Burbank: Hollywood Pictures, 1997: The President orders the bombing of an island to save more lives overall.

Dreyfuss, Richard. *Whose Life Is It Anyway.* DVD. Directed by John Badham. Burbank: Warner Home Video, 2015: A quadriplegic wants to end his life; however, hospital staff is determined to keep the patient alive against his own wishes.

Hanks, Tom. *Saving Private Ryan.* DVD. Directed by Steven Spielberg. Universal City: DreamWorks Pictures, 1999: While searching for Private Ryan, the group questions whether or not saving one person is worth risking the lives of many.

Part II

Absolute Scarcity

Rationing

4 Historical Examples of Rationing

Scarcity is inherent in human life. It is what makes considerations of both justice and economics necessary. With an abundance of food, land, housing, and other goods, there would be no need to worry about how to distribute them to ensure everyone receives what they need. And with an abundance there would be no need for economics to help determine more efficient ways to distribute the goods. But we have both economics and ethics because there are shortages of resources and the shortages are inevitable.

This chapter explores various historical situations in which individuals and institutions were forced to distribute medical resources under conditions of absolute scarcity. Shortages in medicine and medical care are age-old and predate what we would consider effective medical treatments developed beginning in the late 19th century, as explained in Excerpt 1.[1] For instance, triage of wounded soldiers for treatment was a problem that concerned Napoleon's physicians due to limited ability to treat all those who needed care in the midst of a battle. Wounded soldiers were categorized into three groups: those for whom immediate care would improve their chances of survival, those likely to survive even if they did not get treated; and those most likely to die, irrespective of the care they would receive.[2] With the dawn of effective medical treatments in the late 19th century, allocation of scarce resources gave rise to similar life-and-death situations and led to a number of principles that would guide who should get access to treatment.

Excerpt 2 concerns rationing after the discovery of insulin.[3] In 1899, two German researchers discovered that when the pancreas was removed from dogs, they developed diabetes.[4]

---

[1] H. K. Beecher, "Scarce Resources and Medical Advancement," *Daedalus* 98, no. 2 (1969): pp. 275–313.

[2] C. R. Blagg, "Triage: Napoleon to the Present Day," *Journal of Nephrology* 17 (2004): pp. 629–632.

[3] M. Bliss, *The Discovery of Insulin* (Chicago: University of Chicago Press, 1982), pp. 129–153.

[4] L. Rosenfeld, "Insulin: Discovery and Controversy," *Clinical Chemistry* 48, no. 12 (2002): p. 2271.

Multiple groups tried to isolate the pancreatic substance that seemed to control the body's modulation of blood sugar. Nothing seemed to work. But in 1920–21, as outlined in the selection from Michael Bliss' book, *The Discovery of Insulin*, a young Canadian surgeon, Frederick Banting, had a new idea about isolating the pancreatic substance.[5] Along with a medical student, Charles Best, they isolated pancreas, added salt, froze it, ground it up, and then filtered the mixture, which they reinjected into a diabetic dog. Surprisingly, the dog got better.[6] A biochemist, Collip joined the group to help isolate, in a sufficiently pure state, the pancreatic substance that had been called "insulin."[7]

In January 1922, the first pure isolates of insulin were tested in a 14-year-old boy who made a miraculous recovery.[8] As the group was trying to scale up production in 1922 for human trials, they found they could not actually produce very much. The trouble led to an "insulin famine."[9] The Banting group then confronted two major issues: one practical and the other ethical.

The practical problem was how to scale up production. Banting and others teamed up with Eli Lilly and Company, a pharmaceutical company, to produce large quantities of insulin. Initially, Lilly could produce some insulin, but it had difficulty producing insulin in large quantities. Money and men were devoted to solving the insulin production problem.[10]

While the isolation procedure was imperfect, Dr. Banting and his team had to confront the ethical question of how to distribute limited supplies of insulin to a large number of patients. Should the life-saving injections be given to those patients on death's door? Should the limited insulin go to children before adults? Should it go to the rich and well-connected who could finance more research? Should the insulin go to Canadians before citizens of the United States?

Interestingly, there was not a lot of discussion about how to distribute insulin. A third was reserved for Banting's private patients. A third went to the Toronto General Hospital and the Hospital for Sick Children. And a third went to Banting's Christie Street clinic that treated veterans. Among those patients, Banting claims he prioritized sick children.[11] But there were many exceptions. The first American patients to receive insulin included the son of a vice president of Kodak camera company and Elizabeth Hughes, the daughter of a US Supreme Court justice who traveled to Toronto to receive some of the very scarce injections.[12] Simultaneously, Banting refused to sell the patent to New York investors who promised to set up insulin clinics and sell the injections, pay Banting a 5% royalty, and provide as much research funding as he desired. Banting, who was not well-off, refused, asking how poor patients would get the injections.[13] Other physicians who received limited supplies often prioritized those who were closest to death. For instance, E. P. Joslin of Boston gave insulin to those who were beginning to fail.[14]

By 1923, the practical problem was solved because Lilly found a way to produce insulin in large quantities and standardized the dosages. Abundance meant that Banting and the other physicians treating diabetic patients no longer had to choose between patients.

But development of other medical interventions faced the same problem that insulin did. The next set of three excerpts outline the dilemmas set forth by the limited availability of penicillin.

In 1928, Alexander Fleming, working at St. Mary's Hospital in London, found that mold that fell on his Petri plate was able to kill *Staphylococcus aureus* bacteria.[15] It turned out that isolating the bacteria-killing substance was difficult. It was hard to grow sufficient

[5] Bliss, *The Discovery of Insulin*.

[6] Rosenfeld, "Insulin: Discovery and Controversy," p. 2274.

[7] Ibid., pp. 2276–2277.

[8] Ibid., p. 2278.

[9] Bliss, *The Discovery of Insulin*, p. 129.

[10] Ibid., pp. 140–141.

[11] Ibid., p. 135.

[12] Ibid., pp. 135–137, 151–153.

[13] Ibid., p. 142.

[14] Ibid., p. 150.

[15] B. L. Ligon, "Penicillin: Its Discovery and Early Development," *Seminars in Pediatric Infectious Diseases* 15, no. 1 (2004): p. 52.

quantities of mold on the plates. What would later be known as penicillin was forgotten as a potential treatment for people. Nearly a decade later, in Oxford, Professor Howard Florey began trying to isolate penicillin. He succeeded sufficiently to test the drug on bacteria-infected mice and then to initiate human experiments. But his team could not produce sufficient quantities for full-scale research trials. Then, with World War II ongoing, Florey and his team came to Peoria, Illinois, where Peoria Labs had developed a method for growing large quantities of fungus in vats rather than on plates.[16] By 1942, numerous pharmaceutical companies were induced to try to produce penicillin in large quantities.[17] By June 1942, enough penicillin was available to treat just 10 patients.[18] In April 1943, the American Surgeon General of the Army arranged for clinical trials at a military hospital.[19] Production was rapidly escalating, and the evolving data showed that penicillin was incredibly effective at treating a number of infections including staph, strep, and gonorrhea.

As Excerpts 3 and 4 illustrate, by the end of 1943, the US Department of Agriculture, the Office of Scientific Research and Development, and the War Production Board funded and coordinated the construction of new production facilities to boost output.[20] But even with increased production, supply was limited compared to demand from sick patients. Decisions had to be made about who should receive the limited supply of penicillin. This was wartime, and so one pressing question was: How much should go to the military versus the civilian population? Within the military, which soldiers should receive the drug: those with infected wounds or those with gonorrhea contracted from sexual intercourse? In the civilian population, who should get the life-saving drug: children who required less, or adults?

The military rationing dilemma is depicted in James Howie's recollection of the debate among high-ranking officials in the British government (Excerpt 5).[21] In the summer of 1943, at the climax of the battles between the Allies and Rommel in North Africa, the British military was confronting the choice about how to allocate penicillin. Professor Florey was involved and argued against treating soldiers infected with gonorrhea. His argument was that it would not add to scientific knowledge about the best use of penicillin, and it would be politically explosive. Conversely, staff at the War Office was for treating soldiers infected with gonorrhea based on military considerations; namely, the soldiers could get back into the battle quickly. A memo was written to Britain's highest officials. In the margin of the memo, in green ink, the Prime Minister wrote: "The valuable drug must on no account be wasted. It must be used to the best military advantage."[22]

In the United States, the majority of the penicillin supply was reserved for military use. The limited supply saved for civilian use was distributed by Dr. Chester Keefer, chairman of the Committee of Chemo-Therapy of the National Research Council. All requests for the drug were sent to him, and he classified cases into three groups: (1) those where penicillin was shown to work, (2) those where using it would increase knowledge, and (3) those where penicillin was ineffective, such as cancer and glaucoma.[23] At least this allocation was more defensible than allocating the drug based upon wealth, connections, or other factors.

---

16 Ibid., pp. 54–55.

17 Ibid., p. 56.

18 A. N. Richards, "Production of Penicillin in the United States (1941–1946)," *Nature* 201, no. 4918 (1964): p. 442.

19 Ibid., p. 443.

20 W. L. Laurence, "More Penicillin: America Speeds Production of This Bacteria Killer," *New York Times*, August 1, 1943; W. L. Laurence, "Set Plans to Rule Penicillin Supply," *New York Times*, September 26, 1943.

21 J. Howie, "Gonorrhea—a Question of Tactics," *BMJ* 2, no. 6205 (1979): pp. 1631–1632.

22 Ibid.

23 D. P. Adams, *The Greatest Good to the Greatest Number: Penicillin Rationing on the American Home Front, 1940–1945* (New York: P. Lang, 1991), pp. 69–71.

Production increased and rationing ended in March 1945, when penicillin became commercially available.[24]

A third case of rationing concerns the early days of dialysis. Working with sausage skins and other recycled products, Dr. Willem Kolff invented dialysis to treat kidney failure in wartime Netherlands.[25] Patients required dialysis at least three times a week.[26] And chronic dialysis was not possible in part because of the inability to reuse arteries and veins over weeks and months.[27] In 1960, Dr. Belding Scribner working in Seattle developed a shunt between arteries and veins that could be reused over and over again.[28] While constituting a tremendous breakthrough, the shunt also intensified the ethical challenge of choosing which people with kidney failure should receive time on the limited and expensive dialysis machines.

The Swedish Hospital in Seattle established a two-stage process for selecting dialysis patients. At the first stage, physicians would make a technical decision of whether patients were medically appropriate for dialysis. A second committee, the Admissions and Policies Committee of the Seattle Artificial Kidney Center, selected among the medically eligible those few who would actually get dialysis (Excerpt 6).[29]

This Committee, which became dubbed the "God Committee" after an article published in 1962 in *Life* magazine, included seven members: a housewife, a banker, a state legislator, a minister, a lawyer, a labor leader, and a physician. The group rejected patients over 45 years of age because they might develop other medical complications. It rejected patients who did not live in Washington state, since all the basic research had been conducted at the University of Washington and was partially funded by state taxes. They evaluated marital status and number of dependents, wanting to be sure that if someone died their children would not be a burden on the state. They emphasized those who were emotionally and socially stable and had a family that could help them through the treatments. They also emphasized those who would go back to work and those who were religious. Ultimately, they could choose only one of every 50 potential candidates.[30]

The *Life* magazine story created a storm of controversy. People were upset about restricting access to dialysis to employed, religious people with families and children. As some commentators argued in the *UCLA Law Review,* the Seattle process was "[polluted by] prejudices and mindless clichés."[31] The selection criteria excluded "creative nonconformists," or as some put it: "The Pacific Northwest is no place for a Henry David Thoreau with bad kidneys."[32]

In 1971, the need to ration who received dialysis and who died of chronic renal failure ended because US Rep. Wilbur Mills introduced—and enacted—legislation that provided Medicare coverage for all Americans, regardless of age, who needed dialysis (see Chapter 8).[33] But ending the need to ration dialysis did not, of course, end the need to make choices about which treatments to pay for and immediately raised the question of which interventions provide most value for money, as expanded in Chapters 8–11.

---

[24] Ibid., p. 131.

[25] J. S. Cameron, *A History of the Treatment of Renal Failure by Dialysis* (New York: Oxford University Press, 2002), pp. 75–77.

[26] E. Lacson and S. M. Brunelli, "Hemodialysis Treatment Time: A Fresh Perspective," *Clinical Journal of the American Society of Nephrology* 6, no. 10 (2011): pp. 2522.

[27] Cameron, *A History of the Treatment,* pp. 79–80.

[28] L. J. McGough, et al., "Which Patients First? Setting Priorities for Antiretroviral Therapy Where Resources Are Limited," *American Journal of Public Health* 95, no. 7 (2005): pp. 1173–1180.

[29] S. Alexander, "They Decide Who Lives, Who Dies: Medical Miracle Puts a Moral Burden on a Small Committee," *Life*, November 9, 1962.

[30] Ibid.

[31] D. Sanders and J. J. Dukeminier, "Medical Advance and Legal Lag: Hemodialysis and Kidney Transplantation," *UCLA Law Review* 15 (1967): p. 377.

[32] Ibid., p. 378.

[33] C. R. Blagg, "The Early History of Dialysis for Chronic Renal Failure in the United States: A View from Seattle," *American Journal of Kidney Diseases* 49, no. 3 (2007): p. 491.

The rationing of scarce medical interventions is a recurrent problem. Even today, there are important cases of scarce resources that need to be rationed. For instance, in the 2013–14 Ebola outbreak in West Africa, places in treatment facilities had to be rationed. And in all developed countries, physicians have to choose who receives organ transplants: in all such cases, determining who gets access to beneficial healthcare interventions—and who loses out—requires ethical justification.

Questions for Discussion

1. As discussed by Bliss in Excerpt 2, Banting discovered insulin and co-produced it with the company Eli Lilly. He reserved around a third for his private patients, a third for the Toronto General Hospital and the Hospital for Sick Children, and a third for a clinic in which he treated veterans. He was a private individual working with a private company. Suppose you campaigned at the time to compel him to adopt a more fair rationing policy: On what grounds should he accept such a mandate, and what alternative policy would you propose?
2. Should the exigencies of wartime have dictated penicillin allocation decisions the way they prioritized soldiers? If you were a member of an allocation committee, who would you argue should receive scarce penicillin?
3. The Admissions and Policies Committee of the Seattle Artificial Kidney Center could only accept one of 50 patients wishing to access dialyses (Excerpt 6). The Committee's criteria were highly controversial. To what extent could they have reduced controversy? Would different principles, or particular processes for identifying principles, have helped increase acceptability?
4. This chapter included historical examples of rationing principles for penicillin, insulin, and dialysis. Are there any common themes that stand out to you? Should there be common principles or norms across different interventions?

EXCERPTS

Note: The following excerpts have generally been edited for length, and omissions are indicated with ellipses. Editing includes footnotes and endnotes, which have also been renumbered. For citation and related purposes, the full original source texts should be used.

EXCERPT 1

Abridged text from:

H. K. Beecher, "Scarce Resources and Medical Advancement," *Daedalus* 98, no. 2 (1969): pp. 275–313.

Scarce Resources and Medical Advancement

Henry Beecher

Among the recurring problems in the history of medicine, from ancient times to the present, is that of the sound allocation of scarce resources. . . .

Scarce resources in the advancement of medicine are attributable to a variety of causes—some are deliberate, man-made, and some are owing to "natural" scarcities that obtain when a rare and newly discovered drug is found to have great effectiveness, where facilities for its adequate production have to be developed despite almost overwhelming difficulties. Sometimes the difficulty is a costly technique, where the problems are monetary cost and shortages of competent manpower. . . .

Once availability was assured, even though of limited extent, it was often surprisingly difficult or impossible to discover the principles that determined allocation of the new substance or technique to one man while it was withheld from another. . . .

I. A Few Historical Examples from the Last Three Hundred Years

The Chamberlen Forceps

A member of the Chamberlen family (probably Peter, Sr.) developed an obstetrical forceps in the seventeenth century.[1,2] A similar instrument had been suggested by Pierre Franco in 1561. Nonetheless the Chamberlen family kept the secret of their instrument secure for many years.[3,4] At any rate, no outsider saw it until Hugh Chamberlen decided to sell it, for a high price, first in Paris, to Francois Mauriceau, the leading obstetrician of his time. That sale was lost owing to the demonstration's fatal outcome. Eventually Hugh sold the secret in Holland to Roger Roonhuysen and others. Here was limitation on the use of a discovery for private gain.

. . .

The Thyroid Hormone And Myxoedema

Until the latter part of the nineteenth century, myxoedema was considered to be an incurable disease. Observations in man and experimentation in animals led to the suggestion by Victor Horsley that a sheep's thyroid be transplanted into a patient suffering from myxoedema. . . . G. R. Murray cut up a sheep's thyroid and placed it in a little glycerine and 0.5% solution of carbolic acid.[5] After standing for twenty-four hours, the juice was filtered off and injected into a woman suffering from myxoedema, twice weekly

---

[1] F. H. Garrison, *An Introduction to the History of Medicine* (Philadelphia: W. B. Saunders Company, 1921), p. 208.

[2] A. Castiglioni and E. B. Krumbhaar, *A History of Medicine* (A. A. Knopf, 1941), p. 554.

[3] Garrison, *An Introduction to the History of Medicine,* p. 208.

[4] Castiglioni, *A History of Medicine*, p. 554.

[5] G. R. Murray, "Note on the Treatment of Myxoedema by Hypodermic Injections of an Extract of the Thyroid Gland of a Sheep," *British Medical Journal* 2, no. 1606 (1891): p. 796.

at first and later at two- or three-week intervals. Over three months' time, two and a half sheep's thyroid glands were used. The recovery of the patient was spectacular. The tedious and other unsatisfactory aspects of this procedure led to the isolation by Kendall of thyroxine from the thyroid gland. Its chemical structure was established, and finally it was prepared synthetically. Thus the remedy that had been so successful for one patient became easily available, through physiological and chemical studies, to all who need it.

Insulin

Ever since von Mehring and Minkowski had produced diabetes by excision of the pancreas in dogs in 1889, a number of attempts had been made to isolate the pancreatic substance that controlled carbohydrate metabolism. Finally this was accomplished by F. G. Banting and Charles H. Best in 1920 (published in 1922). They isolated the secretion of the islands of Langerhans and called it insulin.

Professor Best has recently had this to say:

> The general principle involved in the early days of the clinical use of insulin was that only severe cases, who were desperately in need of some better treatment, would receive insulin. . . .

In 1922, six distinguished physicians from the United States were invited to Toronto and fully briefed on the available information concerning insulin, and a revolution in medical care was launched. One of these six was Dr. E. P. Joslin of Boston. . . . Dr. Joslin's first concern was for those who were beginning to fail, especially children where the mortality was 100%. They got first priority. Other considerations in the use of the scarce insulin were psychological stamina and "people who could take the routine and not break."

Penicillin

Investigations of the therapeutic usefulness of penicillin and measures to increase its supply were carried out by the Committee on Medical Research of the Office of Scientific Research and Development, by the Division of Medical Sciences of the National Research Council, and by certain commercial companies. These studies were initiated and continued as a phase of the war effort, *primarily for the benefit of the Armed Forces.*[6]

. . .

The first clinical tests of penicillin in this country were reported in 1941. In June of 1942, the Committee on Chemotherapeutic and Other Agents of the National Research Council, under the chairmanship of Dr. Chester S. Keefer, was invited to organize and to supervise clinical investigations in selected hospitals, the records to be coordinated by Dr. Keefer and his Committee.

In April 1943, the Surgeon General of the Army arranged for clinical tests to be made at the Bushnell General Hospital in Utah. There were many soldiers in that hospital who had returned from the Pacific area with unhealed compound fractures, osteomyelitis, and wounds containing long-established infections. The results of treatment with penicillin were so encouraging that within a matter of weeks similar studies were planned in ten General Army Hospitals and venereal studies in six. . . .

By the time Dr. Richards' report was made (May 22, 1943), more than three hundred patients were being treated with penicillin despite the great production problems. . . . At the time of his report, Dr. Richards foresaw that the supply for civilian medical needs would be extremely limited.

On August 28, 1943, Dr. Keefer and his Committee reported on five hundred cases of infection treated with penicillin. Twenty-two groups of investigators were involved. Penicillin was then a scarce resource, and the situation urgent. In order to conserve material and time, the use of penicillin was restricted to a limited number of infectious states. After penicillin had been established as effective in treating staphylococcus and streptococcus infections, its use was soon extended to pneumonia and pneumococcal infections. Then it was shown to have an almost miraculous effect on gonorrhea and later a similar effect on syphilis, and a considerable number of other infections.[7] . . .

Allocation of penicillin within the Military was not without its troubles: When the first sizable

---

[6] A. N. Richards, "Penicillin," *Journal of the American Medical Association* 122 (1943): p. 235.

[7] A. Fleming, *Penicillin, Its Practical Application* (Blakiston, 1946).

shipment arrived at the North African Theatre of Operations, U. S. A., in 1943, decision had to be made between using it for "sulfa fast" gonorrhea or for infected war wounds. Colonel Edward D. Churchill, Chief Surgical Consultant for that Theatre, opted for use in those wounded in battle. The Theatre Surgeon made the decision to use the available penicillin for those "wounded" in brothels. Before indignation takes over, one must recall the military manpower shortage of those days. In a week or less, those overcrowding the military hospitals with venereal disease could be restored to health and returned to the battle line. . . .

Adrenocorticotropic Hormone (A. C. T. H.) And Cortisone

Dr. John R. Mote, while associated with the Armour Laboratories, had control of the distribution of A. C. T. H. Although the hormone had been isolated in an impure form from the pituitary gland in 1925 by Dr. Herbert Evans, it was not until later that it had been purified enough to permit clinical studies. Mote took the purified A. C. T. H. to university hospitals where trained investigators, especially young ones "who had not yet been trapped by their previous training," were given supplies for study. His "guiding principle was to give A. C. T. H. to any competent individual of any age in an accredited teaching institution [with] the freedom to explore his ideas be they ever so bizarre in the light of previous medical concepts."

Dr. George W. Thorn comments:

> . . . The extract was reserved for acute crises. Namely, the patient next to death was given the limited amount of adrenal extract.[8]

. . .

II. The Present

The English View

When experimentation in children is for diagnosis or treatment to the direct benefit of the child, the ethical problems are few so long as the consent of the parent or guardian has been obtained. The situation is vastly more complicated when the experimentation is not for the direct benefit of the child. A strict interpretation of English law declares this to be illegal, even with the approval of the parents, according to the Medical Research Council, 1962–63.

The situation in respect of minors and mentally subnormal or mentally disordered persons is of particular difficulty. In the strict view of the [English] law parents and guardians of minors cannot give consent on their behalf to any procedures which are of no particular benefit to them and which may carry some risk of harm. Whilst English law does not fix any arbitrary age in this context, it may safely be assumed that the Courts will not regard a child of 12 years or under (or 14 years or under for boys in Scotland) as having the capacity to consent to any procedure which may involve him in an injury. Above this age the reality of any purported consent which may have been obtained is a question of fact and as with an adult the evidence would, if necessary, have to show that irrespective of age the person concerned fully understood the implications to himself of the procedures to which he was consenting.

In the case of those who are mentally subnormal or mentally disordered the reality of the consent given will fall to be judged by similar criteria to those which apply to the making of a will, contracting a marriage or otherwise taking decisions which have legal force as well as moral and social implications. When true consent in this sense cannot be obtained, procedures which are of no direct benefit and which might carry a risk of harm to the subject should not be undertaken.

Even when true consent has been given by a minor or a mentally subnormal or mentally disordered person, considerations of ethics and prudence still require that, if possible, the assent of parents or guardians or relatives, as the case may be, should be obtained.

Intermittent Hemodialysis

. . . The main function [of hemodialysis] is the adjustment of the electrolyte and water content

[8] G. W. Thorn, "Personal Communication by Letter on July 9," 1968.

of the body so that they are kept within constant limits and certain wastes derived from protein metabolism are eliminated. If the kidneys cannot do this, the subject will die; life can be maintained even in the absence of kidney function, however, by circulating the blood through an artificial kidney. . . . It requires that the patient be placed on the artificial kidney some twelve to fourteen hours twice weekly. It is customary to carry this out at night in order to interfere as little as possible with normal activities. The patient's liberty is severely curtailed; the site of the arterial and venous connections must be kept absolutely clean and cannot be put into a bath; nor can the subject swim. Vigorous exercise is unwise. The site must be protected from injury. Strict dietary limitations are necessary. In most cases, the procedure much be carried out, at the present time at least, in a hospital.

. . .

In essence, the Seattle screening is done by two committees in which laymen as well as physicians function. In choosing candidates, they consider "worth to the community." For example, a thirty-two-year-old man with a stable history of employment and responsibility, with a family of six to support, was chosen over a forty-five-year-old widow whose children were grown up and had left home. . . .

. . . The first obligation is toward those patients who are already being treated.[9] A new patient is not accepted until the last one has been well launched. . . . To be chosen, the subject must be showing signs of deterioration notwithstanding a low-protein diet. Since hemodialysis facilities are in short supply, a choice must be made among needy candidates. Usually such a choice is made among those between puberty (below this age, they will not mature if on dialysis) and menopause, subjects who are clear mentally and cooperative, and not suffering from some other disease that dialysis will not control. Often patients who have young children are chosen.

A definition of suitability for dialysis depends on a number of factors, some arbitrary, some empirical. For instance, the subject chosen should have the possibility of a prolonged survival. It seems reasonable during the period of establishment of a new technique to choose in the early years those subjects who will probably do best.

. . .

IV. General Comment

It was a considerable disappointment to the writer, after the examination of more than a dozen areas where scarce resources were involved, to find statements of only the most rudimentary principles of procedure. (One must face the fact that this, too, is a kind of principle.)

The guiding factors encountered (rather than principles in most cases) can be summarized: *Avarice* is exemplified in the secrecy surrounding the Chamberlen forceps. Although lemon and orange juice were in short supply, their effectiveness in treating the scurvy was a matter of record; yet decades passed before the general ignorance was overcome. *Self-interest* or dedication to high principle is not clear in the case of anesthesia.

This is not to say that in early times only avarice, ignorance, or self-interest determined the allocation of scarce resources; but it seems evident that these factors were determinants then more often than is now the case.

Continuing with our arbitrary list of examples, the next one, chronologically, is the thyroid hormone. With this, a new and much higher realm of procedure was entered; it could be called a prototype for present action: Myxoedema was recognized as an incurable disease of the thyroid; animals, presumably, had normal thyroids. Seventy-seven years ago the difficulties lying in wait for the transplanter were not known; "transplant" of a sheep's thyroid was carried out. The curative properties of the procedure were evident in a matter of hours, far too soon for grafting to explain the success. It was assumed and later proved true that the infusion of the thyroid "juice" accounted for the good effect.

[9] H. De Wardener, "Some Ethical and Economic Problems Associated with Intermittent Haemodialysis," Wiley Online Library, 1966.

The active element was found to be thyroxine, which was synthesized. The early scarcity of the material and the tedious procedure gave way to the ready availability of the crucial substance as desired for anyone in need. This is a beautiful example of the selfless and effective work of many men, typified also in the triumphs of insulin, penicillin, and the adrenocorticotrophic hormone and cortisone.

There are at the present time plentiful reasons for despairing of mankind, but not in the standards evident in the progress of medicine. In the Western world, at least, the preeminence of the welfare of the individual is recognized as an indispensable component in the welfare of society. (It is inconceivable that a healthy society could be based upon exploitation of individuals, a sick use of individuals.) There is a considerable and growing recognition that science is not necessarily the highest value, that it must be placed in a hierarchy of values.

Some may consider these statements rather too grand. Yet what other conclusion can one come to with such visible evidence for them? Consider some major current concerns of today. May children be used in experimental procedures not for their direct benefit? (The answer seems to be "yes" in certain well-defined children's areas, "no" in others.) Relevant to our present interests is the fact that concern for "yes" or "no" *is* present.

It is now recognized that intermittent hemodialysis, as costly and inadequately available as it is at present, can be given to all who need it, at no greater cost than once was required by tuberculosis, even at less cost than mental disease now exacts. These latter unfortunates can add little to the world; hemodialysis can and does add years of productivity to those with otherwise fatal kidney disease.

Moreover, those who were once a grave and growing burden, the hopelessly comatose, can now be the means of extending life for desperately ill, but still salvageable individuals through a new understanding that the brain can die while other parts of the body remain sound and useful. It is also recognized that to *fail* to utilize this material is far more radical than not to use it.

The current requirements of an ethical approach to the transplantation of tissues and organs are a credit to our present standards of morality. All of these concerns, when contrasted with earlier years, offer heartening evidence of the growth of conscience, the advance in philosophical awareness, the gain in spiritual values, the sound growth of medicine.

EXCERPT 2

Abridged text from:

M. Bliss, *The Discovery of Insulin* (Chicago: University of Chicago Press, 1982), pp. 129–153.

Chapter 6 The Discovery of Insulin

Michael Bliss

"Unspeakably Wonderful"

In 1922, certain of the fact of their discovery and of its therapeutic benefit for human diabetics, the Toronto group had gone ahead with plans to manufacture insulin in large quantities. The Connaught Anti-Toxin Laboratories was to finance and administer production. Collip was to direct insulin manufacture.[1]. . . All the problems with purification, the fights about credit, and the rest of the strains, were surely in the past.

Collip found that he could not make insulin. First he could not make it in large batches using the apparatus set up in the special manufacturing area. Then he started to have trouble making it by any method, even in his own lab. The result of Collip's failure was an insulin famine in Toronto during the spring of 1922. . . .

V.

The rediscovery of a way to make insulin made it possible to consider resuming clinical tests. Banting had played little part in the clinical work at Toronto General Hospital, for he had been denied an appointment to the hospital's staff. . . . It would be unthinkable to deny Dr. Frederick Banting, a licensed physician in good standing, priority in the clinical use of insulin.[2] . . .

Dr. F. G. Banting established an office at 160 Bloor Street West in Toronto and began the private practice of medicine [with] the right to use the facilities of Toronto General Hospital's private patients' pavilion for his private patients. . . . Several weeks later Banting was appointed head of a new diabetes clinic at Toronto's Christie Street Military Hospital.[3]

---

[1] For Collip's responsibilities, see J. J. Macleod, "History of the Researches Leading to the Discovery of Insulin: With an Introduction by Lloyd G. Stevenson," *Bulletins on the History of Medicine* 52, no. 3 (1978): pp. 295–312. A careful reading of Best's various accounts of his work in 1922 indicates that he did not take over direction of insulin production until after Collip left Toronto.

[2] The exact date of the production failure is impossible to determine. F. G. Banting, *Manuscript Account of the Discovery of Insulin, September 1922* (University of Toronto: 1922) states that the supply failed on February 19. This is unlikely, inasmuch as there is no reference to any shortage in F. G. Banting, et al., "Pancreatic Extracts in the Treatment of Diabetes Mellitus," *Canadian Medical Association Journal* 12, no. 3 (1922): pp. 141–146, which has results to February 1922. In a letter written on April 29 (MP, to W. B. Cannon), Macleod states that the production failure developed after publication of that paper, which means after March 22. On the other hand, F. G. Banting, et al., "The Effect Produced on Diabetes by Extracts of Pancreas," *Transactions of the Association of American Physicians* (1922): pp. 1–11, delivered on May 3, states that for two months it had been impossible to secure potent extracts that could be used in the clinic. These confusing statements probably reflect a complex reality, in which the production breakdown was gradual, with the extract supply being inadequate at some times, adequate at others, the small-scale methods working when the large-scale failed (as mentioned in J. J. Macleod and W. R. Campbell, *Insulin. Its Use in the Treatment of Diabetes* [Baltimore: 1925], p. 69), and so on, but with periods when nothing worked at all. April was certainly the cruelest month.

[3] Exactly how the Christie Street situation developed is unclear. An April 3, 1922, Memorandum to the minister, by the Director of Medical Services, Dr. W. C. Arnold, recommending the establishment of the clinic, is in the PAC, RG 32, C2, vol. 13, Banting personnel file. Arnold recommended establishment of the clinic as an excellent and justifiable step by the ministry. But there is some evidence that he had known Banting earlier and wanted to help him out.

About the same time, an agreement was reached with the Connaught Laboratories on the distribution of insulin for clinical use. One-third of the production was to go to Banting for his private practice, one-third was to be used in Banting's Christie Street clinic, and one-third would be available for work at Toronto General and the Hospital for Sick Children.[4] . . .

By mid-May enough insulin was being produced by the new method to permit resumption of limited clinical testing. Dr. Joe Gilchrist received his second injection on May 15. Gilchrist had agreed to work at the Christie Street clinic under Banting, and so served as both physician and patient. In the early months of sporadic production and frequent impurities, Gilchrist became Toronto's self-proclaimed "human rabbit," testing each new batch on himself after it had been tried on the rabbits.[5]

There was also enough insulin in mid-May to allow Banting to meet the urgent request of Dr. John R. Williams, who had come to Toronto from Rochester, New York. Jim Havens, son of a vice-president of Eastman Kodak, had been diagnosed as diabetic seven years earlier at age fifteen. He did fairly well on an Allen diet until 1920 when his capacity began a sharp decline. . . . When news came of the discovery in Toronto a year later, James Havens, Jr., was a 73½-pound skeleton, living on 820 calories a day, barely able to lift his head from his pillow, crying most of the time from pain, hunger, and despair. . . .

Havens got his first insulin on the evening of May 21, 1922. He was the first person treated with it in the United States.[6]. . . On May 26 Banting went to Rochester to examine Havens. He advised doubling and then tripling the dosage. Within a day or so Havens' urine was sugar-free, his blood sugar was down to normal, and his clinical condition greatly improved. Banting agreed to have fresh supplies of insulin sent by train from Toronto. Two weeks after first receiving insulin, Jim Havens was able to rise from his bed and walk. . . .

Williams had come to Toronto personally to plead for insulin. Others, alerted by the May 3 paper in Washington, were beginning to do the same or to write Banting or Macleod asking when the new treatment would be available. . . .

Toronto's decision to collaborate with his company was a triumph for and testimony to the persistence of G. H. A. Clowes. . . .

In 1922 Eli Lilly and Company had been making and selling pharmaceuticals for forty-six years from their base in Indianapolis, Indiana. It was a family-owned "ethical" drug company (no patent medicines, no extravagant claims, and advertising and sales to doctors and pharmacists only), which had grown to become a major, though not dominant factor in the industry. In 1921 Lilly employed about eleven hundred people and did just over $5 million worth of business. The firm was managed, according to the founder's son and president, J. K. Lilly, with the aim of being "conservatively progressive." Part of the house's progressiveness in the early 1900s had been the creation of a substantial research facility. At the end of the First World War the Lilly family had decided to strengthen further the firm's links with the scientific community, even though the short-term returns from such ventures might be minimal. As part of this continuing policy G. H. A. Clowes was hired as a special research chemist in

[4] No copy of this agreement has been found, but it is referred to in the Insulin Committee Minutes, Aug. 17, 1922.

[5] J. A. Gilchrist, C. H. Best and F. G. Banting, "Observations with Insulin on Department of Soldiers; Civil Re-Establishment Diabetics," *Canadian Medical Association Journal* 13, no. 8 (1923): pp. 565–572; F. G. Banting, "The History of Insulin," *Edinburgh Medical Journal* (1929): pp. 1–18.

[6] All of the documents from this time suggest that Havens was the first. In a letter to Best on March 13, 1939 (BI, Best Papers, Historical file), however, Williams casually mentioned that he began giving extract to one Lyman Bushman, a veteran, on May 14, 1922. The Havens family correspondence shows this cannot have been true, and was a slip of Williams' pen or memory. Circumstantial evidence suggests that Bushman was first given insulin in June or July.

1919 and appointed director of research the next year.

. . .

Macleod had known Clowes for some years, was impressed by his stature as a scientist, and by his company's enlightened support of research. He and the other Torontonians were probably also impressed by the plans Clowes outlined to them for the development of insulin. The firm had recently been very active in work on glandular products, and had a good team of chemists ready to work on insulin. It wanted an exclusive licence for an "experimental period" of one year, during which there would be a complete pooling of knowledge between Toronto and Indianapolis. There would be a several-stage development of the product involving large-scale clinical tests in Toronto and the United States, with Lilly supplying extract free of charge in the initial stages and then selling it at cost. Lilly would share any improvements it made in the manufacturing process with Toronto, and if any improvements were patentable would pool the patent rights for all territory outside of the United States. At the end of the experimental period, Lilly wanted a licence to manufacture insulin on the same terms as Toronto would license other manufacturers. As Clowes had proposed in earlier letters, the firm thought it would be appropriate for insulin licensees to pay Toronto royalties on all insulin sold.

. . .

The Toronto group was anxious to get policies for developing insulin in place during May, not only because of the demand from doctors and diabetics, but also because of the imminent break-up of the group. Collip's appointment at Toronto expired on May 31. Such negotiations as there may have been about his staying on seem to have dissolved in the quarrels with Banting and then the difficulties making insulin. . . .

On June 2 and 3 [Best and Collip] told the Lilly chemists all they knew about making insulin and helped with the first attempt to extract it. The process worked." His time in Toronto over, J. B. Collip went back to his job at the University of Alberta.

VII.

Beginning work immediately, the Lilly company poured men and money into insulin production. But they were not the first to make insulin in the United States. Dr. W. D. Sansum of the Potter Metabolic Clinic in Santa Barbara, California, had noticed Banting and Best's first publication and in April had written Banting to ask about progress. When Banting told him of the delays, Sansum decided to try making pancreatic extract himself. . . . The Potter group found they could make potent extracts. On May 31 they began administering insulin to an adult male patient, and soon succeeded in making him sugar free. They tried to increase their supply of the extract early in June, collecting the pancreases from sixteen hundred sheep. Just as had happened in Toronto, they found that the attempt to scale up production failed completely. . . .

To meet the clinicians' demand, while at the same time usefully spreading out the research job, Toronto and Lilly had agreed that a select group of physicians and institutions would be given the extract for testing purposes as soon as it became available. Until then, the Torontonians saw no reason why other researchers should not be able to make insulin. Macleod sent both Sansum and Woodyatt details of the method. To honour the Lilly agreement, he required them not to divulge the method to anyone likely to produce the extract commercially.[7]

[7] IC, Potter file, Macleod to Sansum, June 21, 1922; Woodyatt file, Macleod to Woodyatt, June 21. Macleod may have bad second thoughts about this policy, for a week later, replying to Allen's request, he did not send details, but simply promised a reprint of the paper giving the method when it was published. This became his standard reply to similar requests in the next several months. Of course it was also possible to learn the method from Collip. It is said, for example, that Woodyatt actually learned how to make insulin from a conversation with Collip.

Of course experimental and clinical work would continue in Toronto, with the Connaught Laboratories, small and makeshift as its facility was, doing everything possible to increase insulin production for the city and for Canada. . . .

VIII.

. . . [Banting] was beginning to get offers, some of them princely. [He describes one offer]:

I was called to the phone and a man asked if he could see me. He said he would come up immediately. A few minutes later he arrived. He was a big man and there seemed hardly room for him. He looked about and his first words were, "Well for God's sake."

I sat at my desk and he sat on the only other chair, which was of the hard stiff back kitchen variety. "So this is where you live." "Well you are a damned fool." "Now listen to me" and he proceeded to tell me how the wife of a friend of his had been under the care of the best Doctors in New York and despite the diet treatment she got worse and worse. She had been given insulin and she felt entirely different. He knew the woman. She had tried everything and "knew them all," you could not fool her. She was all for insulin. That was good enough for him. All I had to do was to hand over the patents to a group on Wall Street and he would guarantee me $1,000,000 cash. Insulin would be patented in every country in the world. Ten percent royalty would be collected. The company would keep five & I would be given 5% royalty in addition to the $1,000,000 cash. A chain of clinics would be established across the United States and Canada one or two in every large City. I would be Medical Director and would have all the clinical cases for study and could have all the laboratories I desired. I would thus be relieved of financial responsibilities, being independently wealthy, and could devote myself to scientific research.

. . .

IX.

. . . During July, [Banting] was being deluged with requests for insulin from physicians, diabetics, diabetics' families, people who had come to Toronto, people wondering if they should come to Toronto, people wondering if insulin could come to them. . . . Diabetics were literally camping at the doors of the lab trying to get insulin.[8]

The standard reply to all inquiries was that insulin was still in the experimental stage, supplies were severely limited, and the inquirer would be informed when the situation changed. All available production was going to Jim Havens in Rochester and to Gilchrist and a handful of diabetic soldiers at Christie Street Hospital. Thinking the supply situation was improving, Banting gave in to some of the most desperate pleas; in mid-June and early July he agreed to treat a few private patients who were otherwise about to die. Four living skeletons, three children and one adult, were brought to Toronto from points in the United States and Canada.

Elizabeth Hughes was not among them. The fourteen-year-old diabetic had clung to life through the winter of 1921–22, a pathetically starved little girl, five feet tall but weighing no more than 52 to 54 pounds. In the spring of 1922 she was taken to Bermuda with her nurse to enjoy the climate. She contracted the diarrhea epidemic on the island. Both her weight and her carbohydrate tolerance slipped further. From May 19 to June 2, 1922, Elizabeth received less than 300 calories of nourishment a day. Her weight, fully clothed, fell below 50 pounds. . . . She continued to exercise every day and made it a personal triumph to walk up the ramp to the ship that brought her home from Bermuda.

[8] Best family papers, M. M. Best scrapbook, Banting to Best, July 15, 1922; Toronto *Star*, Feb. 24, 1923.

Elizabeth's mother, Antoinette Hughes, had learned about the discovery in Toronto. Allen and other doctors told her that in this case the newspapers were right; there was something to it. On July 3 she wrote Banting to ask whether anything could be done for her "pitifully depleted and reduced" daughter. Banting's answer on July 10 was the standard discouragement. All the Hughes family could do was try to keep Elizabeth going, hoping she would last until insulin was beyond the experimental stage. In fact it was impossible to build up her tolerance, and Elizabeth continued her drift towards death from starvation. A friend of J. J. R. Macleod's, whose moving appeal on behalf of a poor fisherman on Prince Edward Island had met with the same response, wrote, "It is pitiful that so great a boon should be in sight, yet not in reach."[9]

X.

The insulin situation was a nightmare. Every attempt to increase the quantity of extract being produced in Toronto failed. When Best left on holidays, there were problems procuring pancreas. Then there was a shortage of acetone. Worse still, the quality of extract that was being produced was not good. Protein impurities caused abscesses in many of the patients; salts still in the solution made many injections excruciatingly painful.[10] Strong extract seemed to have the worst side-effects, but weak extract had to be injected in painfully large doses to do any good. . . .

By mid-July, production at the Connaught Laboratories was apparently at the point of failing completely once again. Williams, who had come to Toronto in desperation to get something pure enough to use on Havens, later wrote that "Toronto insulin had become intolerable." Banting was beside himself, Peter Moloney remembered, to get insulin to keep his patients alive.[11]

Could Eli Lilly and Company come to the rescue? When the firm's work on insulin began early in June, Clowes planned to run ongoing small-scale experimental programs in tandem with a series of factory-scale attempts at mass production. . . .

Lilly's preparations, made from pork pancreas, were potent from the beginning. As always, however, it proved painfully difficult to increase the yield. . . .

Banting decided to go to Indianapolis to study Lilly's method for himself. "I have a hunch that Clowes is holding out on us since he would not tell us how that [first Lilly] batch was made," Banting wrote to Best. "And furthermore since the extract we're making here is 'pretty rough', I think they might supply us with some for the patients are needing it very badly."[12] On the 23rd he went to Indianapolis with D. A. Scott, Connaught's latest addition to its insulin team.

Banting's suspicions about Clowes were groundless, for the Lilly group went out of their way to help the Canadians. In fact Clowes and the Lilly family took an instant liking to Fred Banting and decided to support him every way they could. Banting and Scott were shown complete details of the production facility, and the insulin supplies Clowes had promised were waiting for Banting. . . .

---

[9] BP, Elizabeth Hughes file. A. Hughes to Banting, July 3, 16, 1922; MP, A. S. Ferguson to Macleod, July 31, Aug. 9, 1922.

[10] Havens papers, Banting to James Havens, Sr., July 10, 18, 1922; Gilchrist, "Observations with Insulin"; F. G. Banting, W. R. Campbell and A. A. Fletcher, "Insulin in the Treatment of Diabetes Mellitus," *Journal of Metabolic Research* (1922): p. 550; also Lilly archives, XRDc, John R. Williams to G. H. A. Clowes, Jan. 27, 1958: "One day Fred Banting took me up to the Christie Street military hospital where there were 8 soldiers each suffering horribly with large abscesses in hips-buttocks. I was having same trouble with Jim Havens and 3 other cases I had here."

[11] Lilly archives, XRDc, Williams to Clowes, Jan. 27, 1958; interview with Moloney.

[12] Best family papers, M. M. Best scrapbook, Banting to Best, July 21, 1922.

XII.

. . . Lilly was ready to begin supplying Joslin, Allen, and other leading diabetologists with insulin. . . . Clowes and Banting discussed how to go about this in a way that would protect Toronto's—and Banting's—priority in the work. Clowes' idea, consistent with his original plan, was to form a small coordinating committee to plan the course of the testing, with a view to the results being published in a special issue of Allen's *Journal of Metabolic Research*. Banting would be a member of the committee, an editor of the Journal, and at the head of the list of authors in the special issue. Clowes thought the issue could be published by the end of 1922; Lilly would bear the expense of distributing it throughout the United States. "And if this were done," Clowes wrote Banting on August II, 1922, "you would not only get full credit for your work but it would be the first step toward securing the Nobel Prize in medicine for you and your associates."[13] . . .

But insulin did not come easily to the Lilly company either. Just as the Americans thought they had mastered the process and were proceeding in a straight line towards commercial production, unforeseen problems started to develop. Every lot was not coming out at full strength. In early August several lots were not successful at all, apparently because the United States government had forced a change in the kind of alcohol the company was allowed to use. Having just made a commitment to supply the clinicians with more than seven hundred and fifty units of insulin a week (of which Banting was to get five hundred), Lilly found itself "right on the ragged edge" of a serious supply problem.[14] . . . This greatly distressed Clowes, who persuaded Banting to cut back his allotment from five hundred to three hundred and fifty. . . . Banting's cutback enabled Williams in Rochester to begin receiving Lilly "Iletin" to use on Jim Havens instead of the painful Toronto stuff.[15]

Clinical tests began at the Methodist Hospital in Indianapolis on August 3." In Boston, Elliott Joslin received his first insulin on August 6. Thinking about the trials he would begin the next day, Joslin was too excited to sleep that night. It is said he was too nervous to make the first injection himself, so it was given by his associate, Dr. Howard Root. The patient as a forty-two-year-old former nurse, Miss Mudge, who in five years of diabetes had starved herself down to 69 pounds—"just about the weight of her bones and a human soul," Joslin put it.[16] Miss Mudge was an invalid from her diabetes; only once in the past nine months had she found strength to go out on the street. The immediate effect of her first injection of insulin was not that dramatic, Joslin remembered. But six weeks later Miss Mudge was walking four miles daily." . . .

XIII.

. . . By August 12 it had been decided to bring Elizabeth [Hughes] to Toronto. Allen told Banting he would find her a model patient for treatment. "There could not be a child, who for her own self deserved your care more than Elizabeth, in addition to any consideration due on account of her family." . . .

He began insulin treatment at once. The first injections, one cc. twice a day, cleared the sugar from Elizabeth's urine. Banting immediately began increasing her diet. It had been 889 calories (actually 789 through July, but on the 29th Allen had allowed an extra 100 calories off at daily, probably to hold off death from starvation). At the end of the first week's treatment Banting had Elizabeth up to 1,220 calories;

[13] BP, 1, Clowes to Banting, Aug. 8, 11, 1922.

[14] Lilly archives, XBLk, J. K. Lilly to Clowes, Aug. 8, 1922.

[15] Lilly archives, XBLk, J. K. Lilly to Clowes, Aug. 8, 11, 1922.

[16] Lilly archives, Joslin address at the dedication of the Lilly Research Laboratories, Indianapolis, October 1934.

another week and she was on a normal girl's diet of 2,200 to 2,400 calories. . . .

[Banting's] clinic at Christie Street had not gone well, for the first patients had been plagued by pain and abscesses, reactions which discouraged other diabetic veterans from volunteering. But the situation suddenly changed dramatically. One of the "faithful" asked for a weekend's leave and permission to take his insulin supplies with him, Banting remembered. The doctors consented. The soldier returned to the hospital on Monday all smiles. "For the first time in three years I am a man again." Insulin had restored his sexual desire and potency. "By night," Banting wrote, "every diabetic in the hospital was asking for insulin."[17] It was mostly Lilly insulin they were getting, but by the 22nd the Connaught facility, newly equipped with the special vacuum apparatus, was about to produce its first substantial batch of truly potent insulin."[18]

In Rochester Jim Havens had already been switched to the American product. In Toronto Mrs. Charlotte Clarke was learning how to use her new artificial leg. In her rooms at the Athelma Apartments, on Grosvenor Street just next to Toronto General Hospital, little Elizabeth Hughes found herself slowly awakening from her nightmare of diabetes, diet, and starvation. "Isn't that unspeakably wonderful?" she exclaimed to her mother.[19]

---

[17] F. G. Banting, *Banting Papers: The Story of Insulin*, unpublished manuscript (University of Toronto: 1940); with telling, Banting's one suit became shabbier and shabbier, covered with dog hairs and dung.

[18] EH to her mother, Aug. 22, 1922.

[19] EH to her mother, Oct. 6, 1922.

EXCERPT 3

Abridged text from:

W. L. Laurence, "More Penicillin: America Speeds Production of This Bacteria Killer," *New York Times*, August 1, 1943.

More Penicillin: America Speeds Production of this Bacteria Killer

William L. Laurence

One of the great contributions of American scientific genius to the war is the development of relatively large-scale means for the production of penicillin, the chemical manufactured by the cheese mold, penicillin notatum, which has proved to be the most potent bacteria killer so far to be discovered—much more potent than any of the chemicals of the sulfa family. While it was only a laboratory curiosity last year, the large American chemical and pharmaceutical houses went to work on it with the same zeal as the rest of the American industry, with the result that many millions of units are now being made available for our armed forces.

Last week the Winthrop Chemical Company announced plant for a new plant of 20,000 square feet at Renseelaer, N. Y., to be devoted exclusively to the manufacture of penicillin. The new plant, it was announced, will increase the present Winthrop output 100 per cent. Winthrop is only one of a large number of pharmaceutical firms to manufacture this substance. Others include Merk & Co., E. R. Squibb & Sons, Charles A. Pfizer & Co., New York; the Abbott Laboratories Chicago; the Commercial Solvents Corporation; the American Home Products Company, the Frederick Stearns Company of Detroit, the regional laboratory of the United States Department of Agriculture at Peoria, Ill., and many others. The work is under the auspices of the Committee on Medical Research of the Office of Scientific Research and Development, the National Research Council and the Department of Agriculture culture.

Output a Military Secret

The exact amount being extracted from the cheese mold is a military secret, but it certainly is not going to give any comfort to our enemies to state that enough will be made to save thousands of lives among our wounded and sick fighting men. And after the war the chemical will be available to heal the sick of the civilian population. . . .

English Discoverer

Penicillin was first discovered by Dr. Alexander Fleming, English scientist in 1929. . . . He set to work and prepared crude extracts of penicillin, but it was used only for laboratory purposes because of the very minute amounts available.

In 1939 Dr. Howard Florey of Oxford set to work to prepare pure extracts of the substances, and after a set of experiments on mice the substance was tried on human beings, with amazing results. . . . But the difficulty of extracting it from the mold in any sizeable amounts was still there and it took the entry of the United States into the war to break the bottleneck.

Millions of units are now supplied weekly to our fighting men. . . .

Amounts Used in Treatment

One million units weigh approximately one-fifth of an ounce. Yet one ounce is sufficient for treatment of many cases of gonorrhea, for example, Sulfonamide-resistant cases of gonorrhea can be cured by as little as 100,000 units of penicillin (one fiftieth of an ounce) in two days. Larger doses are usually needed for osteomyelitis (infection of the bone marrow) and other bacterial infections.

. . .

Penicillin is now under strict allocation of the War Production Board for national defense, and there is no prospect that a surplus will soon be available for civilian use.

EXCERPT 4

Abridged text from:

W. L. Laurence, "Set Plans to Rule Penicillin Supply," *New York Times*, September 26, 1943.

Set Plans to Rule Penicillin Supply

Laurence W.

Federal Agencies Tell Drug Makers How It May Be Made Available to Civilians
17 Companies Involved
Medical Men Must Give Dr. Keefer at Boston Full Case Histories on Patients' Cases

Washington, Sept. 25 [1943]—The seventeen companies which are either producing or are about to produce penicillin, the new drug which has been found better for some infections than the sulfa drugs, were informed at a meeting with interested Government agencies here of the procedure to be followed in making it available to civilians.

Doctors handling cases which might be benefited by the use of penicillin, it was announced, should submit complete medical and bacteriological case histories to Dr. Chester S. Keefer, chairman of the Committee of Chemo-Therapy of the National Research Council and consultant to the Office of Scientific Research and Development, at Evans Memorial Hospital, 65 East Newton Street, Boston.

Disposition of the request will be determined by policies adopted and frequently reviewed by the Committee of Chemo-Therapy. Much time, it was said, would be saved if doctors in charge of cases would get in touch directly with Dr. Keefer.

Program Moves Rapidly

The penicillin programs was progressing rapidly, it was said, owning to the combined efforts of producers, the Office of Scientific Research and Development and the War Production Board. It will be many months before production will reach planned capacity, but the program outlined at the meeting has been scheduled to meet expected civilian requirements. . . .

EXCERPT 5

Abridged text from:

J. Howie, "Gonorrhea—a Question of Tactics," *BMJ* 2, no. 6205 (1979): pp. 1631–1632.

Gonorrhea—A Question of Tactics

James Howie

In May 1943 the defeat of Rommel's army in North Africa opened the way for the allied invasion of Sicily and Italy. Unhappily, during the period of preparation, several soldiers destined to lead the assault acquired gonorrhoea. Unhappily, also, the gonorrhea was caused by gonococci obstinately resistant to sulphonamides. As more and more assault troops spent their time being ineffectively treated with permanganate douches instead of training for the difficult operation that lay ahead of them, the question naturally was asked whether penicillin would cure the condition.

At that time supplies of penicillin for the British Army were very short, and the issue of the drug was rigidly controlled. The efforts of Howard Florey and Hugh Cairns were concentrated on discovering how penicillin could be most effectively used in the prevention and treatment of infection in war wounds-work whose value was to be firmly established during the invasion of Western Europe a year later. In 1943, however, the effort was understandably concentrated on learning what could be expected from using penicillin to deal with wounds of the limbs, trunk, chest, and head.

Florey and Cairns . . . could never get their hands on all the allocation of penicillin and, therefore, was subject to critical scrutiny. Obviously, with this unknown drug, laboratory control of the observations was essential; thus allocation of the scarce supplies inevitably required an assurance from the director of pathology at the War Office (Major-General Leo Poole of AMD7) that adequate laboratory control was available, that the projected use was important, and that the plans of the inquiry were satisfactory. In addition to the views of the appropriate War Office consultants, General Poole had the immensely wise help of Lieutenant-Colonel Harold Bensted, another regular soldier of great experience and a real understanding of micro biology. In May 1943 I had the interesting experience of being posted to the lowly job of deputy director of army pathology in AMD7. As a result I was included in the great debate: should any penicillin be allocated to treat gonorrhoea in the assault troops preparing in North Africa? In one way, the answer was obvious: penicillin was virtually certain to be highly effective in quickly releasing an important group of men for return to their units. But that was not the only issue, as quickly became clear.

The Great Debate

Brigadier Cairns and Professor Florey sought an interview with General Poole to discuss the proposal. Harold Bensted and I were invited to join the discussion. Florey and Cairns were against using penicillin for treating gonorrhoea—even in the circumstances described among the assault troops. They argued, correctly, that the efficacy of penicillin for the treatment of gonorrhoea was well established. Nothing, therefore, would be added to our knowledge of how to use it in war when supplies increased. We still did not know with certainty how best to use penicillin to prevent gas gangrene; in the treatment of burns, head wounds, and wounds of the thorax and abdomen. More over, they argued, think of the political consequences. The proposed use of penicillin to treat gonorrhoea would certainly provoke parliamentary questions. Why were all the gallant wounded men unable to have penicillin, while some scallywags received it to relieve them of the discomforts their own indiscretions had brought on them? Could General Poole not imagine Members of both Houses, including the bishops, reading from letters sent to them from relatives of wounded men?

When the interview ended with the general's promising to consider the matter with great care, our visitors departed. Harold Bensted at once declared himself: the military arguments for using penicillin in gonorrhoea among assault troops in North Africa were clear and strong. But the political consequences, of which we had received a probably accurate forecast, were so important that the issue must at once go to the highest possible level for a decision on whether the politicians were ready and willing to face the music if the War Office gave Algiers the go ahead.

Accordingly, a succinct memo was composed setting out the case for and against, essentially putting up for decision [whether to prioritize treatment of combat soldiers with gonorrhea or those with battle wounds]. . . .

A Political Decision

As I recall it, the file went through the appropriate medical departments at record speed and went to Downing Street. It did not linger long there either, and we had it back in about a week. Plenty had been written by various highly placed civil servants, but none of this seemed to give the kind of unequivocal answer we needed. Alongside one minute, however, there was a marginal note in green ink which said: "This valuable drug must on no account be wasted. It must be used to the best military advantage." There was debate about the exact initials attached to the marginal note, but there was no doubt about the green ink. [The man who writes with green ink is understood to be Winston Churchill].

We debated the exact meaning of our instructions; but the general cut through the discussion by saying characteristically "I've got to carry the can." He promptly invited Hugh Cairns and Howard Florey to visit him again to resume discussion on the issue they had raised. Harold Bensted and I were invited to be present as witnesses to the conversation. Harold and I agreed to listen without speaking, which we did. I recall the general's exact words, which I think he had memorised because I recall his pacing to and fro reciting words to himself before the meeting. "Gentlemen," said the general, "you warned me of the political importance of the advice I should give on this matter. I accepted your warning. Consequently, I referred the issue for a political decision. I asked that this should go right to the top. We have had our answer. It is written in green ink—you know, I take it, what that means. I am now clear about my advice. It is that penicillin should be used to treat gonorrhoea among the assault troops in Algiers."

The interview ended in polite exchanges and, so far as I know, there were no political repercussions. My own view is that Harold Bensted's military and political judgment was right, and that Leo Poole's way of handling the event proved that he was a wise, shrewd, and honest soldier capable of carrying any can that was handed to him.

"I cannot believe," said Bensted, when it was all over, "that the Royal Navy is denying itself the use of penicillin for the treatment of gonorrhoea." "No indeed," said Surgeon Vice-Admiral Sir Sheldon Dudley when the point was put to him, "we are making our own!" They were indeed, under the direction of Cecil Green at Carshalton. A sample was produced and later given for testing to a medical officer of the Canadian Army. "Marvelous stuff," was his verdict. "It did two things: abolished the gonorrhoea like magic and so pained the injected soldier that it cured him also of the idea of risking his health again."

Years later (in 1966), I told Howard Florey about the openended wording of the marginal note in green ink. He laughed and recalled verbatim what Poole had said. "Yes," he admitted, "what you tell me of the minute is entirely credible; and, of course, Poole did not quote the words. He told us only what he decided after reading the note." He paused and laughed again. "Poole was clever," he said, "and of course he was right."

EXCERPT 6

Full text from:

S. Alexander, "They Decide Who Lives, Who Dies: Medical Miracle Puts a Moral Burden on a Small Committee," *Life*, November 9, 1962.

From the pages of

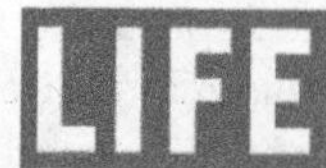

They Decide Who Lives, Who Dies: Medical Miracle Puts a Moral Burden on a Small Committee

Shana Alexander

John Myers has known about his kidney trouble ever since a routine physical examination at the time of his Army discharge in 1945. But until two years ago he felt fine. Then the headaches began and his blood pressure began to rise. By last summer there were days when he could barely drag himself out of bed to get to his office. He was 37 years old. Neither he nor his wife Kari had any idea that he had come, irrevocably, to the terminal stage of his disease. But a glance at his case history was enough to tell any physician that John Myers death would be ugly and soon.

Last Christmas morning when Myers awakened at his home in Bremerton, Wash, his heart was pounding violently. He could not stop coughing. Blood was running from his nose. He had an indescribable headache, a horrible taste in his mount, dreadful nausea. His face and limbs were grossly swollen. He was rushed to a hospital where it seemed certain he would be dead within a matter of hours. But today, 11 months later, Myers is still alive. He is no longer even an invalid in the usual sense of the word. He is back at his old desk with an oil company, and he is living comfortably at home with Kari and their three young children. To the casual observer, John Myers looks and acts just like everybody else. But he is different, in a very special way. There is now a small U-shaped plastic tube sutured into the blood vessels of his left forearm.

Every Monday and Thursday afternoon Myers takes an hour long ferryboat ride across Puget Sound from Bremerton to downtown Seattle. By 6 p.m. he is making his way down a short flight of steps to an unmarked basement door in an annex of Swedish Hospital. Inside, he exchanges his business suit for a green hospital gown and climbs into bed. A compact hunk of medical plumbing which looks like a stainless steel washing machine is wheeled to Myers' bedside. From its innards a technician unfurls a pair of clear plastic tentacles six feet long. A nurse connects these to the little tube in Myers' forearm, and twiddles a few controls. Suddenly, in one bright spurt, one of the tentacles becomes red as John Myers' blood rushes out to fill the beside machine.

The machine is an artificial kidney. Because it can be coupled at will to the U-shaped tube in Myers' forearm, it has become the first true artificial organ in medical history. For the rest of his life Myers will spend two nights a week joined by a plastic umbilical cord to this machine which keeps him alive.

At present the miraculous machine requires 10 to 12 hours to cleanse Myers' blood of accumulating poisons which otherwise would kill him. The procedure is quite painless, and Myers has now become so accustomed to the whole idea of surrendering his life's blood to a medical Laundromat twice a week that during the cleansing he just goes to sleep. A nurse monitors the blood-flow and makes sure he does not roll over and kink the tubing.

Every Tuesday and Friday morning his nurse brings Myers his breakfast—jam, tea, ersatz bread—checks his blood pressure, and unhooks him. He carefully weighs himself (he usually finds he has lost two to four pounds of excess fluids overnight), showers, drives back to the ferryboat and sails off to work.

John Myers knows that so long as he keeps his regular rendezvous with the machine, and so long as he sticks faithfully to a diet consisting chiefly of cornstarch mixtures, leafy vegetables and fruit, and so long as he takes scrupulous care of what is in effect a permanent open wound in his forearm, he should be able to live the semblance of a normal life. He knows too that without regular access to the machine he would die within a week or two.

Talking about his unique way of life. Myers today says, "When you go on the machine you feel absolutely nothing at all. You just watch the gal hook you up. I have no emotional reaction, and I'm glad I don't. I don't feel I'm a prisoner of the system—even though I know perfectly well I am." In the opinion of Myers' continuing good health as a diet and the rest of his strict regime.

The cause of John Myers' multiple agonies last Christmas is properly known as uremic poisoning and congestive heart failure due to end-stage kidney disease. Each year it kills about 100,000 people in the U. S. alone. Of these 100,00 doomed patients, only one in 50 at present can be considered a suitable candidate for wearing Seattle's new U-shaped tubes. These few have kidney disease in a fairly pure form, uncomplicated by other afflictions. They are both physically strong and emotionally mature enough to endure the treatment.

Today Seattle's Swedish Hospital cares regularly for five patients who wear the tubes. In addition to Myers, they are a car salesman, a physicist, and engineer and an aircraft worker. By the end of this year there will be five more. All 10 will be part of an unprecedented two-year trial program to determine whether and how the rugged and expensive new treatment—at present the cost is $15,000 a year per patient—can be made feasible on a mass, nationwide basis.

Until the results of the trial in Seattle are known, many doctors feel it would be premature to set up additional treatment centers elsewhere, even if unlimited funds were available. The same treatment which keeps John Myers and his four companions gratefully alive has driven less carefully selected patients to pray for a swift and merciful death.

As medicine advances and invents assorted other mechanical organs, millions of people with "fatal" diseases may be given the same second chance at life which John Myers was one of the first men in the world to receive. But the Brave New World in which people may literally have hearts of gold or nerves of steel is not yet at hand. In the interim, agonizing practical decisions must be made. For the present, someone must choose which one patient out of 50 shall be permitted to hook up to Seattle's life-giving machines and which shall be denied.

There is in Seattle a small little-known group of quite ordinary people who have now made this choice five times, and will make it five times more before this year is out. For John Myers and his fellow patients were not chosen by lot. They were not even chosen by physicians. Each was selected individually by an organization named "The Admissions and Policies Committee of the Seattle Artificial Kidney Center at Swedish Hospital." Behind this magnificent polysyllabic façade stand seven humble laymen. They are all high-minded, good-hearted citizens, much like the patients themselves, who are selected as a microcosm of society-at-large. They were appointed to their uncomfortable post by Seattle's King County Medical Society, and for more than a year now they have remained there voluntarily, anonymously and without pay.

These seven citizens are in fact a Life or Death Committee. With no moral or ethical guidelines save their own individual consciences, they must decide, in the words of the ancient Hebrew prayer, "Who shall live and who shall die; who shall attain the measure of man's days and who shall not attain it; who shall be at ease and who shall be afflicted." They do not much like the job.

In the summer of 1961 the seven members of Seattle's Life or Death Committee met for the first time. They were a lawyer, a minister, a banker, a housewife, an official of state government, a labor leader and a surgeon. Few of them know any of the others, and most had only a sketchy idea of their committee's true purpose. Needless to add, none of them had ever heard of John Myers, with whose life they would soon be so intimately involved.

At this first meeting the committee was briefed by two physicians, both kidney specialists, who described the new Artificial Kidney Center then under construction, and explained why some grim life-or-death choices would soon have to be made. The doctors explained that the committee would never be asked to make medical decisions. All prospective patients would be prescreened by a board of physicians which would weed out all medically or psychiatrically unsuitable candidates. This medical board in fact already made certain rather arbitrary decisions designed to lighten the committee's burden as much as possible.

For example, the doctors recommended that the committee begin by passing a rule to reject automatically all candidates over 45 years of age. Older patients with chronic kidney disease are too apt to develop other serious complications, the medical men explained. Also, the doctors thought that the committee should arbitrarily reject children. The nature of the treatment itself might cruelly torment and terrorize a child, and there were other purely medical uncertainties, such as whether a child forced to live under the dietary restrictions would be capable of growth. In any case, the doctors believed it would be a mistake to accept children and thereby be forced to reject heads of families with children of their own.

Finally, the two doctors conducting this initial briefing offered to sit in on all the committee's future meetings in an advisory capacity. "We told them frankly that there were no guidelines, they were on their own. We really dumped it on them," one of these doctors has since said.

Before this first session broke up, the seven stunned committee members gratefully voted to accept the doctors' offer of future guidance. They also voted to keep their own names strictly anonymous. At their second session, they decided they did not want to know the names of the patients either. They will be reading John Myers' real name for the first time in this article. Then they drew up a list of all the factors which they would weigh in making their selection: age and sex of patient; marital status and number of dependents; income; net worth; emotional stability, with particular regard to the patient's capacity to accept the treatment; educational background; nature of occupation, past performance and future potential; and name of people who could serve as references.

At the committee's third meeting they finally got around to facing the problem of choice head-on. Somehow they must drastically narrow the field of candidates. "Where do we begin—the universe? the solar system? the earth?" one committee member asked wryly. Finally they agreed to consider only those applicants who were residents of the state of Washington at the time the feasibility trial got under way. They justified this stand on the grounds that, since the basic research to develop the U-shaped tube had been done at the University of Washington Medical School and at its new University Hospital—both state-supported institutions—the people whose taxes had paid for the research should be its first beneficiaries. "This was arbitrary too," one committee member admits, "but we had to start somewhere!"

Six months after the first meeting, the Kidney Center was complete, special medical crews were trained, and the committee had hammered out its bylaws. In the same six months John Myers had changed from a healthy-appearing young executive to a tottering invalid too weak to stand up in the shower. The net effect of the preliminary committee bylaws had been to reduce the number of candidates for treatment that the odds for each remaining eligible, such as Myers, to be selected had increased from one in 50 to about one in four. At least these new odds could be rationally comprehended, the laymen felt.

The meetings of the Life or Death Committee are held in the small, ground-floor library of a nurse's residence hall in downtown Seattle. The room is actually only a few hundred feet away from the three-bed Kidney Center where John Myers and his fellow patients come to be hooked up to their life-giving machines. But save for the comings and goings of the white coated doctors, there is absolutely no traffic between the two rooms. Neither the patients nor the committee wish any such confrontations. Their relationship is far too intimate for casual informality. To protect the integrity of their work, the members of the committee do not disclose exactly how many meetings they have held or how many patients they have considered. But neither do they wish to conceal the way they try to reach a decision, and all seven members have contributed to the preparation of the following facsimile. The dialog has been pieced together from the memories of the people who spoke it. If the exchanges as recorded here seem stilted, the people are nonetheless real, as are the five patients under discussion, and the dynamics of the debate are wholly accurate. The lawyer, who is the committee's chairman, has just called the meeting to order.

LAWYER: The doctors have told us they will soon have two more vacancies at the Kidney Center, and they have submitted a list of five candidates for us to choose from.

HOUSEWIFE: Are they all equally sick?

Dr. MURRAY: (John A. Murray, M. D., Medical Director of the Kidney Center.) Patients Number One and Number Five can last only a couple more weeks. The others probably can go a bit longer. But for purposes of your selection, all five cases should be considered of equal urgency, because none of them can hold out until another treatment facility becomes available.

LAWYER: Are there any preliminary ideas?

BANKER: Just to get the ball rolling, why don't we start with Number One—the housewife from Walla Walla.

SURGEON: This patient could not commute for the treatment from Walla Walla, so she would have to find a way to move her family to Seattle.

BANKER: Exactly my point. It says here that her husband has no funds to make such a move.

LAWYER: Then you are proposing we eliminate this candidate on the grounds that she could not possibly accept treatment if it were offered?

MINISTER: How can we compare a family situation of two children, such as this woman in Walla Walla, with a family of six children such as patient Number Four—the aircraft worker?

STATE OFFICIAL: But are we sure the aircraft worker can be rehabilitated? I note he is already is too ill to work, whereas Number Two and Number Five, the chemist and the accountant, are both still able to keep going.

LABOR LEADER: I know from experience that the aircraft company where this man works will do everything possible to rehabilitate a handicapped employee. . . .

HOUSEWIFE: If we are still looking for the men with the highest potential of service to society, I think we must consider that the chemist and the accountant have the finest educational backgrounds of all five candidates.

SURGEON: How do the rest of you feel about Number Three—the small businessman with three children? I am impressed that his doctor took special pains to mention this man is active in church work. This is an indication to me of character and moral strength.

HOUSEWIFE: Which certainly would help him conform to the demands of the treatment. . . .

LAWYER: It would also help him to endure a lingering death. . . .

STATE OFFICIAL: But that would seem to be placing a penalty on the very people who perhaps have the most provident. . . .

MINISTER: And both these families have three children too.

LABOR LEADER: For the children's sake, we've got to reckon with the surviving parents opportunity to remarry, and a woman with three children has a better chance to find a new husband than a very young widow with six children.

SURGEON: How can we possibly be sure of that? . . .

The central problem of such a Life or Death Committee is, of course, that nobody can be sure of anything. But at the end of an hour-and-a-half's discussion two patients actually were chosen. Both are alive and well today. One is the aircraft worker. The other is the small businessman, John Myers.

Because of the careful groundwork by the trustees of the medical society in appointing the seven members, Seattle's Life or Death Committee has functioned smoothly in its precedent-setting tasks. If the members have had private doubts, they have tried not to inflict them on one another or on their two doctor-advisers. But in private, the members do not shrink from facing or discussing their delicate assignment. On the contrary, they seem rather to welcome the opportunity to speak out about their uneasy doubts and hopes. THE LAWYER is prosperous, soft-spoken, and dead sure. One would not like to face him in court. He says, "When I was first invited to be on this committee, I said I would prefer not to serve. But I knew I was capable and I felt I would be impartial. We are dealing in this work with life that is being artificially sustained for experimental purposes. The so-called "rejected" patients would have died with or without the committee—as, of course, we all will some day. I cannot honestly say I am overwrought by the plight of the patients we do not choose—the ones we do choose have an awfully rugged life to look forward to. Not all men would wish it.

"As human beings ourselves, we rejected the idea instinctively of classifying other human beings in pigeonholes, but we realized we had to narrow the field somehow. Well, we didn't know it then, of course, but the very first rule we made—to take only candidates from the state of Washington—actually eliminated our very first candidate. She was a doctor's wife, from a neighboring state.

"Then I raised the question: what do we do if someone of great wealth says to us. "Take my candidate, and I'll finance your whole program here"? I tried to point out that this is a two-sided problem: special attention to one candidate might well work out for the greatest benefit to all. But the others couldn't see it that way.

"We soon realized that our committee was of such a totally new nature that it was useless to try to anticipate our problems; we would only be borrowing trouble. The fact is that progress in this world comes about through the existence of crises, not the anticipation of them. For example, how much chance would a great artist or composer have before our committee? In theory, I believe that a man's contribution to society should determine our ultimate decision. But I'm not so doggone sure that a great painting or a symphony would loom larger in my own mind than the needs of a woman with six children."

THE MINISTER is young and only rarely wears his collar. But when he doesn't, he has an incomplete look. He says, "I went into this thing with a sense of bewilderment. I had never heard of this research or met any of these other people before I was asked to serve. After our first meeting, I was very bothered. I felt I was forced to make decisions I had no right to make, and I felt that, of necessity, our selections would have to be made on the basis of inadequate information. Yet oddly enough, in the choices I have made, the correct decision appeared quite clear to me in each case. The principle of this thing has bothered me more than the practice.

"As we tried to work out our ground rules for selection, I felt a deep sense of awe, almost that we were going beyond our domain. As a clergyman, I have to deal a great deal with life and death, and there has been something helpful to me in recognizing life with some degree of reverence. I know that even with the best of care, there comes a time when life—physical life, as we know it—ceases to be. The realization that each of us is going to die suggests to me that, so long as we are a part of life, we are in a position of responsibility to use that life to help others.

"In the years since my ordination, I find too that my own viewpoint toward death has changed. Death itself is not the worst thing that can happen to a man, and just to live is not the greatest blessing. I've often lain awake nights wondering: would I want to take this treatment, if it became a medical necessity for me? But then I've thought: well, wouldn't refusing treatment be a sorry admission of cowardice—an easy way to escape my responsibility to my wife and children?

"In my work on the committee, I tend to favor those candidates who have younger children. My thinking on this is—a child who is older has had the privilege of a parent longer, and ought to be better prepared to face life alone. But I often wonder—suppose I should somehow meet a man I had voted against? What would I say to him? I believe I would face it. I would tell him my reasons. The purpose of our committee is to protect the medical men from just such highly emotional situations. If they have to go through emotional stress, they cannot conserve their energies for their own work. A doctor's job is the practice of medicine. My job is to help people form a set of life values. And to help them accept the fact that, like birth, death itself is a part of life—not, wham, the door slams!"

THE HOUSEWIFE is an uncommonly pretty grandmother and she is no fool. She says, "All my life I have always been disgustingly healthy. Perhaps for that reason, I am not at all medically minded. In fact, the truth is that I think doctors are apt to be terribly stuffy—especially about new things. So it is wonderful to me to have a chance to help in a real breakthrough. This is not something like cancer, where you still don't know. This treatment works! That gives me terrific hope.

"I realize the doctors must use people, not animals, for this research, and I think in a funny way that actually helps me to serve on the committee. Because I do like people so much. I feel our own anonymity is vitally important too, because it is only if we are truly unknown that we really can be a buffer for the medical profession.

"At the same time I do wish we could somehow see the patient and get a personal impression. It is so hard to judge from a sheet of paper whether or not a man could take the treatment and hold-on. I know he'd have to be an optimist by nature because it does limit your life.

"You know, the doctors usually give us their estimate of how long a patient will live without treatment, and this information affects our thinking a good deal. We always have hope that by some miracle the facilities can be enlarged in time to save the patient who has some chance of living longer without this treatment."

THE BANKER is direct and peppery. He looks like a retired general. He says, "I've never had any idea how a kidney works, and I still don't. But I do have reservations about the moral aspects, the propriety of choosing A and not B. for whatever reason. I have often asked myself—as a human being, do I have that right? I don't really think I do. I finally came to the conclusion that we are not making a moral choice here—we are picking guinea pigs for experimental purposes. This happens to be true: it also happens to be the way I rationalize my presence on this committee.

"The situation, as I see it, is life and death, complicated by limitations of money. In this situation our function is to take the pressure off the doctors. I don't know if we're doing the right thing or not. Maybe this whole deal is futile. Probably it is, in a sense, now, but maybe some economics of operation can come out of it so that everyone who needs treatment can have it, without becoming a burden on society. It costs $15,000 a year to keep each of these patients alive. And once you put a man on the artificial kidney, it's for life. His life. Where is the money coming from?

"We have limited funds, we take whom we can, and that's it. So far, fortunately, we have not had to make a choice between two absolutely equal candidates. I suspect that somehow the doctors started us out this way deliberately, to make things easier on us until we got used to the idea of choosing. But what happens when we get two men with the same job, the same number of children, the same income, and so forth? We could face that dilemma at any moment.

"I have asked myself—suppose I got this kidney disease, would I apply for treatment? Well, I think I would, like a shot! And if I was denied it, I'd feel bitter. I'd think society would owe it to me if they owe it to another individual.

"We send billions of dollars overseas to people we know nothing about, many of whom despise us. If Congress or somebody wanted to provide the money, we could take care of all our kidney people. But where do we stop? Who decides who needs treatment? The federal government would soon be treating the medically ill, alcoholics, old people, blind people, deaf people, people who need false teeth—everybody! Is this what we really want? I frankly don't know."

THE STATE OFFICIAL acts so meek and mild he almost manages to conceal his flashing intellect. He says, "The central problem here is that medicine has moved forward so rapidly it has advanced beyond the community's support. Our committee must try to bridge the gap. Our chief problem so far has been inadequate information. We have forced ourselves to make life-or-death decisions on a virtually intuitive basis. I do have real faith in the ability of kindly, conscientious, intelligent people to do a good job guided simply by their instincts, but we ought not to go on this way.

"Up to now, our only source of information has been the patient's personal physician, and he is in no position to ask the questions we want answered because he knows we might turn his patient down. In any case, a physician isn't geared to this approach. He is under the pressure of urgent medical problems. The committee needs its own staff of private investigators; a social worker, a vocational guidance counselor and a psychiatrist. We agreed to set up such a staff at our last meeting. We did not do this sooner because for a long time we feared that going directly to the patient for information would cruelly raise false hopes.

"I have come to believe we can tell the patient, if we say something like this: In order to help you best—a person who has a chronic illnesses, and who may be expected to have it for a long time—it is necessary to know as much about you as possible. I believe patients will understand our attitude. The resources of the human spirit in adversity are truly remarkable. These people can face more than we give them credit for.

THE LABOR LEADER wears an old-fashioned gold watch chain and the scrubbed, pragmatic expressions of a railroad conductor with long tenure. He says, "The way I look at it, if the Seattle trial is to be a pilot for other committees, we cannot afford any human failures. Also, we just haven't got the funds. So I want to pick the man with the most will power, the fellow who is least likely to give up.

"Suppose we take someone on the program, keep him going for three months, and then he blows up on us? Suppose he fails to take care of himself, or follow his diet, or gets depressed and tries to take his own life? That can happen in these cases, you know. Well, this would deprive another patient of the opportunity we can offer. That's why knowing about a candidate's past life would rate so heavily with me—it's an indication of character. A man's job, his education, his wealth—that means nothing to me. But I do think a man ought to have some religion, because that indicates character. And I imagine a large family would be a great help—a lot of kids help keep a man from letting down even when the going gets rough.

"The wonderful thing to me about this work is that we are finally past the stage of experiment. We know we can prolong life. These doctors got an idea and they made it work. With the mass production facilities we have in the country, I believe we can eventually take care of everybody. Meanwhile we say to these patients, in effect, "We're going to help you prolong your life by choosing to put you on this machine. Now, what can you do for us?"

THE SURGEON is an enormous man with a tiny voice, a courtly air and great patience. He says, "Medically speaking. I am not a disciple of this particular approach to kidney disease. But in the larger view, this project will not just benefit one disease—it will benefit all aspects of medicine. We are hoping someday to learn how to transplant live organs. So far, the body will not accept foreign tissue from another person, but eventually we will find a way to break this tissue barrier. Meanwhile I serve on this committee not as a doctor but as a citizen and, I hope, a humanitarian.

"You know, at our committee's first meeting we seriously discussed selecting candidates by drawing straws. We were going to make it easy on ourselves by having a human lottery! Frankly, I was almost ready to vote for the lottery idea myself. In the practice as a surgeon, the responsibility of making life-or-death choice faces me practically every day, and I can tell you this: I do sleep better at night after deciding on one of these committee cases than I sleep after deciding a case of my own. I'm awfully glad, too, that we just know these candidates by number, not their actual names.

"Being a medical man, I sometimes hear it via the grapevine when a patient whom we have passed over dies. Each time this happens there always comes a feeling of deep regret, and then the dreadful doubt—perhaps we chose the wrong man. One can just never face these situations without feeling a little sick inside. . . ."

The concept of the little U-shaped tube that started it all germinated two years ago in the mind of a deceptively mild professor of medicine at the University of Washington Medical School named Belding H. Scribner. Within a week the first experimental tube was made and sutured into the arm of a patient who was on his deathbed from Bright's disease. It worked—the man is alive today—and within a month it was successful again then three more "hopeless" cases. Then abruptly for 13 months, the entire experiment was shut down. Before taking on any more patients it was necessary to perfect certain practical techniques. In the beginning, the tubes wore out too fast, or clotted, or became infected and had to be removed and resewn into other parts of the body. The early machines themselves were tricky to handle. The primary need was to simplify the entire technique from a complicated "operating room" type of procedure to a relatively simple routine, like making ex-rays. Until this was done, the technique would remain more a research triumph than a new treatment.

The problem was solved literally in the bodies of the four original patients at the University Hospital. The very first was Clyde Shields, a 42-year-old machinist, who has now survived the implantation of 11 successive sets of U-shaped tubes and has lived totally without any natural kidney function for over two years. Despite his ordeal as a human guinea pig, Shields says he feels better now than at any time since his treatment began.

The most battle-scarred of the original patients is a high-spirited shoe salesman named Harvey Gentry. One month after his treatments, Gentry felt so well he decided to go clam-digging. He got sand in his first set of tubes, lost others through infections, and is now on his 13th set. "I've given the docs a pretty bad time, but they've learned a lot from me and they always manage to keep ahead somehow," he says with apparently indestructible optimism.

Another of these research patients is 37-year-old Kathy Curtiss. Between visits to University Hospital for treatments, she is able to carry on a full schedule of cooking and housekeeping for her husband and two teenage sons. These patients and the dedicated University of Washington medical team which works with them have now proved that the new technique can be made to work. At the same time these patients are living proof that the possibilities of mass treatment must be determined at once.

During the 13-month moratorium on the experimental program, no new patients were accepted, and truly cloak-and-dagger measures were taken to keep the story out of the newspapers. Already, as word of the experiment circulated within the medical fraternity, the doctors were receiving agonizing appeals from colleagues to take on more patients than they could possibly care for. To avoid such intolerable pressures, the novel double-screening device of a medical board back-stopped by a lay committee was proposed in the application for a $250,000 research grant which was made to the John A. Hartford Foundation. Then, even before they were sure the money would come through, the doctors went to the trustees of their own medical association and asked them to appoint members of both the board and the committee.

The trustees agreed to act. This was a crucial decision. It meant acceptance of the principle that all segments of society, not just the medical fraternity, should share the burden of choice as to which patients to treat and which to let die. Otherwise society would be forcing the doctors alone to play God.

As a buffer between the doctors and the public, the committee has functioned well. It has protected doctors from having to make intolerable choices among their own patients. But in the 11 months of its operation a host of new problems has arisen to plague both doctors and laymen which neither group anticipated at the outset.

What happens to the kidney patient who has been maintained in good health by the machine for some time and then suddenly has a stroke or gets cancer? Is he now removed from the machine in favor of a "healthier" patient who only has one fatal disease, not two? Who decides? The patient? The doctor? The committee?

Compared to other vital organs, the kidney is relatively simple in function. It is a filter. What happens when, sooner or later, medicine learns to manufacture other artificial organs? Are we moving, in the name of science and mercy, toward a nightmare world in which a segment of our population is kept alive by being hooked up to ingenious machines operated by the other half? In such a world the most fit individuals would devote their lives to keeping the least fit alive.

Consider, also, a few of the strictly practical problems which have actually arisen in the committee's recent sessions. The patient's case history is written up by his own physician. Some doctors write better than others. How should the committee avoid being swayed by the inadequacy or excellence of the presentation?

In any event, the facts at the past meetings have seemed inadequate. But in the future, when a committee has in its employ a professional social worker, a vocational counselor and a psychologist to report on each patient, how can the relative abilities of these three staff members—say, their ability to write up case reports—be judges? And won't they have unconscious prejudices? And won't they have to be anonymous too? And if all these questions are fairly answered, then won't the committee be abdicating its own responsibilities and making the little three man subcommittee bear the dreadful burden of choice?

No matter who decides, aren't the final choices all shaky, all arbitrary, all relative? They depend on a patient's unique worth, but on his comparative position in a particular slate of candidates. Who really is the more suitable patient under the present committee rules—the man who, if he is permitted to continue living, can make the greatest contribution to society; or the man who by dying would leave behind the greatest burden on society?

On the basis of the past year's record, a candidate who plans to come before this committee would seem well-advised to father a great many children, then to throw away all his money, and finally to fall ill in a season when there will be minimum of competition from other men dying of the same disease.

As the shock waves of each new committee decision reverberate further and wider over our moral and social landscape, we can look back to John Myers' hospital room the afternoon following Christmas Day. The delicate two and-a-half-hour operation to implant the tube in his arm was done at his bedside, under local anesthetic. As soon as the surgeon finished, the artificial kidney was wheeled into the room and hooked up. Myers' long, slow physical decline had unexpectedly accelerated so rapidly that there was no time to wait for the wounds in his arm to heal. Such sudden speedups and slowdowns are characteristic of the disease. They explain why, though by the committee, Myers' arm had not yet been prepared for the machine.

The kidney as set up at the head of Myers' bed, and he asked for his wife Kari and her compact so he could watch in its little mirror what happened to his blood. But what he mainly remembers is staring at the frightening sight of his own face. "My skin had turned funny, dark-gray color, my eyes were pink, and I looked exactly like a very sick seal."

By mid-January, Myers was able to return home, and soon he went back to work, though only for an hour at a time. Now he is up to a seven-hour day and he feels better than he has in two years. "Of course I never feel like running a race or staying up all night," he admits. "Like all the patients, I still have high blood pressure, and I still get tired easily. But at least I'm like other people again."

Like the other patients, Myers is a veteran of many grimly efficient hospitals and he is greatly impressed by the easygoing, casual atmosphere at the Kidney Center. Indeed, at times he finds the whole place almost impossible to believe. So do outside visitors who happen to drop in. While their blood percolates through the machines alongside them, the patients read, chat, eat, watch TV or simply drift off to sleep. All the patients and the medical personnel call each other by their first names, and they all appear as cheery and relaxed and downright folksy as the customers and the attendants at an exclusive health spa. Says Myers, "What a terrific experience this has been"! Even if we were paying through the nose, we wouldn't expect this kind of attention. The personal care they give you here—it borders on affection."

Though all the patients at the center are now aware that they owe their lives as much to a committee of unknown laymen as they do to the doctors and nurses and machines, they find the committee a far more difficult subject to talk about. John Myers says, "I guess that as long as facilities are not unlimited, somebody has to pick and choose. And then they have to go home and sleep at night. What a dreadful decision! It's like trying to play God. Frankly, I'm surprised the doctors were able to round up seven people who were willing to take the job."

Further Resources

Relevant Organizations

Governmental

Social Security Administration: The United States Old-Age, Survivors, and Disability Insurance federal program. Additional information can be found at www.ssa.gov/

Medical Research Council: Coordinates and funds research across the biomedical spectrum in the United Kingdom. Additional information can be found at www.mrc.ac.uk

Nongovernmental

United States Renal Data System: Collects, analyzes, and distributes information about chronic kidney disease and end-stage renal disease. Additional information can be found at https://www.usrds.org/

Literature

Greene, Jeremy A., and Kevin R. Riggs. "Why Is There No Generic Insulin? Historical Origins of a Modern Problem." *New England Journal of Medicine* 372, no. 12 (2015): 1171–1175.

Lax, Eric, *The Mold in Dr. Florey's Coat: The Story of the Penicillin Miracle* (New York: Holt Paperbacks, 2005).

Liverpool Medical Institution. Recent exhibitions: Battlefield Surgery: Baron Dominique-Jean Larrey (1766–1842).

National Archives and Record Administration. "Records of the War Production Board." http://www.archives.gov/research/guide-fed-records/groups/179.html

Romm, Cari. "The World War II Campaign to Bring Organ Meats to the Dinner Table," *The Atlantic*, September 25, 2014.

Social Security Administration. "1972 Social Security Amendments." https://www.ssa.gov/history/1972amend.html

The Library of Congress. "The Office of Scientific Research and Development (ORSD) Collection." https://www.loc.gov/rr/scitech/trs/trsosrd.html

Other Media

Alda, Alan. *M*A*S*H*. DVD. Directed by Robert Altman. Los Angeles: 20th Century Fox, 2009: US soldiers in the Korean War face medical and food supply scarcity

Broderick, Matthew. *Glory*. DVD. Directed by Edward Zwick. Culver City: Sony Pictures Home Entertainment, 1989: During the US Civil War, both medical staff and soldiers face issues of scarcity.

Kitchen, Michael. *Foyle's War*. DVD. Directed by Stuart Orme and Andy Hay. London: Acorn DVD, 2015: A WW II era detective series includes examples of historical rationing.

West, Dominic. *Breaking The Mould—The Story of Penicillin*. DVD. Directed by Peter Hoar. London: Digital Classics DVD, 2009: The story of the development of penicillin.

Woods, Grahame, "Glory Enough for All," Directed by Eric Till. Television Movie. PBS, 1988: Depicts the discovery of insulin.

5

Theories and Principles of Rationing

The recurrent and persistent scarcity of medical interventions creates an imperative to allocate those resources fairly. History, from the discovery of insulin to the manufacture of penicillin to the development of chronic dialysis, has revealed some progress in these allocation decisions. The revelation of the so-called God Committee in Seattle and its method of selecting people for chronic dialysis—and the criticism of its allocation decisions—indicates that we needed a more defensible approach to the rationing of absolutely scarce resources. Beginning in the 1960s, there evolved more systematic, ethical approaches.

The first major step was to take equality seriously. In 1969, Nicholas Rescher, a highly respected professor of philosophy, identified five elements that he thought should "figure primarily among the plausible criteria of selection" (Excerpt 1).[1] He groups them into two biomedical factors, a family factor, and two social factors: (1) relative likelihood of success of the procedure itself; (2) life-expectancy (i.e., prognosis of the procedure); (3) family, so that "the mother of minor children must take priority over the middle aged-bachelor"; (4) future contribution or the prospective value of the "services to be rendered by the patient" to society; and (5) reward for past "services rendered."[2] Rescher proposes using these five factors to create a scoring system and then "introduce[s] an element of chance."[3] Specifically, Rescher proposes a "lottery of life and death" among patients with roughly equal claims based on the five criteria.[4] In his view, this approach would introduce equal chances for people which makes it both "easier for the rejected patient" and the administrators of the selection system.[5] Silverman and Chalmers also

---

[1] N. Rescher, "The Allocation of Exotic Medical Lifesaving Therapy," *Ethics* 79, no. 3 (1969): pp. 173–186.

[2] Ibid., pp. 178–179.

[3] Ibid., p. 183.

[4] Ibid.

[5] Ibid., p. 184.

support a lottery for selection because it is inherently fair (Excerpt 2).[6]

Kamm explores the choice between equal treatment and equal chances (Excerpt 3).[7] She raises the question of whether saving greater numbers of lives can be justified in ways that do not just rely on there being more people saved, but are also being able to independently convince the fewer people why the more people should be saved. This abstract thought applies directly to organ transplantation. Often, there's a choice, in principle, between transplanting two organs—such as a kidney and liver—to save one person or to use them in separate surgeries to save two people. The question Kamm addresses is: Is it possible to give the single person who needs two organs a good reason why two people should be saved that does not just count on there being two?

Kamm's answer is that we do not just count people's lives, but we count "equally each individual's preferences" for who should get the scarce resource. This respects each person by counting his or her preferences regarding the optimal allocation system. Presumably, each individual will want to be saved, and thus two people's preferences will be to not transplant more than one organ in each recipient. But Kamm notes that it is possible that each person's preference is to give the organs to the person who needs both the liver and kidney. If that was the case, we would not save the greatest number, as individuals who needed organs agreed it was better to save fewer people.

Kamm also examines the situation in which we need to save one person in order to save many other people. The example she explores is whether it is ethical to use a scarce drug to save a surgeon whose operations would save 100 others, or, instead, to save 5 people who all need the scarce drug (but cannot directly save further lives). She seems to believe the surgeon's instrumental role in savings others counts as a reason to give him preference over saving the 5 people. We could save 101 rather than 5. Here, Kamm suggests that equal treatment allows us to consider a person's instrumental role in saving others.

Many people are not satisfied by giving people equal chances for scarce resources. And they are not convinced that providing equal treatment to everyone is the right approach. They ask whether it is ethical to treat young people and old people the same. Should the young and the old somehow count equally when we are rationing a scarce medical resource like an organ for transplantation? Or is there a reason to give preference to the younger person?

Daniel Callahan argues for limiting health-care resources to the old (Excerpt 4).[8] He wants to restrict "life extending high technology care for those who have lived out a natural lifespan," which he says is somewhere between the early 70s and early 80s.[9] It is important for people to live a good life, he argues, but once they have reached that "natural lifespan" society should not invest more in trying to find life-extending treatments or in giving the old life-extending treatments. Older people past the natural lifespan should get treatments to relieve their symptoms and the physical limitations of chronic illness, but the fight against inevitable death should not be a priority for either research or care. According to Callahan "a society in which all were assisted to live out a full life span was more tolerable and humane" than one focused on prolonging life no matter what.[10]

Similarly, British health economist Alan Williams defends a "fair innings" view to allocating scarce resources (Excerpt 5).[11] "Everyone is entitled to some 'normal span' of health. . . . [A]nyone failing to achieve this has in some

[6] W. A. Silverman and I. Chalmers, "Casting and Drawing Lots: A Time Honoured Way of Dealing with Uncertainty and Ensuring Fairness," *BMJ* 323, no. 7327 (2001): pp. 1467–1468.

[7] F. M. Kamm, "Equal Treatment and Equal Chances," *Philosophy & Public Affairs* 14, no. 2 (1985): pp. 177–194.

[8] D. Callahan, *Setting Limits: Medical Goals in an Aging Society* (Georgetown University Press, 1995), pp. 133–158.

[9] Ibid., p. 148.

[10] Ibid., p. 156.

[11] A. Williams, "Intergenerational Equity: An Exploration of the 'Fair Innings' Argument," *Health Economics* 6, no. 2 (1997): pp. 117–132.

sense been cheated."[12] Thus, Williams argues, younger people should receive priority over older people for scarce medical resources. Williams points out several advantages of "fair innings." Unlike a lottery that focuses on a fair process, "fair innings" seeks to equalize outcomes. In addition, it evaluates "a person's whole life-time experience" rather than a moment in time.[13] That is, it does not ask who is sickest now, but who has had a worse life overall. And living a short life is worse than living a long life. "Fair innings" is quantifiable; it is easy to assess age in ways that make sense. "Death at 25 is viewed very differently from death at 85."[14] Finally, it might be noted, there appears to be strong public support for giving preference to the younger person over the older person for scarce medical resources.[15]

John Harris asks whether "fair innings" is ageist (Excerpt 6).[16] After all, each of us wishes to live. By not getting an organ or other potentially life-saving medical intervention, each person will lose the same valuable thing: "the rest of our lives." As Harris argues: "However short or long my life will be, so long as I want to go on living it then I suffer a terrible injustice when that life is prematurely cut short."[17] Harris also points out counterarguments and begrudgingly seems to accept that while dying as an older person is a misfortune, it is not a tragedy—whereas dying as a younger person is both a misfortune and a tragedy. Ultimately, he wants to restrict the use of the "fair innings" approach to moments of "despair, when it is clearly impossible to postpone the deaths of all those who wanted to go on living" and choices have to be made—that is, cases of absolute scarcity.[18]

[12] Ibid., p. 119.

[13] Ibid.

[14] Ibid.

[15] A. Tsuchiya, P. Dolan, and R. Shaw, "Measuring People's Preferences Regarding Ageism in Health: Some Methodological Issues and Some Fresh Evidence," *Social Science & Medicine* 57, no. 4 (2003): pp. 687–696.

[16] J. Harris, *The Value of Life: An Introduction to Medical Ethics* (New York: Routledge, 1990), pp. 87–110.

[17] Ibid., p. 89.

Erik Nord offers a different critique of "fair innings" and favoring the young (Excerpt 7).[19] He notes that fair innings determines who should receive scarce resources by assessing their health losses over a lifetime; that is, in the past, present, and future. Nord advocates ignoring past health losses and only focusing on present and future losses. His "severity approach is meant to encapsulate a concern for those who are worse off *now and/or in the future*."[20] In some ways, Nord's argument is a version of giving priority to the sickest first. He points out that, in some cases, his severity of illness approach and fair innings will give the same result, but in others, they will diverge. In particular, people who have lived a long time, say to 70 years of age, and then have a significant decline in their health, are given priority by the severity of illness approach. Fair innings, by contrast, would give these people less priority, as they have already lived close to a "normal life span."

Moss and Siegler address the question initially raised by the Seattle God Committee and Rescher about how people's past—specifically their past medical behavior—should be considered in rationing scarce medical resources (Excerpt 8).[21] Many seem to believe that people should be held responsible for their past conduct in regards to health. If they contributed to their ill health, they should therefore receive lower priority. Moss and Siegler argue that alcoholics should "not compete equally with other candidates for liver transplantation. . . . [They] should be lower on the list than others with [end-stage liver disease]."[22] While alcoholism is a disease, they argue, it is a chronic disease,

[18] Ibid., p. 94.

[19] E. Nord, "Concerns for the Worse Off: Fair Innings Versus Severity," *Social Science & Medicine* 60, no. 2 (2005): pp. 257–263.

[20] Ibid., p. 259.

[21] A. H. Moss and M. Siegler, "Should Alcoholics Compete Equally for Liver Transplantation?", *JAMA* 265, no. 10 (1991): pp. 1295–1298.

[22] Ibid., p. 1296.

unlike, say mushroom poisoning. Thus, patients have had a long time to accept the diagnosis and assume responsibility for seeking and implementing treatment for their disease. For an alcoholic to need a liver transplant indicates that he has not accepted this responsibility. Therefore, he should not receive priority for an absolutely scarce resource, denying other people who could not have avoided their need for treatment in this way a life-saving chance.

Ubel and colleagues decided to test the public's judgments about personal responsibility and rationing decisions (Excerpt 9).[23] They found that prognosis was important. As prognosis declined, people were less willing to give patients organs for transplantation. Consistent with Moss and Siegler's view, past behaviors did influence how people ration scarce medical resources. Intravenous drug users received significantly fewer organs even when they had a better long-term prognosis. People justified their answer by saying that the drug abusers "cause their own illness."[24]

Over time, it has become clear that no single principle, not prognosis, not equality of chances, not prioritizing younger people fully captures the values people think should inform decisions about how to allocate absolutely scarce medical resources. Multiple values are important. Persad and colleagues aim to delineate all the principles that might be considered relevant to rationing scarce resources and then explore how to integrate them into a multiprinciple framework (Excerpt 10).[25] Synthesizing the previous work, they argue that there are four primary ethical values that should influence the allocation of scarce medical resources: equality, priority for the worst off, utility, and social value. Each of these values can be interpreted and realized by two principles. For instance, equality can be realized by the principles of lottery or first-come, first served. Priority for the worst-off can be realized by the principles of sickest-first or youngest-first.

Persad and colleagues then note that no single principle is sufficient. People believe prognosis is important, but they also believe that the youngest should get priority, too. They propose a multiprincipled allocation framework they call the *complete lives account* that integrates five principles. It emphasizes that younger people should receive priority. But, unlike fair innings, the complete lives account argues against a strict youngest-first principle and instead emphasizes giving priority to adolescents and young adults. Younger children have less attachment to the future, have invested less in developing their skills and life plans, and society has invested less in cultivating their abilities and talents. The complete lives account then integrates prognosis—saving the most life years—and saving the most lives. A lottery can be introduced when there is a tie among potential recipients of scarce resources (after using youngest-first, prognosis, and saving the most lives). Finally, Persad and colleagues argue that in public health emergencies, when saving a health care worker or first responder will save more lives, it is appropriate to give them priority. Using the complete lives account, they offer criticism of the current American policy of allocating livers based upon the Model for End-Stage Liver Disease (MELD) score that heavily emphasizes sickest-first, as well as other organ transplantation and ICU bed allocation policies that emphasize first-come, first-served.

Kerstein and Bognar criticize the complete lives account (Excerpt 11).[26] They argue that it fails in part because some of the principles, such as the modified youngest-first principle, do not have secure moral foundations. More importantly, it fails to provide practical guidance in critical cases. Kerstein and Bognar raise a number of cases that, they argue, show tensions between the principles that make up the complete lives account with no way to resolve

[23] P. A. Ubel, J. Baron, and D. A. Asch, "Social Acceptability, Personal Responsibility, and Prognosis in Public Judgments and Transplant Allocation," *Bioethics* 13, no. 1 (1999): pp. 57–68.

[24] Ibid., p. 62.

[25] G. Persad, A. Wertheimer, and E. Emanuel, "Principles for Allocation of Scarce Medical Interventions," *Lancet* 373, no. 9661 (2009): pp. 423–431.

[26] S. J. Kerstein and G. Bognar, "Complete Lives in the Balance," *American Journal of Bioethics* 10, no. 4 (2010): pp. 37–45.

the conflicts. For instance, three 18-year-olds all need transplants. One needs a heart and lung. The other two each needs a heart or lung. Transplanting the heart and lung into one patient might allow that patient to live a complete life, while transplanting each individual organ will save two people but only for a few years. This principle of save-the-most-people conflicts with the principle of allowing people to live a complete life. Which should be determinative? Kerstein and Bognar suggest the complete lives account does not offer guidance on how to resolve this conflict. Instead, they offer a "balancing" approach in which it is determined how much each person realizes of a principle: "We begin by determining the proportion between the values relative to each principle that are manifested in the sets of person who are in competition for the resources. . . . The set that contributes the higher value to the proportion relative to a principle is 'favored' on that principle."[27] Then, by adding up the proportions, Kerstein and Bognar determine who gets the scarce resource.

Reviewing the history of ethical theories for allocating absolutely scarce medical resources indicates that there has been an important evolution. Increasingly, the set of important ethical values and principles that play a role in allocating these resources has become clearer. In addition, the importance of having to integrate and use multiple principles has also become clearer. Which ethical principles should ultimately be incorporated into any multiprinciple theory, and how these multiple principles are integrated and balanced, remains controversial.

[27] Ibid., p. 43.

Questions for Discussion

1. Multicriteria sets of principles such as Nicholas Rescher's or those by Persad, Wertheimer, and Emanuel raise the question of whether principles should be ordered hierarchically. Defend doing so or refraining from doing so.
2. Alan Williams defends a "fair innings" view to allocating scarce resources in Excerpt 5. How would you implement this in practice?
3. In their discussion of the allocation of scarce medical interventions (Excerpt 10), Persad, Wertheimer, and Emanuel reject the principle of first-come, first-served. In practice, this could mean that, all other things being equal, a 70-year-old person in an ICU would need to give way to a 30-year-old. Argue in favor or against dropping the principle of first-come, first-served, paying particular attention to the consequences for how patients perceive hospitals.
4. Some of the authors in this section and some of the cited policy documents draw on public opinion research. In what way is it important to consider the public's views when it comes to identifying and justifying principles for allocating absolutely scare resources?

EXCERPTS

Note: The following excerpts have generally been edited for length, and omissions are indicated with ellipses. Editing includes footnotes and endnotes, which have also been renumbered. For citation and related purposes, the full original source texts should be used.

EXCERPT 1

Abridged text from:

N. Rescher, "The Allocation of Exotic Medical Lifesaving Therapy," *Ethics* 79, no. 3 (1969): pp. 173–186.

The Allocation of Exotic Medical Lifesaving Therapy

Nicholas Rescher

I. The Problem

Technological progress has in recent years transformed the limits of the possible in medical therapy. However, the elevated state of sophistication of modern medical technology has brought the economists' classic problem of scarcity in its wake as an unfortunate side product. The enormously sophisticated and complex equipment and the highly trained teams of experts requisite for its utilization are scarce resources in relation to potential demand. The administrators of the great medical institutions that preside over these scarce resources thus come to be faced increasingly with the awesome choice: Whose life to save?

A (somewhat hypothetical) paradigm example of this problem may be sketched within the following set of definitive assumptions: We suppose that persons in some particular medically morbid condition are "mortally afflicted": It is virtually certain that they will die within a short time period (say ninety days). We assume that some very complex course of treatment (e.g., a heart transplant) represents a substantial probability of life prolongation for persons in this mortally afflicted condition. We assume that the facilities available in terms of human resources, mechanical instrumentalities, and requisite materials (e.g., hearts in the case of a heart transplant) make it possible to give a certain treatment—this "exotic (medical) lifesaving therapy," or ELT for short—to a certain, relatively small number of people. And finally we assume that a substantially greater pool of people in the mortally afflicted condition is at hand. The problem then may be formulated as follows: How is one to select within the pool of afflicted patients the ones to be given the ELT treatment in question; how to select those "whose lives are to be saved"? Faced with many candidates for an ELT process that can be made available to only a few, doctors and medical administrators confront the decision of who is to be given a chance at survival and who is, in effect, to be condemned to die.

. . .

The selection problem, as we have said, is in substantial measure not a medical one. It is a problem for medical men, which must somehow be solved by them, but that does not make it a medical issue. . . . As a problem it belongs to the category of philosophical problems—specifically a problem of moral philosophy or ethics. Structurally, it bears a substantial kinship with those issues in this field that revolve about the notorious whom-to-save-on-the-lifeboat and whom-to-throw-to-the-wolves-pursuing-the-sled questions. But whereas questions of this just-indicated sort are artificial, hypothetical, and far-fetched, the ELT issue poses a genuine policy question for the responsible administrators in medical institutions, indeed a question that threatens to become commonplace in the foreseeable future.

. . .

IV. The Basic Screening Stage: Criteria of Inclusion (and Exclusion)

Three sorts of considerations are prominent among the plausible criteria of inclusion/exclusion at the basic screening stage: the constituency factor, the progress-of-science factor, and the prospect-of-success factor.

A. THE CONSTITUENCY FACTOR

. . .

It is a "fact of life" that ELT can be available only in the institutional setting of a hospital or medical institute or the like. Such institutions generally have normal clientele boundaries.

C. THE PROSPECT-OF-SUCCESS FACTOR

It may be that while the ELT at issue is not without some effectiveness in general, it has been established to be highly effective only with patients in certain specific categories (e.g., females under forty of a specific blood type). This difference in effectiveness in the absolute or in the probability of success is (we assume) so marked as to constitute virtually a difference in kind rather than in degree. In this case, it would be perfectly legitimate to adopt the general rule of making the ELT at issue available only or primarily to persons in this substantial promise-of-success category. . . .

V. The Final Selection Stage: Criteria of Selection

Five sorts of elements must figure primarily among the plausible criteria of selection: the relative-likelihood-of-success factor, the life expectancy factor, the family role factor, the potential-contributions factor, and the services-rendered factor. The first two represent the biomedical aspect, the second three the social aspect.

A. THE RELATIVE-LIKELIHOOD-OF-SUCCESS FACTOR

It is clear that the relative likelihood of success is a legitimate and appropriate factor in making a selection within the group of qualified patients that are to receive ELT. This is obviously one of the considerations that must count very significantly in a reasonable selection procedure.

. . . If the therapy at issue is not a once-and-for-all proposition and requires ongoing treatment, cognate considerations must be brought in. Thus, for example, in the case of a chronic ELT procedure such as haemodialysis it would clearly make sense to give priority to patients with a potentially reversible condition (who would thus need treatment for only a fraction of their remaining lives).

B. THE LIFE-EXPECTANCY FACTOR

Even if the ELT is "successful" in the patient's case he may, considering his age and/or other aspects of his general medical condition, look forward to only a very short probable future life. This is obviously another factor that must be taken into account.

C. THE FAMILY ROLE FACTOR

A person's life is a thing of importance not only to himself but to others—friends, associates, neighbors, colleagues, etc. But his (or her) relationship to his immediate family is a thing of unique intimacy and significance. The nature of his relationship to his wife, children, and parents, and the issue of their financial and psychological dependence upon him, are obviously matters that deserve to be given weight in the ELT selection process. Other things being anything like equal, the mother of minor children must take priority over the middle-aged bachelor.

D. THE POTENTIAL FUTURE-CONTRIBUTIONS FACTOR (PROSPECTIVE SERVICE)

In "choosing to save," one life rather than another, "the society," through the mediation of the particular medical institution in question—which should certainly look upon itself as a trustee for the social interest—is clearly warranted in considering the likely pattern of future services to be rendered by the patient (adequate recovery assumed), considering his age, talent, training, and past record of performance. In its allocations of ELT, society "invests" a scarce resource in one person as against another and is thus entitled to look to the probable prospective "return" on its investment.

It may well be that a thoroughly egalitarian society is reluctant to put someone's social contribution into the scale in situations of the sort at issue. One popular article states that "the most difficult standard would be the candidate's value to society," and goes on to quote someone who said: "You can't just pick a brilliant painter over a laborer. The average citizen would be quickly eliminated." But what if it were not a brilliant painter but a brilliant surgeon or medical researcher that was at issue? One wonders if the author of the obiter dictum that one "can't just pick" would still feel equally sure of his ground. In any case, the fact that the standard is difficult to apply is certainly no reason for not attempting to apply it. The problem of ELT selection is inevitably burdened with difficult standards.

Some might feel that in assessing a patient's value to society one should ask not only who if permitted to continue living can make the greatest contribution to society in some creative or constructive way, but also who by dying would leave behind the greatest burden on society in assuming the discharge of their residual responsibilities.[7] Certainly the philosophical utilitarian would give equal weight to both these considerations. Just here is where I would part ways with orthodox utilitarianism. For I should be prepared to argue that a civilized society has an obligation to promote the furtherance of positive achievements in cultural and related areas even if this means the assumption of certain added burdens.[1]

E. THE PAST SERVICES-RENDERED FACTOR (RETROSPECTIVE SERVICE)

A person's services to another person or group have always been taken to constitute a valid basis for a claim upon this person or group—of course a moral and not necessarily a legal claim. Society's obligation for the recognition and reward of services rendered—an obligation whose discharge is also very possibly conducive to self-interest in the long run—is thus another factor to be taken into account. This should be viewed as a morally necessary correlative of the previously considered factor of prospective service. It would be morally indefensible of society in effect to say: "Never mind about services you rendered yesterday—it is only the services to be rendered tomorrow that will count with us today." We live in very future-oriented times, constantly preoccupied in a distinctly utilitarian way with future satisfactions. And this disinclines us to give much recognition to past services. But parity considerations of the sort just adduced indicate that such recognition should be given on grounds of equity. No doubt a justification for giving weight to services rendered can also be attempted along utilitarian lines. ("The reward of past services rendered spurs people on to greater future efforts and is thus socially advantageous in the long-run future.") In saying that past services should be counted "on grounds of equity"—rather than "on grounds of utility"—I take the view that even if this utilitarian defense could somehow be shown to be fallacious, I should still be prepared to maintain the propriety of taking services rendered into account. The position does not rest on a utilitarian basis and so would not collapse with the removal of such a basis.[2]

These five factors fall into three groups: the biomedical factors A and B. the familial factor C, and the social factors D and E. . . . Factors A and B are ethically uncontroversial factors—their legitimacy and appropriateness are evident from the very nature of the case.

Greater problems arise with the familial and social factors. They involve intangibles

[1] Moreover a doctrinaire utilitarian would presumably be willing to withdraw a continuing mode of ELT such as haemodialysis from a patient to make room for a more promising candidate who came to view at a later stage and who could not otherwise be accommodated. I should be unwilling to adopt this course, partly on grounds of utility (with a view to the demoralization of insecurity), partly on the non-utilitarian ground that a "moral commitment" has been made and must be honored.

[2] Of course the difficult question remains of the relative weight that should be given to prospective and retrospective service in cases where these factors conflict. There is good reason to treat them on a par.

that are difficult to judge. How is one to develop subcriteria for weighing the relative social contributions of (say) an architect or a librarian or a mother of young children? And they involve highly problematic issues. (For example, should good moral character be rated a plus and bad a minus in judging services rendered?) And there is something strikingly unpleasant in grappling with issues of this sort for people brought up in times greatly inclined towards maxims of the type "Judge not!" and "Live and let live!" All the same, in the situation that concerns us here such distasteful problems must be faced, since a failure to choose to save some is tantamount to sentencing all. Unpleasant choices are intrinsic to the problem of ELT selection; they are of the very essence of the matter.[3]

. . . Why should the social aspect of services rendered and to be rendered be taken into account at all? The answer is that they must be taken into account not from the medical but from the ethical point of view. Despite disagreement on many fundamental issues, moral philosophers of the present day are pretty well in consensus that the justification of human actions is to be sought largely and primarily—if not exclusively—in the principles of utility and of justice." But utility requires reference of services to be rendered and justice calls for a recognition of services that have been rendered. Moral considerations would thus demand recognition of these two factors. . . .

VII. The Inherent Imperfection (Non-Optimality) of Any Selection System

. . .

These five factors are clearly insufficient for the construction of a reasonable selection system, since that would require not only that these factors be taken into account (somehow or other), but—going beyond this—would specify a specific set of procedures for taking account of them. The specific procedures that would constitute such a system would have to take account of the inter-relationship of these factors (e.g., B and E), and to set out exact guidelines as to the relevant weight that is to be given to each of them. . . .

In fact, I should want to maintain that there is no such thing here as a single rationally superior selection system. The position of affairs seems to me to be something like this: (1) It is necessary (for reasons already canvassed) to have a system, and to have a system that is rationally defensible, and (2) to be rationally defensible, this system must take the factors A–E into substantial and explicit account. But (3) the exact manner in which a rationally defensible system takes account 'of these factors cannot be fixed in any one specific way on the basis of general considerations. Any of the variety of ways that give A–E "their due" will be acceptable and viable. One cannot hope to find within this range of workable systems some one that is optimal in relation to the alternatives. There is no one system that does "the (uniquely) best"—only a variety of systems that do "as well as one can expect to do" in cases of this sort . . .

. . .

[3] This in the symposium on "Selection of Patients for Haemodialysis," *British Medical Journal* (March 11, 1967), pp. 622–624. F. M. Parsons writes: "But other forms of selecting patients [distinct from first come, first served] are suspect in my view if they imply evaluation of man by man. What criteria could be used? Who could justify a claim that the life of a mayor would be more valuable than that of the humblest citizen of his borough? Whatever we may think as individuals none of us is indispensable." But having just set out this hard-line view he immediately backs away from it: "On the other hand, to assume that there was little to choose between Alexander Fleming and Adolf Hitler . . . would be nonsense, and we should be naive if we were to pretend that we could not be influenced by their achievements and characters if we had to choose between the two of them. Whether we like it or not we cannot escape the fact that this kind of selection for long-term haemodialysis will be required until very large sums of money become available for equipment and services [so that everyone who needs treatment can be accommodated]."

VIII. A Possible Basis for a Reasonable Selection System

Having said that there is no such thing as the optimal selection system for ELT, I want now to sketch out the broad features of what I would regard as one acceptable system. The basis for the system would be a point rating. The scoring here at issue would give roughly equal weight to the medical considerations (A and B) in comparison with the extramedical considerations (C = family role, D = services rendered, and E = services to be rendered), also giving roughly equal weight to the three items involved here (C, D, and E). The result of such a scoring procedure would provide the essential starting point of our ELT selection mechanism. I deliberately say "starting point" because it seems to me that one should not follow the results of this scoring in an automatic way. I would propose that the actual selection should only be guided but not actually be dictated by this scoring procedure, along lines now to be explained.

IX. The Desirability of Introducing an Element of Chance

The detailed procedure I would propose would combine the scoring procedure just discussed with an element of chance. The resulting selection system would function as follows:

. . . If this group is relatively homogeneous as regards rating by the scoring procedure—that is, if there are no really major disparities within this group then the final selection is made by random selection of n persons from within this group.

This introduction of the element of chance—in what could be dramatized as a "lottery of life and death"—must be justified. The fact is that such a procedure would bring with it three substantial advantages.

First, as we have argued above, any acceptable selection system is inherently non-optimal. The introduction of the element of chance prevents the results that life-and-death choices are made by the automatic application of an admittedly imperfect selection method.

Second, a recourse to chance would doubtless make matters easier for the rejected patient and those who have a specific interest in him. It would surely be quite hard for them to accept his exclusion by relatively mechanical application of objective criteria in whose implementation subjective judgment is involved. But the circumstances of life have conditioned us to accept the workings of chance and to tolerate the element of luck (good or bad): human life is an inherently contingent process. Nobody, after all, has an absolute right to ELT—but most of us would feel that we have "every bit as much right" to it as anyone else in significantly similar circumstances. The introduction of the element of chance assures a like handling of like cases over the widest possible area that seems reasonable in the circumstances.

Third, such a recourse to random selection does much to relieve the administrators of the selection system of the awesome burden of ultimate and absolute responsibility.

These three considerations would seem to build up a substantial case for introducing the element of chance into the mechanism of the system for ELT selection in a way limited and circumscribed by other weightier considerations, along some such lines as those set forth above.[4]

It should be recognized that this injection of man-made chance supplements the element of natural chance that is present inevitably and in any case. . . . Life is a chancy business and even the most rational of human arrangements can cover this over to a very limited extent at best.

---

[4] One writer has mooted the suggestion that: "Perhaps the right thing to do, difficult as it may be to accept, is to select [for haemodialysis] from among the medical and psychologically qualified patients on a strictly random basis" (S. Gorovitz, "Ethics and the Allocation of Medical Resources," *Medical Research Engineering*, no. 5 [1966], p. 7). Outright random selection would, however, seem indefensible because of its refusal to give weight to considerations which, under the circumstances, deserve to be given weight. The proposed procedure of superimposing a certain degree of randomness upon the rational-choice criteria would seem to combine the advantages of the two without importing the worst defects of either.

Bibliography

S. Alexander, "They Decide Who Lives, Who Dies: Medical Miracle Puts a Moral Burden on a Small Committee," *Life*, November 9, 1962.

C. Doyle, "Spare-Part Heart Surgeons Worried by Their Success," *Observer* May 12, 1968.

J. Fletcher, *Morals and Medicine* (Princeton, N.J.: Princeton University Press, 1954).

L. Lader, "Who Has the Right to Live?", *Good Housekeeping*, January, 1968.

N. Nabarro, et al., "Selection of Patients for Haemodialysis," *BMJ* (1967): pp. 622–624.

H. M. Schmeck, "Panel Holds Life-or-Death Vote in Allotting of Artificial Kidney," *New York Times*, May 6, 1962.

EXCERPT 2

Abridged text from:

W. A. Silverman and I. Chalmers, "Casting and Drawing Lots: A Time Honoured Way of Dealing with Uncertainty and Ensuring Fairness," *BMJ* 323, no. 7327 (2001): pp. 1467–1468.

Casting and Drawing Lots: A Time Honoured Way of Dealing with Uncertainty and Ensuring Fairness

William A. Silverman and Iain Chalmers

The lot causeth disputes to cease, and it decideth between the mighty.

—Proverbs 18:18

. . .

An Age Old Custom

Jewish law and the early Christian church outlawed the casting lots for divination—at least by the faithful masses, if not by God's authorities on earth.[1] By contrast, casting or drawing lots to assure fairness in allocating duties or rewards has been acceptable for millennia. Human societies have used pebbles, nuts, barleycorn, bones, twigs, yarrow stalks, polished sticks, cards, coins, and dice—the list goes on and on—to make decisions that are transparently fair.

In the Book of Numbers the tribes of Israel are instructed to "Divide the land by lot, for an inheritance among your families"; and at the time of the second temple priests drew lots from the temple urn when differences arose in civil and everyday life.[2] At the end of the 18th century, when Britain was preparing for an expected French invasion of Ireland, each county and county borough was asked to provide a certain number of men for defensive militias. Lists of eligible men were drawn up by parish constables. Names were then randomly selected from the list until the quota for each district was complete.[3] Military draft lotteries were used in Austria-Hungary in 1889–1914 and in the United States and Australia during the Vietnam war.

Seen to Be Fair

Lotteries have been accepted as a fair, democratic way of making difficult choices.[4] The US secretary of the war department, speaking at the beginning of the 1917 military draft lottery, captured the essence of this idea: "This is an occasion of great dignity and some solemnity. It represents the first application of a principle believed by many of us to be thoroughly democratic, equal and fair in selecting soldiers to defend the national honor abroad and at home."[5]

Legal judgments have sometimes emphasised the fairness of drawing lots to decide matters of life and death. In considering a charge of manslaughter brought against a sailor in the 19th century, an American judge concluded, "When the ship is in no danger of sinking, but all sustenance is exhausted, and a sacrifice of one person is necessary to appease the hunger of others, the selection is by lot. This mode is resorted to as the fairest mode . . . we can conceive of no mode so consonant both to humanity and to justice."[6]

From solemn to less solemn uses, there are many uses of lots to ensure fairness these days. These range from deciding who should

---

[1] W. A. Silverman and I. Chalmers, "Casting and Drawing Lots: A Time Honoured Way of Dealing with Uncertainty and Ensuring Fairness," *British Medical Journal* 323, no. 7327 (2001): pp. 1467–1468.

[2] Ibid.

[3] MacAtasney Leitrim and the croppies, "1776–1804. Carrick-on-Shannon,C," Carrick-on-Shannon and District Historical Society, 1998.

[4] S. E. Fienberg, "Randomization and Social Affairs: The 1970 Draft Lottery," *Science* 171, no. 3968 (1971): pp. 255–261.

[5] Ibid.

[6] United States v. Holmes. 26 Fed Cas 360 (No 15383) (Cir Ct E Dist Pa), 1842.

be allocated limited quotas of immigration visas and university places to who should be allocated which dormitory rooms at university and who shall receive the sum of the separate investments of the millions of people who buy lottery tickets.

Lotteries in Health Care

Lottery has been used and is still used to ensure fairness in health care. In the 17th century, to settle a dispute he was having with orthodox practitioners who used bloodletting and purging for treatment, the Flemish physician John Baptiste Van Helmont made the following proposition: "Let us take out of the hospitals. . . 200 or 500 poor people, that have fevers, pleurisies. Let us divide them into halves, let us cast lots, that one halfe of them may fall to my share, and the other to yours; I will cure them without bloodletting and sensible evacuation; but you do, as ye know. . . . We shall see how many funerals both of us shall have."[7]

Van Helmont's point was that when uncertainty and disputes exist about the relative merits of alternative treatments, fair comparisons would result from allowing chance to decide who should receive which treatments. Examples of the adoption of this principle in practice (by using alternate allocation to different treatments) began to appear at least as early as the 19th century.[8] A nice example of patients themselves drawing lots to decide which treatment they would receive was reported by a British obstetrician in the Lancet the following century: "An equal number of blue and white beads were placed in a box. Each woman accepted for the experiment was asked to draw a bead from the box. Those who drew blue beads were placed in group A while those who drew white beads were placed in group B."[9]

A decade later, in a celebrated study by the Medical Research Council reported in the BMJ,[10] lottery in the form of random sampling numbers was used to decide which patients with pulmonary tuberculosis would receive streptomycin as well as bed rest, and which bed rest alone. This randomised study is often seen as having ushered in a new era in making fair comparisons of alternative treatments. Using lottery (random allocation) to decide who shall receive which treatments when uncertainty exists about their relative merits and demerits has now become a widely accepted component of efforts to increase knowledge in therapeutics.

The randomised trial of streptomycin also illustrates how lottery has been used to distribute limited supplies of a potentially beneficial intervention.[11] This "democratic" use of lottery continues to be used today—for example, in a randomised trial of preschool day care in Hackney.[12]

. . .

Contributors: Both authors have been involved in background research and in drafting this paper.

Competing interests: None declared.

[7] J. B. Van Helmont, *Oriatrike, or, Physick Refined the Common Errors Therein Refuted, and the Whole Art Reformed & Rectified: Being a New Rise and Progress of Philosophy and Medicine for the Destruction of Diseases and Prolongation of Life* (London: Lodowick-Loyd, 1662), p. 526.

[8] I. Chalmers, "Comparing Like with Like: Some Historical Milestones in the Evolution of Methods to Create Unbiased Comparison Groups in Therapeutic Experiments," *International Journal of Epidemiology* 30, no. 5 (2001): pp. 1156–1164.

[9] G. W. Theobald, "Effect of Calcium and Vitamins A and D on Incidence of Pregnancy Toxemia," *The Lancet* 229, no. 5937: pp. 1397–1399.

[10] Medical Research Council, "Streptomycin Treatment of Pulmonary Tuberculosis: A Medical Research Council Investigation," *British Medical Journal* 2 (1948): pp. 769–782.

[11] A. B. Hill, "Suspended Judgment. Memories of the British Streptomycin Trial in Tuberculosis. The First Randomized Clinical Trial," *Control Clinical Trials* 11, no. 2 (1990): pp. 77–79.

[12] T. Toroyan, I. Roberts and A. Oakley, "Randomisation and Resource Allocation: A Missed Opportunity for Evaluating Health Care and Social Interventions," *Journal of Medical Ethics* 26, no. 5 (2000): pp. 319–322.

EXCERPT 3

Abridged text from:
F. M. Kamm, "Equal Treatment and Equal Chances," *Philosophy & Public Affairs* 14, no. 2 (1985): pp. 177–194.

Equal Treatment and Equal Chances

Frances Myrna Kamm

In his article, "Should the Numbers Count?" John Taurek deals with conflict situations in which we can help some, but not all, of the people who need help, and we must choose whom we will help. An example of such a case involves six people who need a drug to save their lives. I have the drug, but I cannot give it to all six. . . . Among my options are to give it either to a group of five people on one island or to one person on another island. The following are among the claims Taurek makes:

(i) (a) If the five die, no one will suffer more of a loss than a single person would suffer if he died. We care about the loss a person suffers, the loss to him, not the loss of him or a summation of individual losses that no single individual ever suffers. Therefore, numbers do not count in deciding whom to save. There is no reason to save the greater number, just because they are the greater number. . . .

(2) If we want to show equal concern for all six people—though perhaps we needn't—we should toss a coin, thereby giving each of the six people an equal (50%) chance of getting the drug.

. . .

I

If Claim (i) were true, and it was not worse for more people to die than for fewer to die in conflict situations, then, on at least one interpretation of Taurek, it would also be true that it was not worse for more people to die when we could save all six people, that is, in conflict-free situations.

The interpretation of Taurek which would have this implication takes him to be arguing that, in general, what happens to people may be important to them, but it is not impersonally good or bad.[1] It might be suggested, therefore, that Taurek's argument against automatically saving the five in conflict situations also implies that it makes no moral difference whether we save all six or just one in conflict-free situations. If his argument had this result it would seem even more problematic.

I believe his argument does not have this result. . . . The concern for persons, which is part of equal concern, will lead one to want for each person that he live. A concern for equal treatment alone would be satisfied by tossing a coin to decide whether to save six or one, and then, if need be, throwing a six-sided die to decide on the one. But concern for the loss to each person would lead to saving all six. . . .

Another way to put this is that the empathetic point of view which Taurek favors as grounds for saving a life (that is, concern for the loss to a person if he dies, rather than concern for the loss of the person)[2] would lead him to save all six rather than just one. Yet he would still be free to claim that it was only better for each person who was saved that he

---

[1] There is a good interpretation of Taurek, presented by Thomas Nagel in his paper, "Equality," reprinted in his *Mortal Questions*, p. ii6 (Cambridge: Cambridge University Press, 1979), according to which Taurek means only that so long as a state of affairs is contrary to the interests of at least one person, it is not an impersonally good state of affairs. However, states of affairs which are in everyone's interest are impersonally good states of affairs. (A decision to save the greatest number is contrary to the interests of the one in conflict situations, but not in conflict-free situations.) I believe the first interpretation is the correct one, though I do not believe Taurek maintains it consistently. However, I shall not defend these points here.

[2] Taurek, "Should the Numbers Count?", p. 307.

was saved, not impersonally better. In conflict cases, this ground for saving more rather than fewer lives could be overridden by the desire to show equal concern, which on Taurek's view, requires us to give each person an equal chance to be saved.

. . .

II.

Can we offer a justification for saving the greater number in conflict situations, a justification which any reasonable person should accept as consistent with treating him empathetically as an equal? Can we provide a reason for saving the greater number, which does not depend on any assumption that a situation is worse if more die?

A. Taurek suggests that if we want to show equal concern in a conflict case involving at least two possible outcomes (that five are saved or that one is saved) we should toss a coin. This view requires that we give an equal chance of coming about to all the different, realistically possible outcomes that are preferred by the people involved, at least when the people have equal stakes in the outcomes. In the conflict case in which either one person survives or five people survive, there are among the six people desires for two outcomes—one in which five live, and another in which one lives. . . . The first outcome is desired by five people, but since the object of their preference is the same it is counted only once. When the object of this preference gets an equal chance, each of the people involved gets an equal chance. (Suppose 5000 people prefer policy B and one person prefers policy C, and they each have equal stakes in the outcome. Then in Taurek's view showing equal concern and respect for all 5001 people would involve a procedure like tossing a coin. . . .

I believe, however, that there is an interpretation of equal treatment of all concerned, which does not require equal chances, and yet does not depend on the view that it is worse if more people go unsatisfied in conflict cases. This interpretation requires that we count equally each individual's preference, understood not as the object of his preference but as the fact that he prefers it. It is not enough just to count the object of his preference. . . . If we count only objects of preferences, then a person's preference will be superfluous whenever one other person shares it. When we follow this policy, we "count each person's preference" only in the minimal sense that (a) we examine his preference to see what it is, whether it is different from that of others, and (b) if his preference differs from anyone else's then the state of affairs which is its object will be among those which are given an equal chance.

The reason for counting each person's preference need not be that this will result in more being saved and it is better if more are saved in a conflict case. The reason may simply be that treating people as equals involves counting each one's preference; this is something we simply owe each individual as part of treating him as an equal. Indeed, it might be that the greater number of individuals actually preferred that the single person be saved instead of themselves. In such a case the view for which I am arguing could recommend that the single person be saved even if it were in some sense impersonally better that the greater number be saved. Since what we would be doing in this case would be based on counting each person's preference even when this conflicts with saving the greater number, letting each person's preference count cannot be based on the value of the greater number being saved. . . .

I have argued that if we want to treat people as equals, and we do this when we count someone's preferring an option, rather than just the object of his preference, we should not toss a coin in Taurek's conflict case. . . .

Does equal treatment in deciding who will win when more than one can win require depriving someone of a baseline chance? The answer to this question seems to depend on whether the model of balancing, or what I shall refer to as the model of combat, is the best way to treat individuals in opposing groups as equals. "Combat" involves two opposing equals confronting each other, with one of the two coming out victorious, and, perhaps, going on to confront another opponent. On the other hand, in a balancing procedure opposing individuals cancel each other out; neither "survives."[3]

Of the two procedures, balancing seems to better express the equality of opposing individuals, and hence to be fairer. This is because combat calls upon some morally irrelevant differences between the individuals (in battle), or on some unequal factor outside of them (as in a coin toss), that can distinguish the winner from the loser.

So if equality is best expressed by balancing, and if we give equal chances in a situation where only one can win only because we want to treat all equally, then majority rule would be preferable to the retention of baseline and chances propositional to numbers chances in a situation in which more than one can win. . . .

The heart of the CPN and majority rule analysis is that in conflict situations a procedure reflecting equal treatment is one in which individuals confront other individuals as individuals. . . . When only one can win in a conflict situation, an equal chance for each is derived from the confrontation of each with all. Equal chance for each, then, is not a goal which must be maintained in all situations. Rather, it is a goal subsidiary to the goal of having individuals with opposing preferences confront one another as individuals. When more than one can win, it is still required that those grouped on one side of the preference line be confronted as individuals by someone on the other side. If confrontation by balancing is a better reflection of the equality of the individuals than combat, then balancing is preferred. So to give the one and the opposing five equal chances would ignore the individuality of each of the five, to submerge each into the group, and to treat the group as a single unit.[4]

. . .

III.

Having suggested that numbers should be counted in some cases I will now consider a case in which counting numbers may be more problematic. Consider the Surgeon Case, in which we must distribute a scarce drug. We can use it to save five people in one part of the country or one person in another part of the country, but we cannot save all six. Suppose the single person is about to perform surgery that will save the lives of 100 different people suffering from another disease. He is irreplaceable in the surgery and they will die without him. To whom should we give the drug?

It might be suggested that we handle such a case by giving extra weight to the single person. This is because he has some sort of relationship to other people which the five don't have. Some may object that giving the surgeon extra weight would deny equal treatment to

[3] Balancing is used when calculations of military strength are made: The strength of each side is measured by balancing off soldiers and/or weapons. Real battles, however, involve combat. This is why one side could win a war in reality that it had lost on paper.

[4] In this article I am concerned with procedures for deciding cases in which on one occasion we must decide between the many and the few. There may, however, be repeated conflict cases, that is, cases in which we must decide between the many and the few on several occasions. For example (a case suggested to me by Kenneth Alpem) suppose five people are on one island and one on another. We can deliver ice cream to them once a month for several months, but we cannot go to both islands in any given month. It may be true that in multiple conflict cases we would not apply either majority rule or CPN on each of the several occasions of choice; rather we would deliver ice cream an equal number of times to each island. Does this show that there is something wrong with the use of majority rule or CPN in one-time conflict cases? If we could only deliver the ice cream once should we replicate as chances of each winning the proportions we maintained over the series, that is, equality achieved by tossing a coin?

him and the five. This objection depends on the claim that equal treatment is owed to each individual regardless of his relationships to others, regardless of his instrumental role. It is not clear that this is true, however. An alternative to saying that we are in this case giving the surgeon greater weight would be to claim that while each of the six individuals counts equally, we must also count equally the 100 who will be lost if the surgeon is not saved. That is, we should treat this case as though it involved a choice between saving five people and saving 101. Could there be a reason for not counting the 100 people as 100 separate individuals on the side of the surgeon, though we should count the five confronting him? I am not sure that there is a reason. . . . In this case the 100 people do not directly need the drug which we must distribute. At most, if they could try to buy the drug to give it to the surgeon, they could claim that they need it in order to give it to the surgeon whom they need. That is, they need the drug, but only because someone they need needs it. Their survival is dependent on his, and their need for the drug is dependent on his need. In cases where they could not buy the drug for him, they could only be said to need his having the drug, rather than the drug itself.

To provide equal treatment for all individuals who *directly* need something when only one of them can acquire it requires us to give each an equal chance in virtue of his direct need. . . .

But the 100 do not have a direct need for the drug. If this meant that each on his own would have no claim to confront those who did have a direct need for the drug, how could the pooling of chances occur?: One cannot pool chances that do not exist. If the pooling cannot occur because there are no chances to pool, then there is no ground for giving each of the 101 people a 101/106 chance to win. And it won't be correct to count the 100 on the side of the surgeon as we count the five who directly need the drug. It is only if an indirect need can give each of the 100, on his own, a right to compete with the five, that we can construct an argument for allowing all the numbers to count. . . .

Another way to make this point is to consider a version of this case in which the five need the drug to save their lives, and the surgeon needs the drug to cure a splitting headache that prevents his performing surgery. He himself would not die if he didn't receive the drug, though the one hundred people he could help would. Should he be a candidate to receive the drug nevertheless?[5]

It seems to me that our current social policy in distributing scarce resources would count the one hundred to some degree but would not count them as individuals, strictly speaking. . . .

---

[5] This way of making my point was suggested to me by Deborah Helmers. Versions of this paper were read at the New York Institute for the Humanities Philosophy and Law Seminar (1981), the Economics, Philosophy and Politics Seminar of the City University of New York Graduate Center (1982), and the American Philosophical Association, Western Division, meeting in Chicago (1983). I am grateful to those who commented at these meetings, to my official commentator in Chicago, Kenneth Alpern, and for the philosophical and editorial suggestions made by Thomas Nagel, Derek Parfit, and the Editors of Philosophy & Public Affairs.

EXCERPT 4

Abridged text from:

D. Callahan, *Setting Limits: Medical Goals in an Aging Society* (Georgetown University Press, 1995), pp. 133–158.

Setting Limits: Medical Goals in an Aging Society

Daniel Callahan

Setting Limits

. . .

How might we devise a plan to limit health care for the aged that is fair, humane, and sensitive to the special requirements and dignity of the aged? . . . [N]either in moral theory nor in the various recent traditions of the welfare state is there any single and consistent basis for health care for the elderly. . . . While the need and dependency of the elderly would appear to be the strongest basis of the obligation, it has never been clear just how medical "need" is to be understood or the extent of the claim that can be drawn from it. Minimal requirements for food, clothing, shelter, and income for the aged can be calculated with some degree of accuracy and, if inflation is taken into account, can remain reasonably stable and predictable. Medical "needs," by contrast, admit of no such stable calculation. Forecasts about life expectancy and about health needs have, as noted, consistently been mistaken underestimates in the past. Constant technological innovation and refinement means not only that new ways are always being found to extend life or improve therapy, but also that "need" itself becomes redefined in the process. New horizons for research are created, new desires for cures encouraged, and new hopes for relief of disability engendered. Together they induce and shape changing and, ordinarily, escalating perceptions of need. Medical need is not a fixed concept but a function of technological possibility and regnant social expectations.

If this is true of medical care in general, it seems all the more true of health care for the aged: it is a new medical frontier, and the possibilities for improvement are open, beckoning, and flexible. Medical need on that frontier in principle knows no boundaries; death and illness will always be waiting no matter how far we go. . . . For the aged, however, the forestalling of bodily deterioration and an eventually inevitable death provide the motivation for a constant, never-ending struggle. That struggle will turn on the meaning of medical need, an always malleable concept, and will move on from there to a struggle about the claims of the elderly relative to other age groups and other social needs. That these struggles are carried on in a society wary about the propriety of even trying to achieve a consensus on appropriate individual needs does not help matters.

For all of its difficulties, nonetheless, only some acceptable and reasonably stable notion of need is likely to provide a foundation for resource allocation. The use of merit, or wealth, or social worth as a standard for distributing lifesaving benefits through governmental mechanisms would seem both unfair at best and morally outrageous at worst. We must try, then, to establish a consensus on the health needs of different age groups, especially the elderly, and establish priorities to meet them. At the same time, those standards of need must have the capacity to resist the redefining, escalating power of technological change; otherwise they will lack all solidity. The nexus between need and technological possibility has to be broken. . . .

In the case of the aged, I have proposed that our ideal of old age should be achieving a life span that enables each of us to accomplish the ordinary scope of possibilities that life affords, recognizing that this may encompass a range of time rather than pointing to a precise age. On the basis of that ideal, the aged would need only those resources which would allow them a solid chance to live that long and, once they had passed that stage, to finish out their years free of pain and avoidable suffering. I will, therefore, define need in the old as primarily to achieve a natural life span and thereafter to have their suffering relieved.

The needs of the aged, as so defined, would therefore be based on a general and socially established ideal of old age and not exclusively, as at present, on individual desires—even the widespread desire to live a longer life. That standard would make possible an allocation of resources to the aged which rested upon criteria that were at once age-based (aiming to achieve a natural life span) and need-based (sensitive to the differing health needs of individuals in achieving that goal). . . .

Norman Daniels has helpfully formulated a key principle for my purposes: the concept of a "normal opportunity range" for the allocation of resources to different individuals and age groups. The foundation of his idea is that "meeting health-care needs is of special importance because it promotes fair equality of opportunity. It helps, guarantee individuals a fair chance to enjoy the normal opportunity range for their society." A "fair chance," however, is one that recognizes different needs and different opportunities for each stage of life; it is an "age-relative opportunity range."[1] Even though fairness in this conception is based upon age distinctions, it is not unfairly discriminatory: it aims to provide people with that level of medical care necessary to allow them to pursue the opportunities ordinarily available to those of their age. Everyone needs to walk, for example, but some require an artificial hip to do so. It also recognizes that different ages entail different needs and opportunities. Yet there are two emendations to this approach that would help it better serve my purposes. For one thing, moral and normative possibilities of what *ought* to count as "normal opportunity range" are left unaddressed. For another, the concept should be extended to encompass what I will call a normal "life-span opportunity range"—what opportunities is it reasonable for people to hope for over their lifetimes?—and we will need to know what *ought* to count as "normal" within that range also. For those purposes we will have to resist the implications of the modernizing view of old age, which would deliberately make it an unending frontier, constantly to be pushed back, subject to no fixed standards of "normal" at all. . . .

Where Daniels uses the term "normal" in a statistical sense, it should instead be given a normative meaning; that is, what counts as morally and socially adequate and generally acceptable. That is the aim of my standard of a natural life span, one that I believe is morally defensible for policy purposes. Such a life can be achieved within a certain, roughly specifiable, number of years and can be relatively impervious to technological advances. The minimal purpose is to try to bring everyone up to this standard, leaving any decision to extend life beyond that point as a separate social choice (though one I think we should reject, available resources or not). Daniels recognizes that his strategy has the implication that it "would dictate giving greater emphasis to enhancing individual chances of reaching a normal lifespan than to extending the normal lifespan."[2] But I think that that implication, to me highly desirable, really follows only if taken in conjunction with some theory of what *ought* to count as a "normal opportunity range" and not simply what happens to so count at any given historical and technological moment. The notion of a natural life span fills that gap. With those general points as background, I offer these principles:

1. Government has a duty, based on our collective social obligations, to help people live out a natural life span, but not actively to help extend life medically beyond that point. By life-extending treatment, I will mean any medical intervention, technology, procedure, or medication whose ordinary effect is to forestall the moment of death, whether or not the treatment affects the underlying

[1] N. Daniels, *Just Health Care* (Cambridge University Press, 1985), pp. 104–105.

[2] Ibid., p. 106.

life-threatening disease or biological process.[3]

2. Government is obliged to develop, employ, and pay for only that kind and degree of life-extending technology necessary for medicine to achieve and serve the end of a natural life span; the question is not whether a technology is available that can save a life, but whether there is an obligation to use the technology.
3. Beyond the point of a natural life span, government should provide only the means necessary for the relief of suffering, not life-extending technology.

These principles both establish an upper age limit on life-extending care and yet recognize that great diversity can mark the needs of individuals to attain that limit or, beyond it, to attain relief of suffering.

Age or Need?

The use of age as a principle for the allocation of resources can be perfectly valid.[4] I believe it is a necessary and legitimate basis for providing health care to the elderly. It is a necessary basis because there is not likely to be any better or less arbitrary criterion for the limiting of resources in the face of the open-ended possibilities of medical advancement in therapy for the aged.[5] . . . Age is a legitimate basis because it is a meaningful and universal category. It can be understood at the level of common sense, can be made relatively clear for policy purposes, and can ultimately be of value to the aged themselves if combined with an ideal of old age that focuses on its quality rather than its indefinite extension.

This may be a most distasteful proposal for many of those trying to combat ageist stereotypes and to protect the deepest interests of the elderly. The main currents of gerontology (with the tacit support of medical tradition) have moved in the opposite direction, toward stressing individual needs and the heterogeneity of the elderly. . . . A consensus seems to be emerging—clearly contrary to what I propose—that need is a preferable direction for the future. "Perhaps," as the Neugartens have written, "the most constructive ways of adapting to an aging society will emerge by focusing, not on age at all, but on more relevant dimensions of human needs, human competencies, and human diversity."[6] . . .

The common objections against age as a basis for allocating resources are varied. If joined, as it often is, with the prevalent use of cost-benefit analysis, an age standard is said to guarantee that the elderly will be slighted; their care cannot be readily justified in terms of their economic productivity.[7] The same can be said more generally of efforts to measure the social utility of health care for the old in comparison with other social needs; the elderly will ordinarily lose in comparisons of that kind. By fastening on a general biological trait, age as a standard threatens a respect for the value and inherent diversity of individual lives. There is the hazard of the bureaucratization of the aged, indifferent to their differences.[8]

[3] This general definition is drawn from *S. Wolf, et al., eds, Guidelines on the Termination of Life-Sustaining Treatment and the Case of Dying* (Briarcliff Manor, NY: The Hastings Center, 1987), Introduction.

[4] One of the first articles to explore the idea of an age basis for allocation was Harry R. Moody's "Is It Right to Allocate Health Care Resources on Grounds of Age?", in *Bioethics and Human Rights*, edited by E. L. Bandman and B. Bandman (Boston: Little, Brown, 1978), pp. 197–201.

[5] For a good general discussion of age as an allocation principle, see L. P. Francis, "Poverty, Age Discrimination, and Health Care," in *Poverty, Justice, and the Law*, edited by G. R. Lucas Jr. (Lanham, MD: University Press of America, 1986), pp. 117–129.

[6] B. L. Neugarten and D. A. Neugarten, "Age in the Aging Society," *Daedalus* 115, no. 1 (1986): p. 47.

[7] J. J. Avorn, "Benefit and Cost Analysis in Geriatric Care. Turning Age Discrimination into Health Policy," *New England Journal of Medicine* 310, no. 20 (1984): pp. 1294–1301.

[8] Carole Haber has written well on this problem in *Beyond Sixty-Five: The Dilemma of Old Age in America's Past* (Cambridge University Press, 1985), especially pp. 125–129.

Since age, like sex and race, is a category for which individuals are not responsible, it is unfair to use it as a measure of what they deserve in the way of benefits.[9] The use of an age standard for limiting care could have the negative symbolic significance of social abandonment.[10] Finally, its use will run counter to established principles of medical tradition and ethics, which focus on individual need, and will instead, in an "Age of Bureaucratic Parsimony. . . . be based upon institutional and societal efficiency, or expediency, and upon cost concerns—all emerging rapidly as major elements in decision making."[11]

These are weighty objections, and the hazards perfectly plausible. But all of them fail, or are sharply neutralized in their power. . . . My principle of age-based rationing is not founded on the demeaning idea of measuring "productivity" in the elderly. The use of age as a standard treats everyone alike, aiming that each will achieve a natural life span, productive or not. Far from tolerating social abandonment, it will aim at improving care for the elderly, though not life-extending care. A standard of allocation rooted not in dehumanizing calculations of the economic value or productivity of the elderly, but in a recognition that beyond a certain point they will already have had their fair share of resources does not degrade the elderly or lessen the value of their life. It is only a way of recognizing that the generations pass and that death must come to us all. Nor does it demean the aged as individuals, or signal indifference to the variations among them, to note that they share the trait of being old. It is only if society more generally devalues the aged for being aged—by failing, most notably, to provide the possibility of inherent meaning and significance in old age (as is the case with the modernizing project)—that their individual lives are treated as less valuable. There is nothing unfair about using age as a category if the purpose of doing so is to achieve equity between the generations, to give the aged their due in living out a life-span opportunity range, and to emphasize that the distinctive place and merits of old age are not nullified by aging and death.

That a society could be mature enough to limit care for the aged with no diminution of respect, or could recognize the claims of other age groups without an implication that the elderly are less valuable than they are, seems rarely to be considered. By contrast, the motives I have been advancing reject not the elderly, but a notion of the good of the elderly based on pretending that death and old age can be overcome or ignored, that life has value only if it continues indefinitely, and that there is nothing to be said for the inherent value and contributions of the elderly as elderly. A society that adopts a wholly modernizing approach to old age must necessarily find the possibility of any limitation on care for the elderly a threat. It has robbed old age of all redeeming significance, and only constant efforts to overcome it are acceptable. To pick on the aged for "bureaucratic parsimony," to use Mark Siegler's term, would surely be wrong if done because they were perceived as weak and defenseless, a nice target-of-opportunity for cost containment. That is a very different matter from a societal decision that the overall welfare of the generations, the proper function of medicine, and a fitting understanding of old age and death as part of the life cycle justify limitation on some forms of medical care for the elderly.

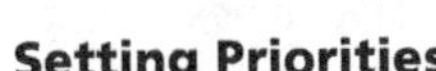

Setting Priorities

There is no task in the fashioning of health policy more intimidating than establishing priorities; yet that is close to the essence of even having a policy. A policy might most concisely be defined as a set of priorities for

[9] US Congress, "Life-Sustaining Technologies and the Elderly," (US Government Printing Office Washington, DC, 1987), p. 11.

[10] J. F. Childress, "Ensuring Care, Respect, and Fairness for the Elderly," *Hastings Center Report* (1984): pp. 27–31.

[11] M. Siegler, "Should Age Be a Criterion in Health Care?", *Hastings Center Report* 14, no. 5 (1984): p. 25.

action and the allocation of resources oriented toward achieving a goal. In this case, we are looking for a policy of allocating resources to the elderly consistent, with acceptable and appropriate goals for their health and welfare. I want to present the outline of an allocation policy and priority system. It will be based on age as a legitimate principle of allocation, and will focus—in setting health-care goals for the elderly—on the averting of a premature death and the relief of suffering. . . .

1 *High Technology Medicine: Finding an Antidote.* The great advances in health care in recent years have come from developments in high-technology medicine. Once the infectious diseases had been controlled or eliminated, further improvements in health have heavily depended upon technology (although changes in lifestyle, particularly in the case of heart disease, have made a contribution also). If any strong reins are to be put on the costs of health care for the elderly, high-technology medicine is one important place to begin. Most of the technological advances of recent decades have come to benefit the old comparatively more than the young (as an instance, dialysis) and the older segment of the old more than any other (as an instance, critical-care units).[12] Those same advances have also been heavily responsible for the increase in life expectancy that developed after the 1960s and continues to the present. . . .

Where there is now a powerful bias in favor of innovative medical technology, and a correspondingly insatiable appetite for more of it, that will have to be replaced by a bias in the other direction where the aged are concerned. The alternative bias, should be this: that no new technologies should be developed or applied to the old that are likely to produce only chronic illness and a short life, to increase the present burden of chronic illness, or to extend the lives of the elderly but offer no significant improvement in their quality of life. Put somewhat differently, no technology should be developed or applied to the elderly that does not promise great and inexpensive improvement in the quality of their lives, no matter how promising for life extension . . .

While it would now be cruel to terminate federal kidney-dialysis support for the elderly, dialysis represents precisely the kind of technology that should not be sought or developed in the future. It does not greatly increase the life expectancy of its users (an average of only five years), and for most, that gain is at the price of a doubtful or poor quality of life and an inability to achieve earlier levels of functioning.[13] That it was originally developed with younger patients (aged 15 to 50) in mind, but soon saw an age creep of great proportions (with some 30%—25,000—of those on dialysis now over 65), is another part of the story to be remembered for the future.[14] . . .

An obvious dilemma here is that most technologies will benefit the young as well and are developed with them often primarily in mind. If technological development is discouraged, will that not damage the health interests of the young, even their chances to avoid a premature death? That is a hazard, but its effects could be lessened by a technology assessment that examined whether, if it were developed for the young, its primary or disproportionate use might be among the elderly, and whether alternative means could be found to meet the needs of the young. I leave these as difficult problems for the trajectory I am proposing.

2 *Providing Equitable Security.* The greatest fear about old age seems to be not death but frailty, the loss of independence and self-direction, declining mental capacities, and impoverishment. The failure of present entitlement programs to cope with the fear of

[12] J. L. Avorn, "Medicine, Health, and the Geriatric Transformation," *Daedalus* (1986): p. 213.

[13] R. B. Freeman, "Treatment of Chronic Renal Failure: An Update," *The New England Journal of Medicine* 312, no. 9 (1985): p. 577; see also R. W. Evans, et al., "The Quality of Life of Patients with End-Stage Renal Disease," *New England Journal of Medicine* 312, no. 9 (1985): pp. 553–559.

[14] A. L. Caplan, "Organ Transplants: The Costs of Success," *Hastings Center Report* 13, no. 6 (1983): pp. 23–32.

impoverishment as a result of old age and attendant ill health remains as a major flaw in the system.[15]

A point not often sufficiently stressed is the insecurity that the present system breeds, even for those who are at the start better off. Though only a minority of the elderly are now in the poverty or near-poverty group, no younger person can be sure he or she will not be in that group, and no older person, even if well off at the moment, can be assured that some medical catastrophe will not put him or her into the group as well. Stories of the economic devastation wrought by catastrophic illnesses—or simply chronic illnesses that last for many expensive years—can be found in almost any family now. . . .

Many years will be required to bring about the kind of shift in values needed to change attitudes and practices pertinent to the provision of life-extending technologies to the elderly. That is the long-term solution. In the meantime, while we are working toward that goal, an intensified effort to provide better basic health-care coverage for the elderly will most effectively demonstrate that there is no lessening of commitment to their well-being. It is that move—and no other—which will neutralize the kind of threat posed by a restriction of life-extending care. I cannot responsibly propose to limit that kind of care without simultaneously proposing to improve other forms of care. I will be the first to object to any effort to deny life-extending care before the other reforms are well under way and assured of success. A denial of the one without the flourishing of the other would indeed be a grave threat to the elderly.

3 *Priorities for Care.* A societal decision deliberately to limit life-extending high-technology care for those who have lived out a natural life span is not meant to be a recipe for, or symbol of, abandonment. It is meant to be an affirmation of the diverse needs of different age groups and an acceptance of the inevitable place of death at the end of life. It can be a tolerable basis for social policy only if that policy strikingly seeks to provide the elderly with an honorable and bearable life in their remaining years. This will entail first working to avert a premature death, and then seeking to minimize pain and suffering.

Any attempt to specify a "premature death" must have a certain arbitrary quality. I define it as a death prior to the living out of a natural life span, something that would ordinarily occur in the early 70s but could extend through the late 70s to early 80s. It is the latter range I will use as the basis for my discussion here. This is actually a more liberal standard than that used by the federal Centers for Disease Control (CDC), which uses the concept of "years-of-life-lost" prior to age 65 in determining premature death. That concept came into use during the 1970s and was incorporated into the CDC's *Morbidity and Mortality Weekly Report* in 1982. A focus on conventional death rates, by simply counting deaths in the population, emphasizes deaths occurring in older age groups. The "years-of-life-lost" calculation, by contrast, highlights the potentially preventable mortality occurring earlier in life and permits a more precise focus for health-care goals. . . . Whether this or some similar method of reckoning is used, the first goal in care for the aged will be to go after the causes of premature death.

Beyond avoiding a premature death, what do the elderly need from medicine to complete their lives in an acceptable way? They need to be as independent as possible, freed from excess worry about the financial or familial burdens of ill, health, and physically and emotionally positioned to seek whatever meaning and significance can be found in old age. Medicine can only try to maintain the health which facilitates that latter quest, not guarantee its success. That facilitation is enhanced by physical mobility, mental alertness, and emotional stability. Chronic illness, pain, and suffering are all major impediments and of course appropriate targets for medical research and improved health-care delivery.

Major research priorities should be those chronic illnesses which so burden the later years

---

[15] *"Aging America: Trends and Projections, 1985," US Government Printing Office, Washington, DC (1986)*; J .L. Palmer and S. G. Gould, "The Economic Consequences of an Aging Society," *Daedalus* (1986): pp. 295–323.

and which have accompanied the increase in longevity. They encompass, in addition to a number of physical problems (particularly multiple organic diseases), a variety of major mental disorders, including schizophrenia, affective disorders, various senile brain diseases, arteriosclerosis, and epilepsy. The OTA study of aging and technology centered on five chronic conditions endemic among the elderly, of which only the first receives any great public attention (or, for that matter, sympathy): dementia, which characterizes Alzheimer's disease—a source first of humiliation, then of a loss of basic human potentials, then death; urinary incontinence—also a humiliating condition and a malodorous symbol of the loss of physical control; hearing impairment—embarrassing, isolating, and frustrating; osteoporosis (thinning of the bones)—because of the greatly enhanced incidence of fractures, a source of constant fear and danger for the old-old in particular; osteoarthritis—painful, sometimes disabling, and pervasive (affecting 16–20 million elderly).

As with the correction of inequities in health care for the elderly, there is no guarantee that the necessary research and future amelioration of such conditions would be inexpensive. Even law-technology approaches to noncurable chronic problems can be enormously expensive if used by enough people; and some of the therapeutic solutions to some of the conditions are clearly of the high-technology variety (e.g., hip and joint replacement at an average cost of $50,000 to victims of osteoarthritis). The most troubling problems in that, respect may well be posed by advances in rehabilitation. Even now, rehabilitation for stroke is labor-intensive, difficult, and often of uncertain outcome, and the moral dilemma of choosing those patients most likely to benefit often wrenching. While rehabilitation has in the past been thought of as a low-technology, a caring-rather-than-curing field, it is also moving in a technological direction and, simultaneously, working to rid itself of the reputation of indifference to and pessimism about rehabilitation for the elderly.[16] The ongoing development of sophisticated prosthetic devices and computer-assisted methods of helping the partially paralyzed, paraplegic and quadriplegic do not promise to lower costs, and neither does their likely extension to use among the elderly. If such developments as these are even to be possible, it is hard to envision how they can financially coexist with continuing investment in life-extending treatments.

The prevention of illness has long been promoted as the best way in the long run to improve the health of the elderly (along with the health of everyone else) and to reduce health-care costs. Its primary virtue from any perspective is that it can help avoid a premature death and enhance physical well-being through an ordinary life span; illness and death would be pushed beyond the normal lifetime-opportunity-range boundary. That it will actually reduce costs is not, however, necessarily true as a flat generalization. Whether the sum total of the direct costs (to mount and implement a program of prevention) and the indirect expenses (time and other social resources) will equal the savings will vary from one disease category to another.[17] In some cases, moreover, it will be no more expensive to cure a disease than to prevent it—for example, the choice between bypass surgery and a preventive regimen for the hypertension that would have led to it.[18] "This means," Louise Russell has written, "that choosing investments in health is more difficult than some of the claims for prevention would suggest. Sometimes prevention buys more health for the money; sometimes cure does. . . . the issue most often is what mix of prevention and therapy is best. It is a rare preventive measure that, like smallpox vaccine, eradicates the condition altogether."[19] Yet even if economic savings are uncertain in each case, prevention programs can have many health benefits, helping to avoid some conditions altogether (cancer most notably through such changes in behavior as the cessation of smoking) and ameliorating the impact of others (as in a reduction of obesity among diabetics). . . .

16 I am particularly indebted for that information to Janet F. Haas, M.D. and other colleagues who were part of a Hastings Center project on ethical issues in rehabilitation medicine 1985–87.

17 L. B. Russell, *Is Prevention Better Than Cure?* (Brookings Institution, 1986).

18 Ibid., p. 111.

19 Ibid.

Changing Expectations

The justification I have proposed for the limitation of life-extending resources for the elderly would make little sense, and be unconscionably harsh, apart from the context of an altered vision of the ends of medicine and of aging. I would reiterate my objection to a rationing scheme that in the name of cost containment would cut back on lifesaving care to the elderly without offering a justification based upon some intrinsic benefit for the elderly themselves and some rich understanding of the place of old age in human life. . . . Would it not be regressive to use age as a rationing standard since, evidently enough, age criteria would not take account of individual variations among the elderly? Would it not be equally regressive to have the government cease providing life-extending care to the elderly when we could predict, with great certainty, that the wealthy (or the desperate of lesser financial means) would seek to buy that care on the private (or black) market?

Each of those questions turns, in its own way, on our present expectations about what old age is (or at least ought to be). Assuming it is desirable to do so, can those expectations be changed without a sense of severe loss, even tragedy? The only possible answer is that it could not be done easily or quickly and would probably require a generation or more for a new understanding, and new expectations, to take hold. The three objections just stated lend themselves to imagining how that might take place, and I will consider them in turn, using each to build upon the last.

We might begin by recalling two points, one historical and the other contemporary. The first is that a century and more ago, there was no human expectation whatever that medicine could significantly extend individual life or effectively combat the infirmities of old age. It was understood that old age was a part of life relatively brief in duration and was followed by death (and usually a relatively swift death, not the lingering one over a period of years that has now become common—for example, the present average of three years in the case of cancer). That set of facts was not taken to be a fundamental indictment of life itself, nor, so far as I can make out, were old age and death feared any more then than they are now. Hence, we know it is perfectly possible psychologically to have a different, more accepting set of expectations toward aging and death; they are, not fixed by human nature. The second point is the near-universal report that, as noted above, it is not aging as such that is feared but the loss of social significance and personal independence with which it has become associated. It is not death in itself that evokes dread so much as a humiliating, oppressive death—either a high-technology death amidst machines and tubes in a modern hospital, or a drawn-out loss of one's faculties in a nursing home, where death seems too long in coming.

Our present expectations about aging and death, it turns out, may not indeed be unambiguously reassuring: we are by no means sure that modern medicine promises us so much better an aging and death, even if some features appear improved and the process begins later. It is not therefore inconceivable that, over time, most people could be persuaded that a different, more limited set of expectations promised to be as satisfying as the present ones. That would be all the more possible if there were a greater assurance than at present that one would live out a full life span, that one's chronic illnesses would be better supported by government programs, and that long-term and home care would be given a more powerful societal backing than is now the case. . . .

Would we not, however, have bought those developments at a high price, that of systematically excluding the great variation among the aged from consideration? In particular, since it is well known that only a small proportion of the elderly have very high health-care costs and needs, why not focus our rationing efforts on them? By limiting life-extending care to everyone, would we not indiscriminately sweep up many in otherwise fine shape who, with one or two timely medical interventions, might have remaining a number of years of good life? The answer is that we would indeed, in a sense, penalize the latter group; or more precisely, we would not benefit them, despite the fact that they would gain much more from life-extending treatment than those in poor condition. But I see no way to avoid, at some point, a choice that will cause anguish, shorten some lives, and possibly appear unjust.

Recall that the main policy goal would be to assure everyone a chance to live out a natural life span. To deny those in poor health a chance to achieve that goal—particularly in order that others, in better health, might be assisted to live well beyond that point—would be unfair. And I assume that we cannot expect for much longer to pay for both. To deny care to those in poor health would be a denial of a basic good that ought to be available to all and, beyond that, the heaping of additional misery on those whose elderly years are already blighted by illness. But those in good health, by contrast, have already had a natural advantage. Their later years have already been superior years in comparison with their afflicted peers'. A restriction of their care would not be as unfair as a restriction of care for those who have not been so fortunate. With such a shift in priorities, the young could look forward to their old age with less anxiety if assured a vigorous societal commitment to give them a full and natural life span; they would know they would not be abandoned prior to that stage if their health-care costs were too heavy. The use of age as a standard for terminating care would be regressive only if used alone, with no other modifications being made in benefits given the elderly. But it could be the fairest possible means of allocation if combined with an improvement in other benefits. For all would have a guarantee that a minimal and common baseline of accessible health care up through a normal life span would be theirs; only thereafter would differences appear.

By refusing the healthy life-extending care beyond a certain age, we would not, however, be denying them a benefit to which they had a special claim. We would instead be saying that a society in which all were assisted to live out a full life span was more tolerable and humane, both to the old who lived in it and to the young who had it to look forward to in their old age, than our present situation. Since the young cannot know in advance whether they will be in the minority who will require heavy and expensive care in their old age to preserve their lives, their prudence would seem to better justify a health-care system that would support such care through (but not beyond) a full life span than one which "did not, even if the latter might extend one's years a bit more beyond that point should one be lucky enough to get that far.[20]

That such a priority system would invite some abuses and create some new problems should not be denied or minimized. A government policy of denying Medicare support for life-extending treatment beyond a certain age would favor those elderly who could afford personally to pay for such care. It could also severely tempt many middle-class families to sacrifice their less-than-ample resources to save the life of a loved one they are not yet ready to relinquish. It would no less tempt physicians, motivated by kindness and a commitment to save life, to evade reimbursement restrictions on life-extending treatment. They could well exploit the often fine, and sometimes indistinguishable, line between the relief of suffering and the extension of life. . . .

There would be no simple solution to problems of that kind, and they would occasion sorrow and anguish. As the British and other Europeans have come to learn, many people are not prepared to stay within a health-care system that imposes limitations on care; they are willing to pay personally for private care. That possibility does favor the wealthy and (though the evidence is not yet in) may do harm to the general health-care system. Yet a rigorous effort to enforce egalitarian solutions is a good prescription for an authoritarian society. The benefits of the unfairness (if such it is) of the system I propose would be limited to those beyond a certain age, and precisely because of that advanced age would for most be a limited benefit, to be terminated shortly by death. I do

---

[20] I profited in thinking about this issue from reading the manuscript of Norman Daniels' new book *Am I My Parents' Keeper?* particularly his notion of "the prudential lifespan account."

not believe a society would be made morally intolerable by that kind of imbalance.

As for the possible, even likely, resistance of many physicians to tolerate a Medicare system that denied life-extending treatment to patients they felt could benefit from it, only a different understanding of their role would suffice to reduce that resistance. Such an understanding could come only from recognizing, on the one hand, that a continuation of the present attitude toward the open-ended use of medical technology to extend the lives of the aged poses a threat to adequate health care for younger generations; and, on the other, that a plausible (even proper) view of the social ends of medicine and aging provides independent grounds for limiting health care. That recognition will require a major effort to reorient medicine away from its captivity by the modernizing, technology-driven, borderless "medical need" model of care for the aged. It will no less require a parallel reorientation of the general public, who will be as reluctant to give it up as will physicians. . . .

EXCERPT 5

Abridged text from:

A. Williams, "Intergenerational Equity: An Exploration of the 'Fair Innings' Argument," *Health Economics* 6, no. 2 (1997): pp. 117–132.

Intergenerational Equity: An Exploration of the "Fair Innings" Argument

Alan Williams

Centre for Health Economics, University of York, UK

. . .

Background

. . .

The general concept of efficiency used here

I shall here take efficiency to mean maximizing health gain as measured in some standardized way [e.g. in life-years or in quality-adjusted lifeyears (QALYs)]. . . . The kind of equity issue in which I am interested is one that adduces some personal characteristic of the beneficiary as a relevant consideration in the estimating the social value of a particular health gain.[1] But a careful distinction needs to be drawn here between personal characteristics of the beneficiary which affect the quantum of benefit to be expected from a treatment and personal characteristics which affect the value attached to any given quantum of benefit. For instance, being old may reduce the number of extra life years gained from an intervention (a quantum effect related to age), but being old may also affect the value that is given to each life year gained (a valuation effect related to age).

Some relevant equity principles

. . . In various surveys[2] that have been conducted to elicit people's views as to who should be given priority over others, there are some recurring themes. One is that the young should in general be given priority over the old (though not infants over slightly older children). Another is that those looking after young children should have priority over those without that responsibility. Many people also believe that priority should be given to those who have cared for their own health over those who have not (e.g. by smoking, drug abuse or heavy drinking).

I have also noted another recurring theme, namely that those who have had a hard life (either specifically to do with health, or more broadly to do with life in general) should not be further penalised in health-care priority-setting by applying to them the full rigours of

---

[1] Here I shall ignore the efficiency and equity issues that attend the method of financing health care provision. Van Doorslaer and colleagues have demonstrated that that is also important to any overall judgement about the equitability of any health care system (especially between rich and poor). E. van Doorslaer, A. Wagstaff and F. Rutten, *Equity in the Finance and Delivery of Health Care: An International Perspective* (OUP/Commission of the European Communities, 1993).

[2] See, for instance, M. C. Charny, P. A. Lewis and S. C. Farrow, "Choosing Who Shall Not Be Treated in the NHS," *Social Science and Medicine* 28, no. 12 (1989): pp. 1331–1338. C. R. Bråkenhielm, "Vå Rd På Lika Villkor," in *VåR dens Pris*, edited by J. Calltorp and C. R. Bråkenhielm (Stockholm: Verbum, 1990). S. Bjork and P. Rosen, *Prioritizing in Health Care: An Empirical Study of the Views of Health Care Politicians on Resource Allocation* (Lund: Swedish Institute of Health Economics, 1993). J. J. van Busschbach, D. J. Hessing and F. T. de Charro, "The Utility of Health at Different Stages in Life: A Quantitative Approach," *Social Science and Medicine* 37, no. 2 (1993): pp. 153–158. Australians and Norwegians seem to be different, however; see E. Nord, et al., "Maximizing Health Benefits Vs Egalitarianism: An Australian Survey of Health Issues," *Social Science and Medicine* 41, no. 10 (1995): pp. 1429–1437.

the efficiency calculus. Rawls's advocacy of the rule that policy should be guided solely by its effects on the worstoff member(s) of a community is the most extreme manifestation of this kind of argument.[3] It also manifests itself in a slightly less extreme form as a "double jeopardy" argument,[4] where it is said that those who have already experienced significant misfortune should not have further tribulations imposed upon them because they are not good candidates (within the efficiency calculus) for the receipt of health care.

The "Fair Innings" Argument

The argument stated in general terms

One version of this general approach centres on people's supposed entitlement to a "fair innings." This reflects the feeling that everyone is entitled to some "normal" span of health (usually expressed in terms of life years. The implication is that anyone failing to achieve this has in some sense been cheated, whilst anyone getting more than this is "living on borrowed time." Thus whereas the "double jeopardy" argument directs attention only to those on the down-side, the "fair innings" argument considers both those on the down-side and those on the up-side.

. . .

It is worth noting four important characteristics of the "fair innings." First of all, it is a notion of equity that is outcome based, not process-based or resource-based. Secondly, it is about a person's whole life-time experience, not about their state at any particular point in time. Thirdly, it reflects an aversion to inequality. And fourthly, it is quantifiable and even in common parlance it has strong numerical connotations. Death at 25 is viewed very differently from death at 85 and age at death is the key variable which is most often focused upon. In my view, age at death should be no more than a first approximation, however, because the quality of a person's life is important as well as its length.

. . .

The "fair innings" argument applied to life expectancy

A powerful part of the rhetoric about equity in health care employs the notion of equality applied to people's whole lifetime experiences and not just to their current situation. Adopting that broad perspective and looking first at life expectancy, we find considerable variation both between countries and within countries. If we take life expectancy at birth as defining a "fair innings" within any society, then in the UK the differences in male survival rates between the professional and managerial groups (social classes 1 and 2) on the one hand and the semi-skilled and unskilled manual workers (social classes 4 and 5) on the other, has been estimated to differ by about 5 years (72.5 compared with 67.7).[5] The equalization of life chances in terms of life expectancy seems to require some changes in public policy, though not wholly confined to health care. But limited though the contribution of health care may be, it could be exploited more fully by weighting additional life years gained from the various health care activities according to the social class of the potential recipient. These same weights might also be applied to other relevant social programmes, so that their combined effect might be coordinated.

---

[3] J. Rawls, *A Theory of Justice* (Oxford: Oxford University Press, 1972).

[4] As promoted, for instance, by J. Harris, "Qualifying the Value of Life," *Journal of Medical Ethics* 13, no. 3 (1987): pp. 117–123, and challenged by P. Singer, et al., "Double Jeopardy and the Use of QALYs in Health Care Allocation," *Journal of Medical Ethics* 21, no. 3 (1995): pp. 144–150.

[5] D. S. F. Bloomfield and S. Haberman, "Male Social Class Mortality Differences around 1981: An Extension to Include Childhood Ages," *Journal of the Institute of Actuaries (1886–1994)* 119, no. 3 (1992): pp. 545–559.

The "fair innings" argument applied to quality-adjusted life expectancy

But if it is to capture the full flavour of this kind of thinking, the concept of a "fair innings" needs to be extended beyond simple life expectancy to embrace quality-adjusted life expectancy. Otherwise it will not be possible to reflect the view that a lifetime of poor quality health entitles people to special consideration in the current allocation of health care, even if their life expectancy is normal.

. . .

It is clear from these data that surviving members of social classes IV and V have noticeably worse health than their contemporaries in social classes I and II, especially once they are past the age of 40 years. When these data are combined with the differences in survival rates we find that the quality-adjusted life expectancy at birth of someone in social classes 1 and 2 is nearly 66 QALYs, but for someone in social classes 4 and 5 it is only about 57 QALYs.[6] To achieve the mean value of about 61.5 QALYs (a "fair innings" for a pure egalitarian) they would need to live to be 65 and 71 years old, respectively, a feat achieved by about 76% of social classes 1 and 2, but by only 46% of social classes 4 and 5.

Aversion to inequality

How should we respond to such data, assuming that it is approximately true? Clearly that depends on (i) how convinced you are that the "fair innings" argument is a good basis for making equity adjustments in the allocation of health care, (ii) how convinced you are that QALE at birth is a good indicator in any country of what constitutes a "fair innings" (and of departures from it) and (iii) on how far you are willing to have the overall level of health of the community reduced in order to reduce inequalities in the distribution of health.

. . .

[6] Obviously this assumes that a person remains in the same social class throughout their lives. Movement between social classes will make these differences less clear cut at individual level.

The equity-efficiency trade-off then consists in discovering the answer to the question, "how big a sacrifice in the overall health of the population would you be prepared to accept in order to eliminate the disparities in health between A and B?"

. . .

Returning to social class differentials between males in the UK, suppose people were prepared to sacrifice 6 months of life expectancy at birth, in order to eliminate the disparity of 5 years. . . . The mean life expectancy (69.5 years) and the equal life expectancy that people would settle for if the 5 year disparity could be eliminated ("equal at 69"). . . .

It is, of course, quite likely that people will regard different discrepancies with differing degrees of concern according to their size, nature (e.g. whether it is a difference in life expectancy or in quality-adjusted life expectancy) and likely causes (e.g. whether due to inherited factors or freely chosen lifestyle).

Fine-tuning the "fair innings" argument

There are two respects in which it might be desirable to "fine tune" the crude version of the "fair innings" argument that I have presented so far. One would be to make it more dynamic and the other would be to individualize it. I will sketch out each possibility in turn.

. . .

Age-weights as well?

. . .

The World Bank has published[7] the set of "age-weights" and has used these weights when measuring the "burden of disease" in different countries. The authors of the *World Development Report 1993* observe that

> "Most societies attach more importance to a year of life lived by a young or middle-aged adult than to a year of life lived by a child or an elderly person."

[7] *World Development Report* 1973. Box Fig. 1.3 on p. 26 and further discussion on p. 213.

So in their table of age-weights a weight of zero is attached to newborns, the weights peak in the late 20s and then decline to fall below 1 in the early 50s. [See also Figure [5.1.]] These age-weights are important social judgements, which may well be appropriate to the conditions in the countries with which the World Bank mainly deals in the field of health. Thus too high a birth rate may justify the low weight given to infants; the peak productivity of manual workers in countries living near subsistence may justify the high weights in the range 15–40; and the low level of real income in such countries may justify the weight less than 1 given after the age of about 50. In richer countries things may be different. For example, with a low birth-rate the starting values will be higher. If the productivity of a largely non-manual workforce peaks later, the peak will be later. And with greater real income an ageing population is more supportable so the age at which the age-weights fall below 1 will come later.

. . .

But the age-weights emerging from the "fair innings" argument and those emerging from the World Bank's argument, are picking up different things. The World Bank's age-weights are designed to reflect the view that people of different ages have a different (social) value (which in turn reflects their likely life stage). The years between 20 and 50 are particularly valuable to society because those are the years of procreation and child-rearing and the years in which the rest of society gets the maximum economic return from earlier investments in an individual's education and training, etc. Even at individual level this period is frequently referred to as "the best years of my life" or the "prime of life" and the marked lack of enthusiasm with which my younger colleagues celebrate their 40th and 50th birthdays seems to reinforce the view that these achievements are seen as "millstones" rather than "milestones."

The age-weights relating to the "fair innings" argument have a different rationale. They are linked to the likelihood that over your lifetime you will achieve a certain target number of life years or QALYs. . . .

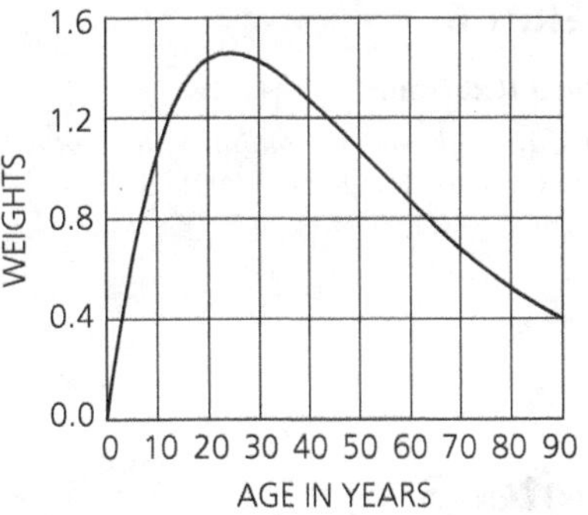

Figure [5.1] Relative value of a year of life (*World Development Report 1993*).

Conclusions for Policy and for Research

Intergenerational equity

But these "fair innings" equity weights have particular salience for the issue of intergenerational equity. If what we wish to equalize is lifetime experience of health, then it indicates that those who have had a "fair innings" (like me) should not expect to have as much spent on a health improvement for them as would be spent to generate the same benefit for someone who is unlikely ever to attain what we have already enjoyed. It calls for self-restraint by us elderly and especially by those of us who have flourished in health terms throughout our lives. Otherwise we may find that demands are being made on the health care system which will deny health improvements to the less fortunate. Unfortunately, that restraint will be called for at a time when our current health is declining and when it would be perfectly possible to spend vast resources on us in the vain pursuit of healthy immortality. The advantage of these "fair innings" generated equity weights is that they will not rule out the offering of very efficient procedures that help improve the QALE of the elderly, but they will establish a variable cut-off point depending on the previous history of the potential beneficiary. This is what a "fair innings" is all about and this is what we need to explore more carefully.

EXCERPT 6

Abridged text from:

J. Harris, *The Value of Life: An Introduction to Medical Ethics* (New York: Routledge, 1990), ch. 5.

Chapter 5

The Value of Life: An Introduction to Medical Ethics

John Harris

The Value of Life

Suppose that only one place is available on a renal dialysis programme or that only one bed is vacant in a vital transplantation unit or that resuscitation could be given in the time and with the resources available to only one patient. Suppose further that of the two patients requiring any of these resources, one is a 70-year-old widower, friendless and living alone, and the other a 40-year-old mother of three young children with a husband and a career.

. . . Suppose further and finally that all candidates stand an equal chance of maximum benefit from any of the available treatments. Whom should wee treat and what justifies our decision?

Many will think that in the first case preference should be given to the young mother rather than the old friendless widower, that this is obviously the right choice. There might be a number of grounds for such a decision. Two of these grounds have to do with age. One indicates a preference for the young on the grounds that they have a greater expectation of life if they are restored to health. The other favours the young simply because their life is likely to be fuller and hence more valuable than that of the older person. Another consideration to which many will want to give some weight is that of the number of people dependent on or even caring about a potential victim. It is sometimes also considered relevant to give weight to the patient's probable usefulness to the community or even their moral character before a final decision is made. And of course these considerations may be taken together in various combinations.

In the case of a major disaster related problems arise. If say a policy of triage[1] has identified the only group of victims to be treated, those for whom medical intervention will make the difference between life and death, but there are still not enough resources to help all such persons, then, again, many will hold that the right thing to do is help the young or those with dependants and so on first.

Those who believe that they ought to select the patient or patients to be saved on any of the above criteria will believe that they must show preference for some types or conditions of person over others. Another available strategy is of course to decline to choose between people in any way that involves preferring one patient, or one sort of person, to another. Perhaps the easiest way of declining to show such a preference is to toss a coin or draw lots to decide who shall be helped. I want to consider what might count as a good reason for preferring to help some patients rather than others where all cannot be helped and also whether our intuitive preference for saving the younger and more useful members of society can be sustained.

---

[1] Triage is a policy for coping with disasters where resources are insufficient to provide the normal standard of care for all. It involves dividing survivors into three groups: those who will die in any event, those who will live in any event, and those for whom care will make the difference between life and death. Care is then given only to this latter group. The argument is that this is the most economical use of resources where resources are insufficient to help all.

I. The Moral Significance of Age

Many, perhaps most, people feel that, in cases like the one with which we began, there is some moral reason to save the 40-year-old mother rather than the 70-year-old widower. A smaller, but perhaps growing, group of people would see this as a sort of "ageist" prejudice which, in a number of important areas of resource allocation and care, involves giving the old a much worse deal than the younger members of society. . . .

The anti-ageist argument

All of us who wish to go on living have something that each of us values equally although for each it is different in character. This thing is of course "the rest of our lives." So long as we do not know the date of our deaths then for each of us the "rest of our lives" is of indefinite duration. Whether we are 17 or 70, in perfect health or suffering from a terminal disease we each have the rest of our lives to lead. So long as we each fervently wish to live out the rest of our lives, however long that turns out to be, then if we do not deserve to die, we each suffer the same injustice if our wishes are deliberately frustrated and we are cut off prematurely. Indeed there may well be a double injustice in deciding that those whose life expectation is short should not benefit from rescue or resuscitation. Suppose I am told today that I have terminal cancer with only approximately six months or so to live, but I want to live until I die, or at least until I decide that life is no longer worth living. Suppose I then am involved in an accident and because my condition is known to my potential rescuers and there are not enough resources to treat all who could immediately be saved I am marked among those who will not be helped. I am then the victim of a double tragedy and a double injustice. I am stricken first by cancer and the knowledge that I have only a short time to live and I'm then stricken again when I'm told that because of my first tragedy a second and more immediate one is to be visited upon me. Because I have once been unlucky I'm now no longer worth saving.

The point is a simple but powerful one. However short or long my life will be, so long as I want to go on living it then I suffer a terrible injustice when that life is prematurely cut short. Imagine a group of people all of an age, say a class of students all in their mid-20s. If fire trapped all in the lecture theatre and only twenty could be rescued in time should the rescuers shout "youngest first!"? Suppose they had time to debate the question or had been debating it "academically" before the fire? It would surely seem invidious to deny some what all value so dearly merely because of an accident of birth? It might be argued that age here provides no criterion precisely because although the lifespans of such a group might be expected to vary widely, there would be no way of knowing who was most likely to live longest. . . .

It is important to be clear that the anti-ageist argument denies the relevance of age or life expectancy as a criterion absolutely. It argues that even if I know for certain that I have only a little space to live, that space, however short, may be very precious to me. Precious, precisely because it is all the time I have left, and just as precious to me on that account as all the time you have left is precious to you, however much those two timespans differ in length. So that where we both want, equally strongly, to go on living, then we each suffer the same injustice[2] when our lives are cut short or are cut further short.[3]

It might seem that someone who would insist on living out the last few months of his life when by "going quietly" someone else might have the chance to live for a much longer time would be a very selfish person. But this would be true only if the anti-ageist argument is false.

---

[2] This may be a rash assumption because of the voluntary nature of many risks.

[3] Of course if I don't value it because it is so short as to be scarcely worth having then the point does not apply in such a case.

I think the anti-ageist argument has much plausibility. It locates the wrongness of ending an individual's life in the evil of thwarting that person's desire to go on living and argues that it is profoundly unjust to frustrate that desire merely because some of those who have exactly the same desire, held no more strongly, also have a longer life expectancy than the others. . . .

The fair innings argument

One problem with the anti-ageist argument is our feeling that there is something unfair about a person who has lived a long and happy life hanging on grimly at the end, while someone who has not been so fortunate suffers a related double misfortune, of losing out in a lottery in which his life happened to be in the balance with that of the grim octogenarian. It might be argued that we could accept the part of the anti-ageist argument which focusses on the equal value of unelapsed time, if this could be tempered in some way. How can it be just that someone who has already had more than her fair share of life and its delights should be preferred or even given an equal chance of continued survival with the young person who has not been so favoured? One strategy that seems to take account of our feeling that there is something wrong with taking steps to prolong the lives of the very old at the expense of those much younger is the fair innings argument.

The fair innings argument takes the view that there is some span of years that we consider a reasonable life, a fair innings. Let's say that a fair share of life is the traditional three score and ten, seventy years. Anyone who does not reach 70 suffers, on this view, the injustice of being cut off in their prime. They have missed out on a reasonable share of life; they have been shortchanged. Those, however, who do make 70 suffer no such injustice, they have not lost out but rather must consider any additional years a sort of bonus beyond that which could reasonably be hoped for. The fair innings argument requires that everyone be given an equal chance to have a fair innings, to reach the appropriate threshold but, having reached it, they have received their entitlement. The rest of their life is the sort of bonus which may be cancelled when this is necessary to help others reach the threshold.

The attraction of the fair innings argument is that it preserves and incorporates many of the features that made the anti-ageist argument plausible, but allows us to preserve our feeling that the old who have had a good run for their money should not be endlessly propped up at the expense of those who have not had the same chance. We can preserve the conclusion of the anti-ageist argument, that so long as life is equally valued by the person whose life it is, it should be given an equal chance of preservation, and we can go on taking this view until the people in question have reached a fair innings.

There is, however, an important difficulty with the fair innings argument. It is that the very arguments which support the setting of the threshold at an age which might plausibly be considered to be a reasonable lifespan, equally support the setting of the threshold at any age at all, so long as an argument from fairness can be used to support so doing. Suppose that there is only one place available on the dialysis programme and two patients are in competition for it. One is 30, and the other 40 years of age. The fair innings argument requires that neither be preferred on the grounds of age since both are below the threshold and are entitled to an equal chance of reaching it. If there is no other reason to choose between them we should do something like toss a coin. However, the 30-year-old can argue that the considerations which support the fair innings argument require that she be given the place. After all, what's fair about the fair innings argument is precisely that each individual should nave an equal chance of enjoying the benefits of a reasonable lifespan. The younger patient can argue that from where she's standing, the age of 40 looks much more reasonable a span than that of 30, and that she should be given the chance to benefit from those ten extra years.

This argument generalised becomes a reason for always preferring to save younger rather than older people, whatever the age difference, and makes the original anti-ageist argument begin to look again the more attractive line to take. For the younger person can always argue that the older has had a' fairer innings, and should now give way. It is difficult to stop whatever span is taken to be a fair innings collapsing towards zero under pressure from those younger candidates who see their innings as less fair than that of those with a larger share.

But perhaps this objection to the fair innings argument is mistaken? If seventy years is a fair innings it does not follow that the nearer a span of life approaches seventy years, the fairer an innings it is. This may be revealed by considering a different sort of threshold. Suppose that most people can run a mile in seven minutes, and that two people are given the opportunity to show that they can run a mile in that time. They both expect to be given seven minutes. However, if one is in fact given only three minutes and the other only four, it's not true that the latter is given a fairer running time: for people with average abilities four minutes is no more realistic a time in which to run a mile than is three. Four minutes is neither a fair threshold in itself, nor a fairer one than three minutes would be.

Nor does the argument that establishes seven minutes as an appropriate threshold lend itself to variation downwards. For that argument just is that seven is the number of minutes that an average adult takes to run a mile. Why then is it different for lifespans? If three score and ten is the number of years available to most people for getting what life has to offer, and is also the number of years people can reasonably expect to have, then it is a misfortune to be allowed anything less however much less one is allowed, if nothing less than the full span normally suffices for getting what can *be* got out of life. It's true that the 40-year-old gets more time than the 30-year-old, but the frame of reference is not time only, but time normally required for a full life.[4]

This objection has some force, but its failure to be a good analogy reveals that two sorts of considerations go to make an innings fair. For while living a full or complete life, just in the sense of experiencing all the ages of man,[5] is one mark of a fair innings, there is also value in living through as many ages as possible. Just as completing the mile is one value, it is not the only one. Runners in the race of life also value ground covered, and generally judge success in terms of distance run.

What the fair innings argument needs to do is to capture and express in a workable form the truth that while it is always a *misfortune* to die when one wants to go on living, it is not a *tragedy* to die in old age; but it is on the other hand, both a tragedy and a misfortune to be cut off prematurely. Of course ideas like "old age" and "premature death" are inescapably vague, and may vary from society to society, and over time as techniques for postponing death improve. We must also remember that while it may be invidious to choose between a 30- and a 40-year-old on the grounds that one has had a fairer innings than the other, it may not be invidious to choose between the 30- and the 65-year-old on those grounds.

If we remember, too, that it will remain wrong to end the life of someone who wants to live or to fail to save them, and that the fair innings argument will only operate as a principle of selection where we are forced to choose between lives, then something workable might well be salvaged.

While "old age" is irredeemably vague, we can tell the old from the young, and even the old from the middle-aged. So that without attempting precise formulation, a reasonable form of the fair innings argument might hold; and might hold that people who had achieved old age or who were closely approaching it would not have their lives further prolonged when this could only be achieved at the cost of the lives of those who were not nearing old age. These categories could be left vague, the idea being that it would be morally defensible to prefer to save the lives of those who "still had their lives before them" rather than those who had "already lived full lives." The

[4] I owe this objection to Tom Sorrel and am greatly in his debt here and elsewhere in this chapter for his generous and penetrating criticisms and comments.

[5] No non-sexist form is available here nor is one desirable since a different formulation would lose the resonance of the phrase.

criterion to be employed in each case would simply be what reasonable people would say about whether someone had had a fair innings. Where reasonable people would be in no doubt that a particular individual was nearing old age *and* that that person's life could only be further prolonged at the expense of the life of someone that no reasonable person would classify as nearing old age, then the fair innings argument would apply, and it would be justifiable to save the younger candidate.

. . .

But again it must be emphasised that the fair innings argument would only operate as a counsel of despair, when it was clearly impossible to postpone the deaths of all those who wanted to go on living. . . .

Numbers of lives and numbers of years

One immediate problem is that although living as long as possible, however long that turns out to be, will normally be very important to each individual, it seems a bad basis for planning health care or justifying the distribution of resources.

Suppose a particular disease, cancer, kills 120,000 people a year. Suppose further that a drug is developed which would prolong the lives of all cancer victims by one month but no more. Would it be worth putting such a drug into production? What if, for the same cost, a different drug would give ten years' complete remission, but would only operate on a form of cancer that affects 1,000 people? If we cannot afford both, which should we invest in? Or, what if there is only one place on a renal dialysis programme and two patients who could benefit, but one will die immediately without dialysis but in six months in any event. The other will also die immediately without dialysis but with such help will survive for ten years. Although each wants the extra span of life equally badly, many would think that we ought to save the one with the longer life expectancy, that she is the "better bet."

All of these cases are an embarrassment for the anti-ageist argument, for our reaction to them implies that we do value extra years more. But how much more?

Extra life-time versus extra lives

. . .

One consequence of this is that we should think it more important to save one 10-year-old rather than five 60-year-olds (if we take 70 as an arbitrary maximum).[6] Equally, it would be better to save one 20-year-old rather than two 50-year-old people, for we would again save ten life years by so doing. Or one 15-year-old rather than two 45-year-olds (a saving of five life years) and so on.

It is just at this point that the anti-ageist argument seems to require resuscitation, for there is surely something invidious about sacrificing two 45-year-olds to one 15-year-old. To take the "life years" view seems to discount entirely the desires and hopes and life plans of people in middle age, whenever an importunate youngster can place herself in the balance against them. But we do not normally think it better to save a 15-year-old rather than a 45-year-old when we cannot save both, so why should we think it better to save a 15-year-old rather than *two* 45-year-olds?

. . .

Unfortunately the force of the comparison between extending the lives of 120,000 people for one month or 1,000 for ten years was to encourage us to think that life-time saved was more important than numbers of lives saved. Its support for this conclusion now seems less decisive. What it seems to indicate is a very complicated calculus in which allocation of resources would be dependent on the amount of life-time such allocation could save. It would also lead to some bizarre orderings of priority, and not necessarily to those envisaged by enthusiasts of such a scheme.

. . .

Threshold of discrimination

It is tempting to think that we might be able to get over some of the problems of the

[6] I'm assuming 70 as the full measure of life expectancy of healthy people and that all candidates are healthy in the sense that there is no reason to regard their life expectancy as less than average.

life-time position by arguing that we can discount small gains in time as below the level of discrimination, in the sense that the benefit to the individual which accrued from living for a comparatively short period of extra time was nugatory. This might solve a few of the problems for the life-time position which arise from the necessity it imposes of favouring one group of people over another, wherever and whenever they are sufficiently numerous that the total life-time saved by rescuing them, even for a negligibly short period, exceeds that which might be saved by rescuing another smaller group who would live longer individually, but shorter collectively. . . .

The fallacy of life-time views

Suppose various medical research teams to be in competition for all research funds available and that one team could demonstrate that it was capable of producing an elixir of life that would make anyone taking it immortal. Suppose further that the entire world medical research budget, if applied to this end would produce just enough elixir for one dose, and that nothing less than a full dose would have any effect at all. The life-time view suggests that all the money should go to making one person immortal rather than say to an alternative project by which another team could make everyone on earth live to a flourishing 80![7]

But there is an obvious fallacy in this argument which reveals a defect in the whole life-time approach. Making one person immortal will produce a saving of no more life years than would the alternative of making everyone on earth live to a flourishing 80. So long as the world itself and its population lasts as long as the immortal (and how—and where—could he last longer?) there would be no net increase in life years lived. Indeed so long as there is either a stable or an increasing world population, from the life years point of view, it matters not at all who lives and who dies, nor does it matter how many years anyone survives. For, so long as those who die are replaced on a one-for-one, or better than a one-for-one basis, there will be no loss of life years. Nor will there be any gain in life years when particular individuals live for longer. For if the overall world population is stable, then prolonging the life of particular individuals does not increase the total number of life years the world contains. And if the world population is increasing then it is highly unlikely that prolonging the lives of particular people will fuel that increase. Indeed the reverse is more likely to be the case with the survival of people beyond child-bearing age having a retarding effect on the rate of increase.

In the context of a stable or of an increasing world population, any idea that any policy which did not have the effect of increasing the population in fact made any contribution to the amount of life-time saved would be an illusion.

We do not then have always to calculate the probable net saving in life-time of any particular policy or therapy, before knowing what to do, and can revert to the more customary consideration of the numbers of lives that might be saved or lost. This, however, highlights once again the problems of whether lives that can only be saved for relatively short periods of time (that can only be prolonged by a few months say) are as worth saving as those for whom the prognosis in terms of life expectancy is much longer. A manoeuvre that seems to capture our intuitions here involves modifying the life-time view into a worthwhile life-time view.

Worthwhile life-time

While to many just staying alive may be the most important consideration, and while they may even wish to continue to live even at appalling cost in terms of pain, disability and so on even, as we have seen, where their lives are hardly worth living, they of course prefer to live worthwhile lives. So that while any life might be better than no life, people generally expect medical care of concern itself not simply with preventing death but with restoring worthwhile existence.

[7] The elixir of life example which prompted this argument about the fallacy of life-time views in stable or increasing populations I owe to Tom Sorrel whose formulation of it I largely use.

Many sorts of thing will go to diminish the worth of life just as many and various considerations go to make life valuable—and these will differ from individual to individual. For the moment we are just concerned with the question of how life expectancy operates as one of these.

If someone were sentenced to death and told that the execution would take place at dawn the next day, they would not, I imagine, be excessively overjoyed if they were then informed that the execution had been postponed for one month. Similarly if the prognosis for a particular disease were very accurate indeed, to be told that one had only seven months to live would not be dramatically less terrible than to be told one had six months to live. There are two related reasons for this. The first is simply that the prospect of imminent death colours, or rather discolours, existence and leaves it joyless. The second is that an almost necessary condition for valuing life is its open-endedness. The fact that we do not normally know how long we have to live liberates the present and leaves us apparently free to plan the future without having to be constantly aware of the futility of so doing.[8] If life had a short and finite (rather than indefinite) future, most things would not seem to be worth doing and the whole sense of the worth of life as an enterprise would evaporate.[9]

In the light of these considerations many people would not much value such short periods of remission, and support for policies which could at best produce such small gains might well be slight. However, some might well value highly the chance of even a small share of extra time. So far from emptying their life of meaning, it might enable them to "round it off" or complete some important task or settle or better arrange their affairs. It might, so far from being of no value, be just what they needed to sort their life out and make some sort of final sense of it.

We have frequently noted the extreme difficulty involved in discounting the value of someone's life where we and they disagree about whether or not it is worth living, and we have also noted the injustice of preferring our assessment to theirs when so much is at stake for them. In view of all this it would be hard to prefer our judgment to theirs here.

. . .

Fair innings or no ageism?

We have then two principles which can in hard cases pull in opposite directions. What should we do in the sorts of hard cases we have been considering? First, we should be clear that while the very old and those with terminal conditions are alike, in, that they both have a short life expectancy, they may well differ with respect to whether or not they have had a fair innings. I do not believe that this issue is at all clear cut but I am inclined to believe that where two individuals both equally wish to go on living for as long as possible our duty to respect this wish is paramount. It is, as I have suggested, the most important part of what is involved in valuing the lives of others. Each person's desire to stay alive should be regarded as of the same importance and as deserving the same respect as that of anyone else, irrespective of the quality of their life or its expected duration.

This would hold good in all cases in which we have to choose between lives, except one. And that is where one individual has had a fair innings and the other not. In this case, while both equally wish to have their lives further prolonged one, but not the other, has had a fair innings. In this case, although there is nothing to choose between the two candidates from the point of view of their respective will to live and both would suffer the injustice of having their life cut short when it might continue, only one would suffer the further injustice of being

[8] Many people have argued of course that it is always futile to plan for the future because the inevitability of our world's ultimate destruction makes everything futile.

[9] For the record we should note that small gains in life-time will only seem to be worthless to those who gain them if it is known that they will be short. If the potential beneficiaries are kept in ignorance of the fact that they can be granted only a short remission then the extra time will not be clouded by the futility deriving from its short duration and the gain, though small, will be as worthwhile as any other segment of their lives of comparable duration. Of course the deception may not be justified.

deprived of a fair innings—a benefit that the other has received.

It is sometimes said that it is a misfortune to grow old, but it is not nearly so great a misfortune as not to grow old. Growing old when you don't want to is not half the misfortune that is not growing old when you do want to. It is this truth that the fair innings argument captures. So that while it remains true, as the anti-ageist argument asserts, that the value of the unelapsed possible lifespan of each person who wants to go on living is equally valuable however long that span may be, the question of which person's premature death involves the greater injustice can be important. The fair innings argument points to the fact that the injustice done to someone who has not had a fair innings when they lose out to someone who has is significantly greater than in the reverse circumstances. It is for this reason that in the hopefully rare cases where we have to choose between candidates who differ only in this respect that we should choose to give as many people as possible the chance of a fair innings.

. . .

IV. The Moral Advantage of Usefulness

There are two sorts of usefulness, usefulness in saving lives and any other kind of usefulness. Usefulness in saving lives is in a class of its own simply because to fail to give extra value to the life of someone whose continued existence will save the lives of others is to discount entirely the value of those extra lives that will be lost if the life-saver dies. However the circumstances in which it is clear that others will die unless a particular individual is preserved will be very exceptional.

Heads of state, members of governments, chiefs of police and the like clearly believe that their usefulness is of this type since they arrange for themselves secure billets in fall-out shelters against the outbreak of nuclear war. Whether other citizens would take the value of these office-holders at their own estimation of it is more doubtful. It is sometimes said that "leading surgeons" are a clear example of the sorts of people who have what might be called class-one usefulness,[10] although, again, this would not be an entirely uncontroversial classification. All that can safely be said is that all whose continued existence is clearly required so that others might live have a good claim to priority. Whether any other sort of usefulness is so important that those who possess it could claim to live on at the cost of the lives of others seems to me to be more doubtful.

. . .

V. Moral Worth

. . .

We all, of course, have a duty to encourage and promote morality, but to do so by choosing between candidates for treatment on moral grounds is to arrogate to ourselves not simply the promotion of morality but the punishment of immorality. And to choose to let one person rather than another die on the grounds of some moral defect in their behaviour or character is to take upon ourselves the right not simply to punish, but capitally to punish, offenders against morality. Even in the, I hope unlikely event of our being satisfied that we were entitled or obliged to do this we would be attempting to discharge a quasi-judicial function without any of the safeguards or rigour of legal proceedings. What standards of proof would be required or discharged in such investigations, what right of reply or defence would be offered? Indeed, what would constitute moral crimes for these purposes? The morality of choosing between candidates for rescue on moral grounds would itself be much more likely to be profoundly immoral than anything any of the candidates is likely to be guilty of.

---

[10] J. Glover, *Causing Death and Saving Lives: The Moral Problems of Abortion, Infanticide, Suicide, Euthanasia, Capital Punishment, War and Other Life-or-Death Choices* (Penguin Books Limited, 1990), p. 223.

EXCERPT 7

Full text from:

E. Nord, "Concerns for the Worse Off: Fair Innings Versus Severity," *Social Science & Medicine* 60, no. 2 (2005): pp. 257–263.

Concerns for the Worse Off: Fair Innings Versus Severity

Erik Nord

Introduction

Distributive fairness is an important goal in health care, to be taken duly account of in the pursuit of allocative efficiency.[1,2,3,4,5] Concerns for fairness are of various kinds. This paper addresses one of them. A common feature of different theories of fairness[6,7] and of the thinking of ordinary people about fairness[8] is a special concern for the worse off members of society. The concern implies that benefits are considered to have greater weight the worse off those who receive them are. Concerns for the worse off thus run counter to the utilitarian idea that resources should be allocated simply with a view to maximising overall health benefits. Parfit refers to concerns for the worse off as "The Priority View."[9] Brock[10] offers a number of possible justifications for the view, including the argument that the worse off suffer undeserved relative deprivation, and/or that the worse off have more urgent needs.

If priority in health care is to be given to the worse off, there is first a question of whether one should be concerned about those worse off in health or those worse off overall, i.e. in their global life situation. While some would argue in favour of the latter, there is probably less agreement about this than about giving priority to those who are worse off in terms of health. I shall therefore restrict myself to discussing who is worse off in terms of health only. This is at any rate of interest in priority setting across groups who are equal on other aspects of life than health.

To decide who is worse of with respect to health is on the one hand a matter of determining the relative weights to be attached to different aspects of illness (pain, discomfort, bodily impairments, loss of capabilities, etc.) in judgements of the "badness" of different conditions.

---

[1] P. Anand, A. Wailoo and O. U. E. Department, *Utilities Vs. Rights to Publicly Provided Goods: Arguments and Evidence from Health-Care Rationing* (Economics Department, Open University, 2000).

[2] J. Broome, "Good, Fairness and QALYs," *Royal Institute of Philosophy Supplements* 23 (1988): pp. 57–73.

[3] G. Mooney and J. A. Olsen, "QALYs: Where Next?", in *Providing Health Care: The Economics of Alternative Systems of Finance and Delivery*, edited by A. McGuire et al. (New York: Oxford University Press, 1991).

[4] A. Sen, *Inequality Reexamined* (Oxford University Press, 1992).

[5] A. Williams, "Ethics and Efficiency in the Provision of Health Care," *Royal Institute of Philosophy Supplements* 23 (1988): pp. 111–126.

[6] N. Daniels, "Rationing Fairly: Programmatic Considerations," *Bioethics* 7, no. 2–3 (1993): pp. 224–233.

[7] J. Rawls, *A Theory of Justice* (Cambridge: Harvard University Press, 1971).

[8] E. Nord, et al., "Incorporating Societal Concerns for Fairness in Numerical Valuations of Health Programmes," *Health Economics* 8, no. 1 (1999): pp. 25–39.

[9] D. Parfit and U. K. D. Philosophy, *Equality or Priority?: The Lindley Lecture, University of Kansas, November 21, 1991* (University of Kansas, 1991).

[10] D. W. Brock, "Priority to the Worse Off in Health Care Resource Prioritization," in *Medicine and Social Justice: Essays on the Distribution of Health Care*, edited by R. Rhodes, M. P. Battin, and A. Silvers (New York: Oxford University Press, 2002).

This question has been widely addressed in the health-related quality of life literature and is not the theme of this paper. Instead I address a question that has to do with the time perspective of "worse-offness": Is being worse off a matter of being in a bad state at a given point in time, or of having a bad prognosis, or of having had a poor history of health, or perhaps all of these, i.e. of having poor health as judged over a whole lifetime?

British economist Alan Williams has strongly advocated the latter view. He relates the notion of being worse off to the idea that resources should be allocated such as to ensure everybody a "fair innings" of health over their life time. According to Williams, one is worse off the less quality adjusted life years one is expected to enjoy from birth till death.

Surprisingly few writers have discussed this proposition. One of the few is Amartya Sen.[11] He regards Williams' approach as an interesting and potentially powerful one, particularly since it seems to deal with social class inequality in a fulsome way. But he also stresses its limitations for policy making. For example, Williams claims that men are not getting their fair innings, insofar as their health adjusted life expectancy is significantly lower than that of women. While acknowledging the latter fact, Sen suggests that giving preference to male patients "cannot but lack some quality that we would tend to associate with the *process* (my italicising) of health equity" (p. 21). Sen thus warns against approaches that insist on taking a single-dimensional view of health equity, stating that "it is possible to accept the significance of a perspective, without taking that perspective to be ground enough for rejecting other ways of looking at health equity, which too can be important."

This paper is written in a somewhat similar vein. It compares the fair innings approach to encapsulating concerns for the worse off with one that focuses on the severity of a patient's condition as an independent determinant of society's valuation (appreciation) of an intervention.[12,13,14,15,16] Williams has claimed that the former approach subsumes the latter and encapsulates distributive concerns in a more sensible way.[17,18] In the following I examine this claim. I first explain the two approaches. I then point out their similarities and differences in terms of implications for social choice in a set of hypothetical health programs. Finally, I discuss briefly the extent to which the partly conflicting implications from each of the approaches are supported by moral argument, political documents and public opinion surveys.

Fair Innings

The fair innings approach centres initially on the feeling that everyone is entitled to some "normal" number of life years, say 70–75. The implication is that anyone failing to achieve this has in some sense been cheated, whilst anyone getting more than this is "living on borrowed time."[19] Williams

[11] A. K. Sen. *Keynote Address to IHEA Conference* (2001).

[12] P. Menzel, *Strong Medicine* (New York: Oxford University Press, 1990).

[13] E. Nord, "The Trade-Off Between Severity of Illness and Treatment Effect in Cost-Value Analysis of Health Care," *Health Policy* 24, no. 3 (1993): pp. 227–238.

[14] J. L. Pinto Prades, "Is the Person Trade-Off a Valid Method for Allocating Health Care Resources?", *Health Economics* 6, no. 1 (1997): pp. 71–81.

[15] J. Richardson, *Critique and Some Recent Contributions to the Theory of Cost Utility Analysis* (Citeseer, 1997).

[16] P. A. Ubel, "How Stable Are People's Preferences for Giving Priority to Severely Ill Patients?", *Social Science and Medicine* 49, no. 7 (1999): pp. 895–903.

[17] A. Williams, "Book Review," *Health Economics* 9 (2000): pp. 739–742.

[18] A. Williams, "The 'Fair Innings Argument' Deserves a Fairer Hearing! Comments by Alan Williams on Nord and Johannesson," *Health Economics* 10, no. 7 (2001): pp. 583–585

[19] A. Williams, "Intergenerational Equity: An Exploration of the 'Fair Innings' Argument," *Health Economics* 6, no. 2 (1997): pp. 117–132.

proposes that gained life years in people facing less than a fair innings should be valued more highly (be assigned a larger weight) than life years gained in people expecting to have a fair innings or more.

Williams furthermore argues that in order to "capture the full flavour of this kind of thinking, the concept of a 'fair innings' needs to be extended beyond simple life expectancy to embrace quality-adjusted life expectancy. Otherwise it will not be possible to reflect the view that a lifetime of poor quality health entitles people to special consideration in the current allocation of health care, even if their life expectancy is normal" (p. 121). So for instance, if quality-adjusted life expectancy (QALE) is 70 QALYs in a population as a whole, and this is considered to be a fair innings, and QALE is 73, 67 and 64 QALYs in subgroups A, B and C, respectively, then (according to Williams) QALYs gained in subgroup C should be weighted more than QALYs gained in subgroup B, which in turn should be weighted more than QALYs gained in subgroup A.

The fair innings approach thus takes into account health losses both in the past and the future in its operationalisation of being worse off.

Severity

The basic hypothesis of the severity approach is that the societal value (appreciation) of a health improvement of a given size is greater the greater the severity of the patient's initial condition. For instance, if person A can be taken from 0.4 to 0.6 on a scale of individual utility with interval scale properties, and person B can be taken from 0.6 to 0.8 on the same scale, then society will value the former improvement more than the latter, due to a preference for giving priority to the worse off when all else is equal. Whether or not this is true, is of course a question for empirical testing. If the proposition is true, it is possible to encapsulate it in numerical valuation models, either by multiplying utility gains in the conventional QALY model by weights reflecting the severity of the start point, or by replacing conventional utilities for health states by values with a strong compression to the upper end of the 0–1 scale.[20]

The severity approach takes into account not only severity at the time of intervention, but also expected severity—including being dead—in future years in case of non-intervention. This follows from the fact that QALY gains from an intervention are calculated as the sum of benefits, i.e. utility gains, in each of the life years affected by the intervention. For instance, if a person's utilities in the next five years in case of non-intervention are expected to be 0.7, 0.7, 0.6, 0.5 and 0.0 (dead), and the utilities would be 0.8 in all 5 years (and then dead) in case of intervention, then the benefit from the intervention would be 0.1 + 0.1 + 0.2 + 0.3 + 0.8 = 1.5 QALYs. The severity approach implies the application of severity weights (or upper end compression of utilities) to *each* of these annual utility gains. Similarly, if a person gets to live 5 years at a utility level of 0.8 instead of dying, then each of these five annual utility gains of 0.8 will be multiplied by the severity weight for the state "dead." I return to this point below.

Comparing Fair Innings and Severity

My focus in the following is on Williams' expansion of the fair innings approach to include quality of life considerations, which is also what the severity approach purports to capture. I do not dispute the validity of the original fair innings approach, which is restricted to length of life considerations. The severity approach does not purport to encapsulate such considerations.

The fair innings approach and the severity approach both require procedures for weighting utility gains in terms of QALYs.

[20] Nord, "Incorporating Societal Concerns."

The weights need to be at a cardinal level of measurement. Various measurement techniques are available in both approaches, including direct questions about severity–efficiency trade-offs[21,22] and willingness-to-pay and person trade-off questions.[23,24] I see no grounds for claiming that one of the two competing approaches is more amenable to measurement than the other.

The fair innings approach and the severity approach are based on different arguments as to who is worse off. To some extent they therefore have different implications when it comes to ranking interventions in terms of societal value or priority. Let us first look at the differences in arguments.

Arguments

As noted above, the severity approach is meant to encapsulate a concern for those who are worse off *now and/or in the future*. In the fair innings approach there is no such concern per se. Present and future severity are of interest only to the extent that they affect life time QALYs. Present and future illness are on a par with past illness.

The fair innings argument is, furthermore, actually not one argument, but two. First, it says that everybody should have the same number of QALYs over their life time. I shall call this the *"equal innings argument."* Second, it says that QALYs beyond a certain threshold should count very little. I shall call this the *sufficient innings argument.*

These two arguments are logically independent of each other. For instance, based on the *equal* innings argument one could say that QALY gains should be weighted proportionally to the difference between a persons QALE and a potential maximum of, say, 100 QALYs. QALY gains for 85-year-olds with a QALE of 84 would then be given only two-thirds of the weight of QALY gains for 70-year-olds with a QALE of 76 ((100 − 84)/(100 − 76) = 2/3). The QALY gains of the 85-year-olds would nonetheless be given greater weight than if for instance 75 QALYs were introduced as a threshold above which QALY gains were to be strongly devalued. Similarly, it would be possible to argue on the basis of the *sufficient* innings argument that QALY gains above a QALE of for instance 75 should count less, without at all assigning different weights to QALY gains for people with a QALE of 50 and 60, respectively.

So the ethical basis of the fair innings approach consists of two distinct arguments—which I call equal innings and sufficient innings—both of which are different from the severity argument of the severity approach. I return to this when I later discuss the claim that the fair innings approach is better than the severity approach.

Implications for priority setting

In some cases the severity approach and the fair innings approach will lead to much the same results with respect to weighting QALYs. In other cases the results will be quite different. In Tables [5.1] and [5.2] I show six hypothetical patient groups that may give us some idea of the degree of overlap and difference between the implications of the two approaches.

In Table [5.1], patients A–C have a life time of 80 years. A- and B-patients are healthy until they are 70, whereafter A-patients drop to a utility level of 0.9 (mild), while B-patients drop to 0.5 (severe). C-patients have a history of illness at utility level 0.8, and drop to 0.7 (moderate) at the age of 70. D-patients are healthy until they are 80, whereafter they live ten more years at utility level 0.9. QALEs without intervention are 79 (A), 75 (B), 63 (C) and 89 (D) QALYs, respectively.

Now, imagine the appearance of a new medical technology that lends itself to treating

[21] P. Dolan, "The Measurement of Individual Utility and Social Welfare," *Journal of Health Economics* 17, no. 1 (1998): pp. 39–52.

[22] A. Wagstaff, "QALYs and the Equity-Efficiency Trade-Off," *Journal of Health Economics* 10, no. 1 (1991): pp. 21–41.

[23] J. A. Olsen, "Aiding Priority Setting in Health Care: Is There a Role for the Contingent Valuation Method?", *Health Economics* 6, no. 6 (1997): pp. 603–612.

[24] Nord, "Incorporating Societal Concerns."

Table [5.1]
Utilities at different times, and life time QALYs, for four hypothetical patient groups, without and with intervention

Patient Group		Years 0–70	Years 70–80	Years 80–90	>90	QALY
A	Without intervention	1.0	0.9	Dead	Dead	79
	With intervention at 70	1.0	1.0	Dead	Dead	80
B	Without intervention	1.0	0.5	Dead	Dead	75
	With intervention at 70	1.0	0.6	Dead	Dead	76
C	Without intervention	0.8	0.7	Dead	Dead	63
	With intervention at 70	0.8	0.8	Dead	Dead	64
D	Without intervention	1.0	1.0	0.9	Dead	89
	With intervention at 80	1.0	1.0	1.0	Dead	90

all these four different types of patients. All four groups can right after the health loss (at 70 for A–C, at 80 for D) be helped one decimal point up on the utility scale by the new technology. In all groups the benefit will be enjoyed for 10 years, corresponding to 1 QALY. How should one prioritise between the groups if the technology is in scarce supply?

Consider first groups A–C. The purpose of the *severity approach* is to capture the difference in current and future severity. It thus gives additional weight to the QALY gains of B-patients relative to A-patients. It also gives additional weight to C-patients relative to A-patients, and to B-patients relative to C-patients.

The *equal innings* argument does the same in the comparison of A with B: Since B-patients have a lower QALE at 70 than A-patients, their QALY gains will be given greater weight. Similarly, the equal innings argument, like the severity argument, suggests priority to C-patients over A-patients.

On the other hand, in the comparison of B and C the two approaches differ. The severity argument suggests priority to B-patients over C (since only current and future severity counts), while the equal innings argument suggests priority to C over B (since the QALE of C is lower).

Consider also A- and D-patients. Assume that 80 QALYs is considered to be a *sufficient* innings in the fair innings approach. The severity argument suggests equal priority to these two groups. The fair innings approach, on the other hand, would give lower weight to D-patients than to A-patients. Their health improvement during their last years of life might in fact receive quite little weight. This would be different from what the severity argument would suggest.

Consider furthermore Table [5.2]. The severity approach would make no difference between E and F, i.e. between life extension for people at different (in this case moderate) ages, while the fair innings approach would give priority to E on account of the lower expected life time QALYs.

Table [5.2]
Life and death at different times, and life time QALYs, for two hypothetical patient groups, without and with intervention

Patient Group		Years 0–50	Years 51–60	Years 61–70	>70	QALY
E	Without intervention	Healthy	Dead	Dead		50
	With intervention	Healthy	Healthy			60
F	Without intervention	Healthy	Healthy	Dead	Dead	60
	With intervention	Healthy	Healthy	Healthy		70

So clearly the severity approach and the fair innings approach may also yield some very *different* results.

Discussion

The hypothesis addressed in this paper is that the fair innings approach is a better way of encapsulating concerns for the worse off in economic evaluation in terms of QALYs than the severity approach. My response to this is that both approaches are technically feasible. But they are based on different ethical arguments and therefore lead to somewhat different results. The crucial question is which of these conflicting results is morally more defensible. To judge this, it is of interest to draw on both careful ethical reflection and societal preferences as observed in political documents and public opinion surveys.

For judging defensibility, cases of pairwise comparisons of interventions in which the two approaches yield similar results are of less interest. Our focus must be on cases in which the two approaches lead to different results. In Table [5.1] there are three examples of such pairwise comparisons: B versus C, A versus D and E versus F. Let us look at these in turn.

B versus C

B-patients are currently severely ill people with a life time in normal health behind them. C-patients are moderately ill people with a life time of moderate illness behind them. The two groups can be helped equally much. Which group should have priority?

The question is: How should current severity be weighted against life time QALYs? I am not aware of any publications in medical ethics that provide a theoretical answer to this question in terms of moral argument. Nor do I know of any studies of population preferences that shed light on the issue.

The only evidence I am aware of is of an indirect nature: Current and future severity are emphasised as the most important criteria for priority setting in government publications on priority setting in Norwegian and Swedish health care.[25,26] In none of these publications is past illness mentioned as a criterion.

If population preferences studies were conducted to shed further light on the issue, my own hypothesis would be that most people would tend to focus more on the present and the future than on the past if asked to prioritise across patient groups. There are two reasons why this may be the case. First, it seems likely that current suffering makes a stronger impression on people than past suffering. That is, it seems likely that current suffering triggers people's compassion and sense of obligation to help (cfr. the "Rule of Rescue") more than past suffering does. This is akin to the myopia component of positive time preference, only looking backwards in time rather than forwards. Second, the past cannot be changed. Past suffering is "sunk costs." It is the present and the future that a society can do anything about. This may affect choices in priority setting. But I stress that these are only hypotheses. They need to be examined empirically.

A versus D

A-patients and D-patients are equally ill. They can be helped equally much in terms of improved functioning and quality of life, but they present themselves for care at different ages, namely at 70 and 80 years, respectively. Should A-patients have priority on the grounds that D-patients have had their fair innings of "well-life"?

Here we need to distinguish between the fair innings argument in its original form and the *generalised* fair innings argument, which incorporates concerns for quality of life. It is one thing to say that very old people cannot expect to have their *lives extended* by costly

---

[25] Norwegian Commission for Prioritising in Health Care, "Retningslinjer for Prioritering Innen Helsevesenet. (Guidelines for Prioritising in Health Care.)," Universitetsforlaget, 1987.

[26] Swedish Health Care and Medical Priorities Commission, "No Easy Choices—the Difficulties of Health Care," The Ministry of Health and Social Affairs, 1993.

interventions when the same resources can be used to prevent death in people who have not even enjoyed an average length of life. It is a different thing to say that society should care more about *suffering*—for instance in terms of pain—in young people than in old people.

It is an interesting task for moral philosophy to explore and assess the various arguments pertaining to the latter issue. In terms of surveys of public preferences, the picture is unclear. Some researchers have found support for giving priority to the young over the elderly, while others have not.[27] The variation in results is partly explained by variation in the problem contexts that subjects were asked to address. In official guidelines in Norway, age per se is explicitly declared as being of little importance in priority setting. Costly life saving organ transplants for old people is an exception—much because the outcome, in terms of gained life years, is much smaller for old people than for younger people. By contrast, in Norwegian guidelines relief of suffering in old patients is regarded as just as important and worthy of funding as similar interventions in younger people.[28] Official guidelines are similar in Sweden.[29] My own hypothesis is that both ethicists and the general public would agree completely with these government positions.

E versus F

E-patients and F-patients are both fatally ill. They can be helped equally much, in terms of getting ten extra years, but they present themselves for care at different ages, namely at 50 and 60 years, respectively. The severity approach makes no difference between these two programmes, while the fair innings approach says that E-patients should have priority on the grounds that they are being more "cheated" of a normal length of life than F-patients.

I believe many people here would tend to support the fair innings view. But this preference would be on the grounds of the *original* fair innings argument, which focuses on entitlement to a fair number of *life years*. It is independent of Williams' generalization of the argument to include quality of life considerations.

The severity approach does not reject the original fair innings argument. It just does not purport to cover it. To cover the original fair innings argument an approach using severity weights would have to also use age weights in the evaluation of life extending programs.[30]

The different conclusions I reach in the case of E versus F and B versus C demonstrate the need to distinguish between the original, life time oriented fair innings argument and the generalised, QALY oriented one. The distinction is important when one judges Williams' recent response to articles by Magnus Johannesson and myself on fairness in valuing life.[31,32,33] Johannesson suggests that QALY gains in a given group of patients be weighted more the greater the difference between (a) the group's QALE without intervention and (b) QALE in the general population of the same sex and age. For instance, if 60-year-old male patients of a given kind face an expected 10 QALYs in case of no intervention, and 60-year-old men in general expect to get 15 more QALYs, then every QALY gained in that patient group should be given a weight of 1,5 (15:10). While I believe there are various problems with this proposal[34] (I do not think Williams' way of "defeating" it is tenable. Williams constructed an example in which a small QALY gain in a 70-year-old person would get more weight than the same small QALY gain in a 50-year-old person, given that the prognosis of the 70-year-old person *compared*

---

[27] E. Nord, *Cost-Value Analysis in Health Care: Making Sense out of QALYS* (Cambridge University Press, 1999).

[28] Norwegian Commission for Prioritising in Health Care, "Retningslinjer."

[29] Swedish Health Care and Medical Priorities Commission, "No Easy Choices."

[30] Nord, "Incorporating Societal Concerns."

[31] M. Johannesson, "Should We Aggregate Relative or Absolute Changes in QALYs?", *Health Economics* 10, no. 7 (2001): pp. 573–577.

[32] E. Nord, "The Desirability of a Condition Versus the Well Being and Worth of a Person," *Health Economics* 10, no. 7 (2001): pp. 579–581.

[33] Williams, "The 'Fair Innings Argument' Deserves a Fairer Hearing!"

[34] E. Nord, P. Menzel and J. Richardson, "The Value of Life: Individual Preferences and Social Choice. A Comment to Magnus Johannesson," *Health Economics* 12, no. 10 (2003): pp. 873–877.

to 70-year-olds in general was poorer than the prognosis of the 50-year-old person *compared to 50-year-olds in general*. Williams argued that this result was counterintuitive, inasmuch as the 50-year-old had lived much shorter than the 70-year-old and would get less QALYs in total over his lifetime than the 70-year-old even if he/ she were to be given priority. I agree that Johannesson's proposal would lead to an unjust result in Williams' example. But that is because Johannesson's proposal in itself does not purport to capture differences in age, i.e. the issue of the original fair innings argument. I presume that Johannesson's approach, just like the severity approach, could be supplemented with age weights in the evaluation of life extending programmes. The problematic part of Williams' proposal lies in the inclusion of quality of life adjustment in the calculation of the number of innings a person is getting over his or her whole life time. Of course such inclusion also captures current and future severity, as Williams shows in one of this tables. That is plain arithmetic logic. But the question is to what extent health-related quality of life losses *in the past* should count. Williams personally seems very convinced that they should count heavily, and that both Johannesson and I are leading the world astray by not counting them. But he offers no arguments or evidence. My own doubts are explained in the section above on 'B versus C. At the end of the day Williams and I seem to agree that further investigations are needed to determine who is right.

Summary and Conclusion

There is a need to incorporate concerns for fairness in economic evaluation of health care. Such concerns are of several kinds. One of them is the concern for the worse off. The severity approach and the generalised fair innings approach—which includes considerations of quality of life—are two ways of incorporating this particular moral concern. They are both technically feasible, but they are based on different ethical arguments and therefore partly lead to different results. The crucial question is which of these results are more consistent with moral arguments and intuitions and observable societal values and preferences.

Both approaches incorporate concerns for current and future severity. There is strong support for this in formal theories of justice and government guidelines and a number of public surveys even indicate the strength of these concerns.[35]

The fair innings approach *additionally* incorporates concerns for past suffering. Intuitively, this is not unreasonable, but there is at this point little ethical theory or empirical evidence to suggest the strength of such concerns.

The fair innings approach furthermore implies that young people should have priority over old people when it comes to functional improvements and symptom relief for nonfatal conditions. For example, it implies that an 80-year-old who has led a good life but now has pain has less moral claims on pain relief than a 50-year-old with the same amount of pain. This runs counter to both moral intuitions and official government guidelines in Norway and Sweden. In my view it is a serious problem with the generalised fair innings approach as it has been proposed by Williams.

I conclude that while the severity approach is less comprehensive than the generalised fair innings approach, it rests on safer theoretical and empirical grounds. At the same time I stress that the generalised fair innings approach needs to be distinguished from the original fair innings argument, which is about individuals' right to a reasonable length of life. Even if the generalised approach has some unresolved problems, the original argument is compelling. It could for instance justify some age weighting in the evaluation of life extending programmes. The generalised fair innings approach, on the other hand, needs further theoretical clarification and empirical research.

[35] E. Nord, "Severity of Illness Versus Expected Benefit in Societal Evaluation of Healthcare Interventions," *Expert Review of Pharmacoeconomics & Outcomes Research* 1, no. 1 (2001): pp. 85–92.

EXCERPT 8

Abridged text from:

A. H. Moss and M. Siegler, "Should Alcoholics Compete Equally for Liver Transplantation?", *JAMA* 265, no. 10 (1991): pp. 1295–1298.

Should Alcoholics Compete Equally for Liver Transplantation?

Alvin H. Moss and Mark Siegler

. . .

Until recently, liver transplantation for patients with alcohol-related end-stage liver disease (ARESLD) was not considered a treatment option. Most physicians in the transplant community did not recommend it because of initial poor results in this population and because of a predicted high recidivism rate that would preclude long-term survival.[1] In 1988, however, Starzl and colleagues[2] reported one-year survival rates for patients with ARESLD comparable to results in patients with other causes of end-stage liver disease (ESLD). Although the patients in the Pittsburgh series may represent a carefully selected population,[3,4] the question is no longer, Can we perform transplants in patients with alcoholic liver disease and obtain acceptable results? But, Should we? . . .

[1] S. Kumar, et al., "Orthotopic Liver Transplantation for Alcoholic Liver Disease," *Hepatology* 11, no. 2 (1990): pp. 159–164.

[2] T. E. Starzl, et al., "Orthotopic Liver Transplantation for Alcoholic Cirrhosis," *Journal of the American Medical Association* 260, no. 17 (1988): pp. 2542–2544.

[3] Starzl, "Orthotonic Liver Transplantation."

[4] M. Olbrisch and J. L. Levenson, "Liver Transplantation for Alcoholic Cirrhosis," *Journal of the American Medical Association* 261, no. 20 (1989): pp. 2958–2958.

Should Patients with ARESLD Receive Transplants?

At first glance, this question seems simple to answer. Generally, in medicine, a therapy is used if it works and saves lives. But the circumstances of liver transplantation differ from those of most other lifesaving therapies, including long-term mechanical ventilation and dialysis, in three important respects:

Nonrenewable Resource

First, although most lifesaving therapies are expensive, liver transplantation uses a nonrenewable, absolutely scarce resource—a donor liver. In contrast to patients with end-stage renal disease, who may receive either a transplant or dialysis therapy, every patient with ESLD who does not receive a liver transplant will die. This dire, absolute scarcity of donor livers would be greatly exacerbated by including patients with ARESLD as potential candidates for liver transplantation. . . .

Comparison with Cardiac Transplantation

. . .

The allocational decisions for heart transplantation differ from those for liver transplantation in two ways: determining a cause for end-stage heart disease is less certain, and patients with a history of alcoholism are usually rejected from heart transplant programs.

Expensive Technology

Third, a unique aspect of liver transplantation is that it is an expensive technology that has become a target of cost containment in health care.[5] It is, therefore, essential to maintain the

[5] H. G. Welch and E. B. Larson, "Dealing with Limited Resources," *New England Journal of Medicine* 319, no. 3 (1988): pp. 171–173.

approbation and support of the public so that organs continue to be donated under appropriate clinical circumstances—even in spite of the high cost of transplantation.

General Guideline Proposed

In view of the distinctive circumstances surrounding liver transplantation, we propose as a general guideline that patients with ARESLD should not compete equally with other candidates for liver transplantation. We are not suggesting that patients with ARESLD should never receive liver transplants. Rather, we propose that a priority ranking be established for the use of this dire, absolutely scarce societal resource and that patients with ARESLD be lower on the list than others with ESLD.

Objections to Proposal

We realize that our proposal may meet with two immediate objections. . . .

Alcoholism: How Is It Similar to and Different from Other Diseases?

We do not dispute the reclassification of alcoholism as a disease.[6] Both hereditary and environmental factors contribute to alcoholism, and physiological, biochemical, and genetic markers have been associated with increased susceptibility.[7] Identifying alcoholism as a disease enables physicians to approach it as they do other medical problems and to differentiate it from bad habits, crimes, or moral weaknesses. More important, identifying alcoholism as a disease also legitimizes medical interventions to treat it.[8]

. . .

Like other chronic diseases . . . alcoholism requires the patient to assume responsibility for participating in continuous treatment. Two key elements are required to successfully treat alcoholism: the patient must accept his or her diagnosis and must assume responsibility for treatment. The high success rates of some alcoholism treatment programs indicate that many patients can accept responsibility for their treatment.[9,10] . . . In view of the years, even decades, required to develop ARESLD, and the availability of effective alcohol treatment, attributing personal responsibility for ARESLD to the patient seems all the more justified. We believe, therefore, that even though alcoholism is a chronic disease, alcoholics should be held responsible for seeking and obtaining treatment that could prevent the development of late-stage complications such as ARESLD. Our view is consistent with that of Alcoholics Anonymous: alcoholics are responsible for undertaking a program for recovery that will keep their disease of alcoholism in remission.[11]

Are We Discriminating Against Alcoholics?

Why should patients with ARESLD be singled out when a large number of patients have health problems that can be attributed to

[6] J. H. Mendelson and N. K. Mello, *The Diagnosis and Treatment of Alcoholism* (McGraw-Hill, 1979).

[7] K. Blum, et al., "Allelic Association of Human Dopamine D2 Receptor Gene in Alcoholism," *Journal of the American Medical Association* 263, no. 15 (1990): pp. 2055–2060.

[8] H. N. Barnes, et al., *Alcoholism: A Guide for the Primary Care Physician* (Springer-Verlag, 1987).

[9] B. Johnson and W. Clark, "Alcoholism," *Journal of General Internal Medicine* 4, no. 5 (1989): pp. 445–452.

[10] J. A. Bigby, "Negotiating Treatment and Monitoring Recovery," in *Alcoholism: A Guide for the Primary Care Physician*, edited by H. N. Barnes, M. D. Aronson and T. L. Delbanco (New York: Springer-Verlag, 1987).

[11] R. W. Thoreson and F. C. Budd, "Self-Help Groups and Other Group Procedures for Treating Alcohol Problems," in *Treatment and Prevention of Alcohol Problem: A Resource Manual*, edited by W. M. Cox (Orlando, FL: Academic Press, 1987), pp. 157–181.

so-called voluntary health-risk behavior? Such patients include smokers with chronic lung disease; obese people who develop type II diabetes; some individuals who test positive for the human immunodeficiency virus; individuals with multiple behavioral risk factors (inattention to blood pressure, cholesterol, diet, and exercise) who develop coronary artery disease; and people such as skiers, motorcyclists, and football players who sustain activity-related injuries. We believe that the health care system should respond based on the actual medical needs of patients rather than on the factors (e.g., genetic, infectious, or behavioral) that cause the problem. We also believe that individuals should bear some responsibility—such as increased insurance premiums—for medical problems associated with voluntary choices. The critical distinguishing factor for treatment of ARESLD is the scarcity of the resource needed to treat it. The resources needed to treat most of these other conditions are only moderately or relatively scarce, and patients with these diseases or injuries can receive a share of the resources (i.e., money, personnel, and medication) roughly equivalent to their need. In contrast, there are insufficient donor livers to sustain the lives of all with ESLD who are in need.[12] This difference permits us to make some discriminating choices—or to establish priorities—in selecting candidates for liver transplantation based on notions of fairness. . . .

Reasons Patients with ARESLD Should Have a Lower Priority on Transplant Waiting Lists

Two arguments support our proposal. . . .

Fairness

Given a tragic shortage of donor livers, what is the fair or just way to allocate them? We suggest that patients who develop ESLD through no fault of their own (e.g., those with congenital biliary atresia or primary biliary cirrhosis) should have a higher priority in receiving a liver transplant than those whose liver disease results from failure to obtain treatment for alcoholism. In view of the dire, absolute scarcity of donor livers, we believe it is fair to hold people responsible for their choices, including decisions to refuse alcoholism treatment, and to allocate organs on this basis.

It is unfortunate but not unfair to make this distinction.[13] When not enough donor livers are available for all who need one, choices have to be made, and they should be founded on one or more proposed principles of fairness for distributing scarce resources.[14,15] We shall consider four that are particularly relevant:

- *To each, an equal share of treatment.*
- *To each, similar treatment for similar cases.*
- *To each, treatment according to personal effort.*
- *To each, treatment according to ability to pay.*

It is not possible to give each patient with ESLD an equal share, or, in this case, a functioning liver. . . . But what is fair need not be equal. Although a first-come, first-served approach has been suggested to provide each patient with an equal chance, we believe it is fairer to give a child dying of biliary atresia an opportunity for a first normal liver than it is to give a patient with ARESLD who was born with a normal liver a second one.

. . . Outka[16] stated it this way: "If we accept the case for equal access, but if we simply cannot, physically cannot, treat all who are in

[12] G. R. Winslow, *Triage and Justice* (University of California Press, 1982).

[13] H. T. Engelhardt, "Allocating Scarce Medical Resources and the Availability of Organ Transplantation," *New England Journal of Medicine* 311, no. 1 (1984): pp. 66–71.

[14] G. Outka, "Social Justice and Equal Access to Health Care," *Journal of Religious Ethics* 2, no. 1 (1974): pp. 11–32.

[15] T. L. Beauchamp and J. F. Childress, *Principles of Biomedical Ethics* (Oxford University Press, 1994).

[16] Outka, "Social Justice and Equal Access."

need, it seems more just to discriminate by virtue of categories of illness, rather than between rich ill and poor ill." This principle is derived from the principle of formal justice, which, roughly stated, says that people who are equal in relevant respects should be treated equally and that people who are unequal in relevant respects should be treated differently.[17] We believe that patients with ARESLD are unequal in a relevant respect to others with ESLD, since their liver failure was preventable; therefore, it is acceptable to treat them differently.

Our view also relies on the principle of, To each, treatment according to personal effort. Although alcoholics cannot be held responsible for their disease, once their condition has been diagnosed they can be held responsible for seeking treatment and for preventing the complication of ARESLD. The standard of personal effort and responsibility we propose for alcoholics is the same as that held by Alcoholics Anonymous. We are not suggesting that some lives and behaviors have greater value than others—an approach used and appropriately repudiated when dialysis machines were in short supply.[18,19,20,21,22] But we are holding people responsible for their personal effort.

. . .

To each, treatment according to ability to pay has also been used as a principle of distributive justice. Since alcoholism is prevalent in all socioeconomic strata, it is not discrimination against the poor to deny liver transplantation to patients with alcoholic liver disease. In fact, we believe that poor patients with ARESLD have a stronger claim for a donor liver than rich patients, precisely because many alcohol treatment programs are not available to patients lacking in substantial private resources or health insurance. Ironically, it is precisely this group of poor and uninsured patients who are most likely not to be eligible to receive a liver transplant because of their inability to pay. We agree with Outka's view of fairness that would discriminate according to categories of illness rather than according to wealth.

Policy Considerations Regarding Public Support for Liver Transplantation

. . .

Much of the initial success in securing public and political approval for liver transplantation was achieved by focusing media and political attention not on adults but on children dying of ESLD. The public may not support transplantation for patients with ARESLD in the same way that they have endorsed this procedure for babies born with biliary atresia. . . .

Should Any Alcoholics Be Considered for Transplantation? Need for Further Research

Our proposal for giving lower priority for liver transplantation to patients with ARESLD does not completely rule out transplantation for this group. Patients with ARESLD who had not previously been offered therapy and who are now abstinent could be acceptable candidates. In addition, patients lower on the waiting list, such as patients with ARESLD who have been treated and are now abstinent, might be eligible for a donor liver in some regions because of the increased availability of donor organs there. Even if only because of these possible conditions for transplantation, further research is needed to determine which patients with ARESLD would have the best outcomes after liver transplantation. . . .

In the recently proposed Medicare criteria for coverage of liver transplantation, the HCFA acknowledged that the decision to

---

[17] Beauchamp, *Principles of Biomedical Ethics*.

[18] Outka, "Social Justice and Equal Access."

[19] Beauchamp, *Principles of Biomedical Ethics*.

[20] P. Ramsey, *The Patient as Person: Explorations in Medical Ethics* (Yale University Press, 2002).

[21] R. R. C. Fox and J. P. Swazey, *The Courage to Fail: A Social View of Organ Transplants and Dialysis* (Transaction Publishers).

[22] G. J. Annas, "The Prostitute, the Playboy, and the Poet: Rationing Schemes for Organ Transplantation," *American Journal of Public Health* 75, no. 2 (1985): pp. 187–189.

insure patients with alcoholic cirrhosis "may be considered controversial by some."[23] As if to counter possible objections, the HCFA listed requirements for patients with alcoholic cirrhosis: patients must meet the transplant center's requirement for abstinence prior to liver transplantation and have documented evidence of sufficient social support to ensure both recovery from alcoholism and compliance with the regimen of immunosuppressive medication.

Further research should answer lingering questions about liver transplantation for ARESLD patients: Which characteristics of a patient with ARESLD can predict a successful outcome? How long is abstinence necessary to qualify for transplantation? What type of a social support system must a patient have to ensure good results? . . . Until the answers are known, we propose that further transplantation for patients with ARESLD be limited to abstinent patients who had not previously been offered alcoholism treatment and to abstinent treated patients in regions of increased donor liver availability, and that it be carried out as part of prospective research protocols at a few centers skilled in transplantation and alcohol research. . . .

[23] Health Care Financing Administration, "Medicare Program: Criteria for Medicare Coverage of Adult Liver Transplants," *Federal Register* 55 (1990): pp. 3545–3553.

EXCERPT 9

Abridged text from:

P. A. Ubel, J. Baron, and D. A. Asch, "Social Acceptability, Personal Responsibility, and Prognosis in Public Judgments and Transplant Allocation," *Bioethics* 13, no. 1 (1999): pp. 57–68.

Social Acceptability, Personal Responsibility, and Prognosis in Public Judgments About Transplant Allocation

Peter A. Ubel, Jonathan Baron, and David A. Asch

. . .

The scarcity of transplantable life saving organs has forced the transplant community to make difficult decisions about which patients should receive available organs. . . .

In this paper, we explore the role that social acceptability, personal responsibility, and prognosis play in people's judgments about how to allocate scarce transplantable organs.

Subjects

We surveyed prospective jurors in the Philadelphia County Courthouse. . . . Surveys were distributed to prospective jurors after announcing that those who filled out a survey would receive a candy bar.

Questionnaire Design

We presented subjects with three scenarios in which they were asked to distribute 100 transplantable hearts among two groups of 100 patients needing transplant. . . .

We chose three scenarios in order to vary the social acceptability of the behaviors distinguishing the two groups of transplant patients. In one scenario, subjects were asked to divide the 100 organs between 100 patients with and 100 patients without a history of intravenous drug use, in another between patients with and without a history of cigarette smoking, and in another between patients with and without a history of eating high fat diets against a doctor's recommendation.

By random allocation, subjects received one of five questionnaire versions (see Table [5.3]). The versions differed according to the post-transplant prognoses of the two groups of patients. In all versions, patients not displaying the behavior were said to have a 70% chance of surviving five years after transplant. Different questionnaire versions reported different prognoses for those patients displaying the behavior. In version 1, for example, the prognosis between the two transplant groups was equal for all three scenarios. In contrast, for version 2 and version 4 the intravenous drug users were said to have better transplant prognoses, 90% versus 70% five year survival. . . .

For version 3 and version 5, intravenous drug users were said to have worse prognoses.

The versions also differed according to whether the behavior distinguishing the two groups of patients was said to be responsible for their primary heart failure. . . .

Results

A total of 283 subjects completed the survey. Their mean age was 43 years (sd 13), mean number of years of education was 14 (sd 3). Sixty two percent were female. Fifty seven percent were Caucasian and 34% African-American. . . .

Type of Behaviour

. . . Across all five questionnaire versions, and regardless of prognosis, subjects gave significantly fewer organs to intravenous drug users

Table [5.3]
Descriptions of prognosis and personal responsibility across questionnaire versions

Questionnaire version

Behavior		Version 1 ($n = 55$)	Version 2 ($n = 58$)	Version 3 ($n = 63$)	Version 4 ($n = 49$)	Version 5 ($n = 58$)
Intravenous drug use	Prognosis – % surviving 5 years*	70	90	50	90	50
	Behavior responsible for illness?	yes	yes	yes	no	no
Cigarette smoking	Prognosis – % surviving 5 years*	70	50	90	50	90
	Behavior responsible for illness?	yes	yes	yes	no	no
High-fat diets	Prognosis – % surviving 5 years*	70	50	90	50	90
	Behavior responsible for illness?	yes	yes	yes	no	no

*Compared to the group of patients without the behavior, who were always said to have a 70% chance of 5-year survival.

than to either cigarette smokers or people eating high fat diets ($F(2) = 47.763$, $p < 0.0005$). This reluctance to give organs to intravenous drug users was true even for versions 2 and 4, where intravenous drug users had a better transplant prognosis than any other group of patients, with intravenous drug users receiving 33% of the organs in these questionnaire versions and cigarette smokers and people eating high fat diets receiving 36% and 40% respectively ($F(2) = 4.711$, $p = 0.01$).

Justifications for Allocation Decisions

. . . The most common justification subjects gave for giving fewer organs to these patients, provided by 27% of the subjects, was that people who cause their own illness should not receive equal priority for organs. . . .

Prognosis and Responsibility

Prognosis was also important in influencing subjects' allocation decisions. As shown in Table [5.4], as the prognosis of the group with the behavior in question increased, so too did the percent of organs they received. In no case, however, was the mean percent of organs allocated to those with the behavior greater than 50%. . . . In contrast, subjects' allocation decisions were not influenced, for any of the three behaviors, by whether the behavior in question was said to be causally responsible for patients' initial organ failure (all p's > 0.8).

Table [5.4]
Mean percent of organs distributed to patients with behaviors of interest, according to their prognosis

Behavior	Prognosis of group with behavior* (percent chance of 5-year survival)		
	90	70	50
Intravenous drug use	33	33	26
Cigarette smoking	45	43	36
High fat diet	48	47	41

*For each behavior, the remainder of the organs were given to patients without the behavior in question, who had a 70% chance of 5-year survival

Discussion

. . .

We found that subjects were less likely to give organs to patients as their post-transplant prognosis diminished. Previous studies also show that people think prognosis should be important in transplant allocation.[1,2,3,4] We found no relationship between subjects' allocation choices and whether patients' behaviors were said to cause original heart failure. Most importantly, however, across all five questionnaires, we found a strong relationship between patients' behaviors and subjects' willingness to give them organs. Subjects were less willing to give organs to people with a history of intravenous drug use than to patients with a history of cigarette smoking or of eating high fat diets against a physician's advice. Even when the intravenous drug users were said to have a better chance of transplant success than other patients, and were said not to have caused their own heart failure with intravenous drug use, subjects were only willing to give them one third of the transplant organs, while giving the other two-thirds to patients with worse transplant prognoses but no history of intravenous drug use.

While subjects were quite reluctant to give organs to intravenous drug users, they were also somewhat reluctant to give them to smokers and people eating high fat diets; even when these patients were said to have a better prognosis than people without those behaviors, on average subjects gave them less than half of the organs. Thus, while many subjects responded that prognosis and causality were important in their allocation decisions, the most important factor influencing subjects' allocation decisions was the specific behavior of the patients needing transplant (i.e. intravenous drug use, cigarette smoking, or high fat diets).

. . .

Ethical Implications

. . .

It is not uncommon for people to argue in favor of allocating resources on the basis on personal responsibility. What our study shows is that these arguments may be convenient ways to support what otherwise merely reflect social desirability judgments. In other words, for some people, because a behavior is socially undesirable, they look for other reasons to direct resource toward other patients. Alternatively, this social desirability judgment may be subconscious. When thinking about allocation decisions, people may not consciously want to divert resources away from patients who engage in socially undesirable behaviors. However, their behavior may cause people to pay more attention to other relevant allocation criteria. People notice when they see a policeman eating a doughnut, but do not pay much attention when they see other people eating doughnuts. . . . Similarly, people might notice when people engaging in socially undesirable behaviors have worse transplant prognoses and, therefore, may pay attention to their prognosis more than they do for other patients with similar prognoses. . . .

Acknowledgments

The authors gratefully acknowledge Ellen Wise for assistance in manuscript preparation, Christine Weeks, Dave Weeks, and Andrea Gurmankin for research assistance, and to the prospective jurors who responded to our questionnaire.

---

[1] L. J. Skitka and P. E. Tetlock, "Allocating Scarce Resources: A Contingency Model of Distributive Justice," *Journal of Experimental Social Psychology* 28 (1992): pp. 491–522.

[2] P. A. Ubel and G. Loewenstein, "Distributing Scarce Livers: The Moral Reasoning of the General Public," *Social Science and Medicine* 42, no. 7 (1996): pp. 1049–1055.

[3] P. A. Ubel and G. Loewenstein, "The Efficacy and Equity of Retransplantation: An Experimental Survey of Public Attitudes," *Health Policy* 34, no. 2 (1995): pp. 145–151.

[4] P. A. Ubel and G. Loewenstein, "Public Perceptions of the Importance of Prognosis in Allocating Transplantable Livers to Children," *Medical Decision Making* 16, no. 3 (1996): pp. 234–241.

EXCERPT 10

Full text from:

G. Persad, A. Wertheimer, and E. Emanuel, "Principles for Allocation of Scarce Medical Interventions," *Lancet* 373, no. 9661 (2009): pp. 423–431.

Principles for Allocation of Scarce Medical Interventions

Govind Persad, Alan Wertheimer, and Ezekiel J. Emanuel

Allocation of very scarce medical interventions such as organs and vaccines is a persistent ethical challenge. We evaluate eight simple allocation principles that can be classified into four categories: treating people equally, favouring the worst-off, maximising total benefits, and promoting and rewarding social usefulness. No single principle is sufficient to incorporate all morally relevant considerations and therefore individual principles must be combined into multiprinciple allocation systems. We evaluate three systems: the United Network for Organ Sharing points systems, quality-adjusted life-years, and disability-adjusted life-years. We recommend an alternative system—the complete lives system—which prioritises younger people who have not yet lived a complete life, and also incorporates prognosis, save the most lives, lottery, and instrumental value principles.

In health care, as elsewhere, scarcity is the mother of allocation.[1] Although the extent is debated,[2,3] the scarcity of many specific interventions—including beds in intensive care units,[4] organs, and vaccines during pandemic influenza[5]—is widely acknowledged. For some interventions, demand exceeds supply. For others, an increased supply would necessitate redirection of important resources, and allocation decisions would still be necessary.[6]

Allocation of scarce medical interventions is a perennial challenge. During the 1940s, an expert committee allocated—without public input—then-novel penicillin to American soldiers before civilians, using expected efficacy and speed of return to duty as criteria.[7] During the 1960s, committees in Seattle allocated scarce dialysis machines using prognosis, current health, social worth, and dependants as criteria.[7] How can scarce medical interventions be allocated justly? This paper identifies and evaluates eight simple principles that have been suggested.[8,9,10,11,12] Although some are better than others, no single principle allocates interventions justly. Rather, morally relevant simple principles must be combined into multi-principle allocation systems. We evaluate three existing systems and then recommend a new one: the complete lives system.

---

[1] J. Rawls, *A Theory of Justice, Revised Edition* (Cambridge: Harvard University Press, 1999).

[2] J. Harris, "Qualifying the Value of Life," *Journal of Medical Ethics* 13, no. 3 (1987): pp. 117–123.

[3] A. L. Caplan, "Organ Transplant Rationing: A Window to the Future?", *Health Progress* 68, no. 5 (1987): pp. 40–45.

[4] R. D. Truog, et al., "Rationing in the Intensive Care Unit," *Critical Care Medicine* 34, no. 4 (2006): pp. 958–963; quiz 971.

[5] E. Emanuel and A. Wertheimer, "Who Should Get Influenza Vaccine When Not All Can?", *Science* 312, no. 5775 (2006): pp. 854–855.

[6] R. M. Veatch, "Disaster Preparedness and Triage: Justice and the Common Good," *Mt Sinai Journal of Medicine* 72, no. 4 (2005): pp. 236–241.

[7] L. J. McGough, et al., "Which Patients First? Setting Priorities for Antiretroviral Therapy Where Resources Are Limited," *American Journal of Public Health* 95, no. 7 (2005): pp. 1173–1180.

[8] F. M. Kamm, *Morality, Mortality: Death and Whom to Save from It* (Oxford University Press, 1998).

[9] R. Cookson and P. Dolan, "Principles of Justice in Health Care Rationing," *Journal of Medical Ethics* 26, no. 5 (2000): pp. 323–329.

[10] J. D. Arras, 'Rationing Vaccine During an Avian Influenza Pandemic: Why It Won't Be Easy', *Yale Journal of Biology and Medicine* 78, no. 5 (2005): pp. 287–300.

[11] N. Rescher, "The Allocation of Exotic Medical Lifesaving Therapy," in *Biomedical Ethics and the Law*, edited by J. Humber and R. Almeder (Springer US, 1976), pp. 447–463.

[12] T. L. Beauchamp and J. F. Childress, *Principles of Biomedical Ethics* (Oxford University Press, 1994).

Simple Allocation Principles

Eight simple ethical principles for allocation can be classified into four categories, according to their core ethical values: treating people equally, favouring the worst-off, maximising total benefits, and promoting and rewarding social usefulness (Table [5.5]). We do not regard ability to pay as a plausible option for the scarce life-saving interventions we discuss.

Some people wrongly suggest that allocation can be based purely on scientific or clinical facts, often using the term "medical need."[13,14] There are no value-free medical criteria for allocation.[15,16] Although biomedical facts determine a person's post-transplant prognosis or the dose of vaccine that would confer immunity, responding to these facts requires ethical, value-based judgments.

When evaluating principles, we need to distinguish between those that are insufficient and those that are flawed. Insufficient principles ignore some morally relevant considerations. Conversely, flawed principles recognise morally irrelevant considerations: inherently flawed principles necessarily recognise irrelevant considerations, whereas practically flawed principles allow irrelevant considerations to affect allocation. Principles that are individually insufficient could form part of an acceptable multiprinciple system, whereas systems that include flawed principles are untenable because they will always recognise irrelevant considerations.

Treating People Equally

Many scarce medical interventions, such as organ transplants, are indivisible. For indivisible goods, benefiting people equally entails providing equal chances at the scarce intervention—equality of opportunity, rather than equal amounts of it.[17] Two principles attempt to embody this value.

Lottery

Allocation by lottery has been used, sometimes with explicit judicial and legislative endorsement, in military conscription, immigration, education, and distribution of vaccines.[18,19,20]

Lotteries have several attractions. Equal moral status supports an equal claim to scarce resources.[21] Even among only roughly equal candidates, lotteries prevent small differences from drastically affecting outcome.[22] Some people also support lottery allocation because "each person's desire to stay alive should be regarded as of the same importance and deserving the same respect as that of anyone else."[23] Practically, lottery allocation is quick

[13] M. J. Langford, "Who Should Get the Kidney Machine?", *Journal of Medical Ethics* 18, no. 1 (1992): pp. 12–17.

[14] P. E. Liss, "Hard Choices in Public Health: The Allocation of Scarce Resources," *Scandinavian Journal of Public Health* 31, no. 2 (2003): pp. 156–157.

[15] T. Hope, D. Sprigings and R. Crisp, '"Not Clinically Indicated": Patients' Interests or Resource Allocation?', *British Medical Journal* 306, no. 6874 (1993): pp. 379–381.

[16] D. W. Brock, "The Misplaced Role of Urgency in Allocation of Persistently Scarce Life-Saving Organs," in *Ethical, Legal, and Social Issues in Organ Transplantation*, edited by T. Gutmann, et al. (Lengerich, Germany: Pabst Science Publishers, 2004), pp. 41–48.

[17] Rawls, *A Theory of Justice*.

[18] Arras, "Rationing Vaccine During an Avian Influenza Pandemic."

[19] W. A. Silverman and I. Chalmers, "Casting and Drawing Lots: A Time Honoured Way of Dealing with Uncertainty and Ensuring Fairness," *British Medical Journal* 323, no. 7327 (2001): pp. 1467–1468.

[20] J. Broome, "Selecting People Randomly," *Ethics* 95, no. 1 (1984): pp. 38–55.

[21] P. Ramsey, *The Patient as Person: Explorations in Medical Ethics* (Yale University Press, 2002).

[22] Broome, "Selecting People Randomly."

[23] J. Harris, *The Value of Life: An Introduction to Medical Ethics* (New York: Routledge, 1990).

Table [5.5]
Simple principles and their core ethical values

	Advantages	Disadvantages	Examples of use	Recommendation
Treating people equally				
Lottery	Hard to corrupt; little information about recipients needed	Ignores other relevant principles	Military draft; schools; vaccination	Include
First-come, first-served	Protects existing doctor–patient relationships; little information about recipients needed	Favors wealthy, powerful, and well-connected; ignores other relevant principles	ICU beds; part of organ allocation	Exclude
Favoring the worst-off: prioritarianism				
Sickest first	Aids those who are suffering right now; appeals to "rule of rescue"; makes sense in temporary scarcity; proxy for being worst-off overall	Surreptitious use of prognosis; ignores needs of those who will become sick in future; might falsely assume temporary scarcity; leads to people receiving interventions only after prognosis deteriorates; ignores other relevant principles	Emergency rooms; part of organ allocation	Exclude
Youngest-first	Benefits those who have had least life; prudent planners have an interest in living to old age	Undesirable priority to infants over adolescents and young adults; ignores other relevant principles	New NVAC/ACIP pandemic flu vaccine proposal	Include
Maximizing total benefits: utilitarianism				
Number of lives saved	Saves more lives, benefiting the greatest number; avoids need for comparative judgments about quality or other aspects of lives	Ignores other relevant principles	Past ACIP/NVAC pandemic flu vaccine policy; bioterrorism response policy; disaster triage	Include
Prognosis or life-years saved	Maximizes life-years produced	Ignores other relevant principles, particularly distributive principles	Penicillin allocation; traditional military triage (prognosis) and disaster triage (life-years saved)	Include
Promoting and rewarding social usefulness				
Instrumental value	Helps promote other important values; future oriented	Vulnerable to abuse through choice of prioritized occupations or activities; can direct health resources away from health needs	Past and current NVAC/ACIP pandemic flu vaccine policy	Include but only in some public health emergencies
Reciprocity	Rewards those who implemented important values; past-oriented	Vulnerable to abuse; can direct health resources away from health needs; intrusive assessment process	Some organ donation policies	Include only irreplaceable people who have suffered serious losses

and requires little knowledge about recipients.[24] Finally, lotteries resist corruption.[25]

The major disadvantage of lotteries is their blindness to many seemingly relevant factors.[26,27] Random decisions between someone who can gain 40 years and someone who can gain only 4 months, or someone who has already lived for 80 years and someone who has lived only 20 years, are inappropriate. Treating people equally often fails to treat them as equals.[28] Ultimately, although allocation solely by lottery is insufficient, the lottery's simplicity and resistance to corruption suggests that it could be incorporated into a multiprinciple system.[29]

First-come, first-served

Within health care, many people endorse a first-come, first-served distribution of beds in intensive care units[30] or organs for transplant.[31] The American Thoracic Society defends this principle as "a natural lottery—an egalitarian approach for fair [intensive care unit] resource allocation."[32] Others believe it promotes fair equality of opportunity,[33] and allows physicians to avoid discontinuing interventions, such as respirators, even when other criteria support moving those interventions to new arrivals.[34] Some people simply equate it to lottery allocation.[35]

As with lottery allocation, first-come, first-served ignores relevant differences between people, but in practice fails even to treat people equally. It favours people who are well-off, who become informed, and travel more quickly, and can queue for interventions without competing for employment or childcare concerns.[36] Queues are also vulnerable to additional corruption. As New York State's pandemic influenza planners stated, "Those who could figuratively (and sometimes literally) push to the front of the line would be vaccinated and stand the best chance for survival".[37] First-come, first-served allows morally irrelevant qualities—such as wealth, power, and connections—to decide who receives scarce interventions, and is therefore practically flawed.

Favouring the Worst-Off: Prioritarianism

Franklin Roosevelt argued that "the test of our progress is not whether we add more to the abundance of those who have much; it is whether we provide enough for those who have too little."[38] Philosophers call this preference

[24] Broome, "Selecting People Randomly."

[25] Ibid.

[26] M. S. Stein, "The Distribution of Life-Saving Medical Resources: Equality, Life Expectancy, and Choice Behind the Veil," *Social Philosophy Policy* 19, no. 2 (2002): pp. 212–245.

[27] E. Elhauge, "Allocating Health Care Morally," *California Law Review* 82, no. 6 (1994): pp. 1449–1544.

[28] R. Dworkin, *Sovereign Virtue: The Theory and Practice of Equality* (Harvard University Press, 2002).

[29] Elhauge, "Allocating Health Care Morally."

[30] American Thoracic Society Bioethics Task Force, "Fair Allocation of Intensive Care Unit Resources," *American Journal of Respiratory Critical Care Medicine* 156, no. 4 Pt 1 (1997): pp. 1282–1301.

[31] J. F. Childress, "Putting Patients First in Organ Allocation: An Ethical Analysis of the US Debate," *Cambridge Quarterly of Healthcare Ethics* 10, no. 4 (2001): pp. 365–376.

[32] American Thoracic Society Bioethics Task Force, "Fair Allocation of Intensive Care Unit Resources."

[33] Childress, "Putting Patients First."

[34] B. Lo and D. B. White, "Intensive Care Unit Triage During an Influenza Pandemic: The Need for Specific Clinical Guidelines," 2007.

[35] Ramsey, *The Patient as Person*.

[36] N. Daniels, "Fair Process in Patient Selection for Antiretroviral Treatment in WHO's Goal of 3 by 5", *Lancet* 366, no. 9480 (2005): pp. 169–171.

[37] A. J. Billittier, "Who Goes First?", *Journal of Public Health Management and Practice* 11, no. 4 (2005): pp. 267–268.

[38] F. D. Roosevelt, *Second Inaugural Address* (Washington, DC, 1937).

for the worst-off prioritarianism.[39] Some define being worst-off as currently lacking valuable goods, whereas others define it as lacking valuable goods throughout one's entire life.[40] Two principles embody these two interpretations.

Sickest first

Treating the sickest people first prioritises those with the worst future prospects if left untreated. The so-called rule of rescue, which claims that "our moral response to the imminence of death demands that we rescue the doomed," exemplifies this principle.[41] Transplantable livers and hearts, as well as emergency-room care, are allocated to the sickest individuals first.[42]

Some people might argue that treating the sickest individuals first is intuitively obvious.[43] Others claim that the sickest people are also probably worst off overall, because healthier people might recover unaided or be saved later by new interventions.[44] Finally, sickest-first allocation appeals to prognosis if untreated—a criterion clinicians frequently consider.[45]

On its own, sickest-first allocation ignores post-treatment prognosis: it applies even when only minor gains at high cost can be achieved. To circumvent this result, some misleadingly claim that sick people with a small but clear chance of benefit do not have a medical need.[46] Sick recipients' prognoses are wrongly assumed to be normal, even though many interventions—such as liver transplants—are less effective for the sickest people.[47]

If the failure to take account of prognosis were its only problem, sickest-first allocation would merely be insufficient. However, it myopically bases allocation on how sick someone is at the current time—a morally arbitrary factor in genuine scarcity.[48] Preferential allocation of a scarce liver to an acutely ill person unjustly ignores a currently healthier person with progressive liver disease, who might be worse off when he or she later suffers liver failure.[49,50] Favouring those who are currently sickest seems to assume that resource scarcity is temporary: that we can save the person who is now sickest and then save the progressively ill person later.[51,52] However, even temporary scarcity does not guarantee another chance to save the progressively ill person. Furthermore, when interventions are persistently scarce, saving the progressively ill person later will always involve depriving others. When we cannot save everyone, saving the sickest first is inherently flawed and inconsistent with the core idea of priority to the worst-off.

Youngest first

Although not always recognised as such, youngest-first allocation directs resources to those who have had less of something supremely valuable—life-years.[53] Dialysis machines and scarce organs have been allocated to younger recipients first,[54] and proposals for allocation in

---

[39] D. Parfit, "Equality and Priority," *Ratio* 10, no. 3 (1997): pp. 202–221.

[40] Kamm, *Morality, Mortality*.

[41] A. R. Jonsen, "Bentham in a Box: Technology Assessment and Health Care Allocation," *Law Medicine and Health Care* 14, no. 3-4 (1986): pp. 172–174.

[42] Stein, "The Distribution of Life-Saving Medical Resources."

[43] D. McKerlie, "Justice Between the Young and the Old," *Philosophy & Public Affairs* 30, no. 2 (2001): pp. 152–177.

[44] R. M. Veatch, "Equity in Liver Allocation: Professor Veatch's Reply," *Medical Ethics* (2001).

[45] Liss, "Hard Choices in Public Health."

[46] Langford, "Who Should Get the Kidney Machine?"

[47] D. H. Howard, "Hope Versus Efficiency in Organ Allocation," *Transplantation* 72, no. 6 (2001): pp. 1169–1173.

[48] Brock, "The Misplaced Role of Urgency."

[49] Kamm, *Morality, Mortality*.

[50] E. Elhauge, "Allocating Health Care Morally," *California Law Review* 82, no. 6 (1994): pp. 1449–1544.

[51] Kamm, *Morality, Mortality*.

[52] Elhauge, "Allocating Health Care Morally."

[53] Kamm, *Morality, Mortality*.

[54] G. W. Rutecki and J. F. Kilner, "Dialysis as a Resource Allocation Paradigm: Confronting Tragic Choices Once Again?", *Seminars on Dialysis* 12 (1999): pp. 38–43.

pandemic influenza prioritise infants and children.[55] Daniel Callahan[56] has suggested strict age cut-off s for scarce life-saving interventions, whereas Alan Williams[57] has suggested a system that allocates interventions based on individuals' distance from a normal life-span if left unaided.

Prioritising the youngest gives priority to the worst-off—those who would otherwise die having had the fewest life-years—and is thus fundamentally different from favouritism towards adults or people who are well-off[58,59] Also, allocating preferentially to the young has an appeal that favouring other worst-off individuals such as women, poor people, or minorities lacks: "Because [all people] age, treating people of different ages differently does not mean that we are treating persons unequally."[60] Prudent planners would allocate life-saving interventions to themselves earlier in life to improve their chances of living to old age.[61] These justifications explain much of the public preference for allocating scarce life-saving interventions to younger people.[62,63]

Strict youngest-first allocation directs scarce resources predominantly to infants. This approach seems incorrect.[64] The death of a 20-year-old young woman is intuitively worse than that of a 2-month-old girl, even though the baby has had less life.[65] The 20-year-old has a much more developed personality than the infant, and has drawn upon the investment of others to begin as-yet-unfulfilled projects. Youngest-first allocation also ignores prognosis,[66] and categorically excludes older people.[67] Thus, youngest-first allocation seems insufficient on its own, but it could be combined with prognosis and lottery principles in a multiprinciple allocation system.[68]

Maximising Total Benefits: Utilitarianism

Maximising benefits is a utilitarian value, although principles differ about which benefits to maximise.

Save the most lives

One maximising strategy involves saving the most individual lives, and it has motivated policies on allocation of influenza vaccine[69] and responses to bioterrorism.[70] Since each life is valuable, this principle seems to need no special justification. It also avoids comparing individual lives. Other things being equal, we should always save five lives rather than one.[71]

---

55 United States Department of Health and Human Services, *Guidance on Allocating and Targeting Pandemic Influenza Vaccine* (Washington, DC: US Government Printing Office, 2008).

56 D. Callahan, *Setting Limits: Medical Goals in an Aging Society* (Georgetown University Press, 1995).

57 A. Williams, "Intergenerational Equity: An Exploration of the 'Fair Innings' Argument", *Health Economics* 6, no. 2 (1997): pp. 117–132.

58 Kamm, *Morality, Mortality*.

59 R. Cookson and P. Dolan, "Principles of Justice in Health Care Rationing," *Journal of Medical Ethics* 26, no. 5 (2000): pp. 323–329.

60 N. Daniels, *Am I My Parents' Keeper?: An Essay on Justice Between the Young and the Old* (Oxford University Press, 1988).

61 Ibid.

62 J. McKie and J. Richardson, "Neglected Equity Issues in Cost-Effectiveness Analysis, Part 1: Severity of Pre-Treatment Condition, Realisation of Potential for Health, Concentration and Dispersion of Health Benefits, and Age-Related Social Preferences" (Melbourne: Centre for Health Program Evaluation, 2005).

63 A. Tsuchiya, P. Dolan and R. Shaw, "Measuring People's Preferences Regarding Ageism in Health: Some Methodological Issues and Some Fresh Evidence," *Social Science and Medicine* 57, no. 4 (2003): pp. 687–696.

64 Emanuel, "Who Should Get Influenza Vaccine."

65 McKie, " Neglected Equity Issues."

66 D. W. Brock, "Children's Rights to Health Care," *Journal of Medical Philosophy* 26, no. 2 (2001): pp. 163–177.

67 Howard, "Hope Versus Efficiency."

68 Ibid.

69 Emanuel, "Who Should Get Influenza Vaccine."

70 S. Phillips, "Current Status of Surge Research," *Academy of Emergency Medicine* 13, no. 11 (2006): pp. 1103–1108.

71 N. Hsieh, A. Strudler and D. Wasserman, "The Numbers Problem," *Philosophy & Public Affairs* 34, no. 4 (2006): pp. 352–372.

However, other things are rarely equal. Some lives have been shorter than others; 20-year-olds have lived less than 70-year-olds.[72] Similarly, some lives can be extended longer than others. How to weigh these other relevant considerations against saving more lives—whether to save one 20-year-old, who might live another 60 years if saved, or three 70-year-olds who could only live for 10 years each—is unclear.[73] Although insufficient on its own, saving more lives should be part of a multiprinciple allocation system.

Prognosis or life-years

Rather than saving the most lives, prognosis allocation aims to save the most life-years. This strategy has been used in disaster triage and penicillin allocation, and motivates the exclusion of people with poor prognoses from organ transplantation waiting lists.[74,75,76] Maximising life-years has intuitive appeal. Living more years is valuable, so saving more years also seems valuable.[77]

However, even supporters of prognosis-based allocation acknowledge its inability to consider distribution as well as quantity.[78] Making a well-off person slightly better off rather than slightly improving a worse-off person's life would be unjust; likewise, why give an extra year to a person who has lived for many when it could be given to someone who would otherwise die having had few?[79,80] Similarly, giving a few life-years to many differs from giving many life-years to a few.[81] As with the principle of saving the most lives, prognosis is undeniably relevant but insufficient alone.

Promoting and Rewarding Social Usefulness

Unlike the previous values, social value cannot direct allocation on its own.[82] Rather, social value allocation prioritises specific individuals to enable them to promote other important values, or rewards them for having promoted these values.

In view of the multiplicity of not legislate socially conventional, mainstream values,[83] when Seattle's dialysis policy favoured parents and church-goers, it was criticised: "The Pacific Northwest is no place for a Henry David Thoreau with kidney failure."[84] Allocators must also avoid directing interventions earmarked for health needs to those not relevant to the health problem at hand, which covertly exacerbates scarcity.[85,86] For instance, funeral directors might be essential to preserving health in an influenza pandemic, but not during a shortage of intensive-care beds.[87]

---

72 McKie, "Neglected Equity Issues."

73 J. Glover, *Causing Death and Saving Lives: The Moral Problems of Abortion, Infanticide, Suicide, Euthanasia, Capital Punishment, War and Other Life-or-Death Choices* (Penguin Books Limited, 1990).

74 L. J. McGough, et al., "Which Patients First? Setting Priorities for Antiretroviral Therapy Where Resources Are Limited," *American Journal of Public Health* 95, no. 7 (2005): pp. 1173–1180.

75 Stein, "The Distribution of Life-Saving Medical Resources."

76 L. B. Russell, et al., "Cost-Effectiveness Analysis as a Guide to Resource Allocation in Health: Roles and Limitations," in *Cost-Effectiveness in Health and Medicine*, edited by M. R. Gold, et al. (New York: Oxford University Press, 1996), pp. 3–24.

77 Kamm, *Morality, Mortality.*

78 Russel, "Cost-Effectiveness Analysis."

79 Kamm, *Morality, Mortality.*

80 K. Kappel and P. Sandoe, "QALYs, Age and Fairness," *Bioethics* 6, no. 4 (1992): pp. 297–316.

81 Kamm, *Morality, Mortality.*

82 Harris, *The Value of Life.*

83 Rawls, *A Theory of Justice.*

84 D. Sanders and J. Dukeminier, "Medical Advance and Legal Lag: Hemodialysis and Kidney Transplantation," *UCLA Law Review* 15 (1968): pp. 357–419.

85 Kamm, *Morality, Mortality.*

86 D. W. Brock, "Separate Spheres and Indirect Benefits," *Cost Effective Resour Allocation* 1, no. 1 (2003): p. 4.

87 Emanuel, "Who Should Get Influenza Vaccine."

Instrumental value

Instrumental value allocation prioritises specific individuals to enable or encourage future usefulness. Guidelines that prioritise workers producing influenza vaccine exemplify instrumental value allocation to save the most lives.[88] Responsibility-based allocation—eg, allocation to people who agree to improve their health and thus use fewer resources—also represents instrumental value allocation.[89]

This approach is necessarily insufficient, because it derives its appeal from promoting other values, such as saving more lives: "all whose continued existence is clearly required so that others might live have a good claim to priority".[90] Prioritising essential health-care staff does not treat them as counting for more in themselves, but rather prioritises them to benefit others. Instrumental value allocation thus arguably recognises the moral importance of each person, even those not instrumentally valuable.

Student military deferments have shown that instrumental value allocation can encourage abuse of the system.[91] People also disagree about usefulness: is saving all legislators necessary in an influenza pandemic?[92] Decisions on usefulness can involve complicated and demeaning inquiries.[93] However, where a specific person is genuinely indispensable in promoting morally relevant principles, instrumental value allocation can be appropriate.

Reciprocity

Reciprocity allocation is backward-looking, rewarding past usefulness or sacrifice. As such, many describe this allocative principle as desert or rectificatory justice, rather than reciprocity. For important health-related values, reciprocity might involve preferential allocation to past organ donors,[94] to participants in vaccine research who assumed risk for others' benefit,[95] or to people who made healthy lifestyle choices that reduced their need for resources.[96] Priority to military veterans embodies reciprocity for promoting non-health values.[97]

Proponents claim that "justice as reciprocity calls for providing something in return for contributions that people have made."[98] Reciprocity might also be relevant when people are conscripted into risky tasks. For instance, nurses required to care for contagious patients could deserve reciprocity, especially if they did not volunteer.

Reciprocity allocation, like instrumental value allocation, might potentially require time-consuming, intrusive, and demeaning inquiries, such as investigating whether a person adhered to a healthy lifestyle.[99,100] Furthermore, unlike instrumental value, reciprocity does not have the future-directed appeal of promoting important health values. Ultimately, the appropriateness of allocation based on reciprocity seems to depend in a complex way on several factors, such as seriousness of sacrifice and irreplaceability. For instance, former organ donors seem to deserve reciprocity since they make a serious sacrifice and since there is no surplus of organ donors. By contrast, laboratory staff who serve as vaccine production workers do not incur serious risk nor are they irreplaceable, so reciprocity seems less appropriate for them.

---

88 Ibid.

89 E. H. Morreim, "Lifestyles of the Risky and Infamous. From Managed Care to Managed Lives," *Hastings Center Reports* 25, no. 6 (1995): pp. 5–12.

90 Harris, *The Value of Life*.

91 E. W. Burgess, "The Effect of War on the American Family," *American Journal of Sociology* (1942): pp. 343–352.

92 Harris, *The Value of Life*.

93 E. S. Anderson, "What Is the Point of Equality?", *Ethics* 109, no. 2 (1999): pp. 287–337.

94 Kamm, *Morality, Mortality*.

95 R. Macklin, "Ethics and Equity in Access to HIV Treatment: 3 by 5 Initiative," (2004).

96 Morreim, "Lifestyles of the Risky and Infamous."

97 L. Kass. *Session 5: Organ Donation Procurement, Allocation, and Transplantation: Policy Options*, in *The President's Council on Biotethics* (2006).

98 Macklin, "Ethics and Equity."

99 Elhauge, "Allocating Health Care Morally."

100 Anderson, "What Is the Point of Equality?"

Assessing Principles: Allocation Systems

Which principles best embody morally relevant values? First-come, first-served is flawed in practice because it unwittingly allows irrelevant considerations, such as wealth, to affect allocation decisions, whereas a lottery is insufficient but not flawed. Similarly, sickest-first allocation is inherently flawed, whereas the youngest-first principle, though insufficient, recognises the important value of priority to the worst-off. Both utilitarian principles—maximising lives saved and prognosis—are relevant but insufficient, and usefulness and reciprocity are relevant where irreplaceable individuals make serious sacrifices, such as those during public health emergencies.

Ultimately, no principle is sufficient on its own to recognise all morally relevant considerations. Combining principles into systems increases complexity and controversy, but is inevitable if allocations are to incorporate the complexity of our moral values (Figure [5.2]). People disagree about which principles to include and how to balance them. Many allocation systems do not make their content explicit, nor do they justify their choices about inclusion, balancing, and specification.[101] Elucidating, comparing, and evaluating allocation systems should be a research priority.[102]

United Network for Organ Sharing (UNOS) Points Systems

The UNOS points systems are used for organ allocation (Figure [5.2]). They combine three principles: sickest-first (current medical condition); first-come, first-served (waiting time); and prognosis (antigen, antibody, and blood type matching between recipient and donor). UNOS weights principles differently depending on the organ distributed. Kidney and pancreas allocation is mainly by waiting time, with some weight given to sickest-first and prognosis.[103] Conversely, heart allocation weights sickest-first principles heavily and waiting time less so.[104] Lung and liver allocation takes into account waiting time, sickest-first, and prognosis.[105] Historically, no UNOS system has emphasised prognosis, although UNOS's most recent policy discussions on lung allocation suggest such a change.[106]

The UNOS point systems are flexible: conceivably, they could include any simple principle by translating it into a points framework. The systems are easily revisable to weight one principle more heavily than others.

Current UNOS systems incorporate two flawed simple principles: first-come, first-served and sickest first. They are also vulnerable to additional exploitation. Taking advantage of the first-come, first-served principle, well-off patients place themselves on multiple waiting lists.[107] Exploiting the sickest-first element, some transplant centres have temporarily altered or misrepresented their patients' health state to get them scarce organs, making sickest-first both practically and inherently flawed.[108,109]

Furthermore, UNOS points systems do not appropriately consider the benefit-maximising principles, prognosis, and saving the most lives, nor do they include youngest-first allocation. Most dramatically, multiple-organ transplants to one individual are permitted, even

[101]. Rawls, *A Theory of Justice.*

[102] Cookson, "Principles of Justice."

[103] United Network for Organ Sharing (UNOS), "Policies," accessed Sept. 30, 2008, http://www.unos.org/policiesandbylaws/policies.asp.

[104] Ibid.

[105] Ibid.

[106] Organ Procurement and Transplantation Network, "Public Forum to Discuss Kidney Allocation Policy Development Synopsis" (2007).

[107] S. Zink, et al., "Examining the Potential Exploitation of UNOS Policies," *American Journal of Bioethics* 5, no. 4 (2005): pp. 6–10.

[108] T. F. Murphy, "Gaming the Transplant System," *American Journal of Bioethics* 4, no. 1 (2004): p. W28.

[109] E. H. Morreim, "Another Kind of End-Run: Status Upgrades," *Am J Bioeth* 5, no. 4 (2005): pp. 11–12.

	Principles Included	Advantages	Objections
UNOS points systems for organ allocation in the USA	First-come, first-served; sickest-first; prognosis	Can combine all possible principles; flexible	Includes least justifiable principles: first-come, first-served and sickest-first; low priority given to prognosis; vulnerable to bias and manipulation, such as being listed on multiple transplantation lists and misrepresentation of health status; allows multiple organ transplants, thus saving fewer lives
QALY allocation	Prognosis; excludes save the most lives	Maximizes future benefits; considers quality of life; used in many existing, quantitatively sophisticated frameworks	Outcome measure disadvantages disabled people; incorrect conception of equality by focusing on equality of QALYs rather than equality of persons; does not incorporate many relevant principles
DALY allocation	Prognosis; instrumental value; excludes save the most lives	Maximizes future benefits; includes instrumental value, saving people whose productivity is key to a flourishing society	Outcome measure disadvantages disabled people; age considered as modifying value of individual life-years, rather than from standpoint of distributive justice; definition of instrumental value is too focused on economic worth, and could justify bias towards heads of household and other "traditional" social positions; does not incorporate many relevant principles
Complete lives system	Youngest-first; prognosis; save the most lives; lottery; instrumental value, but only in public health emergency	Matches intuition that death of adolescents is worse than that of infants or elderly; everyone has an interest in living through all life stages; incorporates the largest number of relevant principles; resistant to corruption	Reduced chances for persons who have lived many years; life-years are not a relevant health care outcome; unable to deal with international differences in life expectancy; need lexical priority rather than balancing; complete lives system is not appropriate for general distribution of health care resources

Figure [5.2] Four multiprinciple systems.

UNOS, United Network for Organ Sharing; *QALY*, quality-adjusted life-years; *DALY*, disability-adjusted life-years.

when a heart-lung-liver combination could save three lives if transplanted separately.[110,111] Similarly, policy revisions during the 1990s de-emphasised organ-recipient matching even though poorer matching leads to fewer lives saved.[112]

Attempts to remedy these deficiencies have been covert and haphazard. In an effort to implement prognosis allocation tacitly, ill or old people have been excluded from supposedly first-come, first-served waiting lists.[113] Physicians can misdiagnose comorbidities as contraindications, wrongly implying that transplants will harm recipients, rather than explicitly practising prognosis-based allocation.[114] Some have proposed so-called old-for-old policies that match donor organ age to recipient age—misrepresenting both youngest-first and prognosis-based allocation as biological fact.[115] Others have advocated local rather than national waiting lists to circumvent sickest-first allocation.[116,117] Explicit and public acknowledgment of allocation strategies would be preferable to this surreptitious and piecemeal approach.

Quality-Adjusted Life-Years

Allocation systems based on quality-adjusted life-years (QALY) have two parts (table 2). One is an outcome measure that considers the quality of life-years. As an example, the quality-of-life measure used by the UK National Health Service rates moderate mobility impairment as 0·85 times perfect health.[118] QALY allocation therefore equates 8·5 years in perfect health to 10 years with moderately impaired mobility.[119] The other part of QALY allocation is a maximising assumption: that justice requires total QALYs to be maximised without consideration of their distribution.[120,121] QALY allocation initially constituted the basis for Oregon's Medicaid coverage initiative, and is currently used by the UK's National Institute for Health and Clinical Excellence (NICE).[122,123] Both the ethics and efficacy of QALY allocation have been substantially discussed.[124]

The QALY outcome measure has problems. Even if a life-year in which a person has impaired mobility is worse than a healthy life-year, someone adapted to wheelchair use might reasonably value an additional life-year in a wheelchair as much as a non-disabled person would value an

110 Veatch, "Disaster Preparedness and Triage."

111 Kamm, *Morality, Mortality.*

112 N. Mutinga, D. C. Brennan and M. A. Schnitzler, "Consequences of Eliminating HLA-B in Deceased Donor Kidney Allocation to Increase Minority Transplantation," *American Journal of Transplantation* 5, no. 5 (2005): pp. 1090–1098.

113 G. C. Oniscu, et al., *Equity of Access to Renal Transplant Waiting List and Renal Transplantation in Scotland: Cohort Study* (2003).

114 L. W. Miller, "Listing Criteria for Cardiac Transplantation: Results of an American Society of Transplant Physicians-National Institutes of Health Conference," *Transplantation* 66, no. 7 (1998): pp. 947–951.

115 W. Arns, F. Citterio and J. M. Campistol, "'Old-for-Old'—New Strategies for Renal Transplantation," *Nephrology Dialysis Transplantation* 22, no. 2 (2007): pp. 336–341.

116 Stein, "The Distribution of Life-Saving Medical Resources."

117 G. C. Alexander, R. M. Werner and P. A. Ubel, "The Costs of Denying Scarcity," *Archives of Internal Medicine* 164, no. 6 (2004): pp. 593–596.

118 P. Kind, et al., *UK Population Norms for EQ-5d* (Centre for Health Economics, University of York, 1999).

119 National Institute for Health Care Excellence, *Guide to the Methods of Technology Appraisal* (London: NICE, 2003).

120 Russell, "Cost-Effectiveness Analysis as a Guide to Resource Allocation."

121 M. McGregor, "Cost-Utility Analysis: Use QALYs Only with Great Caution," *Canadian Medical Association Journal* 168, no. 4 (2003): pp. 433–434.

122 M. D. Rawlins and A. J. Culyer, "National Institute for Clinical Excellence and Its Value Judgments," *British Medical Journal* 329, no. 7459 (2004): pp. 224–227.

123 D. C. Hadorn, "The Oregon Priority-Setting Exercise: Quality of Life and Public Policy," *Hastings Center Reports* 21, no. 3 (1991): pp. S11–S16.

124 Russell, "Cost-Effectiveness Analysis as a Guide to Resource Allocation."

additional life-year without disability.[125] Allocators have struggled with this issue.[126]

More importantly, maximising the number of QALYs is an insufficient basis for allocation.

Although QALY advocates appeal to the idea that all QALYs are equal, people, not QALYs, deserve equal treatment.[127] Treatment of a serious disease such as appendicitis gives a few people many more QALYs, whereas treatment of a minor problem like uncapped teeth gives many people a few more QALYs.[128] Even though the two strategies produce equal numbers of QALYs, they treat individuals very differently.[129] Likewise, giving QALYs to someone who has had few life-years differs morally from giving them to someone who has already had many.[130,131] Ultimately, QALY allocation systems do not recognise many morally relevant values—such as treating people equally, giving priority to the worst-off, and saving the most lives—and are therefore insufficient for just allocation.

Disability-Adjusted Life-Years

WHO endorses the system of disability-adjusted life-year (DALY) allocation (table 2).[132] As with QALY allocation, DALY allocation does not consider interpersonal distribution. DALY systems also incorporate quality-of-life factors—for instance, they equate a life-year with blindness to roughly 0·6 healthy life-years.[133] Additionally, DALY allocation ranks each life-year with the age of the person as a modifier: "The well-being of some age groups, we argue, is instrumental in making society flourish; therefore collectively we may be more concerned with improving health status for individuals in these age groups."[134] This argument, although used to justify age-weighting, would equally justify counting the life-years of economically productive people and those caring for others for more.

DALY allocation wrongly incorporates age into the outcome measure, claiming that a year for a younger person is in itself more valuable. Priority for young people is better justified on grounds of distributive justice.[135] Also, the use of instrumental value to justify DALY allocation resembles that used in Seattle's dialysis allocation, which inappropriately favoured wage earners and careers of dependants.[136,137]

The Complete Lives System

Because none of the currently used systems satisfy all ethical requirements for just allocation, we propose an alternative: the complete lives system. This system incorporates five principles (table 2): youngest-first, prognosis, save the most lives, lottery, and instrumental value.[138] As such, it prioritises younger people who have not yet lived a complete life and will be unlikely to do so without aid. Many thinkers have accepted

[125] P. Menzel, et al., "The Role of Adaptation to Disability and Disease in Health State Valuation: A Preliminary Normative Analysis," *Social Science and Medicine* 55, no. 12 (2002): pp. 2149–2158.

[126] P. A. Ubel, et al., "Improving Value Measurement in Cost-Effectiveness Analysis," *Medical Care* 38, no. 9 (2000): pp. 892–901.

[127] P. Pronovost and D. C. Angus, "Economics of End-of-Life Care in the Intensive Care Unit," *Critical Care Medicine* 29, no. 2 Suppl (2001): pp. N46–N51.

[128] Hadorn, "The Oregon Priority-Setting Exercise."

[129] Kamm, *Morality, Mortality*.

[130] Ibid.

[131] Kappel, "QALYs, Age and Fairness."

[132] C. J. Murray and A. K. Acharya, "Understanding DALYs (Disability-Adjusted Life Years)," *Journal of Health Economics* 16, no. 6 (1997): pp. 703–730.

[133] Ibid.

[134] Ibid.

[135] Tsuchiya, "Measuring People's Preferences."

[136] McGough, "Which Patients First?"

[137] D. Sanders and J. Dukeminier, "Medical Advance and Legal Lag: Hemodialysis and Kidney Transplantation," *UCLA Law Review* 15 (1968): pp. 357–419.

[138] Emanuel, "Who Should Get Influenza Vaccine."

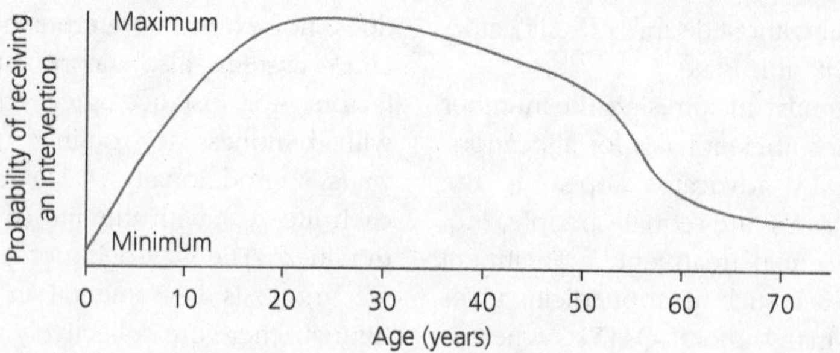

Figure [5.3] Age-based priority for receiving scarce medical interventions under the complete lives system.

complete lives as the appropriate focus of distributive justice: "individual human lives, rather than individual experiences, [are] the units over which any distributive principle should operate."[139,140,141] Although there are important differences between these thinkers, they share a core commitment to consider entire lives rather than events or episodes, which is also the defining feature of the complete lives system.

Consideration of the importance of complete lives also supports modifying the youngest-first principle by prioritising adolescents and young adults over infants (Figure [5.3]). Adolescents have received substantial education and parental care, investments that will be wasted without a complete life. Infants, by contrast, have not yet received these investments. Similarly, adolescence brings with it a developed personality capable of forming and valuing long-term plans whose fulfilment requires a complete life.[142] As the legal philosopher Ronald Dworkin argues, "It is terrible when an infant dies, but worse, most people think, when a three-year-old child dies and worse still when an adolescent does";[143] this argument is supported by empirical surveys.[144,145] Importantly, the prioritisation of adolescents and young adults considers the social and personal investment that people are morally entitled to have received at a particular age, rather than accepting the results of an unjust status quo. Consequently, poor adolescents should be treated the same as wealthy ones, even though they may have received less investment owing to social injustice.

The complete lives system also considers prognosis, since its aim is to achieve complete lives. A young person with a poor prognosis has had few life-years but lacks the potential to live a complete life. Considering prognosis forestalls the concern that disproportionately large amounts of resources will be directed to young people with poor prognoses.[146] When the worst-off can benefit only slightly while better-off people could benefit greatly, allocating to the better-off is often justifiable.[147,148] Some small benefits, such as a few weeks of life, might also be intrinsically insignificant when compared with large benefits.[149] Saving the most lives is also included in this system because enabling more people to live complete lives is better than enabling fewer.[150,151] In a public health emergency, instrumental value

139 Rawls, *A Theory of Justice*.

140 T. Nagel, *Mortal Questions* (Cambridge University Press, 2012).

141 Aristotle, *Aristotle: Nicomachean Ethics* (Cambridge University Press, 2000).

142 D. Shaffer and K. Kipp, *Developmental Psychology: Childhood and Adolescence* (Cengage Learning, 2006).

143 R. Dworkin, *Life's Dominion: An Argument About Abortion, Euthanasia, and Individual Freedom* (Knopf Doubleday Publishing Group, 2011).

144 Tsuchiya, "Measuring People's Preferences."

145 J. R. J. Richardson and Centre for Health Program Evaluation, *Age Weighting and Discounting: What Are the Ethical Issues?* (Austin & Repatriation Medical Centre, Health Economics Unit, 1999).

146 Brock, "Children's Rights to Health Care."

147 Rawls, *A Theory of Justice*.

148 Parfit, "Equality and Priority."

149 Kamm, *Morality, Mortality*.

150 Ibid.

151 Hsieh, "The Numbers Problem."

could also be included to enable more people to live complete lives. Lotteries could be used when making choices between roughly equal recipients, and also potentially to ensure that no individual—irrespective of age or prognosis—is seen as beyond saving.[152,153] Thus, the complete lives system is complete in another way: it incorporates each morally relevant simple principle.

When implemented, the complete lives system produces a priority curve on which individuals aged between roughly 15 and 40 years get the most substantial chance, whereas the youngest and oldest people get chances that are attenuated (Figure [5.3]).[154] It therefore superficially resembles the proposal made by DALY advocates; however, the complete lives system justifies preference to younger people because of priority to the worst-off rather than instrumental value. Additionally, the complete lives system assumes that, although life-years are equally valuable to all, justice requires the fair distribution of them. Conversely, DALY allocation treats life-years given to elderly or disabled people as objectively less valuable.

Finally, the complete lives system is least vulnerable to corruption. Age can be established quickly and accurately from identity documents. Prognosis allocation encourages physicians to improve patients' health, unlike the perverse incentives to sicken patients or misrepresent health that the sickest-first allocation creates.[155,156]

Objections

We consider several important objections to the complete lives system.

The complete lives system discriminates against older people.[157,158] Age-based allocation is ageism.[159] Unlike allocation by sex or race, allocation by age is not invidious discrimination; every person lives through different life stages rather than being a single age.[160,161] Even if 25-year-olds receive priority over 65-year-olds, everyone who is 65 years now was previously 25 years.[162] Treating 65-year-olds differently because of stereotypes or falsehoods would be ageist; treating them differently because they have already had more life-years is not.

Age, like income, is a "non-medical criterion" inappropriate for allocation of medical resources.[163,164] In contrast to income, a complete life is a health outcome. Long-term survival and life expectancy at birth are key health-care outcome variables.[165] Delaying the age at onset of a disease is desirable.[166,167]

The complete lives system is insensitive to international differences in typical lifespan. Although broad consensus favours adolescents

152 Howard, "Hope Versus Efficiency in Organ Allocation."

153 D. L. Schwappach, "Resource Allocation, Social Values and the QALY: A Review of the Debate and Empirical Evidence," *Health Expect* 5, no. 3 (2002): pp. 210–222.

154 Dworkin, *Life's Dominion*.

155 Murphy, "Gaming the Transplant System."

156 Morreim, "Another Kind of End-Run."

157 N. S. Jecker and R. A. Pearlman, "Ethical Constraints on Rationing Medical Care by Age," *Journal of the American Geriatric Society* 37, no. 11 (1989): pp. 1067–1075.

158 M. M. Rivlin, "Protecting Elderly People: Flaws in Ageist Arguments," *British Medical Journal* 310, no. 6988 (1995): pp. 1179–1182.

159 Ibid.

160 Kamm, *Morality, Mortality*.

161 Daniels, *Am I My Parents' Keeper?*

162 Brock, "The Misplaced Role of Urgency."

163 Liss, "Hard Choices in Public Health."

164 American Medical Association, "Allocation of Limited Medical Resources" (1994), http://www.ama-assn.org/ama/pub/physician-resources/medical-ethics/code-medical-ethics/opinion203.page?

165 C. D. Mathers, et al., "Healthy Life Expectancy in 191 Countries, 1999," *Lancet* 357, no. 9269 (2001): pp. 1685–1691.

166 M. A. Atkinson and G. S. Eisenbarth, "Type 1 Diabetes: New Perspectives on Disease Pathogenesis and Treatment," *Lancet* 358, no. 9277 (2001): pp. 221–229.

167 M. X. Tang, et al., "Effect of Oestrogen During Menopause on Risk and Age at Onset of Alzheimer's Disease," *Lancet* 348, no. 9025 (1996): pp. 429–432.

over very young infants, and young adults over the very elderly people, implementation can reasonably differ between, even within, nation-states.[168,169] Some people believe that a complete life is a universal limit founded in natural human capacities, which everyone should accept even without scarcity.[170] By contrast, the complete lives system requires only that citizens see a complete life, however defined, as an important good, and accept that fairness gives those short of a complete life stronger claims to scarce life-saving resources.

Principles must be ordered lexically: less important principles should come into play only when more important ones are fulfilled.[171] Rawls himself agreed that lexical priority was inappropriate when distributing specific resources in society, though appropriate for ordering the principles of basic social justice that shape the distribution of basic rights, opportunities, and income.[172] As an alternative, balancing priority to the worst-off against maximising benefits has won wide support in discussions of allocative local justice.[173,174,175] As Amartya Sen argues, justice "does not specify how much more is to be given to the deprived person, but merely that he should receive more."[176]

Accepting the complete lives system for health care as a whole would be premature. We must first reduce waste and increase spending.[177,178] The complete lives system explicitly rejects waste and corruption, such as multiple listing for transplantation. Although it may be applicable more generally, the complete lives system has been developed to justly allocate persistently scarce life-saving interventions.[179,180] Hearts for transplant and influenza vaccines, unlike money, cannot be replaced or diverted to non-health goals; denying a heart to one person makes it available to another. Ultimately, the complete lives system does not create "classes of Untermenschen whose lives and well being are deemed not worth spending money on,"[181] but rather empowers us to decide fairly whom to save when genuine scarcity makes saving everyone impossible.

Legitimacy

As well as recognising morally relevant values, an allocation system must be legitimate. Legitimacy requires that people see the allocation system as just and accept actual allocations as fair. Consequently, allocation systems must be publicly understandable, accessible, and subject to public discussion and revision.[182] They must also resist corruption, since easy corruptibility undermines the public trust on which legitimacy depends. Some systems, like the UNOS points systems or QALY systems, may fail this

---

168 E. J. Emanuel, "Finding New Ethical Conceptions through Practical Ethics: Global Justice and the 'Standard of Care' Debates," (University of Toronto Center for Ethics, "Inaugural Conference: Is There Progress in Ethics," 2006).

169 J. Rawls, *The Law of Peoples: With, the Idea of Public Reason Revisited* (Harvard University Press, 2001).

170 Callahan, *Setting Limits.*

171 J. D. Arras, "Rationing Vaccine During an Avian Influenza Pandemic: Why It Won't Be Easy," *Yale Journal of Biology and Medicine* 78, no. 5 (2005): pp. 287–300.

172 Rawls, *A Theory of Justice.*

173 Ibid.

174 Kamm, *Morality, Mortality.*

175 Parfit, "Equality and Priority."

176 A. Sen, *On Economic Inequality* (Clarendon Press, 1973).

177 N. S. Jecker and R. A. Pearlman, "Ethical Constraints on Rationing Medical Care by Age," *Journal of the American Geriatric Society* 37, no. 11 (1989): pp. 1067–1075.

178 P. N. Lanken, P. B. Terry and M. L. Osborne, *Ethics of Allocating Intensive Care Unit Resources* (Baltimore: New Horizons, 1997).

179 Daniels, *Am I My Parents' Keeper?*

180 Schwappach, "Resource Allocation, Social Values and the QALY."

181 J. G. Evans, *The Rationing Debate: Rationing Health Care by Age: The Case Against* (1997).

182 N. Daniels, "Accountability for Reasonableness," *British Medical Journal* 321 (2000): pp. 1300–1301.

test, because they are difficult to understand, easily corrupted, or closed to public revision. Systems that intentionally conceal their allocative principles to avoid public complaints might also fail the test.[183] Although procedural fairness is necessary for legitimacy, it is unable to ensure the justice of allocation decisions on its own.[184,185]

Although fair procedures are important, substantive, morally relevant values and principles are indispensable for just allocation.[186,187]

Conclusion

Ultimately, none of the eight simple principles recognise all morally relevant values, and some recognise irrelevant values. QALY and DALY multiprinciple systems neglect the importance of fair distribution. UNOS points systems attempt to address distributive justice, but recognise morally irrelevant values and are vulnerable to corruption. By contrast, the complete lives system combines four morally relevant principles: youngest-first, prognosis, lottery, and saving the most lives. In pandemic situations, it also allocates scarce interventions to people instrumental in realising these four principles. Importantly, it is not an algorithm, but a framework that expresses widely affirmed values: priority to the worst-off, maximising benefits, and treating people equally. To achieve a just allocation of scarce medical interventions, society must embrace the challenge of implementing a coherent multiprinciple framework rather than relying on simple principles or retreating to the status quo.

183 G. Calabresi and P. Bobbitt, *Tragic Choices: The Conflicts Society Confronts in the Allocation of Tragically Scarce Resources* (New York: Norton, 1978).

184 N. Daniels, "How to Achieve Fair Distribution of Arts in 3 by 5: Fair Process and Legitimacy in Patient Selection" (Geneva: World Health Organization, 2004).

185 J. Mielke, D. K. Martin and P. A. Singer, "Priority Setting in a Hospital Critical Care Unit: Qualitative Case Study," *Critical Care Medicine* 31, no. 12 (2003): pp. 2764–2768.

186 A. Hasman and S. Holm, "Accountability for Reasonableness: Opening the Black Box of Process," *Health Care Analysis* 13, no. 4 (2005): pp. 261–273.

187 A. Friedman, "Beyond Accountability for Reasonableness," *Bioethics* 22, no. 2 (2008): pp. 101–112.

EXCERPT 11

Abridged text from:

S. J. Kerstein and G. Bognar, "Complete Lives in the Balance," *American Journal of Bioethics* 10, no. 4 (2010): pp. 37–45.

Complete Lives in the Balance

Samuel J. Kerstein
University of Maryland, College Park

Greg Bognar
New York University

The allocation of scarce health care resources presents stark problems of distributive justice.[1,2,3] When we must decide how to allocate beds in an intensive care unit, vaccinations during a flu pandemic, or organs for transplant, our choice can determine who lives and who dies. But there is little agreement on principles for such allocation. . . .

. . . Any acceptable "system" of principles must satisfy at least the following two conditions: First, its component principles must rest on secure moral foundations, and second, it must be able to provide practical guidance—especially in cases when different principles conflict and must be balanced. These conditions are necessary (but not sufficient) for any resource allocation scheme to be legitimate. A legitimate scheme can be seen as just and fair by those who are potentially affected by its decisions—that is, all of us—and it is capable of enjoying broad public support.[4,5]

. . . We argue that the complete lives system fails. . . : Some of its main component principles lack adequate moral foundations, and it fails to provide meaningful guidance in a range of central cases. . . .

Complete Lives and Modified Youngest-First

The aim of the complete lives system is to promote complete human lives. In the allocation of scarce life-saving health care resources, we should enable people to live such lives, contend the system's developers. . . .

The notion of a "complete life" is central to Persad and colleagues' proposal. It is unfortunate, therefore, that they never tell us precisely what they mean by it. What they do say is compatible with different and mutually exclusive interpretations.

Consider a related idea, formulated by some philosophers, that focuses on the concept of a life plan. People construct and revise their overarching plans and projects for their lives in the light of how long they expect to live and how much time they expect they will need to carry out their plans. In some views, a system for allocating scarce resources should aim to provide the opportunity to complete life plans. Justice in health care requires equalizing such opportunity.[6]

This is not an unattractive idea, but it does not seem to be what Persad and colleagues have in mind. For them, a complete life seems to consist in a given number of life years—which might vary depending on the typical life span in a given society—rather than in having the opportunity to carry out a life plan.[7] Moreover, they argue that "youngest-first

[1] F. M. Kamm, Morality, *Mortality: Death and Whom to Save from It* (Oxford University Press, 1998).

[2] N. Daniels, *Just Health: Meeting Health Needs Fairly* (Cambridge University Press, 2008).

[3] E. Nord, *Cost-Value Analysis in Health Care: Making Sense out of QALYS* (Cambridge University Press, 1999).

[4] Daniels, *Just Health*.

[5] G. Persad, A. Wertheimer and E. J. Emanuel, "Principles for Allocation of Scarce Medical Interventions," *The Lancet* 373, no. 9661): pp. 423–431.

[6] For an account that develops this idea, see N. Daniels, *Am I My Parents' Keeper?: An Essay on Justice between the Young and the Old* (Oxford University Press, 1988); Daniels, *Just Health*. See also J. Rawls, *A Theory of Justice* (Cambridge: Harvard University Press, 1971).

[7] At one point, Persad and colleagues do say that the fulfillment of long-term plans requires a complete life (428). But they do not seem to endorse the notion that a complete life for a person consists in having the opportunity to fulfill a life plan.

allocation directs resources to those who have had less of something supremely valuable—lifeyears." This suggests that they hold the view that life-years have intrinsic value, independently of what opportunities they provide and what level of well-being they enable people to achieve. Having more life-years is valuable even if life provides few opportunities and contains very little well-being.

But perhaps Persad and colleagues treat life-years merely as a proxy for well-being, rather than as valuable in themselves. . . .

The argument for a modified youngest-first principle is problematic in the context of the complete lives system. For one thing, it seems arbitrary to think of "investment" in a person as limited to formal education and parental care. Why, for example, should not the experience and training that a diplomat or business leader gets on the job also count as societal investment in her? If the greater degree of societal investment in a 20-year-old over an infant gives us reason to prioritize saving the 20-year-old, then it seems that the greater degree of societal investment in a 40-year-old over a 20-year-old would give us reason to prioritize saving the 40-year-old. But in the complete lives system, the 20-year-old would have priority (see Figure 1). To this objection, Persad and colleagues might reply that more investment would be "wasted" in the case of the 20-year-old, since the 40-year-old has already given back to society. But this reply is unconvincing. The societal investment in the 40-year-old (e.g., a surgeon) might be much larger than that in the 20-year-old (e.g., a student), and, as a result of a lengthy training period, she might not yet have had much occasion to produce returns.

In any case, the prioritarian argument Persad and colleagues invoke for the youngest-first principle undermines the modified youngest-first principle. As we have noted, one way that they justify giving priority to the younger is on the grounds that they are worse off than the older in terms of years lived. An infant is obviously worse off than an adolescent in these terms. So if benefits ought to go to the worse off, then they should go to the infant. But according to modified youngest-first, of course, it is the adolescent who should get priority.

Persad and colleagues face yet another problem in embracing the modified youngest-first principle. This principle is incompatible with the argument that they use to defend age discrimination. In order to see why, consider an old person who is denied some life-saving intervention. She cannot argue that she is being treated unfairly, since as a young person she enjoyed (or would have enjoyed if she had been in need) the benefits of an arrangement that gives priority to the young. In other words, she has no legitimate complaint that she is denied a life-saving resource. Consider now a very young child who, according to the complete lives system, is denied a life-saving intervention because priority is given to older children and young adults. It seems that she does have a legitimate complaint (one that someone can advance on her behalf): After all, she has not benefited from an arrangement that gives priority to young adults. In fact, she is being denied a life-saving resource for the sake of those who have had more of that "supremely valuable" thing—life-years. She neither has enjoyed nor ever will enjoy the benefits of the arrangement. She is not even potentially compensated.

In sum, the prioritarian view that younger people ought to get priority on the grounds of being worse off and the modified youngest-first principle undermine one another. Moreover, the argument that age discrimination is not unfair since everyone can expect to live through the same ages is unavailable for those who accept the modified youngest-first principle.

. . .

Does the Complete Lives System Provide Practical Guidance?

. . .

Consider first a case in which we have three 18-year-old patients who will soon die unless they receive transplants. We have one heart and one set of lungs available. If we give the whole heart/lung combination to the first patient, she will live until 70—which, we shall assume, is sufficient for a complete life. If, in contrast, we give the heart to the second and the lungs to the third patient, they will live for 2 years each. Prognosis prescribes that we give the heart/lung combination to the first patient, for that is the way to maximize life-years. However, to act in accordance with the principle of saving the most lives we would obviously have to give the heart to the second and the lungs to the third. Here we have a conflict between prognosis and maximizing the number of lives saved: Should we sacrifice two lives for the sake of a complete one? The complete lives system offers no guidance for how to proceed.[8]

Next imagine that, through a multiple transplant, we can either save one 20-year-old for 4 years or two 55-year-olds for 2 years each. Since either way we preserve the same number of life-years, prognosis does not tip the scale in favor of saving the one or saving the two. The modified youngest-first principle favors saving the 20-year-old, for she is worse off in terms of the extent to which she has lived a complete life. However, the principle of saving the most lives would obviously imply that we should save the two 55-year-olds. The complete lives system leaves us with no clear idea of what we are required to do.

Finally, suppose that we are at an outpost in the midst of a flu pandemic and we have only enough medicine to treat either a 20-year-old who will then live for 5 years or an infant who will then live for 80 years. The complete lives system gives us no help in determining how to distribute the medicine justly. Prognosis requires giving it to the infant, while modified youngest-first demands that we give it to the 20-year-old.[9]

[8] A. Gandjour, "Ethical Criteria for Allocating Health-Care Resources," *The Lancet* 373, no. 9673): p. 1425.

[9] The numbers, of course, are merely illustrations. Depending on the precise weights assigned to different ages on the priority curve, the larger benefit to the infant may outweigh the increased chance of the 20-year-old of receiving the intervention. Evidently, however, there are always going to be cases in which modified youngest-first remains in conflict with the other principles, whatever the precise weights are.

As we mentioned, Persad and colleagues suggest that in cases where there are "roughly equal" candidates for lifesaving interventions, it is legitimate to conduct a lottery. But within our cases do we have such candidates? For example, is the 18-year-old who, if given a heart and lungs, will live for another 52 years roughly equal to the two other 18-year-olds who, if given organs, will live for another 2 years each? We are unsure how Persad and colleagues would answer that question. But even if their view is that the candidates within our cases are roughly equal, it is not clear what sort of lottery we should conduct. In the case of the 18-year-old patients, should each one get a 50% chance of being saved, or should the one who needs a heart/lungs combination receive a 1/3 chance while each of the others gets a 2/3 chance?

. . .

Allocation Systems and Balancing

The practical ineffectiveness of Persad and colleagues' proposal leaves us with an important lesson. In order to develop a just system for the distribution of persistently scarce, lifesaving resources, we need to undertake the arduous task of specifying how to balance allocation principles when they yield conflicting prescriptions. Of course, we also need to determine which principles should figure into allocation decisions in the first place. As our criticisms of the foundations of the complete lives system suggest, we doubt whether there is sufficient warrant to include a principle of modified youngest-first. Indeed, although we cannot discuss our reasons here, we are also skeptical whether we should include any principle that itself demands priority for the youngest.[10]

However, we do agree that a system for just allocation must balance some principle akin to prognosis with some principle akin

[10] G. Bognar and S. J. Kerstein, "Saving Lives and Respecting Persons," 2010.

to maximizing the number of lives saved. A principle akin to prognosis that we defend elsewhere prescribes extending the lives of persons: beings who have certain psychological capacities, including the capacities to set ends and to form, act on, and revise plans for attaining them.[11] Another principle might prescribe extending life, but only when its quality is above a certain threshold. These principles do not demand that we use scarce resources to prolong lives regardless of their quality. But we shall put aside considerations regarding the precise shape that such principles should take and consider how we might balance between the defeasible imperatives to save as many lives as we can and to extend life as much as possible.[12] Such reflection, no matter how helpful, would constitute only one step toward developing a system for scarce, life-saving resource allocation. . . .

Here is a proposal for balancing these principles. We begin by determining the proportion between the values relative to each principle that are manifested in the sets of persons who are in competition for the resources. . . . The value relative to prognosis is the number of additional life-years made possible, while the value relative to life-saving is the number of lives saved. The set that contributes the higher value to the proportion relative to a principle is "favored" on that principle. We then determine which proportion relative to each principle is greater. We preserve the set of persons that is favored by the proportion that yields the higher number.

Our example will help to illustrate the procedure. We must choose between saving one person for 11 years and saving five people for 2 years each. The one person has a higher value relative to prognosis, but the group of five has a higher value relative to life-saving. Regarding prognosis, the proportion between the values possessed by the one versus the group is 11/10 (11 years versus 5 × 2 years). Thus, the one person is favored. In contrast, the proportion between the values possessed by the group and the one regarding life-saving is 5/1 (5 lives saved versus 1 life saved). On this principle, the group is favored. The second proportion is equivalent to a number (5) that is greater than that yielded by the first proportion (1.1). So, according to this method, we should save the group of five persons.[13]

. . .

[11] Ibid.

[12] By a defeasible imperative, we mean simply an imperative that can legitimately be overridden by some other principle in an allocation system. If an imperative to preserve the most lives were categorical, in contrast to defeasible, then, according to it, any allocation that did not maximally preserve lives would be wrong.

[13] A fully developed weighing scheme would have to be sensitive to the uncertainty of a choice regarding both the number of persons preserved and the duration of their preservation. This is a further complication that we set aside.

Further Resources

Relevant Organizations

Governmental

Centers for Disease Control and Prevention (CDC): The CDC conducts research and provides information for US health threats. Additional information can be found at www.cdc.gov

The National Council for Priority Setting in Health Care: Has an advisory role in regard to health care priority setting in Norway. Additional information can be found at http://www.prioritering.no/hjem?language=english

Nongovernmental

National Center for Priority Setting in Health Care: A nonprofit Swedish national resource to support development and transfer of knowledge on priority setting in health are. Additional information can be found at http://www.imh.liu.se/halso-och-sjukvardsanalys/prioriteringscentrum?l=en

Literature

Bramstedt, Katrina A. "Is It Ethical to Prioritize Patients for Organ Allocation According to Their Values About Organ Donation?" *Progress in Transplantation* 16, no. 2 (June 1, 2006): 170–174.

Bickenbach, Jerome, "Disability and Health Care Rationing," The Stanford Encyclopedia of Philosophy (Spring 2016 Edition), Edward N. Zalta (ed.), http://plato.stanford.edu/archives/spr2016/entries/disability-care-rationing/.

Organ Procurement and Transplantation Network. "Ethical Principles in the Allocation of Human Organs." https://optn.transplant.hrsa.gov/resources/ethics/ethical-principles-in-the-allocation-of-human-organs/.

Persad, Govind C., Alan Wertheimer, and Ezekiel J. Emanuel. "Standing by Our Principles: Meaningful Guidance, Moral Foundations, and Multi-Principle Methodology in Medical Scarcity." *The American Journal of Bioethics* 10, no. 4 (2010/04/09 2010): 46–48.

Porter, Eduardo. "Rationing Health Care More Fairly," *New York Times*, August 21, 2012.

The President's Council on Bioethics. "Organ Transplantation: Defining the Ethical and Policy Issues." https://bioethicsarchive.georgetown.edu/pcbe/background/staff_cohen.html.

Selective Service System. "How the Draft Has Changed Since Vietnam." https://www.sss.gov/About/History-And-Records/How-The-Draft-Has-Changed- Since-Vietnam.

6 Organ Transplantation

A tragedy strikes: Susan, a young, newly married woman has died in a terrible car accident. At the same time, a wonderful thing happens: Susan's husband agrees to have her organs donated for transplantation. But, unfortunately, tragedy strikes again. Three people who desperately need a new liver wait in the hospital: Joey, a 3-year-old with acute liver failure; Melissa, a 22-year-old recent college graduate with liver failure due to Wilson's disease; and Charles, a 70-year-old retired electrician with alcoholic cirrhosis who needs a transplant. Who should get the liver?

Organ transplantation goes back to the 19th century with the successful transplantation of thyroid tissue.[1] The first successful cornea transplant dates to 1905 and the Czech republic.[2] But modern organ transplantation can be dated from 1954, when Dr. Joseph Murray of the Brigham Hospital in Boston was the first to successfully transplant a kidney from one identical twin to the other (Table 6.1).[3]

Organ transplantation did not really take off as a successful intervention until doctors solved the problem of immune rejection by the person receiving the donated organ. The discovery of the immune suppressant cyclosporine in 1970 made long-term transplant survival a reality.[4]

The success in organ transplantation created serious ethical problems: What criteria should be used to decide who gets organs, and how should such criteria be implemented? Over the decades, the challenges arising from these questions have not become easier. If anything, things have gotten worse and are likely to continue to get worse. In large measure, this is due to driving becoming much safer, and, therefore,

---

[1] T. Schlich, *The Origins of Organ Transplantation: Surgery and Laboratory Science, 1880–1930* (University of Rochester Press, 2010), p. 37.

[2] S. L. Moffatt, V. A. Cartwright, and T. H. Stumpf, "Centennial Review of Corneal Transplantation," *Clinical & Experimental Ophthalmology* 33, no. 6 (2005): p. 642.

[3] P. K. Linden, "History of Solid Organ Transplantation and Organ Donation," *Critical Care Clinics* 25, no. 1 (2009): p. 167.

[4] Ibid., p. 170.

Table 6.1
OPTN Classification System for Nodules Seen on Imaging of Cirrhotic Livers

Year	Organ	Surgeon	Location
1954	Kidney[a]	Joseph Murray	Boston, Massachusetts, USA
1966	Pancreas[b]	Richard Lillehei	Minneapolis, Minnesota, USA
1967	Liver[a]	Thomas Starzl	Denver, Colorado, USA
1967	Heart[a]	Christian Bernard	Cape Town, South Africa
1981	Heart/lung[a]	Bruce Reitz	Stanford, California, USA

[a]P. K. Linden, "History of Solid Organ Transplantation and Organ Donation," *Critical Care Clinics* 25, no. 1 (2009): p. 167."

[b]J. P. Squifflet, R. W.G. Gruessner and D. E.R. Sutherland, "Surgical History: The History of Pancreas Transplantation: Past, Present and Future," *Acta Chir Belg* 108 (2008): p. 368.

the number of people dying in car accidents declining and continuing to decline. This is a good thing, but it also means that the number of transplantable cadaveric organs will decline.

Consider the situation for liver transplants. Livers are in short supply. As of January 2015, there were 15,449 people on the waiting lists in the United States for a liver.[5] In all of 2014, there were 6,729 livers transplanted in the United States.[6] Each year, more than 10,000 people are added to the transplant lists.[7] The consequence is that the median waiting time for a liver for transplantation is nearly a year—336 days. This is not uniform for all age groups. Children aged 6 to 10 have a median waiting time of around 4.5 months, while adults aged 35–49 have a median waiting time of about 43 months.[8] It also means that nearly 2,000 people die each year waiting for liver transplants.[9] Researchers who have analyzed how often families of potential donors are asked if organs may be taken, and how often families actually consent to organ donation, believe there will never be a time when there will be enough livers for transplantation:

> [E]ven if livers were successfully recovered from all potential donors at the same rate at which they are currently recovered from actual donors, the supply would be insufficient to meet the demand of the annual additions to waiting lists.[10]

If we will always face shortages of livers for transplantation, then who should get Susan's liver? Should it be Joey? Or Melissa? Or Charles? What criteria should we use to choose among them?

Initially, livers were allocated predominantly by time on the waiting list.[11] The problem is that many patients who were becoming sicker died on the waiting list. Then, in 2002, after much discussion, the United Network for Organ Sharing (UNOS) introduced an allocation system based on the MELD score. The MELD—Model for End Stage Liver Disease—score is

[5] Organ Procurement and Transplantation Network, "Data," 2015, accessed January 3, 2015, http://optn.transplant.hrsa.gov/converge/data/.

[6] Ibid.

[7] Ibid.

[8] United Network for Organ Sharing, "Requested Data: Median Time to Deceased Donor Transplant for Liver Registrations Added 01/01/2009–12/31/2013 by Age at Listing," 2015, accessed November 13, 2015, http://optn.transplant.hrsa.gov/converge/data/request_main.asp.

[9] Scientific Registry of Transplant Recipients, "Reported Deaths and Annual Death Rates Per 1,000 Patient-Years at Risk, 2002 to 2011, Liver Waiting List," 2012, accessed June 16, 2015, http://www.srtr.org/annual_Reports/2011/903_age_li.aspx.

[10] E. Sheehy, et al., "Estimating the Number of Potential Organ Donors in the United States," *New England Journal of Medicine* 349, no. 7 (2003): p. 673.

[11] A. P. Martin, et al., "Overview of the MELD Score and the UNOS Adult Liver Allocation System," *Transplantation Proceedings* 39, no. 10 (2007): pp. 3169–3170.

based on three physiological variables and is an accurate but not perfect predictor of a patient's risk of death while waiting for a liver transplant. Excerpts from the UNOS liver allocation policy and an article by Adrian Martin and colleagues explaining the MELD score algorithm appear later in the chapter (Excerpt 1, Excerpt 2).[12,13]

The MELD score ranges from 6 to 40—the higher the score, the higher the risk of death. However, below 15, patients have a higher mortality rate from the transplant than from their liver failure and so are not given a liver.[14] With the adoption of the MELD score, UNOS changed from a waiting time standard to one that prioritizes the sickest patients on the waiting list. This minimizes deaths while waiting.

But is prioritizing sicker patients the right criterion? It is recognized that using the MELD score but allocating organs within a local area still means that some patients with equal MELD scores, but located in different areas, will have very different chances of getting a liver—and of dying on the waiting list. Is it ethical if geography influences who gets Susan's liver?

Furthermore, there is a question of whether prioritizing sicker patients is better than prioritizing patients who would do better—that is, tend to live longer with a new liver. The MELD score does not take into account prognosis with a new liver. Is prognosis an important criterion? Should MELD be replaced or modified by another factor that considers prognosis?

It turns out that not all patients have the same prognosis. Age is an important determinant of prognosis (Table 6.2). Given that younger people have a higher survival rate than older people, should age be a factor in determining who gets the liver? Should Joey receive priority since children his age have the highest survival rate? Or is his higher survival rate compared to Melissa—less than 5% for 5 years—not sufficient to use age?

These are important questions about the formal criteria that should guide the allocation of organs for transplantation. But there are also ethical issues that arise in the implementation of these criteria. Consider the case of Steve Jobs, the late CEO of Apple, as depicted in William Saletan's article (Excerpt 3).[16] He had pancreatic cancer and then received a liver transplant. Jobs lived in the San Francisco area but received his transplant in Memphis, Tennessee. He was able to list himself in more than one place for a liver transplant. UNOS permits multiple listings. But is multiple listings ethical? Only the wealthy who can undergo evaluations at multiple centers can be listed at more than one place. Furthermore, only a person who can get to another center within a few hours can be listed in multiple regions. To be specific, only a person with access to a private plane can really be listed in both Memphis and San Francisco. Is that fair? Should wealth and access to a private plane determine who gets Susan's liver?

There is also the case of Mickey Mantle, a record-setting American Major League Baseball player from the 1950s–60s. Years of alcohol and then hepatitis C caused him to suffer from liver failure and, ultimately, liver cancer. He received a liver transplant within days of being listed.[17] Mark Siegler argues that it is ethical to give a true national hero a liver even

Table 6.2
Age and 5-Year Survival After a Liver Transplant[15]

Age	5-Year Survival Rate
1–5	80.0%
6–10	77.3%
11–17	76.4%
18–34	76.3%
35–49	70.5%
50–64	65.8%
≥65	61.2%

[12] UNOS/OPTN, "OPTN Policies: Section 3.6 Allocation of Livers," 2013.

[13] Martin, "Overview of the MELD Score."

[14] Ibid., pp. 3170–3171.

[15] Organ Procurement and Transplantation Network, "Advanced Data."

[16] W. Saletan, "How Did Steve Jobs Get His Liver?", *Slate Magazine*, January 19, 2001.

[17] J. Randal, "Mantle's Transplant Raises Delicate Issues About Organ Allocation," *Journal of the National Cancer Institute* 88, no. 8 (1996): p. 484.

though he had cancer and had not waited long (Excerpt 4).[18] But who should count as a national hero? Would Steve Jobs also qualify as a hero? And what ethical principle could justify giving heros priority? Should it matter that many people would argue that Mickey Mantle could have avoided being an alcoholic?

Finally, there is the question of whether any person should receive multiple organs for transplantation. There are long waiting lists for every organ. Giving two organs to one patient—for instance, a liver and a kidney—instead of two patients saves half as many lives. Is it ethical to save fewer lives? Is maximizing the number of people saved from organ transplantation a valid ethical principle? But is it discrimination not to give a patient organs just because they have two rather than one failing organ? After all, in most cases, they did not choose or do anything to have multiple organs failing, and it is not self-evident that they should not be treated just like every other person in need of an organ. The case of Jesica Santillon, elucidated in a news article by Sheryl Gay Stolberg and Lawrence K. Altman, raises these and other questions about the ethics of multiorgan transplantation (Excerpt 5).[19]

Without a major breakthrough in synthesizing organs, there will absolute shortages of organs for transplantation. Physicians will have to choose between people, and, unfortunately, every year thousands of people will die waiting for organs. Determining the criteria for who should get the available organs and picking those individuals is a very difficult ethical problem.

---

[18] G. Kolata, "Transplants, Morality and Mickey," *New York Times*, June 11, 1995.

[19] S. G. Stolberg and L. K. Altman, "An Ethical Dilemma with Few Precedents," *New York Times*, February 21, 2003.

Questions for Discussion

1. The history of organ transplantation shows that there have been many different criteria used. For livers, the initial criteria was waiting time, but recently it has shifted to degree of illness. Other criteria that seem relevant include prognosis with the new transplanted organs as well as trying to save the most people. Is there a principle that is clearly more important than others, and, if so, on what grounds?
2. Lung and liver cancer are often linked to excessive consumption of alcohol and smoking, respectively. In what way, if any, should personal responsibility enter as a criterion for access to organs? If you oppose a role for personal responsibility, why?
3. Principles that are set out by organizations such as the United Network for Organ Sharing (UNOS) determine the ranking on transplant lists. In practice, physicians may still need to make judgment calls on who gets an organ. Is this acceptable, or should principles and guidelines be developed and applied in such a way that there is no discretion whatsoever for physicians?
4. Should it ever be ethical to allow people to be listed in multiple locations for organ transplants, such as in the case of Steve Jobs (Excerpt 3)?
5. Each of the following patients are on the Organ Procurement and Transplantation Network waiting list for a liver. According to UNOS liver allocation rules (Excerpt 1), which of the following patients is most likely to get a liver first? In your view, which one should be prioritized?
   a. EE – 57-year-old male, obese, nonalcoholic fatty liver disease; 2 grandchildren; MELD: 32
   b. AS – 46-year-old male, alcohol abuse, cirrhosis but stopped drinking; MELD: 26
   c. KO – 72-year old-female, hepatitis C cirrhosis, well compensated, on anti-hep C drugs; MELD: 11
   d. HS – 59-year old-male, hepatitis C from IV drug abuse, and hepatic carcinoma, still smoking, severe emphysema; MELD: 33

EXCERPTS

Note: The following excerpts have generally been edited for length, and omissions are indicated with ellipses. Editing includes footnotes and endnotes, which have also been renumbered. For citation and related purposes, the full original source texts should be used.

EXCERPT 1

Abridged text from:

UNOS/OPTN, "OPTN Policies: Section 3.6 Allocation of Livers," 2013, accessed August 7, 2014, http://optn.transplant.hrsa.gov/governance/policies/.

3.6. Allocation of Livers

. . . For the purpose of enabling physicians to apply their consensus medical judgement for the benefit of liver transplant candidates as a group, each candidate will be assigned a status code or probability of candidate death derived from a mortality risk score corresponding to the degree of medical urgency. Mortality risk scores shall be determined by the prognostic factors specified and calculated in accordance with the Model for End-Stage Liver Disease (MELD) Scoring System. . . . Candidates will be stratified within MELD or PELD score by blood type similarity as described in Policy 3.6.2. . . .

Livers will be offered to candidates with an assigned Status of 1A and 1B in descending point sequence with the candidate having the highest number of points receiving the highest priority before being offered for candidates listed in other categories within distribution areas as noted below. Following Status 1, livers will be offered to candidates based upon their probability of candidate death derived from assigned MELD scores, in descending point sequence with the candidate having the highest probability ranking receiving the highest priority before being offered to candidates having lower probability rankings. . . .

At each level of distribution, adult livers (i. e., greater than or equal to 18 years old) will be allocated in the following sequence (adult donor liver allocation algorithm):

Adult Donor Liver Allocation Algorithm

Combined Local and Regional

1. Status 1A candidates in descending point order
2. Status 1B candidates in descending order

Local and Regional

3. Candidates with MELD/PELD Scores ≥35 in descending order of mortality risk (MELD) scores, with Local candidates ranked above Regional candidates at each level of MELD score

Local

4. Candidates with MELD/PELD Scores 29–34 in descending order of mortality risk scores (probability of candidate death)

National

5. Liver-Intestine Candidates in descending order of Status and mortality risk scores (probability of candidate death)

Local

6. Candidates with MELD/PELD Scores 15–28 in descending order of mortality risk scores (probability of candidate death)

Regional

7. Candidates with MELD/PELD Scores 15–34 in descending order of mortality risk scores (probability of candidate death)

National

8. Status 1A candidates in descending point order
9. Status 1B candidates in descending point order
10. Candidates with MELD/PELD Scores ≥15 in descending order of mortality risk scores (probability of candidate death)

. . .

3.6.4. Degree of Medical Urgency. Each candidate is assigned a status code or mortality risk score (probability of candidate death) which corresponds to how medically urgent it is that the candidate receive a transplant.

3.6.4.1. Adult Candidate Status. Medical urgency is assigned to an adult liver transplant candidate (greater than or equal to 18 years of age) based on either the criteria defined below for Status 1A, or the candidate's mortality risk score as determined by the prognostic factors specified in Table [6.3] and calculated in accordance with the MELD Scoring System. A candidate who does not have a MELD score that, in the judgment of the candidate's transplant physician, appropriately reflects the candidate's medical urgency, may nevertheless be assigned a higher MELD score upon application by his/her transplant physician(s) and justification to the applicable Regional Review Board that the candidate is considered, by consensus medical judgment, using accepted medical criteria, to have an urgency and potential for benefit comparable to that of other candidates having the higher MELD score. The justification must include a rationale for incorporating the exceptional case as part of MELD calculation. A report of the decision of the Regional Review Board and the basis for it shall be forwarded to for review by the Liver and Intestinal Organ Transplantation and Membership and Professional Standards Committees to determine consistency in application among and within Regions and continued appropriateness of the MELD criteria.

. . .

Status	Definition
1A	A candidate greater than or equal to 18 years of age listed as Status 1A has fulminant liver failure with a life expectancy without a liver transplant of less than 7 days. For the purpose of Policy 3.6, fulminant liver failure shall be defined as described in (i)–(iv). Centers that list candidates not meeting these criteria for Status 1A will be referred to the Liver and Intestinal Organ Transplantation Committee for review. . . .

(i) fulminant hepatic failure defined as the onset of hepatic encephalopathy within 8 weeks of the first symptoms of liver disease. The absence of pre-existing liver disease is critical to the diagnosis. One of three criteria below must be met to list an adult candidate, who must be in the ICU, with fulminant liver failure: (1) ventilator dependence (2) requiring dialysis or continuous veno-venous hemofiltration (CVVH) or continuous veno-venous hemodialysis (CVVD) or (3) INR >2.0, or

(ii) primary non-function of a transplanted liver within 7 days of implantation; as defined by (a) or (b):

(a) AST ≥3,000 and one or both of the following:
an INR ≥2.5
Acidosis, defined as having an arterial pH ≤7.30 or venous pH of 7.25 and/or Lactate ≥4 mMol/L

(b) Anhepatic candidate, or

(iii) hepatic artery thrombosis in a transplanted liver within 7 days of implantation, with evidence of severe liver injury as defined in (ii(a)) and (ii(b)) above; Candidates with HAT in a transplanted liver within 14 days of implantation not meeting the above criteria will be listed at a MELD of 40; or

(iv) acute decompensated Wilson's disease.

. . . Candidates who are listed as a Status 1A automatically revert back to their most recent MELD Score after 7 days unless these candidates are relisted as Status 1A by an attending physician. . . .

Table [6.3]
Short History of First Successful Organ Transplants

Class	Description	Comment
0	**Incomplete or technically inadequate study**	Repeat study required for adequate assessment; automatic priority MELD points cannot be assigned based on a OPTN 0 classified imaging study
5	**Meets radiologic criteria for HCC**	May qualify for automatic exception depending on stage (see 3.6.4.4 section A.)
	5A: > or equal to 1 cm and less than 2 cm measured on late arterial or portal phase images.	Increased contrast enhancement on late hepatic arterial phase AND washout during later contrast phases AND peripheral rim enhancement (capsule/pseudocapsule).
	5A-g: same size as 5A	Increased contrast enhancement on late hepatic arterial phase AND growth by 50% or more documented on serial CT/MRI obtained <or equal to 6 months apart.
	5B: maximum diameter > or equal to 2 cm and less than or equal to 5 cm.	Increased contrast enhancement on late hepatic arterial phase AND either washout during later contrast phases OR peripheral rim enhancement (capsule/pseudocapsule) OR growth by 50% or more documented on serial CT/MRI obtained <or equal to 6 months apart (5B-g).
	5T: prior local regional treatment for HCC	Describes any residual lesion or perfusion defect at site of prior UNOS class 5 lesion.
	5X: maximum diameter > or equal to 5 cm.	Increased contrast enhancement on late hepatic arterial phase AND either washout during later contrast phases OR peripheral rim enhancement (capsule/pseudocapsule)

For descriptions of Classes 1–4, which are not applicable to OPTN policy, please see http://www.acr.org/Quality-Safety/Resources/LIRADS.

All other adult liver transplant candidates on the Waiting List shall be assigned a mortality risk score calculated in accordance with the MELD scoring system. . . . These data must be based on the most recent clinical information (e.g., laboratory test results and diagnosis) and include the dates of the laboratory tests.

. . .

Using these prognostic factors and regression coefficients, the UNet[SM] shall assign a MELD score for each candidate based on the following calculation:

$$\text{MELD Score} = 0.957 \text{ x } \text{Log}_e(\text{creatinine mg/dL}) + 0.378 \text{ x } \text{Log}_e(\text{bilirubin mg/dL}) + 1.120 \text{ x } \text{Log}_e(\text{INR}) + 0.643$$

Laboratory values less than 1.0 will be set to 1.0 for the purposes of the MELD score calculation.

. . .

3.6.4.5. Liver Candidates with Exceptional Cases. Special cases require prospective review by the Regional Review Board. The center will request a specific MELD/PELD score and shall submit a supporting narrative. The Regional Review Board will accept or reject the center's requested MELD/PELD score based on guidelines developed by each RRB. Each RRB must set an acceptable time for Reviews to be completed, within twenty-one days after application; if approval is not given and the physician wishes to pursue the listing, then the physician and the RRB must meet by conference call to review the case. If approval is not given within twenty-one days, the candidate's transplant physician may list the candidate at the higher MELD or PELD score, subject to automatic referral to the Liver and Intestinal Organ Transplantation Committee for review; this review by the Liver and Intestinal Organ Transplantation Committee may result in further referral of the matter to the Membership and Professional Standards Committee for appropriate action in accordance with *Appendix L: Reviews, Actions, and Due Process* of the OPTN Bylaws. Exceptions to the MELD/PELD score must be reapplied every three months; otherwise the candidate's score will revert back to the candidate's current calculated MELD/PELD score. If the RRB does not recertify the MELD/PELD score exception, then the candidate will be assigned a MELD/PELD score based on current laboratory values. Centers may apply for a MELD/PELD score equivalent to a 10% increase in candidate mortality every 3 months as long as the candidate meets the original criteria. Extensions shall undergo prospective review by the RRB. A candidate's approved score will be maintained if the center enters the extension application more than 3 days prior to the due date and the RRB does not act prior to that date (i.e., the candidate will not be downgraded if the RRB does not act in a timely manner). If the extension application is subsequently denied then the candidate will be assigned the laboratory MELD score. Candidates meeting the criteria listed in 3.6.4.5.1–3.6.4.5.6 are eligible for additional MELD/PELD exception points, provided that the criteria are included in the clinical narrative. Unless the applicable RRB has a pre-existing agreement for a higher point assignment for these diagnoses, an initial MELD score of 22/PELD score of 28 shall be assigned. For candidates with Primary Hyperoxaluria meeting the criteria in 3.6.4.5.5, an initial MELD score of 28/PELD score of 41 shall be assigned. These pre-existing agreements must be renewed on an annual basis.

3.6.4.5.1. Liver Candidates with Hepatopulmonary Syndrome (HPS). Candidates with a clinical evidence of portal hypertension, evidence of a shunt, and a PaO_2 <60 mmHg on room air will be listed at a MELD score of 22 without RRB review with a 10% mortality equivalent increase in points every three months if the candidate's PaO2 stays below 60 mmHg. Candidates should have no significant clinical evidence of underlying primary pulmonary disease.

3.6.4.5.2. Liver Candidates with Cholangiocarcinoma. Candidates meeting the criteria listed in Table [6.4] will be eligible for a MELD/PELD exception with a 10% mortality equivalent increase every three months.

3.6.4.5.3. Liver Candidates with Cystic Fibrosis. Liver candidates with signs of reduced pulmonary function, defined as having an FEV1 that falls below 40%,will be eligible for a MELD/PELD exception with a 10% mortality equivalent increase every three months.

3.6.4.5.4. Liver Candidates with Familial Amyloid Polyneuropathy (FAP). Candidates with a clear diagnosis, to include an echocardiogram showing the candidate has an ejection fraction >40%, ambulatory status, and identification of TTR gene mutation (Val30Met vs. non-Val30Met) and a biopsy proven amyloid in the involved organ, will be eligible for a MELD/PELD exception with a 10% mortality equivalent increase every three months.

3.6.4.5.5. Liver Candidates with Primary Hyperoxaluria. Candidates with AGT deficiency proven by liver biopsy (sample analysis and/or genetic analysis), and listed for a combined liver-kidney transplant will be eligible for a MELD/PELD exception with a 10% mortality equivalent increase every three months. Candidates must have a GFR ≤ 25 ml/min for 6 weeks or more by MDRD6 or direct measurement (Iothalamate or iohexol).

3.6.4.5.6. Liver Candidates with Portopulmonary Syndrome. Candidates that meet the following criteria will be eligible for a MELD/PELD exception with a 10% mortality equivalent increase every three months if the mean pulmonary arterial pressure (MPAP) stays

Table [6.4]
Criteria for MELD Exception for Liver Transplant Candidates with Cholangiocarcinoma (CCA)

- Centers must submit a written protocol for patient care to the OPTN/UNOS Liver and Intestinal Organ Transplantation Committee before requesting a MELD score exception for a candidate with CCA. This protocol should include selection criteria, administration of neoadjuvant therapy before transplantation, and operative staging to exclude patients with regional hepatic lymph node metastases, intrahepatic metastases, and/or extrahepatic disease. The protocol should include data collection as deemed necessary by the OPTN/UNOS Liver and Intestinal Organ Transplantation Committee.
- Candidates must satisfy diagnostic criteria for hilar CCA: malignant-appearing stricture on cholangiography and one of the following: carbohydrate antigen 19-9 100 U/mL, or and biopsy or cytology results demonstrating malignancy, or aneuploidy. The tumor should be considered unresectable on the basis of technical considerations or underlying liver disease (e.g., primary sclerosing cholangitis).
- If cross-sectional imaging studies (CT scan, ultrasound, MRI) demonstrate a mass, the mass should be 3 cm or less.
- Candidates must satisfy diagnostic criteria for hilar CCA: malignant-appearing stricture on cholangiography and biopsy or cytology results demonstrating malignancy, carbohydrate antigen 19-9 100 U/mL, or aneuploidy. The tumor should be considered unresectable on the basis of technical considerations or underlying liver disease (e.g., primary sclerosing cholangitis).
- If cross-sectional imaging studies (CT scan, ultrasound, MRI) demonstrate a mass, the mass should be 3 cm.
- Intra- and extrahepatic metastases should be excluded by cross-sectional imaging studies of the chest and abdomen at the time of initial exception and every 3 months before score increases.
- Regional hepatic lymph node involvement and peritoneal metastases should be assessed by operative staging after completion of neoadjuvant therapy and before liver transplantation. Endoscopic ultrasound-guided aspiration of regional hepatic lymph nodes may be advisable to exclude patients with obvious metastases before neoadjuvant therapy is initiated.
- Transperitoneal aspiration or biopsy of the primary tumor (either by endoscopic ultrasound, operative, or percutaneous approaches) should be avoided because of the high risk of tumor seeding associated with these procedures.

. . .

CT, computed tomography; *MRI*, magnetic resonance imaging.

below 35 mmHg (confirmed by repeat heart catheterization).

- Diagnosis should include initial MPAP and pulmonary vascular resistance (PVR) levels, documentation of treatment, and post-treatment MPAP <35 mmHg and PVR <400 dynes/sec/cm^3.
- Transpulmonary gradient should be required for initial diagnosis to correct for volume overload.

. . .

3.6.4.7. Combined Liver-Intestine Candidates. Candidates awaiting a combined liver–intestine transplant who are registered and active on both waiting lists will automatically receive an additional increase in their MELD/PELD score equivalent to a 10% risk of 3-month mortality. Candidates age 0–17 will receive a 23 point increase in their calculated MELD/PELD score instead of the 10% increase. The center must verify that an intestinal transplant is required and took place.

3.6.4.8. Combined Liver-Intestine Allocation. For combined liver-intestine allocation, the liver must first be offered:

- according to the liver match run
- sequentially to **each** potential liver recipient (including all MELD/PELD potential recipients) through national Status 1A and 1B offers.

The liver may then be offered to combined liver-intestine potential recipients sequentially according to the intestine match run.

3.6.5. Center Contact and Acceptance. Livers shall be offered in descending computer print-out order but the offering calls may be made concurrently (e.g., 5 liver teams may be called and given donor information provided that each team is told its priority number for the liver offer). Policy 3.4.1 (Time Limit for Acceptance) assures that each team will know within one hour whether or not another center with a candidate who has higher points has accepted or rejected the offer.

3.6.5.1. Execution of the Liver Match System. The Match System for liver allocation shall be executed within 8 hours prior to the initial liver offer. This match system printout of the liver transplant candidate waiting list shall be utilized by the Host OPO for placement of the donor liver. The liver match system may be re-executed if a previously accepted liver is subsequently turned down because there is a change in specific medical information related to the liver donor. Any re-execution of the liver match system for the same donor for other reasons must be retrospectively reviewed by the Regional Review Board. This policy shall not apply to a donor liver that has been recovered and has not been placed within 2 hours of organ recovery.

. . .

EXCERPT 2

Full text from:

A. P. Martin, et al., "Overview of the MELD Score and the UNOS Adult Liver Allocation System," *Transplantation Proceedings* 39, no. 10 (2007): pp. 3169–3174.

Overview of the MELD Score and the UNOS Adult Liver Allocation System

A. P. Martin, M. Bartels, J. Hauss, and J. Fangmann

Since liver transplantation has become a universally accepted treatment for end-stage liver disease, the number of patients accumulating on the waiting list has gradually outweighed the scarce resources of available organs. Fair allocation of donor livers to patients with end-stage liver disease is a difficult task. The United States and Europe use prioritization systems based on waiting time and on the parameters of the Child-Turcotte-Pugh (CTP) score. However, these systems put too much emphasis on waiting time as a prioritization criterion. The transplant community, as well as the patient population, felt that there was a lack of objective criteria to quantify the severity or progression of liver disease. Indeed, the CTP score was never prospectively validated as an accurate predictor of mortality for patients on the transplant waiting list.[1] Also, it includes 2 subjective variables—ascites and encephalopathy—and does not discriminate between patients with progressively altered laboratory values.

History of the Model for End-Stage Liver Disease

Over time, increasing evidence suggested that a prioritization system should allocate organs based on the need for a transplant, rather than on the waiting time. In 1999, a Liver Disease Severity Score (LDSS) Committee was formed within the Organ Procurement and Transplantation Network (OPTN), an institution administered by the United Network for Organ Sharing (UNOS). This committee was assigned the task to define a model that would accurately predict mortality on the waiting list. The Model for End-Stage Liver Disease (MELD) has been proposed as an objective quantification method. This score had been previously validated as a predictor of mortality among patients with end-stage liver disease undergoing transjugular intrahepatic portosystemic shunt (TIPS) procedures.[2] In the pediatric population, however, the MELD score was not found to be an accurate predictor of mortality. Accordingly, the Pediatric End-Stage Liver Disease (PELD) score has been developed, replacing the creatinine value with albumin, and incorporating variables for age and growth failure in the calculation. After defining transition policies to assure that the implementation of the new allocation system did not affect patients already on the waiting list, the new policy took effect starting February 27, 2002.

What Is MELD?

The MELD score was first reported in 2000[3] to be a predictor of mortality risk among patients undergoing TIPS. It is an equation using 3 clinical laboratory measurements that were observed to have statistical impact on patient mortality risk. The MELD score is currently considered to be the most accurate predictor of 90-day mortality risk for patients on the liver transplant waiting list. Before being validated and introduced in practice, the score was found to accurately predict mortality in

1 R. B. Freeman, et al., "The New Liver Allocation System: Moving Toward Evidence-Based Transplantation Policy," *Liver Transplantation* 8, no. 9 (2002): pp. 851–858.

2 Ibid.

3 M. Malinchoc, et al., "A Model to Predict Poor Survival in Patients Undergoing Transjugular Intrahepatic Portosystemic Shunts," *Hepatology* 31, no. 4 (2000): pp. 864–871.

several cohorts of patients with various disease etiologies.[4,5,6]

UNOS Territory

UNOS is a private, nonprofit organization that was contracted by the US Government to regulate and manage the organ allocation system in the United States. The territory of the United States is divided into 11 UNOS regions. Within each region, there are several Organ Procurement Agencies (OPO). Each OPO serves several transplant centers within their territory. The OPO centralizes the patients from the waiting lists of all centers within its territory and grants them priority by MELD score, so that available organs will first be allocated to the patients in descending order of MELD score within each specific OPO. Organ prioritization is denominated as "local" (within the OPO), "regional" (within a UNOS region), and "national."

How Does the Allocation System Work?

Patients are prioritized on the waiting list within each blood type group by descending MELD score. This implies that the organs are basically allocated to the waitlisted patients with the highest mortality risk at the given time. Within each MELD score, livers are first allocated to blood type-identical patients. To prevent inequitable distribution of organs, blood type O livers may only be attributed to blood type O recipients. The system allows patients with special situations (like very small size adult patients or AB type patients) to be listed for more than one blood type and thus be granted a higher chance of receiving a transplant. MELD scores have to be updated periodically (every 7 days for Status 1 patients and patients with MELD higher than 25).

The UNOS algorithm for liver allocation is shown in Table [6.5]. The organ allocation is first directed to local recipients (listed at centers within the OPO). Should there be no adequate recipient within the OPO, the offer is directed regionally and, ultimately, nationally. The impact of this policy is that cold ischemia time is reduced by shipping the organs within a limited territory. By reducing the cold ischemia time, and thus improving the quality of the transplanted organs, and by lowering the logistical and transportation expenses, the global costs of the procedure are also reduced.

Attributing organs to regional patients with MELD higher than 15 before local patients with lower MELD is a measure that attempts to

Table [6.5]
Adult Donor Liver Allocation Policy

1. Local Status 1 patients in descending point order
2. Regional Status 1 patients in descending point order
3. Local patients with 3 MELD/PELD Scores ≥15 in descending order of mortality risk scores (probability of candidate death)
4. Regional patients with MELD/PELD Scores ≥15 in descending order of mortality risk scores (probability of candidate death)
5. Local patients with MELD/PELD Scores <15 in descending order of mortality risk scores (probability of candidate death)
6. Regional patients with MELD/PELD Scores <15 in descending order of mortality risk scores (probability of candidate death)
7. National Status 1 patients in descending point order

Source: www.unos.org.

[4] R. H. Wiesner, et al., "MELD and PELD: Application of Survival Models to Liver Allocation," *Liver Transplantation* 7, no. 7 (2001): pp. 567–580.

[5] J. A. Hanley and B. J. McNeil, "The Meaning and Use of the Area under a Receiver Operating Characteristic (Roc) Curve," *Radiology* 143, no. 1 (1982): pp. 29–36.

[6] P. S. Kamath, et al., "A Model to Predict Survival in Patients with End-Stage Liver Disease," *Hepatology* 33, no. 2 (2001): pp. 464–470.

remove the inequity of sicker patients waiting longer, while patients with questionable transplant benefit are transplanted.

Even so, differences and inequalities between regions and between OPOs cannot be totally removed. The number, experience, and volume of transplant centers within OPOs, as well as the experience and efficacy of the OPOs themselves, differ within large ranges, resulting in differences of average transplantation MELD scores among OPOs and among regions. Schaffer et al,[7] in a study involving 1 UNOS region with 3 OPOs, mentioned that within OPOs with competing transplant centers, patients received transplants at significantly higher MELD scores and using more MELD exceptions than within OPOs with single-center domination.

Adult Status 1 patients may also be allocated pediatric livers; however, pediatric Status 1 patients have priority. By definition, adult Status 1 patients are those patients who fulfill 1 of the following criteria: (1) fulminant hepatic failure, with a life expectancy less than 7 days without a liver transplant; (2) primary nonfunction (PNF) of a transplanted liver within 7 days of implantation; (3) hepatic artery thrombosis (HAT) in a transplanted liver within 7 days of implantation; or (4) acute decompensated Wilson's disease.

Too Healthy Versus Too Sick

One of the problems that has been raised is the balance between allocating the organs to the sickest patients (with the drawback of poorer post-transplantation outcome) versus allocating them to patients who would benefit most from transplantation by having the best survival rates. The interest of a liver transplant candidate is best served when the expected survival is higher than that without transplantation. It has been shown that among patients with MELD scores under 15, the mortality risk with transplantation is higher than the mortality risk without transplantation.[8,9] There is, however, a certain death rate on the waiting list among these patients: 53 deaths per 1000 patient years. There are also isolated patients with low MELD scores who have significant complications of end-stage liver disease: 17% of transplantations in the period from February 2002 to August 2003 occurred in patients with MELD scores under 15.[10]

Imposing a minimal transplant score has been a widely debated topic. By applying this policy, organs would be directed toward patients with higher MELD scores; also, transplantation with low MELD scores and thus less benefit from the operation would be avoided. Recent UNOS policies have required a minimal transplant score of 15. Exceptions can be granted in selected cases (eg, for AB blood type or direct donation).

At the other end of the disease spectrum, there are patients who are too sick to withstand liver transplantation. Allocating organs to these patients may not benefit them and may also be a waste of valuable organ resources. To limit this, 2 measures have been implemented. The creatinine value has been capped at 4 mg/dL. For patients with values above 4 mg/dL, as well as those undergoing hemodialysis, this maximal value is used in the calculation, and thus, their MELD score cannot further be increased. Also, 40 is the maximal score that can be attributed to a patient; patients with MELD scores higher than 40, while not receiving any extra priority, can still be transplanted if deemed reasonable by the transplant center.

[7] R. L. Schaffer, et al., "The Sickest First? Disparities with Model for End-Stage Liver Disease—Based Organ Allocation: One Region's Experience," *Liver Transplantation* 9, no. 11 (2003): pp. 1211–1215.

[8] R. M. Merion, et al., "The Survival Benefit of Liver Transplantation," *American Journal of Transplantation* 5, no. 2 (2005): pp. 307–313.

[9] D. W. Hanto, et al., "Liver and Intestine Transplantation: Summary Analysis, 1994-2003," *American Journal of Transplantation* 5, no. 4 (2005): pp. 916–933.

[10] K. M. Olthoff, et al., "Summary Report of a National Conference: Evolving Concepts in Liver Allocation in the MELD and PELD Era," *Liver Transplantation* 10, no. S10 (2004): pp. A6-A22.

MELD Exceptions

It is recognized that there are categories of patients whose MELD scores do not reflect the true urgency of their need for transplantation. Several categories of patients qualify under current regulations for various degrees of upgrading of their MELD scores to values that would allow them to undergo transplantation within a predictable time frame. Examples of exceptions include patients with hepatocellular carcinoma (HCC); biliary strictures; recurrent biliary sepsis; refractory upper gastrointestinal and variceal bleeding requiring transfusions and/or Blakemore tube insertion; refractory ascites and/or pleural effusions when TIPS is contraindicated; hepatopulmonary syndrome; metabolic diseases; severe polycystic liver disease; and pulmonary hypertension.

Transplantation of Patients with HCC [Hepatocellular Carcinoma]

Prioritization of patients with hepatocellular cancer—liver cancer—is one of the most debated topics. Under the previous organ allocation system, Yao et al[11] found a 25% yearly dropout rate from the waiting list due to progressive disease. Still, Putting these patients at advantage may diminish the chances of otherwise sicker candidates to receive an organ in time. Currently, T2 tumors (namely, 1 nodule 2.0 to 5.0 cm: 2 or 3 nodules, all <3.0 cm as defined by the American Liver Tumor Study Group Modified Tumor-Node-Metastasis Staging Classification) are allocated 24 MELD points. Considering that T1 patients are at a relatively low risk of being removed from the list because of tumor progression, since April 2004, T1 patients do not receive extra MELD points.[12] Based on data reporting good outcomes among patients transplanted with tumors larger than 5 cm,[13] the review boards can accept well-documented lesions beyond T2 criteria to be granted 24 MELD points.

MELD and Retransplantation

Retransplanted patients tend to have a poorer outcome than patients undergoing a first liver transplantation. Data reported by Edwards and Harper in a study based on OPTN data[14] showed that the MELD scores of retransplanted patients were higher than those of first-transplant patients. Also, in patients with MELD scores higher than 20, the relative risk of death on the waiting list was higher for relisted patients at similar MELD scores. Similar data were reported by other authors.[15] These patients seem to have a greater risk of dying than that reflected by the MELD score, and the accuracy of MELD as a predictor of waitlist mortality is thus somewhat lower in relisted patients.

Improving the Predictive Accuracy of the MELD Score

Several factors have been studied as potential elements to improve the estimation of

---

[11] F. Y. Yao, et al., "Liver Transplantation for Hepatocellular Carcinoma: Analysis of Survival According to the Intention-to-Treat Principle and Dropout from the Waiting List," *Liver Transplantation* 8, no. 10 (2002): pp. 873–883.

[12] P. Sharma, et al., "Liver Transplantation for Hepatocellular Carcinoma: The MELD Impact," *Liver Transplantation* 10, no. 1 (2004): pp. 36–41.

[13] F. Y. Yao, et al., "Liver Transplantation for Hepatocellular Carcinoma: Expansion of the Tumor Size Limits Does Not Adversely Impact Survival," *Hepatology* 33, no. 6 (2001): pp. 1394–1403.

[14] R. M. Merion, R. A. Wolfe and D. E. Schaubel, et al., "Final Analysis for SRTR Data Requests from the OPTN Liver Intestine Transplantation Committee Meeting of May 14-15, 2003."

[15] N. Onaca, et al., "An Outcome Comparison between Primary Liver Transplantation and Retransplantation Based on the Pretransplant MELD Score," *Transplant International* 19, no. 4 (2006): pp. 282–287.

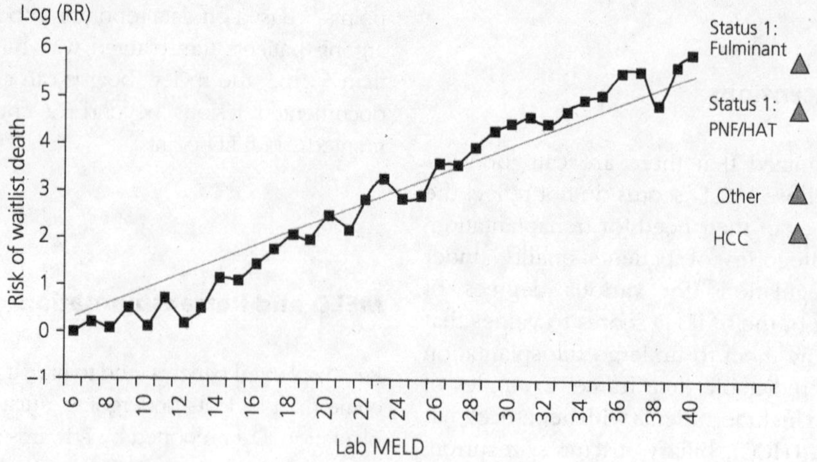

Figure [6.1] Correlation between MELD score and waitlist mortality.

Source: Olthoff et al,[16] with permission.

pre-transplantation mortality. There are data to suggest that the change in MELD or PELD scores over short periods may correlate with higher mortality risk on the waiting list.[17,18] Ascites, encephalopathy, and variceal bleeding do not add significant improvement to the statistical performance of MELD. Serum sodium seems to be a reliable surrogate for ascites. In one single-center study, hyponatremia correlated well with the presence of ascites and was a predictor of 3-month mortality.[19] Adding serum sodium to MELD may improve the predictive value of the score. Further data are needed to assess its practical value.

Transplant Statistics in the MELD Era

After the implementation of MELD as the basis of organ allocation, a large amount of statistical work has been done to follow the results of this change on organ distribution.

Correlation with Waitlist Mortality and Posttransplantation Outcome

Analyzing the correlation of the MELD score on patients listed within 1 year after the implementation of the new allocation system, a linear relationship was observed between MELD score and waitlist mortality (Figure [6.1]). While the MELD score was confirmed as an excellent predictor of waitlist mortality, its relationship with post-transplantation outcome was less consistent.

Still, there was a correlation between the pre-transplantation MELD score and patient survival after transplantation.[20] The 2004

---

16 Olthoff, "Summary Report of a National Conference."

17 R. M. Merion, et al., "Longitudinal Assessment of Mortality Risk among Candidates for Liver Transplantation," *Liver Transplantation* 9, no. 1 (2003): pp. 12–18.

18 "Report of the OPTN/UNOS Liver and Intestinal Organ Transplantation Committee to the Board of Directors," June 26–27, 2003.

19 A. D. Ruf, S. E. Yanrorno and V. I. Descalzi, et al., "Addition of Serum Sodium into the MELD Score Predicts Waiting List Mortality Better Than MELD Alone: A Single Center Experience," *American Journal of Transplantation* 4 (2004): p. 438.

20 Merion, "Final Analysis for SRTR Data Requests."

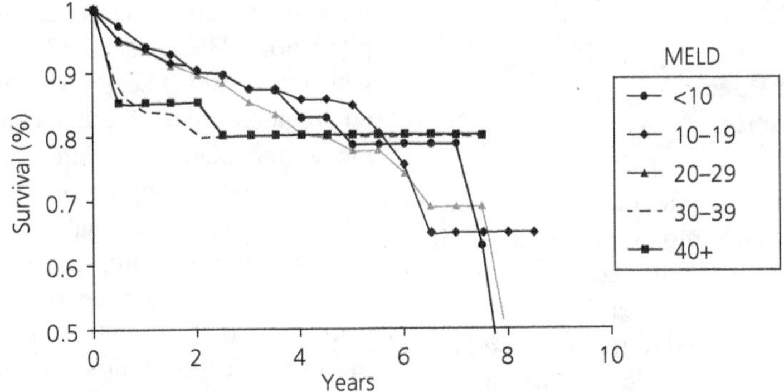

Figure [6.2] Correlation between MELD score and postoperative survival rate.

Source: Olthoff et al,[21] with permission.

OPTN/SRTR Annual Report showed slightly lower 3-month and 1-year survivals for patients with MELD >30.[22]

The same tendency was noted for graft survival. Olthoff et al[23] cited data from The Mayo Clinic (Rochester, Minn) showing that patients with MELD >30 displayed lower survival rates than those with lower MELD. This tendency was based on a steep decrease in survival in the first year, while at 5 years the survival curves for all MELD scores overlapped (Figure [6.2]). Graft survival decreased for patients with MELD >30, while it was fairly equal among patients with lower MELD.

Effects on the Waiting List

Before implementation of the current allocation system, the waiting time for a liver transplant grew constantly from an average of 225 days in 1994 to 1811 days in 1999. Adding patients early on to the transplant list based on the necessity to accrue waiting time, rather than on medical urgency, was one of the main reasons behind the continuous growth of the waiting lists. The new system drastically de-emphasizes the importance of waiting time and imposes minimal criteria for transplantation, leading to a significant reduction in overall waiting time.[24]

Between February 2002 and February 2003, there was a 12% reduction in waiting list registrations, especially among patients with low MELD scores, as an effect of a reduced urge to list patients to accrue waiting time. Thereafter the number of waitlisted patients has again been showing a slowly increasing trend.[25] Among the waitlisted patients in 2003, 96% had MELD scores ≤20 and 43% had MELD <10.[26]

However, after implementation of the new organ allocation policy, the death rate on the waiting list did not significantly decrease. In an analysis of the first "after-MELD" year, Freeman et al[1] found only a 4% (P = .076) decrease in waiting list mortality, possibly as a result of the listing dynamics, which balanced the *quicker transplantation* of sicker patients with an *increased listing* of sicker patients. This also meant a shifting of available organs toward patients in more need for a transplant.

[21] Ibid.

[22] "2004 Annual Report of the US Organ Procurement and Transplantation Network and the Scientific Registry of Transplant Recipients: Transplant Data 1994–2003," 2004.

[23] Olthoff, "Summary Report of a National Conference."

[24] Hanto, "Liver and Intestine Transplantation."

[25] "2005 Annual Report of the US Organ Procurement and Transplantation Network and the Scientific Registry of Transplant Recipients: Transplant Data 1994–2004," 2005.

[26] Hanto, "Liver and Intestine Transplantation."

Effects on the Rate of Transplantation

An overall increased rate of transplantation was observed after implementation of the new allocation policy, in the context of a better rate of usage of cadaveric donors. The response might be related to the increased use of marginal donors in an era when, through the MELD score, one can better assess the probability of a patient to tolerate a less optimal organ. The increased rate of transplanted livers after 2002 cannot simply be attributed to a steadily increasing trend of the transplantation rate. Other factors that need to be taken into account to explain this growth include the higher rate of organ donor referrals and consent to donation. These increased by almost 10% and 5%, respectively, from 2002 to 2003.[27]

Future Trends

Even if the new organ allocation policy is considered to be an improvement in comparison to the waiting time-based prioritization, it is still far from perfect.

There are still many areas of concern and many discrepancies. Inter- and intraregional differences in number and size of transplant centers, as well as in the efficiency of OPOs, make a difference in the patients' chances of receiving a transplant and in the average transplantation MELD scores.[28,29] Thus, patients with equal MELD scores but located in different regions have different chances of receiving a transplant and different waiting times. Intraregional sharing of organs is a feature of interest for a more equitable allocation.

Other areas of improvement are centered on the already mentioned concept of transplant benefit. The ultimate goal of organ allocation would be to allocate organs to patients who would have the best post-transplantation outcome, while at the same time reducing as much as possible the removal rate due to death or severity of sickness from the waiting list. MELD alone does not serve both these goals, and is especially vulnerable in the prediction of post-transplantation outcome. Improving this aspect would require adding donor- and center-dependent factors to the allocation algorithm but further data are necessary to sustain such a change. Future developments may also be directed toward attempting to match donor organs and recipients through an elaborate information network. Such attempts have already been made at the University of Birmingham.[30]

In conclusion, the MELD score has proved to be effective as a predictor of pretransplantation mortality. It is currently the most reliable criterion to select waitlisted patients for liver transplantation. The applicability of MELD exceptions adds versatility and flexibility to the allocation algorithm. As time passes, further efforts to monitor the weaknesses and the strengths of this promising system must be undertaken.

---

27 "2004 Annual Report of the US Organ Procurement and Transplantation Network."

28 Schaffer, "The Sickest First?"

29 "2004 Annual Report of the US Organ Procurement and Transplantation Network."

30 M. R. Lucey, "How Will Patients Be Selected for Transplantation in the Future?", *Liver Transplantation* 10, no. S10 (2004): pp. S90–S92.

EXCERPT 3

Full text from:

W. Saletan, "How Did Steve Jobs Get His Liver?", *Slate Magazine*, January 19, 2001.

How Did Steve Jobs Get His Liver?: Steve Jobs Used His Advantages to Get a Donated Liver. Should It Have Gone to Somebody Else?

William Saletan

What's wrong with Steve Jobs? Apple won't say. On Monday, the company said he was taking a medical leave—his third since 2004—but refused to disclose why. Yesterday Apple touted its market prospects in a conference call but again said nothing about its CEO's health. You can argue that Jobs' medical privacy is more important than the interests of Apple's investors. But there's another reason why he should tell us what's going on, and it's bigger than money. It's life and death.

Two years ago, Jobs gamed the transplant allocation system to get a liver that could have saved somebody else. At the time, skeptics doubted that he should have received the organ, since he'd been treated for pancreatic cancer—in fact, he may have sought the liver because of the cancer—and the likelihood of the cancer's recurrence made him a bad bet for putting the liver to best use. If his health is now failing because of the cancer, that suspicion may be vindicated.

Jobs lives in Northern California, but he got his liver in Tennessee. Why? Different parts of the country have different waiting lists, and the wait in Northern California was three times longer than the wait in Tennessee. In fact, the median wait in the Tennessee area where Jobs snagged his liver was around 15% of the national average. Jobs confirmed last year that this is why he went to Tennessee: "My doctors here advised me to enroll in a transplant program in Memphis, Tennessee, where the supply/demand ratio of livers is more favorable than it is in California here."* Legally, you're allowed to get on multiple waiting lists around the country. That's how you game the system.

So why doesn't everybody do this? Because they can't. First you have to show up for an extensive in-person evaluation. Then you have to be available for a transplant in the area within hours of an organ becoming available. And while one jurisdiction might accept you as a charity case, if you want to play the field you'll have to prove you can pay for the transplant yourself. You also get priority points for being able to guarantee follow-up medical care, since this assures transplant allocators that the organ will be well cared for. Ordinary people can't compete with billionaires at meeting these tests. They can't go to multiple states for evaluations. They don't have private jets. Their insurance doesn't cover multiple evaluations and may not cover much of the half-million dollar transplant, much less the follow-up care.

If Jobs was on multiple lists, he wasn't just multiplying his chances and shortening his projected wait. He was increasing the odds that one of the transplant centers where he was listed would give him a liver despite his cancer history. That's another way to game the system: criteria shopping. "Patients who are smart or who have savvy primary care doctors know that different transplant centers follow different rules in deciding who to admit," Arthur Caplan, an expert in the transplant allocation process, observed two years ago. "Some would view a liver transplant for a person with cancer as a 'waste' of an organ. Some might take a chance on a patient with cancer." Caplan called this a likely factor in the targeting of Tennessee: Jobs had to find a transplant center that would "take him despite his cancer." And, being a CEO, he succeeded.

Jobs never explained the reason for his transplant. But it's hard to believe it was unconnected to his cancer. One expert notes that the kind of cancer Jobs had in 2004 commonly spreads to another organ—the probability of metastasis is 75%—and that organ is usually the liver. Jobs' pre-transplant health problems—weight loss and hormone imbalance—also match the symptom list for a recurrence of his cancer. And doctors sometimes try a liver transplant when the cancer has migrated there.

It's a dubious strategy. Half the time, the cancer comes back. The patient, impaired by immunosuppressive drugs because of the transplant, is often more vulnerable to the cancer. At the time, the Wall Street Journal cited a surgeon's warning that attempting a liver transplant in such a scenario was "controversial because livers are scarce and the surgery's efficacy as a cure hasn't been proved." And Caplan pointed out that:

> "there were roughly 16,000 people on the national liver waiting list when Jobs got a liver. He was one of 1,581 people who got livers in the United States in the first quarter of [2009]. Almost none of those people had any form of cancer. In fact, if Jobs' tumor has spread from his pancreas into his liver as is likely, some transplant surgeons say that they would not recommend a liver transplant because there is no data that shows a transplant will stop or even slow the spread of the cancer. This raises the question: Is this the best use of a liver?"

Caplan posed that question a year and a half ago. Now Jobs is taking yet another unexplained medical leave. Given his symptoms, in the absence of further information, the most likely reason is recurrence or complications of his cancer. If that's the case, then Jobs, having gamed the system to obtain a liver that could have saved somebody else, might soon take that liver to his grave. And he's had it less than two years.

To his great credit, Jobs has used his influence to help others in his situation. As Nicholas Carlson reported in Business Insider, Jobs pressed last year for a new law in California that requires applicants for a driver's license to be asked whether they'd like to be organ donors.*

But now comes the new report of Jobs' illness, and with it, the unresolved question of whether he should have gotten that liver. We don't know what's ailing him, because he won't say. "My family and I would deeply appreciate respect for our privacy," he pleads.

I hear you, Steve. We're all pulling for you. It's your life and your family. But that liver wasn't yours. Somebody died to make it available. And other people who aren't billionaires may have died on waiting lists so you could have it. What was your cancer situation when you got the transplant? Has the cancer returned? You owe us some answers.

* I originally wrote that Jobs "never explained why" he went to Tennessee. But after the article was posted, I found Nicholas Carlson's Business Insider story, which quoted Jobs' comments on this subject at a press conference last year. In these remarks, Jobs confirmed that he went to Tennessee for an easier waiting list. More important, Jobs attended the press conference to promote the California organ-donor legislation, and Carlson detailed Jobs' role in lobbying for the bill. I've added a paragraph to note this contribution by Jobs. It doesn't erase the questions of inequity and judgment in Jobs' transplant, but it does attest to his character.

EXCERPT 4

Full text from:

G. Kolata, "Transplants, Morality and Mickey," *New York Times*, June 11, 1995.

The Nation: Transplants, Morality and Mickey

Gina Kolata

A moralist might be tempted to say that to a large extent Mickey Mantle brought his liver problems upon himself. Granted, his liver cancer probably resulted from the hepatitis C infection he acquired from a blood transfusion years ago. But Mr. Mantle also had been an alcoholic for years and developed alcoholic cirrhosis, which greatly accelerates the course of the virus-initiated cancer. If Mr. Mantle had abstained, the cancer might never have occurred or not have materialized for decades.

So why are Mr. Mantle's doctors so eager to give a precious organ to someone who actively contributed to his disease? Why does any doctor give a liver to an alcoholic, when thousands of other, more temperate people languish on the waiting list or are never listed? The case of Mickey Mantle raises a troubling question about medical desserts: Should alcoholics with liver failure, smokers with lung cancer and obese people with heart disease receive the same treatment as people who have lived lives of moderation?

Doctors and ethicists agonize over this question and have come to very different conclusions. Some argue that it should make no difference how a person became ill; a few go so far as to say that they will even transplant livers to current alcoholics as well as to those with alcoholic cirrhosis.

On the other side are health-care professionals who say that patients whose livers fail through no fault of their own should be given preference over alcoholics.

Yet the most common reason for liver transplant is alcoholic cirrhosis, and nearly 18% of such transplants go to these victims of alcoholism, said Joel Newman, a spokesman for United Network for Organ Sharing, a national group in Richmond, Va., that allocates organs. Hepatitis C is next, followed by biliary atresia, a congenital malformation of the organ; liver cancer is way down on the list.

A national survey in the late 1980's by Dr. James Levenson, professor of psychiatry, medicine and surgery at the Medical College of Virginia, showed that individual transplant policies vary widely for people with alcoholic cirrhosis. While about 80% of them said heavy drinking argues against transplantation, 6.5% said that it was irrelevant to decision-making. Nationwide 117 hospital programs transplant livers.

Dr. Arthur Caplan, director of the Center for Bioethics at the University of Pennsylvania, said that at first glance a transplant to current or former alcoholics appears outrageous. "Spending $300,000 for a liver transplant for somebody who brought harm upon himself is not a prudent use of scarce money and scarce livers," Dr. Caplan said.

"If society wants to pass laws saying no transplants for alcoholics, no transplants for felons or for smokers or for people who drive too fast, then it should," he said. But society, he said, "should not dump the issue of what to do about sin on those who work at the bedside; they're not equipped to make judgments and it violates their professional ethics."

In the transplant program at the University of Chicago School of Medicine, heavy drinkers must demonstrate that they have been alcohol free for six months before they can be placed on a waiting list. The director of the program, Dr. Richard Thistlethwaite, agrees that doctors should not have to decide who deserves a new liver.

I think it's very difficult for physicians to make moral judgments about their patients," Dr. Thistlethwaite said. "There are a lot of traps we could fall into if we start to allocate medical therapies according to if we thought the patient was good or bad or had laudable or deplorable habits."

Dr. Thistlethwaite's colleague, Dr. Mark Siegler, who directs the University of Chicago's clinical ethics program, says all alcoholics should go to the bottom of the transplant list. Because there is a "dire scarcity" of livers, he says, it is justifiable and reasonable to give them first to people whose life styles did not contribute to their disease. "It's not so much blaming people for their disease," he said, "as saying that some are more blameless than others."

Yet Dr. Siegler said he would exempt Mickey Mantle from his rule because the baseball legend is "a real American hero." He said Mr. Mantle, "who captures the imagination of a generation through his skill and ability and personality," should not be lumped in with the rest of the population and perhaps denied a liver so that a more blameless person can live.

"I think we have to give deference to the rare heroes in American life," he added. "We don't have enough of these people in America, and when one comes along, we have got to take them with all their warts and failures and treat them differently."

EXCERPT 5

Full text from:

S. G. Stolberg and L. K. Altman, "An Ethical Dilemma with Few Precedents," *New York Times*, February 21, 2003.

An Ethical Dilemma with Few Precedents

Sheryl Gay Stolberg and Lawrence K. Altman

With the nation facing a dire shortage of human organs, the case of Jésica Santillán renews long-simmering questions in medical ethics: Should surgeons perform second transplants on patients like Ms. Santillán, whose chances of survival are diminished because they have rejected their first organs? Or should others on the waiting list come first?

In the case of Ms. Santillán, the 17-year-old patient at Duke University Hospital who was mistakenly given a heart and lungs that did not match her blood type, the debate is especially poignant. That is because her body rejected the organs because of a medical mistake that her doctors, who gave her a second heart and lungs on Thursday, are furiously trying to correct.

"This is a horrible moral tension," said Arthur Caplan, a professor of bioethics at the University of Pennsylvania who has written extensively about transplant ethics. "Doctors feel an obligation to their patient in any transplant situation. They feel a special obligation when they made a mistake that is causing the death of this patient. Now they are trying to rescue her. This makes perfect sense, but it isn't necessarily the best national policy."

Dr. Caplan argued that if there were another patient waiting whose situation was as dire as Ms. Santillán's, that person had a higher claim to the organs, because statistics show that a second transplant is generally less successful than the first. But others disagreed, saying Ms. Santillán was, in effect, denied her first chance.

"I'd argue she never got the first transplant," said Dr. Joseph J. Fins, an internist and the director of medical ethics at New York Hospital-Cornell Medical Center.

The data on the success of repeat heart-lung transplants is scant, in part because such transplants are extremely rare. According to the United Network for Organ Sharing, an organization based in Richmond, Va., that coordinates organ donations, 793 heart-lung transplants were performed in the United States from January 1988 to Nov. 30, 2002.

Of these, 10 were second transplants. Anne Paschke, the network's spokeswoman, said she did not have statistics on their success.

Ms. Santillán's chances for survival in the next few weeks are about 50-50 at best, experts say. If she does survive, there is about an 80% chance she will have serious medical problems in the future, they said.

But whether there are any other heart-lung transplant patients as close to death as Ms. Santillán is impossible to know; officials at the organ network would not discuss the status of others on the waiting list. That made it hard for medical ethicists to assess whether the second transplant was the best course.

"The devil is in the details here about who didn't get the organ," said Dr. Stuart Youngner, chairman of the department of bioethics at Case Western Reserve University in Cleveland. "Is there a real person? Were they just as sick and going to die? Were their chances much better of doing well than hers?"

Yet even if there were such a person, some said it only seemed fair that Ms. Santillán had been given a second chance. R. Alta Charo, a professor of law and medical ethics at the University of Wisconsin, said she had not formulated a careful, academic opinion about the ethics of Ms. Santillán's second transplant. Still, Professor Charo said, something in her gut told her it was the right thing to do.

"I think there is something phenomenally cruel about the raising of expectations and then the dashing of them this way that gives her a greater entitlement as an individual, even over others who have never had their first shot," Professor Charo said.

Within the transplant community, there is intense debate about even performing heart-lung transplants. One reason they have become so rare over the past decade is that lung transplants are increasingly successful, as are heart transplants, and there is less need to combine them.

Though there are some people like Ms. Santillán who could not survive without a double transplant, such an operation involves organs that could have gone to a total of three people, instead of one, experts say. If the transplant is performed twice, as in Ms. Santillán's case, six organs will have gone to a single patient.

"The real challenge here from an ethical perspective is the realization that you're taking a perfectly good heart and taking a chance now in a very, very high-risk recipient," said Dr. Mehmet Oz, a heart transplant surgeon at New York Presbyterian-Columbia Presbyterian Medical Center in Manhattan. "I understand why they're doing it, and I would probably do the same, but you are gambling with a very scarce resource."

Many transplant surgeons say they would have done the same, despite the ethical hand-wringing and calculations—however imprecise—of survival and success rates.

In the end, said Dr. Kenneth McCurry, director of lung and heart transplantation at the University of Pittsburgh, the decision to give another heart and lungs to Ms. Santillán probably came down to this: "She is a 17-year-old girl who no one wants to see die."

Further Resources

Relevant Organizations

Nongovernmental

United Network for Organ Sharing (UNOS): A private, nonprofit organization that manages the United States organ transplant system under contract with the federal government. Additional information can be found at www.unos.org

American Society of Transplantation (AST): A nonprofit organization of professionals dedicated to advancing the field of transplantation and improving patient care by promoting research, education, advocacy, and organ donation. Additional information can be found at https://www.myast.org/

The Center for the Evaluation of Value and Risk in Health (CEVR): Located within Tufts Medical Center, Boston, a non-profit hospital, analyzes the benefits, risks, and costs of strategies to improve health and healthcare. Additional information can be found at research.tufts-nemc.org/cear4/

The Transplantation Society: A nonprofit organization which serves as an international forum for the worldwide advancement of organ transplantation. Additional information can be found at https://www.tts.org/

Literature

Glassman, Amanda. "Who Gets a New Kidney? Healthier People Could have Priority" *The Atlantic*, March 11, 2011.

Kolata, Gina. "Getting on a Transplant List Is the First of Many Hurdles," *New York Times*, June 10, 1995. http://www.nytimes.com/1995/06/10/sports/getting-on-a-transplant-list-is-the-first-of-many-hurdles.html?pagewanted=all.

National Health Service. "[Organ Donation] Legislative Framework." http://www.odt.nhs.uk/donation/deceased-donation/consent-authorisation/legislative-framework.as.

Oliver, Michael, Alexander Woywodt, Aimun Ahmed, and Imran Saif. "Organ Donation, Transplantation and Religion." *Nephrology Dialysis Transplantation* (October 20, 2010).

Orandi, Babak J., Xun Luo, Allan B. Massie, Jacqueline M. Garonzik-Wang, Bonne E. Lonze, Rizwan Ahmed, Kyle J. Van Arendonk, et al. "Survival Benefit with Kidney Transplants from Hla-Incompatible Live Donors." *New England Journal of Medicine* 374, no. 10 (2016): 940–950.

Rudge, C., R. Matesanz, F. L. Delmonico, and J. Chapman. "International Practices of Organ Donation." *British Journal of Anaesthesia* 108, no. suppl 1 (January 1, 2012): i48–i55.

US Army, Army Medical Department Center and School, US Army Health Readiness Center. "Clinical Practice Guidelines: Mass Casualty and Triage." http://www.cs.amedd.army.mil/FileDownloadpublic.aspx?docid=68aca9a0- 9cd7-4d8f-a17f-a4c01264daef.

University of California, San Francisco, Department of Surgery. "Alcoholic Liver Disease (ALD)." http://www.transplant.surgery.ucsf.edu/conditions-- procedures/alcoholic-liver-disease.aspx.

US Department of Health & Human Services. "Organ Procurement Organizations." http://www.organdonor.gov/materialsresources/materialsopolist.html.

US Department of Health & Human Services. "Proposal to Address the Requirements Outlined in the HIV Organ Policy Equity Act." https://optn.transplant.hrsa.gov/media/1147/0115_04_opo_hope_act.pdf.

United Network for Organ Sharing. "Questions and Answers for Patients and Families About the Regional Review Board Process." https://www.unos.org/wp- content/uploads/unos/RRB_Public_FAQ.pdf.

Yasinski, Emma. "When Donated Organs Go to Waste." *The Atlantic, February 24*, 2016.

Other Media

Ejiofor, Chiwetel. *Dirty Pretty Things*. DVD. Directed by Stephen Frears. Santa Mona: Miramax, 2004: A hotel manager runs an operation where immigrants exchange kidneys for forged passports.

Hanks, Tom. *Cast Away*. DVD. Directed by Robert Zemeckis. Los Angeles: 20th Century Fox, 2002: The main character, while stranded on an island by himself, must find a way to survive off scarce resources.

7

Vaccine Allocations in Emergencies

Every year, a seasonal flu typically spreads through the world in the fall and winter. In seasonal flu, the influenza virus undergoes a small change. But a pandemic occurs when the influenza virus undergoes a significant transformation—technically called *antigenic shift*. This most commonly occurs when genes from birds, pigs, or humans combine into a new virus strain that most people have not encountered and lack antibodies to fight.[1] Such pandemic-producing antigenic shifts have occurred at intervals between 10 and 50 years dating back to the 16th century.[2] In the 20th century, there were three pandemics: the great pandemic of 1918, and two smaller ones in 1957 and 1968.

The 1918 pandemic, also known as the Spanish flu, was caused by an H1N1 influenza virus and is estimated to have killed at least 50 million and as many as 100 million people worldwide.[3] While we will never know for sure, the pandemic probably originated in a small Kansas town and spread to Camp Funston, now Fort Riley in Kansas, in the early spring of 1918. American soldiers being deployed in World War I then brought the virus to other army bases in the eastern United States and eventually to France. With the end of the war in November 1918, returning soldiers of all nationalities brought the virus to their home countries, and displaced refugees brought it to their homes.[4] The most deadly months were the fall of 1918 and the early part of 1919.[5]

---

[1] United States Department of Health and Human Services, *HHS Pandemic Influenza Plan* (Washington DC: US Government Printing Office, 2005), B4–B5.

[2] World Health Organization, *Pandemic Influenza Risk Management: WHO Interim Guidance* (2013), p. 19.

[3] J. Taubenberger and D. Morens, "1918 Influenza: The Mother of All Pandemics," *Emerging Infectious Disease journal* 12, no. 1 (2006): pp. 15–22.

[4] J. M. Barry, "The Site of Origin of the 1918 Influenza Pandemic and Its Public Health Implications," *Journal of Translational Medicine* 2 (2004): p. 3.

[5] Taubenberger, "1918 Influenza: The Mother of All Pandemics," p. 17.

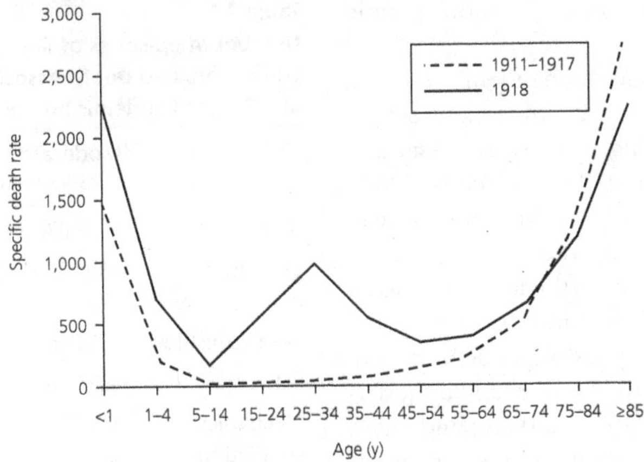

Figure 7.1 U- and W-shaped combined influenza and pneumonia mortality, by age at death, per 100,000 persons in each age group, United States, 1911–1918.[6]
Source: Emerging Infectious Diseases

This pandemic was remarkable for a number of reasons. First, it had a high case-fatality rate of 2.5%, meaning that 2.5 people died of every 100 people infected. The normal case-fatality rate for seasonal flu is about 0.1% or 1 death per 1,000 people infected.[7] More importantly, while seasonal flu is typically most threatening to older people and infants, the 1918 influenza virus killed young adults. What many commentators noticed was that, one day soldiers and other 20-year-olds were in fine health and literally in the next day or two they were dead.[8] The felling of those at the peak of physical fitness was shocking. This created a new epidemiology of influenza, the W-shaped curve (Figure 7.1). Similarly, the number of people in a community who were afflicted was high. It was not that one or two members of the community got the flu, but hundreds at the same time were laid low.

It is estimated that 28% of all Americans were infected with influenza and that at least 500,000 died during the 1918 pandemic.[9] This is much more than the 116,000 American soldiers killed in World War I and even more than the 405,000 American soldiers killed in World War II. So many people, and especially young people, died in the United States that the average life expectancy between 1917–18 declined by 11.8 years.[10]

By comparison, the pandemics of 1957 and 1968 were far less severe. The 1957 pandemic was caused by the H2N2 virus and killed between 1 and 4 million people worldwide.[11] The 1968 pandemic was caused by the H3N2 virus. It originated in Hong Kong and came to the United States with returning Vietnam soldiers.[12]

---

6 Taubenberger, "1918 Influenza: The Mother of All Pandemics," p. 19.

7 Ibid., p. 15.

8 J. K. Taubenberger and D. M. Morens, "The Pathology of Influenza Virus Infections," *Annual review of pathology* 3 (2008): p. 510.

9 A. W. Crosby, *America's Forgotten Pandemic: The Influenza of 1918* (Cambridge: Cambridge University Press, 2003), pp. 205–206.

10 E. Arias, "United States Life Tables, 2009," *National Vital Statistics Reports, HHS* 62, no. 2 (2014): p.46.

11 World Health Organization, *Pandemic Influenza Risk Management: WHO Interim Guidance* (2013), p. 19.

12 K. Rogers, *Infectious Diseases* (The Rosen Publishing Group, 2011), p. 121.

It killed between 1 and 4 million people worldwide.[13]

With the last influenza pandemic in 1968 and with growing concern over new strains of influenza developing in southeast Asia and China during the late 1990s and early 2000s, the US Department of Health and Human Services (HHS) began a process of pandemic preparations. It began by estimating the impact of an influenza pandemic and delineating the best responses.[14] Two types of pandemics were modeled, a severe 1918-like one, and a moderate one more like the 1957 or 1968 pandemics. On the latter scenario, 90 million Americans—between 25% and 35% of the population—would be infected by influenza, with children having the highest rates of infection. About half of those infected—45 million—would go to the doctor's office for healthcare (Table 7.1). About 865,000 Americans would be hospitalized, with 65,000 requiring ventilators and more than 200,000 people dying. In the severe, 1918-like scenario, 9.9 million people would be hospitalized, nearly 1.5 million would require ICU care, and about 750,000 would need ventilators. In the end, nearly 2 million Americans would die. Both types of pandemic would create serious strains on the healthcare system. For instance, there are fewer than 1 million ICU beds in the country and just 62,000 ventilators.[15,16]

Similarly, the DHHS estimated that there would be inadequate supplies of vaccine for the nation. In 2005, it estimated that using all production facilities, after a delay of approximately 3–6 months necessary to develop the vaccine, the US could produce 3–5 million doses per week.[18]

Table 7.1
Number of Episodes of Illness, Healthcare Utilization, and Death Associated with Moderate and Severe Pandemic Influenza Scenarios[a17]

	Moderate (1958/68-like)	Severe (1918-like)
Illness	90 million (30%)	90 million (30%)
Outpatient medical care	45 million (50%)	45 million (50%)
Hospitalization	865,000	9,900,000
ICU care	128,750	1,485,000
Mechanical ventilation	64,875	742,500
Deaths	209,000	1,903,000

[a]Estimates based on extrapolation from past pandemics in the United States. Note that these estimates do not include the potential impact of interventions not available during the 20th-century pandemics.
Source: United States Department of Health and Human Services

Absolute scarcity in the case of an influenza pandemic is obvious: demand for both vaccines and other health services would outstrip supply across countries and individual communities. To address the shortages, the DHHS developed detailed plans for the rationing of influenza vaccine during a pandemic. The initial 2005 proposal for allocating vaccines (Excerpt 1) was based on the principles that "the primary goal of a pandemic response considered was to decrease health impacts including severe morbidity and death; secondary pandemic response goals included minimizing societal and economic impacts."[19] Invoking these two principles, the top priority in the case of an epidemic was to vaccinate personnel at vaccine and antiviral manufacturers and medical workers in direct patient

[13] World Health Organization, *Pandemic Influenza Risk Management,* p. 19.

[14] HHS, *HHS Pandemic Influenza Plan,* pp. 18–21.

[15] N. A. Halpern and S. M. Pastores, "Critical Care Medicine in the United States 2000–2005: An Analysis of Bed Numbers, Occupancy Rates, Payer Mix, and Costs," *Critical Care Medicine* 38, no. 1 (2010): pp. 65–71.

[16] L. Rubinson, et al., "Mechanical Ventilators in US Acute Care Hospitals," *Disaster Med Public Health Prep* 4, no. 3 (2010): pp. 199–206.

[17] United States Department of Health and Human Services, *HHS Pandemic Influenza Plan*, p. 18.

[18] HHS, HHS Pandemic Influenza Plan, p. D-12.

[19] Ibid., p. D-10.

contact. The second group to receive priority were Americans over 65 years of age with one or more high-risk conditions, such as emphysema or diabetes, that increased their risk of dying from influenza, as well as Americans between 6 months and 64 years of age with two or more conditions that increase risks of morbidity or mortality from influenza. Healthy Americans aged 2–64 years of age were given the absolute lowest priority, even lower than funeral directors and embalmers.

After this priority list was disseminated, two events occurred to cause the Department to reconsider its initial prioritization scheme. First, Emanuel and Wertheimer criticized the priorities and ethical values used to justify them (Excerpt 2).[20] Second, the Department engaged in a public outreach "to engage the public and obtain a broader perspective into decisions on priority groups for pandemic vaccine."[21]

Emanuel and Wertheimer argued that minimizing mortality, or "save the most lives," should not be the primary value guiding rationing decisions in a pandemic. Instead, they developed the idea that "each person should have an opportunity to live through all stages of life."[22] This means we should prioritize younger people who could live through all stages of life rather than older people. They argued that almost all of us accept this principle for our own lives—we would rather ensure that we can live to an old age than being struck down in youth or adding more years to our old age. They also emphasized that priority should be given to people in early adolescence rather than younger children because of the investment the young adults have and because they "have more developed interests, hopes, and plans but have not had an opportunity to realize them."[23]

Similarly, when it engaged the public, the DHHS discovered that most people believe that younger patients should be prioritized over older patients. Summarizing the findings, the Department reported that the public thought there was "no single, overriding objective for pandemic vaccination."[24] The public meetings came to the same conclusion, showing also that an important policy objective would be to protect personnel responding to the pandemic, as well as children.

The public response led the Departments of Health and Human Services and Homeland Security in 2008 to issue a new "Guidance on Allocating and Targeting Pandemic Influenza Vaccine" that proposed a new vaccine prioritization scheme with five tiers (Excerpt 3).[25] As in 2005, vaccine production workers and healthcare personnel were granted top priority because they would save others' lives. In the 2008 revision, however, the second tier involved military and other personnel to keep essential services, such as utilities and telecommunications, operating. The third tier encompassed healthy children and teenagers aged 3–18. Older Americans were placed in the fourth tier, while healthy adults were in the final tier.

In 2009, the Centers for Disease Control and Prevention (CDC) issued guidelines about the allocation of ventilators in a severe influenza pandemic (Excerpt 4).[26] As the CDC acknowledged, historically, the principle for allocating ventilators has been to minimize death and hospitalizations. The CDC reviewed a number of principles including sickest first; first-come, first-served; patients most likely to recover; and maximizing lives saved. This

[20] E. Emanuel and A. Wertheimer, "Who Should Get Influenza Vaccine When Not All Can?", *Science* 312, no. 5775 (2006): pp. 854–855.

[21] HHS, HHS Pandemic Influenza Plan, p. D-10.

[22] Ibid.

[23] Emanuel, "Who Should Get Influenza Vaccine," pp. 854–855.

[24] United States Department of Health and Human Services, *Guidance on Allocating and Targeting Pandemic Influenza Vaccine* (Washington, DC: US Government Printing Office, 2008), pp. 2–3.

[25] HHS, *Guidance on Allocation and Targeting,* pp. 2–6.

[26] Ventilator Document Workgroup for the Ethics Subcommittee of the Advisory Committee to the Director, *Ethical Considerations for Decision Making Regarding Allocation of Mechanical Ventilators During a Severe Influenza Pandemic or Other Public Health Emergency* (Centers for Disease Control and Prevention, 2009).

report emphasized that the primary principle during a pandemic should be "preserving the functioning of society" but that while this principle applies to vaccines it "is not as relevant to decision making about distribution of ventilators." The main reason for this conclusion was that those who require ventilator support are not likely to "bounce back" but have a "prolonged recovery," requiring weeks of rehabilitation and producing a long-term reduction in quality of life. In the end, after surveying a number of principles, the report did not endorse a particular criterion, and instead noted that "it will be important to have a broad public deliberation about the various tradeoffs among the principles."

Questions for Discussion

1. When it comes to accessing vaccines and ventilators in a pandemic, who should decide and why?
   a. White House
   b. CDC
   c. Other federal agency
   d. State health department
   e. Local health department
   f. Doctors and nurses
2. Given the difficulties with adjudicating between different principles, would a lottery in which everyone in need would have a fair chance be an appropriate way of allocating vaccines at the peak of a pandemic?
3. The CDC held public meetings to elicit values from the general population to inform the framework for allocating vaccine during an influenza pandemic. In what way is this approach helpful? In what way might it cause problems?
4. What are the driving principles behind the 2005 HHS policy, shown in Excerpt 1?
5. What are the driving principles behind the 2008 HHS policy revision (Excerpt 3)?
6. The findings from the public debate had significant impact on the 2008 policy revisions of Excerpt 3. The ethical issues are deep and complex. How would you have structured public debate about what the right policy is? Would you simply poll people based on the knowledge and attitudes they have at the time? Should participants be given basic information on ethical principles, values, and frameworks?

EXCERPTS

Note: The following excerpts have generally been edited for length, and omissions are indicated with ellipses. Editing includes footnotes and endnotes, which have also been renumbered. For citation and related purposes, the full original source texts should be used.

EXCERPT 1

Abridged text from:
US Department of Health and Human Services, *HHS Pandemic Influenza Plan* (Washington DC: US Government Printing Office, 2005).

HHS Pandemic Influenza Plan

United States Department of Health and Human Services

. . .

The Pandemic Influenza Threat

A pandemic occurs when a novel influenza virus emerges that can infect and be efficiently transmitted among individuals because of a lack of pre-existing immunity in the population. . . .

Although a novel influenza virus could emerge from anywhere in the world at any time, scientists are particularly concerned about the avian influenza (H5N1) currently circulating in Asia and parts of Europe. Outbreaks of influenza H5N1 have occurred among poultry in several countries in Asia since 1997. The H5N1 avian influenza virus is widespread in the region and has become endemic in migratory birds and several other animal species. As of October 2005, cases of human H5N1 infection have been reported in Thailand, Vietnam, Cambodia, and Indonesia. The reported death rate for these cases has been about 50%, although the true number of people who have been exposed to and infected by the H5N1 virus is unknown. . . .

Pandemic Planning Assumptions

. . . Public health experts and government officials are escalating and intensifying their pandemic preparedness planning. . . .

Doctrine for HHS Pandemic Influenza Planning and Response

The ongoing outbreaks of avian influenza in Asia and the progression from the interpandemic period (the period prior to human infections) to a pandemic alert (once human infections have occurred) have prompted HHS to enhance its preparedness planning and activities. In addition to the characteristics of a pandemic noted above, HHS' preparedness planning and response activities are guided by the following principles:

1. Preparedness will require coordination among federal, state and local government and partners in the private sector.
2. An informed and responsive public is essential to minimizing the health effects of a pandemic and the resulting consequences to society.
3. Domestic vaccine production capacity sufficient to provide vaccine for the entire US population is critical, as is development of vaccine against each circulating influenza virus with pandemic potential and acquisition of sufficient quantities to help protect first responders and other critical personnel at the onset of a pandemic.
4. Quantities of antiviral drugs sufficient to treat 25% of the US population should be stockpiled.

5. Sustained human-to-human transmission anywhere in the world will be the triggering event to initiate a pandemic response by the United States.
6. When possible and appropriate, protective public health measures will be employed to attempt to reduce person-to-person viral transmission and prevent or delay influenza outbreaks.
7. At the onset of a pandemic, vaccine, which will initially be in short supply, will be procured by HHS and distributed to state and local health departments for immunization of pre-determined priority groups.
8. At the onset of a pandemic, antiviral drugs from public stockpiles will be distributed to health care providers for administration to pre-determined priority groups.

Key Pandemic Response Elements and Capabilities for Effective Implementation

The nature of the HHS response will be guided by the epidemiologic features of the virus and the course of the pandemic. An influenza pandemic will place extraordinary and sustained demands not only on public health and health care providers, but also on providers of essential services across the United States and around the globe. Realizing that pandemic influenza preparedness is a process, not an isolated event, to most effectively implement key pandemic response actions, specific capabilities must be developed through preparedness activities implemented before the pandemic occurs. This plan outlines key actions for an effective pandemic response, involving surveillance, investigation, protective public health measures; vaccines and antiviral drug production; healthcare and emergency response; and communications and public outreach.

Once sustained human infection is documented, early in a pandemic, especially before a vaccine is available or during a period of limited supply, HHS may implement travel-related and community-based public health strategies. . . .

Part 2—Public Health Guidance to State and Local Partners

. . .

Planning Assumptions

Pandemic preparedness planning is based on assumptions regarding the evolution and impacts of a pandemic. Defining the potential magnitude of a pandemic is difficult because of the large differences in severity for the three 20th-century pandemics. While the 1918 pandemic resulted in an estimated 500,000 deaths in the US, the 1968 pandemic caused an estimated 34,000 US deaths. This difference is largely related to the severity of infections and the virulence of the influenza viruses that caused the pandemics. The 20th century pandemics have also shared similar characteristics. In each pandemic, about 30% of the US population developed illness, with about half seeking medical care. Children have tended to have the highest rates of illness, though not of severe disease and death. Geographical spread in each pandemic was rapid and virtually all communities experienced outbreaks.

Pandemic planning is based on the following assumptions about pandemic disease:

- Susceptibility to the pandemic influenza subtype will be universal.
- The clinical disease attack rate will be 30% in the overall population. Illness rates will be highest among school-aged children (about 40%) and decline with age. Among working adults, an average of 20% will become ill during a community outbreak.
- Of those who become ill with influenza, 50% will seek outpatient medical care.

. . . [see also Table [7.2].]

Table [7.2]
Number of Episodes of Illness, Healthcare Utilization, and Death Associated with Moderate and Severe Pandemic Influenza Scenarios[a]

Characteristic	Moderate (1958/68-like)	Severe (1918-like)
Illness	90 million (30%)	90 million (30%)
Outpatient medical care	45 million (50%)	45 million (50%)
Hospitalization	865,000	9,900,000
ICU care	128,750	1,485,000
Mechanical ventilation	64,875	742,500
Deaths	209,000	1,903,000

[a]Estimates based on extrapolation from past pandemics in the United States. Note that these estimates do not include the potential impact of interventions not available during the 20th-century pandemics.

Risk groups for severe and fatal infections cannot be predicted with certainty

- Risk groups for severe and fatal infections cannot be predicted with certainty. During annual fall and winter influenza season, infants and the elderly, persons with chronic illnesses, and pregnant women are usually at higher risk of complications from influenza infections. In contrast, in the 1918 pandemic, most deaths occurred among young, previously healthy adults.

. . .

- In an affected community, a pandemic outbreak will last about 6 to 8 weeks. At least two pandemic disease waves are likely. Following the pandemic, the new viral subtype is likely to continue circulating and to contribute to seasonal influenza.
- The seasonality of a pandemic cannot be predicted with certainty. The largest waves in the US during 20th century pandemics occurred in the fall and winter. Experience from the 1957 pandemic may be instructive in that the first US cases occurred in June but no community outbreaks occurred until August and the first wave of illness peaked in October.

. . .

Appendix B: Pandemic Influenza Background

E. Impact of influenza and influenza pandemics

An annual influenza season in the US, on average, results in approximately 36,000 deaths, 226,000 hospitalizations, and between $1 billion and $3 billion in direct costs for medical care. This impact occurs because influenza infections result in secondary complications such as pneumonia, dehydration, and worsening of chronic lung and heart problems. Despite the severity of influenza epidemics, it is sobering to understand that the effects of seasonal influenza are moderated because most individuals have some underlying degree of immunity to recently circulating influenza viruses either from previous infections or from vaccination.

Certain modern trends could increase the potential for pandemics to cause more illnesses and deaths than occurred in earlier pandemics

- First, the global population is larger and increasingly urbanized, allowing viruses to be transmitted within populations more easily.
- Second, levels of international travel are much greater than in the past, allowing viruses to spread globally more quickly than in the past.
- Third, populations in many countries consist of increasing numbers of elderly persons and those with chronic medical conditions, thus increasing the potential for more complicated illnesses and deaths to occur.

This combination of factors suggests that the next pandemic may lead to more illnesses occurring more quickly than in the past, overwhelming countries and health systems that are not adequately prepared.

The 1957 pandemic, during an era with much less globalization, spread to the US within 4–5 months of its detection in China, and the 1968 pandemic spread to the US from Hong

Table [7.3]
Effects of Past Pandemics on the United States

Pandemic	Estimated US Deaths	Influenza A Strain	Populations at Greatest Risk
1918–1919	500,000	H1N1	Young, healthy adults
1957–1958	70,000	H2N2	Infants, elderly
1968–1969	34,000	H3N2	Infants, elderly

Kong within 2–3 months. As was amply demonstrated by the SARS outbreak, modern travel patterns may significantly reduce the time needed for pandemic influenza viruses to spread globally to a few months or even weeks. The major implication of such rapid spread of an infectious disease is that many, if not most, countries will have minimal time to implement preparations and responses once pandemic viruses have begun to spread. While SARS infections spread quickly to multiple countries, the epidemiology and transmission modes of the SARS virus greatly helped to contain the spread of this infection in 2003, along with quarantine, isolation, and other control measures. Fortunately, no widespread community transmission took place. By contrast, because influenza spreads more rapidly between people and can be transmitted by those who are infected but do not yet have symptoms, the spread of pandemic influenza to multiple countries is expected to lead to the near simultaneous occurrence of multiple community outbreaks in an escalating fashion. No other infectious disease threat, whether natural or engineered, poses the same current threat for causing increases in infections, illnesses, and deaths so quickly in the US and worldwide (see Table [7.3]).

. . .

Appendix D: NVAC/ACIP Recommendations for Prioritization of Pandemic Influenza Vaccine and NVAC Recommendations on Pandemic Antiviral Drug Use

Advisory Committee recommendations are presented in this report to provide guidance for planning purposes and to form the basis for further discussion of how to equitably allocate medical countermeasures that will be in short supply early in an influenza pandemic.

Two federal advisory committees, the Advisory Committee on Immunization Practices (ACIP) and the National Vaccine Advisory Committee (NVAC), provided recommendations to the Department of Health and Human Services on the use of vaccines and antiviral drugs in an influenza pandemic.

Although the advisory committees considered potential priority groups broadly, the main expertise of the members was in health and public health. The primary goal of a pandemic response considered was to decrease health impacts including severe morbidity and death; secondary pandemic response goals included minimizing societal and economic impacts. However, as other sectors are increasingly engaged in pandemic planning, additional considerations may arise. The advisory committee reports explicitly acknowledge the importance of this, for example highlighting the priority for protecting critical components of the military. Finally, HHS has recently initiated outreach to engage the public and obtain a broader perspective into decisions on priority groups for pandemic vaccine and antiviral drugs. Though findings of the outreach are preliminary, a theme that has emerged is the importance of limiting the effects of a pandemic on society by preserving essential societal functions.

. . .

On July 19, 2005, ACIP and NVAC voted unanimously in favor of the vaccine priority recommendations summarized in Table [7.4]. . . .

A. Critical assumptions

The recommendations summarized in Table [7.4] were based on the following critical assumptions:

Morbidity and mortality. The greatest risk of hospitalization and death—as during the 1957 and 1968 pandemics and annual influenza—will be in infants, the elderly, and those with underlying health conditions. In the 1918 pandemic, most deaths occurred in young adults, highlighting the need to reconsider the recommendations at the time of the pandemic based on the epidemiology of disease.

Healthcare system. . . . CDC models estimate increases in hospitalization and intensive care unit demand of more than 25% even in a moderate pandemic.

Workforce. During a pandemic wave in a community, between 25% and 30% of persons will become ill during a 6 to 8 week outbreak. Among working-aged adults, illness attack rates will be lower than in the community as a whole. A CDC model suggests that at the peak of pandemic disease, about 10% of the workforce will be absent due to illness or caring for an ill family member. . . .

Vaccine production capacity. The US-based vaccine production capacity was assumed at 3 to 5 million 15μg doses per week with 3 to 6 months needed before the first doses are

Table [7.4]
Vaccine Priority Group Recommendations[a]

Tier	Subtier	Population	Rationale
1	A	• Vaccine and antiviral manufacturers and others essential to manufacturing and critical support (~40,000)	• Need to assure maximum production of vaccine and antiviral drugs
		• Medical workers and public health workers[b] who are involved in direct patient contact, other support services essential for direct patient care, and vaccinators (8–9 million)	• Healthcare workers are required for quality medical care (studies show outcome is associated with staff-to-patient ratios). There is little surge capacity among healthcare sector personnel to meet increased demand.
	B	• Persons ≥65 years with 1 or more influenza high-risk conditions, not including essential hypertension (approximately 18.2 million)	• These groups are at high risk of hospitalization and death. Excludes elderly in nursing homes and those who are immunocompromised and would not likely be protected by vaccination
		• Persons 6 months to 64 years with 2 or more influenza high-risk conditions, not including essential hypertension (approximately 6.9 million)	
		• Persons 6 months or older with history of hospitalization for pneumonia or influenza or other influenza high-risk condition in the past year (740,000)	
	C	• Pregnant women (approximately 3.0 million)	• In past pandemics and for annual influenza, pregnant women have been at high risk; vaccination will also protect the infant who cannot receive vaccine.
		• Household contacts of severely immunocompromised persons who would not be vaccinated due to likely poor response to vaccine (1.95 million with transplants, AIDS, and incident cancer × 1.4 household contacts per person = 2.7 million persons)	• Vaccination of household contacts of immunocompromised and young infants will decrease risk of exposure and infection among those who cannot be directly protected by vaccination.
		• Household contacts of children <6 month olds (5.0 million)	

Table [7.4] (Continued)

Tier	Subtier	Population	Rationale
	D	• Public health emergency response workers critical to pandemic response (assumed one-third of estimated public health workforce = 150,000) • Key government leaders	• Critical to implement pandemic response such as providing vaccinations and managing/monitoring response activities • Preserving decision-making capacity also critical for managing and implementing a response
2	A	• Healthy 65 years and older (17.7 million) • 6 months to 64 years with 1 high-risk condition (35.8 million) • 6–23 months old, healthy (5.6 million)	• Groups that are also at increased risk but not as high risk as population in Tier 1B
	B	• Other public health emergency responders (300,000 = remaining two-thirds of public health work force) • Public safety workers including police, fire, 911 dispatchers, and correctional facility staff (2.99 million) • Utility workers essential for maintenance of power, water, and sewage system functioning (364,000) • Transportation workers transporting fuel, water, food, and medical supplies as well as public ground public transportation (3.8 million) • Telecommunications/IT for essential network operations and maintenance (1.08 million)	• Includes critical infrastructure groups that have impact on maintaining health (e.g., public safety or transportation of medical supplies and food); implementing a pandemic response; and on maintaining societal functions
3		• Other key government health decision-makers (estimated number not yet determined) • Funeral directors/embalmers (62,000)	• Other important societal groups for a pandemic response but of lower priority
4		• Healthy persons 2–64 years not included in above categories (179.3 million)	• All persons not included in other groups based on objective to vaccinate all those who want protection

[a]The committee focused its deliberations on the US civilian population. ACIP and NVAC recognize that Department of Defense (DoD) needs should be highly prioritized. DoD Health Affairs indicates that 1.5 million service members would require immunization to continue current combat operations and preserve critical components of the military medical system. Should the military be called upon to support civil authorities domestically, immunization of a greater proportion of the total force will become necessary. These factors should be considered in the designation of a proportion of the initial vaccine supply for the military.

Other groups also were not explicitly considered in these deliberations on prioritization. These include American citizens living overseas, noncitizens in the US, and other groups providing national security services, such as the border patrol and customs service.

[b]This is inclusive of federal healthcare providers to Indian nations and tribes.

produced. Two doses per person were assumed to be required for protection. Subsequent results of an NIH clinical trial of influenza A (H5N1) vaccine suggest that higher doses of antigen will be needed to elicit a good immune response; thus, the assumptions made by the committee could potentially substantially exceed the amount of vaccine that would be produced.

B. Definitions and rationales for priority groups

1. Healthcare workers and essential healthcare support staff

. . .

a) Rationale

The pandemic is expected to have substantial impact on the healthcare system with large increases in demand for healthcare services placed on top of existing demand. HCW will be treating influenza-infected patients and will be at risk of repeated exposures. Further, surge capacity in this sector is low. To encourage continued work in a high-exposure setting and to help lessen the risk of healthcare workers transmitting influenza to other patients and HCW family members, this group was highly prioritized. In addition, increases in bed/nurse ratios have been associated with increases in overall patient mortality. Thus, substantial absenteeism may affect overall patient care and outcomes.

2. Groups at high risk of influenza complications

. . .

a) Rationale

These groups were prioritized based on their risk of influenza-related hospitalization and death and also their likelihood of vaccine response. . . .

3. Critical infrastructure

a) Definitions and rationale

Those critical infrastructure sectors that fulfill one or more of the following criteria: have increased demand placed on them during a pandemic, directly support reduction in deaths and hospitalization; function is critical to support the healthcare sector and other emergency services, and/or supply basic necessities and services critical to support of life and healthcare or emergency services. Groups included in critical infrastructure are needed to respond to a pandemic and to minimize morbidity and mortality. . . .

4. Public health emergency response workers

. . .

a) Rationale

Persons in this sector have been critical for past influenza vaccine pandemics and influenza vaccine shortages and little surge capacity may be available during a public health emergency such as a pandemic.

5. Persons in skilled nursing facilities

. . .

a) Rationale

This group was not prioritized for vaccine because of the medical literature finding poor response to vaccination and occurrence of outbreaks even in the setting of high vaccination rates. Other studies have suggested that vaccination of healthcare workers may be a more effective strategy to prevent influenza in this group.

6. Severely immunocompromised persons

. . .

b) Rationale

These groups have a lower likelihood of responding to influenza vaccination. Thus, strategies to prevent severe influenza illness in this group should include vaccination of healthcare workers and household contacts of severely immunocompromised persons and use of antiviral medications. Consideration should be given to prophylaxis of severely immunocompromised persons with influenza antivirals and early antiviral treatment should they become infected.

7. Children <6 months of age

a) Rationale

Influenza vaccine is poorly immunogenic in children <6 months and the vaccine is currently not recommended for this group. In addition, influenza antiviral medications are not FDA-approved for use in children <1 year old. Thus, vaccination of household contacts and out-of-home caregivers of children <6 months is recommended to protect this high-risk group.

C. Other discussion

There was substantial discussion on priority for children. Four potential reasons were raised for making vaccination of children a priority:

- At the public engagement session, many participants felt that children should have high priority for vaccination.
- Children play a major role in transmitting infection, and vaccinating this group could slow the spread of disease and indirectly protect others.
- Children have strong immune systems and will respond well to vaccine where as vaccination of the elderly and those with illnesses may be less effective.
- Some ethical frameworks would support a pediatric priority.

ACIP and NVAC did not make children a priority (other than those included in tiers, because of their underlying diseases [Tiers 1B and 2A] or as contacts of high-risk persons [Tier 1C]) for several reasons:

- Healthy children have been at low risk for hospitalization and death in prior pandemics and during annual influenza seasons.
- It is uncertain whether vaccination of children will decrease transmission and indirectly protect others. Studies that show this impact or mathematical models that predict it rely on high vaccination coverage that may not be possible to achieve given limited supplies in a pandemic.

. . .

EXCERPT 2

Abridged text from:

E. Emanuel and A. Wertheimer, "Who Should Get Influenza Vaccine When Not All Can?", *Science* 312, no. 5775 (2006): pp. 854–855.

Public Health: Who Should Get Influenza Vaccine When Not All Can?

Ezekiel J. Emanuel and Alan Wertheimer

. . .

The potential threat of pandemic influenza is staggering: 1.9 million deaths, 90 million people sick, and nearly 10 million people hospitalized, with almost 1.5 million requiring intensive-care units (ICUs) in the United States.[1] The National Vaccine Advisory Committee (NVAC) and the Advisory Committee on Immunization Policy (ACIP) have jointly recommended a prioritization scheme that places vaccine workers, health-care providers, and the ill elderly at the top, and healthy people aged 2 to 64 at the very bottom, even under embalmers (Table [7.5]).[2] The primary goal informing the recommendation was to "decrease health impacts including severe morbidity and death"; a secondary goal was minimizing societal and economic impacts.[3] As the NVAC and ACIP acknowledge, such important policy decisions require broad national discussion. In this spirit, we believe an alternative ethical framework should be considered.

[1] United States Department of Health and Human Services, *HHS Pandemic Influenza Plan* (Washington DC: US Government Printing Office, 2005), Supplement E.

[2] Ibid.

[3] Ibid.

The Inescapability of Rationing

Because of current uncertainty of its value, only "a limited amount of avian influenza A (H5N1) vaccine is being stockpiled."[4] Furthermore, it will take at least 4 months from identification of a candidate vaccine strain until production of the very first vaccine.[5] At present, there are few production facilities worldwide that make influenza vaccine, and only one completely in the USA. Global capacity for influenza vaccine production is just 425 million doses per annum, if all available factories would run at full capacity after a vaccine was developed. Under currently existing capabilities for manufacturing vaccine, it is likely that more than 90% of the US population will not be vaccinated in the first year.[6] Distributing the limited supply will require determining priority groups.

Who will be at highest risk? Our experience with three influenza pandemics presents a complex picture. The mortality profile of a future pandemic could be U-shaped, as it was in the mild-to-moderate pandemics of 1957 and 1968 and interpandemic influenza seasons, in which the very young and the old are at highest risk. Or, the mortality profile could be an attenuated W shape, as it was during the devastating 1918 pandemic, in which the highest risk occurred among people between 20 and 40 years of age, while the elderly were not at high excess risk.[7,8] Even during pandemics, the elderly appear to be at no higher risk than during interpandemic influenza seasons.[9]

[4] Ibid.

[5] Ibid.

[6] Ibid.

[7] S. D. Collin, *Public Health Reports* 60 (1945): p. 853.

[8] D. R. Olson, et al., "Epidemiological Evidence of an Early Wave of the 1918 Influenza Pandemic in New York City," *Proceedings of the National Academy of Sciences of the United States of America* 102, no. 31 (2005): pp. 11059–11063.

[9] L. Simonsen et al., in *The Threat of Pandemic Influenza: Are We Ready?*, edited by S. L. K. Knobler et al. (Washington, DC: National Academies Press, 2004).

Table [7.5]
Priorities for Distribution of Influenza Vaccine

Tier*	NVAC and ACIP recommendations (subtier)[†]	Life-cycle principle (LCP)	Investment refinement of LCP including public order
1	Vaccine production and distribution workers Frontline health-care workers **People 6 months to 64 years old with >2 high-risk conditions or history of hospitalization for pneumonia or influenza** Pregnant women Household contacts of severely immunocompromised people Household contacts of children <6 months of age **Public health and emergency response workers** Key government leaders	Vaccine production and distribution workers Frontline health-care workers	Vaccine production and distribution workers Frontline health-care workers
2	Healthy people >65 years old People 6 months to 64 years old with 1 or more high-risk conditions Healthy children 6 months to 23 months old **Other public health workers, emergency responders, public safety workers (police and fire), utility workers, transportation workers, telecommunications and IT workers**	Healthy 6-month-olds **Healthy 1-year-olds** Healthy 2-year-olds **Healthy 3-year-olds** Etc.	People 13 to 40 years old with <2 high-risk conditions, with priority to key government leaders; public health, military, police, and fire workers; utility and transportation workers; telecommunications and IT workers; funeral directors **People 7 to 12 years old and 41 to 50 years old with <2 high-risk conditions with priority as above** People 6 months to 6 years old and 51 to 64 years old with <2 high-risk conditions, with priority as above[††] **People >65 years old with <2 high-risk conditions**
3	Other health decision-makers in government Funeral directors	People with life-limiting morbidities or disabilities, prioritized according to expected life years	People 6 months to 64 years old with >2 high-risk conditions
4	Healthy people 2 to 64 years old		People >65 years old with > high risk conditions

** Tiers determine priority ranking for the distribution of vaccine if limited in supply. [†]Subtiers in bold text establish who gets priority within the tier (starting from the top of the tier) if limited vaccine cannot cover everyone in the tier; prioritization may occur within subtiers as well. [††]Children 6 months to <13 years would not receive vaccine if they can be effectively confined to home or otherwise isolated.*

Clear ethical justification for vaccine priorities is essential to the acceptability of the priority ranking and any modifications during the pandemic. With limited vaccine supply, uncertainty over who will be at highest risk of infection and complications, and questions about which historic pandemic experience is most applicable, society faces a fundamental ethical dilemma: Who should get the vaccine first?

The NVAC and ACIP Priority Rankings

Many potential ethical principles for rationing health care have been proposed. "Save the most lives" is commonly used in emergencies, such as burning buildings, although "women and children first" played a role on the Titanic. "First come, first served" operates in other emergencies and in ICUs when admitted patients retain beds despite the presentation of another patient who is equally or even more sick; "Save the most quality life years" is central to cost-effectiveness rationing. "Save the worst-off" plays a role in allocating organs for transplantation. "Reciprocity"—giving priority to people willing to donate their own organs—has been proposed. "Save those most likely to fully recover" guided priorities for giving penicillin to soldiers with syphilis in World War II. Save those "instrumental in making society flourish" through economic productivity or by "contributing to the well-being of others" has been proposed by Murray and others.[10,11]

The save-the-most-lives principle was invoked by NVAC and ACIP. It justifies giving top priority to workers engaged in vaccine production and distribution and health-care workers. They get higher priority not because they are intrinsically more valuable people or of greater "social worth," but because giving them first priority ensures that maximal life-saving vaccine is produced and so that health care is provided to the sick.[12] Consequently, it values all human life equally, giving every person equal consideration in who gets priority regardless of age, disability, social class, or employment.[13] After these groups, the save-the-most-lives principle justifies priority for those predicted to be at highest risk of hospitalization and dying. We disagree with this prioritization.

Life-Cycle Principle

The save-the-most-lives principle may be justified in some emergencies when decision urgency makes it infeasible to deliberate about priority rankings and impractical to categorize individuals into priority groups. We believe that a life-cycle allocation principle (see table) based on the idea that each person should have an opportunity to live through all the stages of life is more appropriate for a pandemic.[14,15] There is great value in being able to pass through each life stage—to be a child, a young adult, and to then develop a career and family, and to grow old—and to enjoy a wide range of the opportunities during each stage.

Multiple considerations and intuitions support this ethical principle. Most people endorse this principle for themselves.[16,17] We would prioritize our own resources to ensure we could live past the illnesses of childhood and young adulthood and would allocate fewer resources to living ever longer once we reached old age.[18] People strongly prefer maximizing the chance of living until a ripe old age, rather than being struck down as a young person.[19,20]

---

[10] C. J. L. Murray and A. D. Lopez, eds, *The Global Burden of Disease* (Geneva: World Health Organization, 1996).

[11] C. Murray and A. Acharya, *Journal of Health Economics* 16 (1997): p. 710.

[12] R. Dworkin, *Taking Rights Seriously* (Cambridge, MA: Harvard University Press, 1978), pp. 150–205.

[13] Ibid.

[14] A. Williams, "Intergenerational Equity: An Exploration of the "Fair Innings" Argument," *Health Economics* 6, no. 2 (1997): pp. 117–132.

[15] N. Daniels, *Am I My Parents' Keeper?: An Essay on Justice between the Young and the Old* (Oxford University Press, 1988), pp. 66–102.

[16] Williams, "Intergenerational Equity," pp. 117–132.

[17] Daniels, *Am I My Parents' Keeper?*, pp. 66–102.

[18] Ibid.

[19] M. L. Cropper, S. K. Aydede and P. R. Portney, "Preferences for Life Saving Programs: How the Public Discounts Time and Age," *Journal of Risk and Uncertainty* 8, no. 3 (1994): pp. 243–265.

[20] M. Johannesson and P. O. Johansson, "Is the Valuation of a QALY Gained Independent of Age? Some Empirical Evidence," *Journal of Health Economics* 16, no. 5 (1997): pp. 589–599.

Death seems more tragic when a child or young adult dies than an elderly person—not because the lives of older people are less valuable, but because the younger person has not had the opportunity to live and develop through all stages of life. Although the life-cycle principle favors some ages, it is also intrinsically egalitarian.[21] Unlike being productive or contributing to others' well-being, every person will live to be older unless their life is cut short.

The Investment Refinement

A pure version of the life-cycle principle would grant priority to 6-month-olds over 1-year-olds who have priority over 2-year-olds, and on. An alternative, the investment refinement, emphasizes gradations within a life span. It gives priority to people between early adolescence and middle age on the basis of the amount the person invested in his or her life balanced by the amount left to live.[22] Within this framework, 20-year-olds are valued more than 1-year-olds because the older individuals have more developed interests, hopes, and plans but have not had an opportunity to realize them (11,12).[23,24] Although these groupings could be modified, they indicate ethically defensible distinctions among groups that can inform rationing priorities.

One other ethical principle relevant for priority ranking of influenza vaccine during a pandemic is public order. It focuses on the value of ensuring safety and the provision of necessities, such as food and fuel. We believe the investment refinement combined with the public-order principle (IRPOP) should be the ultimate objective of all pandemic response measures, including priority ranking for vaccines and interventions to limit the course of the pandemic, such as closing schools and confining people to homes. These two principles should inform decisions at the start of an epidemic when the shape of the risk curves for morbidity and mortality are largely uncertain.

Like the NVAC and ACIP ranking, the IRPOP ranking would give high priority to vaccine production and distribution workers, as well as health-care and public health workers with direct patient contact. However, contrary to the NVAC and ACIP prioritization for the sick elderly and infants, IRPOP emphasize people between 13 and 40 years of age. The NVAC and ACIP priority ranking comports well with those groups at risk during the mild-to-moderate 1957 and 1968 pandemics. IRPOP prioritizes those age cohorts at highest risk during the devastating 1918 pandemic. Depending on patterns of flu spread, some mathematical models suggest that following IRPOP priority ranking could save the most lives overall.[25]

Conclusions

The life-cycle ranking is meant to apply to the situation in the United States. During a global pandemic, there will be fundamental questions about sharing vaccines and other interventions with other countries. This raises fundamental issues of global rationing that are too complex to address here.

Fortunately, even though we are worried about an influenza pandemic, it is not upon us. Indeed, the current H5N1 avian flu may never develop into a human pandemic. This gives us time both to build vaccine production capacity to minimize the need for rationing and to rationally assess policy and ethical issues about the distribution of vaccines.

[21] Dworkin, *Taking Rights Seriously*, pp. 150–205.

[22] R. Dworkin, *Life's Dominion: An Argument About Abortion, Euthanasia, and Individual Freedom* (Knopf, 1993), pp. 68–101.

[23] Johannesson, "Is the Valuation of a QALY," pp. 589–599.

[24] Dworkin, *Life's Dominion*, pp. 68–101.

[25] M. E. Halloran and I. M. Longini, "Community Studies for Vaccinating Schoolchildren against Influenza," *Science* 311, no. 5761 (2006): pp. 615–616.

EXCERPT 3

Abridged text from:
US Department of Health and Human Services, *Guidance on Allocating and Targeting Pandemic Influenza Vaccine* (Washington, DC: US Government Printing Office, 2008).

Guidance on Allocating and Targeting Pandemic Influenza Vaccine

United States Department of Health and Human Services

Introduction

Effective allocation of pandemic influenza vaccine will play a critical role in preventing influenza and reducing its effects on health and society when a pandemic arrives. The specific type of influenza that causes a pandemic will not be known until it occurs. Developing a new vaccine in response will take several months and pandemic vaccine may not be available when cases first occur in the United States. Moreover, once vaccine production begins, it will not be possible to make enough new vaccine to protect everyone in the early stages of a pandemic.

. . .

How the Guidance Was Developed

The Federal Government developed this guidance through a rigorous and collaborative process that included input from all interested parties. Hearing opinions from persons and organizations with a wide variety of interests and concerns is the best way to ensure that allocation of vaccine in the early stages of a pandemic is fair and provides the best chance for our country to emerge from a pandemic with minimal levels of illness, death, and disruption to our society and economy.

. . .

Meetings with the public and stakeholders, including businesses and community organizations, provided key input on public values and priorities. Participants discussed and rated the importance of potential vaccination program objectives based on a severe pandemic scenario.

. . .

Draft Guidance on Allocating and Targeting Pandemic Influenza Vaccine

Goals and Objectives

The *goal* of the pandemic influenza vaccination program is to vaccinate all persons in the United States who choose to be vaccinated.

It is recognized that vaccine supply to meet this goal will likely not be available all at once, but rather, be produced at a rate that depends on both vaccine characteristics (antigen required) and manufacturing capacity. Given that influenza vaccine supply will increase incrementally as vaccine is produced during a pandemic, allocation decisions will have to be made. Such decisions should be based on publicly articulated and discussed program objectives and principles. The overarching objectives guiding vaccine allocation and use during a pandemic are to reduce the impact of the pandemic on health and minimize disruption to society and the economy.

One of the most important findings of the working group analysis, and the strongest communication from the public and stakeholder meetings, was that there is no single, overriding objective for pandemic vaccination and no single target group to protect at the exclusion of others. Rather, there are several important *objectives* and, thus, vaccine should be allocated simultaneously to several groups (see Figure [7.2]). Each of the

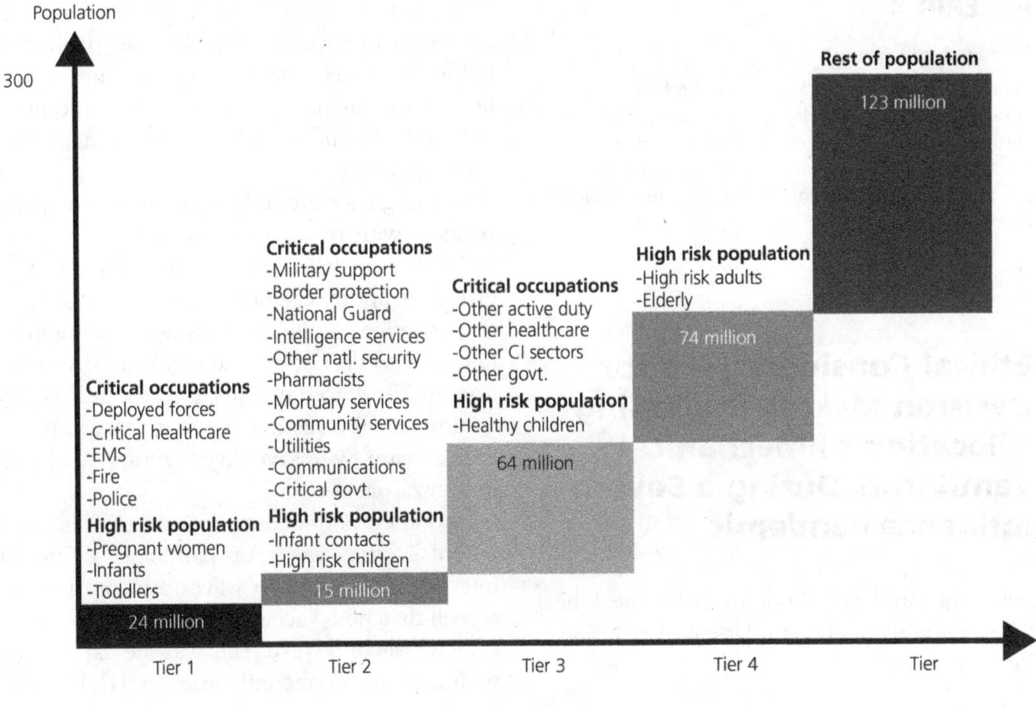

Figure [7.2] Vaccination tiers and target groups for a severe pandemic. This figure illustrates how vaccination is administered by tiers until the entire US population has had the opportunity to be vaccinated, and how tiers integrate target groups across the four categories balancing vaccine allocation to occupationally defined groups and the general population.

meetings came to the same conclusions about which program objectives are most important:

- Protecting those who are essential to the pandemic response and provide care for persons who are ill,
- Protecting those who maintain essential community services,
- Protecting children, and
- Protecting workers who are at greater risk of infection due to their job.

In addition to these, working group discussions highlighted the important Federal objective of maintaining homeland and national security.

. . .

Defining who is included in each target group

The primary objective of vaccinating persons in critical infrastructure sectors is not to reduce absenteeism generally through an incremental reduction in pandemic illness afforded by vaccination. Rather, vaccination is targeted to protect workers with critical skills, experience, or licensure status whose absence would create bottlenecks or collapse of critical functions, and to protect workers who are at especially high occupational risk.

. . .

. . .

EXCERPT 4

Abridged text from:

Ventilator Document Workgroup for the Ethics Subcommittee of the Advisory Committee to the Director, "Ethical Considerations for Decision Making Regarding Allocation of Mechanical Ventilators During a Severe Influenza Pandemic or Other Public Health Emergency," 2009.

Ethical Considerations for Decision Making Regarding Allocation of Mechanical Ventilators During a Severe Influenza Pandemic

Ventilator Guidance Workgroup for the Ethics Subcommittee, Centers for Disease Control and Prevention

Key Assumptions

Use of this document is based on a number of assumptions regarding severity of illness and the availability of resources. It is intended only for circumstances when people with severe acute respiratory failure far outnumber available and adequate mechanical ventilator supply. For most US communities, such extreme imbalances are only anticipated in special circumstances (e.g., an influenza pandemic that is both widespread and severe). . . . Currently the National Ventilator Inventory has revealed that there are approximately 62,000 full-feature mechanical ventilators in the United States. In addition, there are approximately an additional 100,000 devices across a range of categories of respiratory equipment (not including anesthesia machines) at US acute care hospitals which might be used for surge capacity.[1] Almost half of the 100,000 additional devices have enough features to be useful for anticipated surge capacity events. . . . Despite these crucial activities, it is possible that in the event of a particularly virulent pandemic influenza virus, many hospitals and other healthcare facilities will not have adequate numbers of ventilators to support a major disaster response.

[1] Data from unpublished HHS study.

During a severe influenza pandemic, many patients with respiratory failure who are able to receive mechanical ventilation (and all associated supportive critical care components) may survive, while patients with respiratory failure who do not receive mechanical ventilation are likely to die. Thus, a major underlying assumption for this document is that advanced critical care will save lives during a severe influenza pandemic.

Another of the assumptions of this document is that cases of pandemic influenza infection will occur in waves and most likely a well-matched vaccine will not be available until the second wave. This was the experience with 2009 pandemic influenza A (H1N1).

During a severe influenza pandemic it is anticipated that resources will be overwhelmed in the first or second wave of illness because the entire community will be at risk for illness. Equipment for emergency respiratory care, including ventilators, may be in full use and no longer available to additional patients by the first or second wave of a severe influenza pandemic, depending on the geographical spread and timing of the waves, the symptoms of the disease, the availability of pandemic vaccine, and the local effectiveness of community mitigation strategies. This document assumes that ventilators may be in short supply in some communities as early as prior to or during the peak of the first wave of a severe influenza pandemic.

The need to make difficult decisions during a severe influenza pandemic or other public health emergency will most likely occur in an environment of overall limited public health resources. Considerable costs are associated with stockpiling, maintaining reserve ventilators, and funding training of personnel needed to operate ventilators skillfully and safely. The decision by states, regions, healthcare systems, or hospitals to augment mechanical ventilation capacity (and all associated critical care elements) for emergency use during a severe influenza pandemic should be made within the larger context of everyday public health and clinical obligations, as well as broader community-based emergency preparedness and response resource needs. This document assumes that individual communities will need to balance pandemic-preparedness requirements with other healthcare and public health needs.

Priorities for Ventilator Allocation

Historically, during routine clinical practice the organizing principle for ventilator distribution, as well as for the distribution of most therapeutic procedures and interventions has been the minimization of adverse outcomes, including hospitalization and death. Typically all patients who have a medical need for mechanical ventilation and who consent to treatment (or have the concurrence of a surrogate) are provided this type of care. However, during a severe pandemic when there is a shortage of health care resources, it may be necessary to re-evaluate the ethical considerations that govern the usual provision of care.[2] In this and in the next two sections, we explore how the usual ethical considerations that govern allocation to ventilators may need to be modified during a severe influenza pandemic or other public health emergency when there might not be enough ventilators for all who need one.

During a public health emergency, there will be competing priorities for ventilator use from patients whose need for a ventilator is unrelated to influenza. In addition, decisions will need to be made regarding whether patients should be removed from a ventilator to make way for others who may have a better chance of recovery, and whether there should be suspension of non-emergency surgical procedures that might create a need for ventilator therapy.

The principle of *sickest first* is routinely employed to triage patients presenting for care in the emergency department, where staff time is scarce but medical resources are not. Other patients will still receive care, but they must wait. During a severe influenza pandemic that creates a critical shortage of ventilators, however, this strategy may lead to resources being used by patients who ultimately are too sick to survive.

First-come, first-served is used to allocate intensive care unit (ICU) beds during routine clinical circumstances. Once a patient is in the ICU, they are generally not transferred out of the ICU if they still need intensive care unless the patient or surrogate agrees to forego life-sustaining interventions. That is, fiduciary duties to existing patients take priority over potential benefits to other patients. During ordinary clinical care, the healthcare system generally can accommodate patients with a very poor prognosis who require an ICU bed for many days and who ultimately may not survive. Other patients are still able to receive intensive care if needed. However, the situation would be different if ventilators are in extremely short supply during a severe influenza pandemic; other patients, who may have a much better prognosis if they receive intensive care, will not have access to it. After a public health emergency is declared, rules that favor the overall benefit to the population and society may have to be considered.

In order to use scarce resources most efficiently, in some clinical situations where there is a severe shortage of life-saving medical resources, priority is given to those who are *most likely to recover* after receiving them. When treating soldiers with life threatening injuries, medics give priority to those who are most likely to survive with a relatively small amount of scarce resources. Such triage is carried out without regard to rank. Similarly during cholera epidemics in refugee camps, limited supplies of intravenous fluid are given not to those with the most severe dehydration, but instead to those with moderate

---

[2] L. O. Gostin, et al., *Guidance for Establishing Crisis Standards of Care for Use in Disaster Situations: A Letter Report* (National Academies Press, 2009).

dehydration who will likely recover with small amounts of fluid.[3]

In the Ethics Subcommittee's previous document, *Ethical Guidelines in Pandemic Influenza*, which addressed distribution of vaccines and antiviral medications, the *principle of preserving the functioning of society* was given greater priority than preventing serious complications.[4] This is because vaccines and antiviral medications are predominantly used to prevent or lessen illness and thus can be useful in maintaining or restoring health for groups identified as essential for preserving the functioning of society. However, decisions about priorities for ventilator distribution pose a different situation. Ventilators are an essential life-saving intervention. Thus, prioritizing based on preserving the functioning of society is not as relevant to decision making about distribution of ventilators as with vaccines and antiviral medications. The vast majority of patients who required mechanical ventilation due to illness caused by 2009 pandemic influenza A (H1N1) had ARDS. While published data regarding systematic post ICU follow-up of these patients has been limited, patients with ARDS due to bacterial pneumonia and sepsis take a median of one week to recover from requiring mechanical ventilation and then frequently have prolonged recoveries with long-term reduction of quality of life. Therefore, those who are ill enough to require ventilator therapy are unlikely to recover sufficient function to be able to contribute to the preservation of the functioning of society–at least not during the "wave" of the pandemic during which they fell ill.

[3] D. B. White, et al., "Who Should Receive Life Support During a Public Health Emergency? Using Ethical Principles to Improve Allocation Decisions," *Annals of Internal Medicine* 150, no. 2 (2009): pp. 132–138.

[4] K. Kinlaw, D. H. Barrett and R. J. Levine, "Ethical Guidelines in Pandemic Influenza: Recommendations of the Ethics Subcommittee of the Advisory Committee of the Director, Centers for Disease Control and Prevention," *Disaster Medicine and Public Health Preparedness* 3, no. S2 (2009): pp. S185-S192.

What Principles Should Guide Ventilator Allocation?

Basic Biomedical Ethical Principles

A consideration of the basic biomedical ethical principles is a useful starting place for decision making about ventilator allocation. These basic principles include respect for persons and their autonomy, beneficence, and justice.

Specific Ethical Considerations

In addition to the basic biomedical ethical principles discussed above, there are a number of more specific ethical considerations that will be useful in guiding decision making about allocation of ventilators. These considerations focus on differing approaches to maximizing and distributing benefits.

Maximizing Net Benefits

Historically, allocation decisions in public health have been driven by the utilitarian goal of maximizing net benefits.[5] Although this broad principle can be specified in numerous ways (i.e., maximizing the number of lives saved, maximizing years of life saved, maximizing adjusted years of life saved), several recent guidelines for allocating life support during a public health emergency have specified it narrowly as "maximize the number of people who survive to hospital discharge."[6,7,8]

[5] Ohio State University Center for Public Health Practice, "Ohio Pandemic Influenza Public Engagement Demonstration Project: Mass Fatality Management, Final Report," 2009, http://www.ohiopha.org/admin/uploads/documents/OH_Rural_Final_Report_2009.pdf.

[6] S. E. Erickson, et al., "Recent Trends in Acute Lung Injury Mortality: 1996–2005," *Critical Care Medicine* 37, no. 5 (2009): p. 1574.

[7] Burkle, "Mass Casualty Management."

[8] Public Health-Seattle & King Count, "Public Engagement Project on Medical Service Prioritization During an Influenza Pandemic: Health

Maximize the number of lives saved—The utilitarian rule of maximizing the number of lives saved is widely accepted during a public health emergency.[9] Some non-consequentialist views also favor maximizing the number of lives saved, not because this approach produces the most good; but, because each life has an equal claim on being saved. Prioritizing individuals according to their chances for short-term survival also avoids ethically irrelevant considerations, such as race or socioeconomic status. Finally, it is appealing because it balances utilitarian claims for efficiency with egalitarian claims that because all lives have equal value the goal should be to save the most lives.

Working groups in Ontario, Canada and New York State have proposed modifying a relatively simple mortality prediction model—the Sequential Organ Failure Assessment (SOFA) score—to determine an individual's priority for access to a ventilator.[10],[11] No model can predict with perfect accuracy which patients will benefit from mechanical ventilation during a severe influenza pandemic and which will not. When selecting a predictive score model, physicians and policy makers need to take into account several considerations, including whether the scoring system is validated in the populations it is being considered for (e.g. pediatrics, non-influenza patients who will be triaged together with patients with influenza-related critical illness), whether it is a disease-specific or general score, if the score can be used at multiple time points in disease course in addition to feasibility, ease of use, accuracy, validity, objectivity, and transparency. The predictive score model employed should be based on the best available science; hence research needs to be carried out to validate and potentially modify whatever predictive score model is employed.

Any predictive score model yields probabilities of outcomes, which may not accurately predict the outcome for any one individual. This concern has limited the use of probabilistic scoring systems to make treatment decisions during routine clinical practice. However, the rationale for their use is stronger during a severe influenza pandemic, when the goal is to maximize population-level outcomes. Such an objective approach during a severe pandemic may also be viewed by the public as fairer than decisions based on more subjective criteria. No matter which scoring system is utilized within a triage schema, the performance of the score must be reviewed to assess its accuracy and to minimize misclassification of people's predicted outcomes. Ideally this reevaluation should be ongoing during the event, and data collection systems must be planned for and implemented during an event.

Maximizing years of life saved—A broader conceptualization of maximizing net benefits is to consider the *years of life* saved in addition to the *number of lives* saved. Assuming equal chances of short term survival, giving priority to a 60-year-old woman who is otherwise healthy over a 60-year-old woman with a limited life expectancy from severe co-morbidities will result in more "life years" gained. The justification for incorporating this utilitarian claim is simply that, all other things being equal, it is better to save more years of life than fewer.

The principle of maximizing years of life saved has been used in organ transplantation to exclude as recipients persons with such severe co-morbidities that they have a very poor prognosis for survival even if they receive a transplant. Furthermore, this principle has also been invoked in some published guidelines regarding triage of ventilators during a severe influenza pandemic to exclude certain poor-prognosis subgroups of patients from access to ventilator support. For example, one group advocates denying ventilator support to

---

Care Decisions in Disasters," 2009, http://s3.amazonaws.com/propublica/assets/docs/seattle_public_engagement_project_final_sept2009.pdf.

[9] D. E. Vawter, et al., *For the Good of Us All: Ethically Rationing Health Resources in Minnesota in a Severe Influenza Pandemic* (Minneapolis: Minnesota Center for Health Care Ethics and University of Minnesota Center for Bioethics, 2010).

[10] Public Health, "Public Engagement Project."

[11] N. Pesik, M. E. Keim and K. V. Iserson, "Terrorism and the Ethics of Emergency Medical Care," *Annals of Emergency Medicine* 37, no. 6 (2001): pp. 642–646.

persons who are functionally dependent from a neurologic impairment.[12] Another group recommends excluding those older than 85 years of age and those with New York Heart Association Class III or IV heart failure.[13,14] These recommendations have been criticized because the criteria for exclusion (age, long-term prognosis, and functional status) are selectively applied to some patients, rather than to all patients who require life-sustaining interventions. Such selective application violates the principle of justice because patients who are similar in ethically relevant ways are treated differently. Categorical exclusion may also have the unintended negative effect of implying that some groups are "not worth saving," leading to perceptions of unfairness. These concerns might be addressed by keeping as *eligible* all patients who require mechanical ventilation but allowing the availability of ventilators to determine how many eligible patients receive one.

Maximizing adjusted years of life saved—A still more nuanced utilitarian approach would be to maximize years of life after adjusting for the quality of those years. However, predicting quality-adjusted life years (QALYs) or disability-adjusted life years (DALYs) for an individual patient requires considerable clinical information about an individual and would not be feasible when making decisions regarding intubation and mechanical ventilations in an emergency department or ambulance during a public health crisis.[15,16]

Although the utilitarian goal of maximizing net benefits is an important public health principle, we conclude that ethically, allocating scarce resources during a severe pandemic by only considering chances of survival to hospital discharge is insufficient because it omits other important ethical considerations.

Social Worth

Additional principles that have been used to allocate scarce resources are concerned with the distribution of benefits among patients, rather than the aggregate level of benefit. This has included criteria based on social worth and instrumental value.

Broad social value—Broad social value refers to one's overall worth to society. It involves summary judgments about whether an individual's past and future contributions to society's goals merit prioritization for scarce resources.[17] When dialysis was first introduced, social value was a key consideration in allocating scarce dialysis machines. Patients who were professionals, heads of families, and caregivers received priority over others who were perceived as less worthy.[18] The public firestorm in response to revelations that social worth was a key factor in the Seattle Dialysis Committee's deliberations partly led Congress to authorize universal coverage for hemodialysis.[19]

In our morally pluralistic society, there has been widespread rejection of the idea that one individual is intrinsically more worthy of saving than another. Many writers advocate the egalitarian view that all individuals have an equal moral claim to treatment regardless of whether they can contribute measurably to broad social

---

12 M. D. Christian, et al., "Development of a Triage Protocol for Critical Care During an Influenza Pandemic," *Canadian Medical Association Journal* 175, no. 11 (2006): pp. 1377–1381.

13 Erickson, "Recent trends."

14 Public Health, "Public Engagement Project."

15 J. F. Childress, "Triage in Response to a Bioterrorist Attack," *In the Wake of Terror: Medicine and Morality in a Time of Crisis* (2003): pp. 77–93.

16 NYS Workgroup on Ventilator Allocation in an Influenza Pandemic, "NYS Document Allocation of Ventilators in an Influenza Pandemic: Planning Document," 2007, http://www.health.state.ny.us/diseases/communicable/influenza/pandemic/ventilators/docs/ventilator_guidance.pdf.

17 Vawter, *For the Good of Us All.*

18 Utah Hospitals and Health Systems Association Triage Guidelines Workgroup, "Utah Pandemic Influenza Hospital and ICU Triage Guidelines," 2009, http://pandemicflu.utah.gov/plan/med_triage081109.pdf.

19 Minnesota Department of Health, "Mechanical Ventilation Strategies for Scarce Resource Situations," 2010, http://www.health.state.mn.us/oep/healthcare/scarcevent.html.

goals.[20] As one philosopher put it, one's "dignity as a person . . . cannot be reduced to his past or future contribution to society."[21]

Instrumental value: The multiplier effect—Instrumental value refers to an individual's ability to carry out a specific function that is viewed as essential to prevent social disintegration or a great number of deaths during a time of crisis. It has also been described as "narrow social utility"[22] and the "multiplier effect."[23] Federal guidance on prioritization of pandemic vaccines adopted this principle by recommending that priority be given to individuals essential to the pandemic response (including public health and healthcare personnel) and to those who maintain essential community services.[24,25] The ethical justification is that prioritizing certain key individuals will achieve a "multiplier effect" through which more many lives are ultimately saved through their work.

Instrumental value must be distinguished from judgments about broad social worth. Individuals who have instrumental value for one type of public health disaster may not have instrumental value during another type of crisis. For example, vaccine manufacturer workers would not be prioritized during the public health response to a terrorist attack with chemical or nuclear weapons. Individuals are prioritized not because they are judged to hold more "intrinsic worth," but because of their ability to perform a specific task that is essential to society. In this sense, instrumental value is a derivative allocation principle; it is desirable because it ensures an adequate workforce to achieve public health goals. Even critics of allocation based on broad social value accept the use of instrumental value in certain circumstances.[26]

However as indicated previously, using instrumental value may be ethically problematic for decision making about allocation of ventilators. In general, to justify a restrictive public health measure, there must be good evidence that the measure is *necessary* and will be *effective*.[27] Most important, will individuals with respiratory failure who receive priority for mechanical ventilation recover in time to reenter the work force and achieve their instrumental purposes during the pandemic wave? Because of the uncertainty about which key personnel will be in short supply and whether they will recover in time to achieve their instrumental value, this criterion would likely be highly controversial.

The Life Cycle Principle

The life cycle principle grants each individual equal opportunity to live through the various phases of life.[28] This principle has also been called the "fair innings" argument and "intergenerational equity."[29] In practical terms, the life cycle principle gives relative priority to younger individuals over older individuals. The ethical justification of the life cycle principle is that it is a desirable as a matter of justice to give individuals equal opportunity to pass through

---

[20] J. L. Hick and D. T. O'Laughlin, "Concept of Operations for Triage of Mechanical Ventilation in an Epidemic," *Academic Emergency Medicine* 13, no. 2 (2006): pp. 223–229.

[21] N. Daniels, "Fair Process in Patient Selection for Antiretroviral Treatment in WHO's Goal of 3 by 5," *The Lancet* 366, no. 9480 (2005): pp. 169–171.

[22] The Keystone Center, "Citizen Voices on Pandemic Flu Choices. A Report of the Public Engagement Pilot Project on Pandemic Influenza," 2005, http://keystone.org/files/file/about/publications/FINALREPORT_PEPPPI_DEC_2005.pdf.

[23] Ohio State University, "Ohio Pandemic Influenza."

[24] S. E. Shortt, "Waiting for Medical Care: Is It Who You Know That Counts?", *Canadian Medical Association Journal* 161, no. 7 (1999): pp. 823–824.

[25] D. Sanders and J. Dukeminier Jr, "Medical Advance and Legal Lag: Hemodialysis and Kidney Transplantation," *UCLA Law Review* 15 (1967): p. 357.

[26] Hick, "Concept of Operations for Triage."

[27] N. Rescher, "The Allocation of Exotic Medical Lifesaving Therapy," *Ethics* (1969): pp. 173–186.

[28] P. Ramsey, *The Patient as Person: Explorations in Medical Ethics* (Yale University Press, 2002).

[29] J. F. Childress, "Who Shall Live When Not All Can Live?", *Soundings* 53, no. 4 (1970): pp. 339–355.

the stages of life—childhood, young adulthood, middle age, and old age.[30] The justification for this principle does not rely on considerations of one's intrinsic worth or social utility. Rather, younger individuals receive priority because they have had the least opportunity to live through life's stages.

Empirical data suggest that when individuals are asked to consider situations of absolute scarcity of life sustaining resources, most believe younger patients should be prioritized over older.[31] One advocate for a life cycle approach declares: "it is always a misfortune to die . . . it is both a misfortune and a tragedy [for life] to be cut off prematurely."[32] Prioritization based on the life cycle approach is not a simple linear function of a persons' age (that is, the claim of priority does not increase bit by bit as one ages year by year). Instead, this approach appeals to significant age differences rather than small differences of a few years.

Some critics contend that the life cycle principle unjustly discriminates against older individuals. However, others respond that this principle is inherently egalitarian because it seeks to give *all individuals* equal opportunity to live a normal life span. It applies the notion of equality to individuals' *whole lifetime experiences* rather than just to their current situation.[33] In their view, unlike prioritization based on gender or race, everyone faces the prospect of aging and everyone hopes to move through all stages of life.[34] However, when public input was sought in Seattle-King County on values and priorities for delivery of medical services during a severe influenza pandemic, most participants agreed that the number of years a person would live if they survive should only be a factor in the absence of other priority criteria.[35]

Fair Chances versus Maximization of Best Outcomes

Traditionally, public health emergency response has focused on maximizing population health, for example, through saving the most lives. However, some have challenged this assumption and have suggested that fairness considerations be more explicitly included in policy decisions, even if doing so does not maximize population health.[36,37,38] Conflict between providing "fair chances" and maximizing "best outcomes" arises when there are relatively small differences in expected benefits that may be gained by people in different prioritization groups. In the case of access to ventilators, if ventilators are provided only to people with the highest probability of surviving and denied to those with a somewhat less, but still significant chance of survival, then we may save more lives but we do so by asking some individuals to give up all chance of survival. Some argue that this approach is not fair to those who give up their chance of survival, even though more total lives are saved. Some propose an alternative approach (e.g., a "weighted lottery") to provide more people with a fair

[30] Ramsey, *The Patient as Person*.

[31] United States Department of Health and Human Services, *HHS Pandemic Influenza Plan* (Washington DC: US Government Printing Office, 2005).

[32] United States Department of Health and Human Services, *Guidance on Allocating and Targeting Pandemic Influenza Vaccine* (Washington, DC: US Government Printing Office, 2008).

[33] Childress, "Who Shall Live When Not All Can Live?"

[34] Ramsey, *The Patient as Person*.

[35] The Keystone Center, "The Public Engagement Project on Community Control Measures for Pandemic Influenza: Findings and Recommendations from Citizen and Stakeholder Deliberation Days," 2007, http://keystone.org/files/file/about/publications/FinalReport1_CommunityControl5_2007.

[36] L. O. Gostin, et al., "The Model State Emergency Health Powers Act: Planning for and Response to Bioterrorism and Naturally Occurring Infectious Diseases," *Journal of the American Medical Association* 288, no. 5 (2002): pp. 622–628.

[37] E. Emanuel and A. Wertheimer, "Who Should Get Influenza Vaccine When Not All Can?", *Science* 312, no. 5775 (2006): pp. 854–855.

[38] A. Williams, "Intergenerational Equity: An Exploration of the 'Fair Innings" Argument', *Health Economics* 6, no. 2 (1997): pp. 117–132.

chance at survival, even if it would not maximize the number of lives saved.[39,40] Objections to the fair chances approach include: lack of clarity and transparency about what criteria are being used to make choices and practical limitations in applying a complex, weighted lottery in an emergency setting. A deliberative public engagement process may be required to establish appropriate weights.[41]

Incorporating Multiple Principles

Because several different considerations for allocating ventilators during a severe influenza pandemic may be justified, some writers have proposed that several principles be combined into a composite priority score.[42] Although a multi-principle allocation system may be more complex to implement in a timely and practical manner than a single principle allocation system, it may better reflect the diverse moral considerations relevant to these difficult decisions. In addition, this approach avoids the need to categorically deny treatment to certain groups, a problem that one legal scholar calls a "political and legal minefield."[43] This multi-principle approach can take into account the degree of scarcity—patients with lower priorities can receive ventilators until no more remain. However, a multi-principle allocation approach that relies on a composite priority score raises difficult questions regarding what principles should be represented in the composite score and how to weight the various components that contribute to the score. People may legitimately disagree about the weights. It will be important to have a broad public deliberation about the various tradeoffs among the principles in order for such an index to be accepted as legitimate. The values and priorities of community members who will be impacted by decisions about allocation of scarce life-saving resources must be considered in the development of triage plans.

39 Gostin, "The Model State Emergency Health Powers Act."

40 Emanuel, "Who Should Get Influenza Vaccine?"

41 J. Neuberger, et al., "Assessing Priorities for Allocation of Donor Liver Grafts: Survey of Public and Clinicians," *British Medical Journal* 317, no. 7152 (1998): pp. 172–175.

42 Gostin, *Guidance for Establishing Crisis Standards*.

43 J. Harris, *The Value of Life: An Introduction to Medical Ethics* (New York: Routledge, 1990).

Further Resources

Relevant Organizations

Governmental

Advisory Committee on Immunization Practices: Provides guidance on diseases that can be prevented by vaccines to the Centers for Disease Control and Prevention in the US. Additional information can be found at http://www.cdc.gov/vaccines/acip/

European Centre for Disease Prevention and Control: Identifies, assesses, and communicates current and emerging threats to human health posed by infectious diseases. Additional information can be found at http://ecdc.europa.eu/en/Pages/home.aspx

National Vaccine Program Office: An office in the US Department of Health and Human Services that recommends vaccine policies. Additional information can be found at http://www.hhs.gov/nvpo/nvac/

Literature

Barry, John M. *The Great Influenza: The Epic Story of the Deadliest Plague in History.* (New York: Penguin Books, 2005).

Billings, Molly. "The Influenza Pandemic of 1918," *Stanford University*, February 2005.

"Drastic Rule in Chicago: Will Arrest Persons Not Using Handkerchiefs in Sneezing," *New York Times*, October 4, 1918.

European Centre for Disease Prevention and Control. "Priority Risk Groups for Influenza Vaccination." http://ecdc.europa.eu/en/publications/Publications/0808_GUI_Priority_Risk_Gr oups_for_Influenza_Vaccination.pdf.

Shanks, G. D., and J. F. Brundage. Pathogenic responses among young adults during the 1918 influenza pandemic. *Emerging Infectious Diseases.* doi: 10.3201/eid1802.102042. 2012 Feb, visited 2016 May.

Uscher-Pines, Lori, Saad B. Omer, Daniel J. Barnett, Thomas A. Burke, and Ran D. Balicer. "Priority Setting for Pandemic Influenza: An Analysis of National Preparedness Plans." *PLoS Medicine* 3, no. 10 (10/17 2006): e436.

World Health Organization. "Guidelines on the Use of Vaccines and Antivirals During Influenza Pandemics." http://www.who.int/csr/resources/publications/influenza/11_29_01_A.pdf.

Other Media

Cotillard, Marion. *Contagion*. DVD. Directed by Steven Soderbergh. Burbank: Warner Home Video, 2012: Access to a vaccine is determined via lottery, with doctors and government officials being exempt.

Pacino, Al. *Angels in America*. DVD. Directed by Mike Nichols. New York City: HBO Studios, 2006: Scarce resources of new drugs to combat AIDS were administered through carefully regulated trials and via prioritization.

Pandemic: The Case of the Killer Flu, Directed by Elliot Halpern, UK, February 4, 1999: Discusses the 1918 Spanish flu and explores what caused it.

Patterson, Bill. *Spanish Flu: The Forgotten Fallen.* Directed by Justin Hardy. *BBC Four*, August 5, 2009: Deals with Dr. James Niven's attempt to deal with the 1918 flu pandemic.

Part III

Relative Scarcity

Resource Allocation

8

From Rationing to Resource Allocation

Cases of Conversion and Historical Context of Efforts to Ensure Quality and Value of Healthcare

On November 24, 1971, Shep Glazer stood in a corridor of the US Congress, readying himself to testify before the House Ways and Means Committee. He straightened his tie and went over his notes. Then his doctor connected him to an artificial kidney machine. Shep Glazer suffered from renal failure. He was also the vice president of the National Association of Patients on Hemodialysis.[1]

In 1971, approximately 4,000 patients were being kept alive by dialysis.[2] However, dialysis costs were prohibitive for more than 8,000 end-stage kidney disease patients.[3] Hospital-centered dialysis cost $15,000–$25,000 per year, or around twice the median annual household income at the time ($9,027).[4] Home dialysis, at between $5,000 and $7,000 per year and $12,000–$19,000 initial investment for a dialysis machine, was less costly.[5]

Glazer's aim was to persuade the House Ways and Means Committee to cover access to dialysis at home for all Americans who needed it. Connected to the machine, and supported by his wife and a delegation of seven additional advocates of kidney patients, including a medical student on dialysis, he said (Excerpt 1):

> Let me introduce myself personally. I am 43 years old, married for 20 years, with

---

[1] American Association of Kidney Patients, "NAPH Testifies before Congress Shep Glazer Dialyzes," 1971, accessed June 16, 2015, https://www.aakp.org/education/resourcelibrary/ckd-resources/item/naph-testifies-before-congress-shep-glazer-dialyzes.html.

[2] Ibid.

[3] *Congressional Record*, September 30, 1972, pp. 33003–33008.

[4] *Background Information of Kidney Disease Benefits under Medicare*. Report to Subcommittee on Health of the Committee on Ways and Means, US House of Representatives (Washington, DC: US Government Printing Office, June 24, 1975).

See also US Department of Commerce, *Current Population Reports: Consumer Income: Household Money Income in 1971 and Selected Social and Economic Characteristics of Households* (Washington, DC: US Government Printing Office, 1972), p. 1.

[5] *Congressional Record*, September 30, 1972, p. 33004.

> two children, ages 14 and 10. . . . [I] have a major medical [insurance] policy [which pays for dialysis] but the funds [will] soon be consumed by the expensive treatments. . . . I was a salesman until a couple of months ago, until it became necessary for me to supplement my income to pay for the dialysis supplies. I tried to sell a noncompetitive line, was found out, and was fired.
>
> Gentlemen, what should I do? End it all and die? Sell my house for which I worked so hard, and go on welfare? Should I go into the hospital under my hospitalization policy, then I cannot work? Please tell me.
>
> If your kidneys failed tomorrow, wouldn't you want the opportunity to live? Wouldn't you want to see your children grow up?[6]

In October of the following year, President Richard Nixon signed the Social Security Amendments of 1972 (H.R. 1) into law, which included a section that provided Medicare coverage for all Americans who needed dialysis.[7] This approach is remarkable, not least because Medicare is a federal government-funded program that, at that time, only covered healthcare for people 65 years and older.

Glazer's intervention and the response it received was historic. Less than a decade earlier, only 1 in 50 patients could receive dialysis.[8] And, as noted in Chapter 4, hospitals such as Seattle's Swedish Hospital created committees to select patients for dialysis. Both the committees and the criteria they used were highly controversial. The decision to cover dialysis for all patients through Medicare ended the difficult rationing decisions surrounding chronic renal failure. But it also created two other problems.

First, a cost problem. Paying for dialysis has turned out to be extremely expensive. Today, there are about 525,000 Americans receiving dialysis that is paid for by Medicare under the End Stage Renal Dialysis (ESRD) program.[9] On average, patients requiring hemodialysis cost the program in excess of $80,000 per year for their medical care, while the cost is greater than $70,000 for peritoneal dialysis patients.[10] In 2012, their total healthcare costs amounted to more than $28 billion.[11] This means that about 1% of the total Medicare population accounted for about 6% of all Medicare costs.[12]

Then, there is a different type of selection problem. Why dialysis and chronic renal failure? Why shouldn't the government provide comprehensive coverage of treatment of cancer patients, or diabetics, or patients with multiple sclerosis? What is the ethical justification for selecting patients suffering from one type of illness but not other illnesses?

The example of dialysis illustrates that the border between cases of rationing and resource allocation can be fluid and that the nature of the ethical issues that are at stake can change from one sphere to the next. Before universal Medicare coverage for dialysis, rationing choices were inevitable, direct, and often tragic. Given that not everyone could be a winner, the issues were to select who would have access to dialysis and what processes and

---

[6] S. Glazer, *National Health Insurance Proposals, Part 7 House Ways and Means Committee, 92nd Congress* (Washington DC: US Government Printing Office, November 3, 1971), pp. 1524–1546.

[7] R. M. Ball, "Social Security Amendments of 1972: Summary and Legislative History," *Social Security Bulletin*, March 1973.

[8] S. Alexander, "They Decide Who Lives, Who Dies: Medical Miracle Puts a Moral Burden on a Small Committee," *Life*, November 9, 1962.

[9] United States Renal Data System, *2014 USRDS Annual Data Report: An Overview of the Epidemiology of Kidney Disease in the United States* (Bethesda, MD: National Institutes of Health, National Institute of Diabetes and Digestive and Kidney Diseases, 2014), p. 184.

[10] United States Renal Data System, *2013 USRDS Annual Data Report, Volume 2: Atlas of Chronic Kidney Disease and End-Stage Renal Disease in the United States* (Bethesda, MD: National Institutes of Health, National Institute of Diabetes and Digestive and Kidney Diseases, 2014), p. 326. *2014 USRDS Annual Data Report*, p. 184.

[11] USRDS, *2014 Annual Data Report*, p. 184.

[12] Ibid.

people (or groups of people) should make these decisions. Once dialysis became a matter of resource allocation, the central issues present themselves as less tragic but are nonetheless tough and pressing. Is the money used to cover dialysis well spent? While the benefits of dialysis to patients are literally of vital interest, they accrue only to a relatively small number of people at very high cost: would it be more fair—and efficient—to use the same amount of money to pay for other healthcare services for many more people? Even if we would not want to remove dialysis, related issues arise in a number of other contexts. For example, modern cancer chemotherapy can often extend life by a few months but can cost $100,000 or more per patient. Is this worth it? If we cover all such treatments, how can we control total health expenditures?

These considerations are, of course, not limited to cases where the government pays for healthcare. They arise for any system in which pooled funds are used to cover services for eligible populations, whether these are privately insured people, those with coverage through large employers, or those in countries that operate a choice of public insurance programs.

For a systematic decision-making process about whether or not to cover a particular intervention, three questions are fundamental: Can it work in principle (efficacy), does it work in practice (effectiveness), and does it provide good value for the money spent (efficiency)?[13] The first two questions are centered on ensuring that interventions confer benefit to patients by improving meaningful health outcomes such as quality of life and life expectancy. Efficacy and effectiveness considerations mattered at best in a peripheral sense in the case of rationing, where they are largely taken for granted. Intensive care units are clearly beneficial, as are dialysis machines for patients with kidney failure, and organs for patients in need of transplants (even if some patients may benefit more than others because of better basic health status or better organ compatibility). While vaccines for infectious diseases can differ in their effectiveness—for example, because they need to be tailored to each new strain of infectious agent—the central rationing question here, as for scarce ICU beds or organs, is who should have access to the intervention, given that not all needs can be met. In resource allocation, by contrast, efficacy and effectiveness can often not be taken for granted.

As Andrew Stevens, Ruairidh Milne, and Amanda Burls note (Excerpt 2):

> [m]any interventions are seen to be based on conventional wisdom rather than robust science, with perhaps only 50 per cent of health care procedures based on good RCTs [Randomized Controlled Trials]. (Some have reported a figure as low as 15 per cent, although the meaning of such figures has also been disputed).[14]

The existence of interventions with limited or no effectiveness is of ethical relevance in resource allocation decisions. First, it is unethical to expose patients to interventions that have no benefit, particularly where the interventions also entail risks. Second, paying for any intervention—even relatively low-cost ones—has opportunity costs. Covering an intervention with no or very limited effectiveness could preclude covering higher value treatments with superior outcomes for patients' health.

The field of health technology assessment (HTA) has emerged to systematically assess efficacy and effectiveness (and, as Chapter 10 sets out, in some cases also efficiency). Stevens, Milne, and Burls identify three major roots of HTA: empiricism, as it evolved in the mid-18th century; outcomes and variation research in healthcare, starting to emerge in the early 20th century; and pioneering work

---

[13] B. Haynes, "Can It Work? Does It Work? Is It Worth It?: The Testing of Healthcare Interventions Is Evolving," *BMJ: British Medical Journal* 319, no. 7211 (1999): p. 652.

[14] A. Stevens, R. Milne and A. Burls, "Health Technology Assessment: History and Demand," *Journal of Public Health Medicine* 25, no. 2 (2003): p. 99.

by Archie Cochrane and others in the late 20th century, leading to the increasing recognition of RCTs as the "gold standard" to determine effectiveness.[15] The authors suggest that the main forces behind increasing implementation of HTA are awareness about the limited available evidence, a significant rise in consumer expectations for better treatment, and escalating cost attributed to an "apparently exponential increase" of new interventions, higher unit costs of interventions that replace previously existing ones, and more acceptable intervention profiles associated with newer innovations that often make clinicians more likely to encourage tests and treatment.[16]

David Banta and Egon Jonsson trace the beginning of HTA to 1976 and the US Office of Technology Assessment's (OTA) report *Development of Medical Technology, Opportunities for Assessment* (Excerpt 3).[17] This, and subsequent OTA publications, focused on methods around determining efficacy, safety, and cost-effectiveness and "largely determined the general shape of HTA programs around the globe."[18] After a review of a number of mostly short-lived US technology assessment initiatives as well as international initiatives with similar mandates, they observe that despite the initial leadership and landmark contributions to the field, "HTA has not found a home in the US Federal government, especially after the OTA was abolished in 1995."[19] This has changed somewhat with the creation of the Patient-Centered Outcome Research Institute (PCORI) in 2010 in the Affordable Care Act.[20] Nonetheless, their overview illustrates the political nature of the generation, synthesis, and appraisal of evidence of healthcare interventions, an issue revisited in Chapter 10. The authors' principal conclusion is:

> A major challenge for HTA in the future concerns *impact*—to bridge the gap between evidence and health policy and practice. This may require some type of mechanism to hold decision makers accountable for making use of evidence.[21]

Rationing concerns cases of absolute scarcity in which tragic choices need to be made between people, given that everyone's needs could not be met. The case of dialysis illustrates that sometimes conversion is possible and that absolute scarcity—the defining feature of rationing—can be converted into relative scarcity simply by allocating resources to cover interventions for all in need (in this case, through political commitment). How to determine whether interventions represent adequate value more systematically is the subject of the following three chapters. Chapter 9 elucidates the basic elements of cost-effectiveness analysis (CEA)—the dominant overarching theoretical model for making coverage decisions—as well as some of its major criticism. Chapter 10 describes considerable variation between countries in implementing CEA and HTA, further illustrating Banta and Jonsson's observation that evidence from HTA alone does not guarantee impact in policy and practice, in no small part due to disagreement about how to resolve the value judgments that efficiency considerations entail, particularly CEA. Chapter 11 consists of four cases that illustrate the kinds of resource allocation decisions that are at stake: interventions for prostate cancer, colon cancer, Gaucher's disease, and HIV AIDS treatment.

15 Ibid.

16 Ibid., p. 99.

17 D. Banta and E. Jonsson, "History of HTA: Introduction," *International Journal of Technology Assessment Health Care* 25, no. S1 (2009): pp. 1–6.

18 Ibid., p. 2.

19 Ibid.

20 Note that PCORI's term is slated to expire in 2018 unless a law is passed to reauthorize the Institute.

21 Banta, "History of HTA," p. 5.

Questions for Discussion

1. If you heard Shep Glazer's testimony (Excerpt 1) as a member of Congress, would you have provided funding for ESRD?
2. When, if ever, should the government step in and earmark funds to avoid that rationing becomes necessary?
3. In their discussion of health technology assessment in Excerpt 2, Stevens, Milne, and Burls state that only between 15% and 50% of healthcare interventions are based on what is commonly regarded as the best evidence: robust randomized controlled trials. Why might this be so?
4. What is the difference between efficacy, effectiveness, and efficiency? Can you give examples of ethical questions that arise in determining each for given healthcare interventions?
5. Banta and Egon Jonsson argue in Excerpt 3 that although the principal benefits of HTA have been established, the main challenge is to bridge the gap between evidence and health policy and practice. They envisage "some type of mechanism to hold decision makers accountable for making use of evidence". What might such mechanisms look like?

EXCERPTS

Note: The following excerpts have generally been edited for length, and omissions are indicated with ellipses. Editing includes footnotes and endnotes, which have also been renumbered. For citation and related purposes, the full original source texts should be used.

EXCERPT 1

Abridged text from:

S. Glazer, *National Health Insurance Proposals, Part 7 House Ways and Means Committee, 92nd Congress* (Washington DC: US Government Printing Office, November 3, 1971), pp. 1524–1546.

Statement of Shep Glazer, Vice President, National Association of Patients on Hemodialysis

NAPH: Its Origin and Membership

The National Association of Patients on Hemodialysis originated in 1969. The formation of the organization was a natural result of something entirely unique in medical history: individuals facing a terminal disease were restored to life by a dramatic, virtually miraculous product of modern technology, the artificial kidney. The new life given to these individuals by hemodialysis and the problems the treatment presented gave them a common bond. . . .

Hemodialysis and transplant programs have given us the potential to maintain these persons in the mainstream of American life as breadwinners, homemakers, taxpayers and valuable members of their communities. . . .

What NAPH Seeks

NAPH seeks to attain for all Americans, regardless of income, status or other personal limitations, the God-given right to life, now available through advanced medical technology, which is presently denied to a majority of our citizens. . . .

NAPH's Comments

Why were 5,383 people allowed to die? They died because existing health programs have been proven inadequate. . . .

NAPH's Recommendations

We are here today before this committee, to implore you to legislate in accordance with every conceivable standard of justice, equity and humanity. We are here to ask you to give the American people a comprehensive health insurance program which will fully protect them in cases of catastrophic illness. . . .

A catastrophic illness is catastrophic only for those who cannot afford it. Despite the difficult life required of patients with kidney disease, over 5,000 dialysis patients have proven that if financial means are available, they can remain socially productive citizens. The inescapable fact, however, is that this treatment is beyond the reach of persons of average income. The cost of hemodialysis treatment ranges from a mean figure of $5,000 a year for patients on home treatment, to a mean figure of over $20,000 a year for institutionalized care. Initially, the hemodialysis machine costs between $2,500 and $3,300. But, the consumable products for each treatment costs approximately $85.00. The patient must have 2 to 3 treatments a week to survive. (Approximately 15 hours per week.) [The median income in 1971 was $9,027.]

A Matter of Economics

A national health insurance program will systematically lower these costs by inviting more manufacturers to enter the market place in the production of these vital products. This development would lead to expanded medical research, more employment and a new avenue for job training.

Ultimately, the treatment becomes self-supporting. By being able to return to their customary employment, patients can resume their role as taxpayers, circulate their money in the national economy and more than help pay back the cost of their treatment. A federal outlay might even be considered as a short term investment in human life with a guaranteed return.

Social Implications of Hemodialysis

Financial coverage for hemodialysis must be considered a priority. We are addressing ourselves to an issue that involved 50,000 Americans. . . .

A National Health Insurance Program for all would ensure the desired stability of the home life of these 50,000 individuals and their families. It would allow thousands of young persons afflicted by renal failure to realize their potential. . . .

Because of presently limiting finances, dialysis raises many moral issues. Selection committees are forced to choose who shall be allowed to survive. This moral dilemma can be eliminated. . . .

Mr. Glazer: . . .

Kidney disease is the fourth leading cause of death in this country; 100,000 people die from kidney disease each year in the United States. Ten thousand of these people could be saved if they could get artificial kidney treatments.

Kidney disease is unique because unlike other terminal diseases, for all practical purposes the hemodialysis patient can live a relatively normal life. . . .

But we live in constant terror that if these treatments are taken away from us because our money has run out, death will come in a matter of weeks. It is not easy to live with this thought confronting us each and every day.

. . .

There are many problems connected with hemodialysis, the most pressing at this time is the inadequate financial coverage for hemodialysis existing in this country today. . . .

We patients find ourselves confronted with the overwhelming thoughts of either dying or at best becoming welfare recipients.

Hemodialysis affects not only the patient, but the entire family. Not only can we not provide the basic necessities of life to our families but we cannot provide education for our children so as to insure their futures.

What NAPH is requesting in any future federally sponsored health program is the following:

1. Funds to train dialysis attendants.
2. Funds to make dialysis machines available to all kidney patients who need them.
3. Funds to make available the necessary materials to support the dialysis machine.
4. Funds to promote a donor program for patients who do not have access to a live kidney.

We feel that this country is morally obligated to its citizens to provide this treatment to all who need it.

That was Shep Glazer, vice president of the NAPH. Now let me introduce myself personally. I am 43 years old, married for 20 years, with two children, ages 14 and 10. I was a salesman until a couple of months ago until it became necessary for me to supplement my income to pay for the dialysis supplies. I tried to sell a noncompetitive line, was found out, and was fired.

Gentleman, what should I do? End it all and die? Sell my house for which I worked so hard, and go on welfare? Should I go into the hospital under my hospitalization policy, then I cannot work? Please tell me.

If your kidneys failed tomorrow, wouldn't you want the opportunity to live? Wouldn't you want to see your children grow up?

Just before our trip down here we received a letter from the president of the New York Blue Cross. I would like to distribute copies to the committee. I would like to read some passages for the record, and may I quote:

> ***we share their concern for the problem they face, the tremendous cost of maintaining a person with total kidney failure on hemodialysis.
>
> Such a patient is in a unique medical position. The machinery to keep him alive exists but the costs are generally prohibitive. Currently, there is no adequate program for covering the necessary health expense of appropriate hemodialysis.
>
> AHS believes the efforts of the National Association of Patients on Hemodialysis must be supported.
>
> We recognize that we can not do the whole job. The resolution of a health problem of the magnitude of that presented by personas requiring hemodialysis can be solved by the joint efforts of all responsible for financing health care.

The letter is signed "J. Douglas Colman," who is president of the AHS.

Statement of Mrs. Shep Glazer

. . .

The reality of the situation is that kidney disease is competing for the federal health dollar with heart disease, cancer and stroke—which cripple or kill 10 times as many people. Last year, the US Regional Medical Program allocated 26% of its funds to research in heart disease. 13% for cancer, and 12% for stroke. Kidney disease got four per cent.

"When you are dealing with bureaucrats, it's hard to make out a case for fund if the numbers aren't there," one doctor said. Moreover, the public knows comparatively little about kidney disease. Nearly everyone can recall a member of his family stricken or dying from heart disease, cancer or stroke. But far fewer people have had personal experiences with kidney ailments.

. . .

Given this low visibility, the federal agency responsible for coordinating health efforts on Long Island has yet to work out a master plan to expand dialysis facilities. "I wouldn't argue there is a need," said Dr. Glen Hastings, executive director of the Nassau-Suffolk Regional Medical Program. "The question is whether there is a need for these facilities in terms of costs and expenses? And should they be a first priority basis?"

What could be a higher priority item than a life-saving treatment? "Why don't you ask how come migrant workers can be denied primary health care?" Hastings said. "Let's ask how come there still can be malnutrition problems in this affluent area of the country? Let's ask why there aren't any comprehensive mental health services beyond the three western towns in Suffolk?" He paused, then added: "If you want to get morally indignant, I'll get morally indignant. But it goes far beyond renal [kidney] disease."

. . .

EXCERPT 2

Abridged text from:

A. Stevens, R. Milne, and A. Burls, "Health Technology Assessment: History and Demand," *Journal of Public Health Medicine* 25, no. 2 (2003): pp. 98–101.

Health Technology Assessment: History and Demand

Andrew Stevens, Ruairidh Milne, and Amanda Burls

. . .

Origins of HTA

The origins of effectiveness research in western medicine have usually been traced back to the "méthode numérique" of Pierre Louis in Paris in the 1830s and the demonstration that phlebotomy did not after all improve survival for patients with pneumonia.[1] The starting point can, however, plausibly be traced back another 80 years to mid-eighteenth-century Britain and the "arithmetical medicine" associated particularly with graduates of the Edinburgh medical school.[2] One of these, James Lind, memorably conducted a controlled trial of six different treatments for scurvy. Others have looked back to the book of Daniel in the Old Testament.[3]

At the start of the 20th century, Ernest Codman a Boston surgeon called for detailed follow-up of patient outcomes.[4] What is now called health services research dates back in England to the 1930s, when it emerged partly from epidemiological research, a classic case being Glover's findings of a 10-fold variation in tonsillectomy in England and Wales.[5] Glover's work appears not to have been taken further in the United Kingdom until a flurry of studies in the 1970s and 1980s demonstrating wide geographical variations in general medical admissions and in a range of operations (including tonsillectomy, appendicectomy, hysterectomy, cholecystectomy, prostatectomy and caesarean section).[6]

Such variations exposed uncertainty about the "appropriate" rates of a treatment in a population, which in turn raised questions about the treatment's effectiveness and cost-effectiveness. Such questions are best answered by randomized controlled trials (RCTs) and one of the most famous early RCTs, published in 1948, demonstrated the life-saving effects of streptomycin in tuberculosis;[7] but it was by no means the first.[8]

A more recent milestone in the effectiveness revolution was the publication in 1972 of Archie Cochrane's *Effectiveness and efficiency: random reflections on health services.*[9]

---

[1] R. Porter, *The Greatest Benefit to Mankind: A Medical History of Humanity (the Norton History of Science)* (W. W. Norton, 1999).

[2] U. Tröhler and Royal College of Physicians of Edinburgh, *To Improve the Evidence of Medicine: The 18th Century British Origins of a Critical Approach* (Royal College of Physicians of Edinburgh, 2000).

[3] A. R. Jadad and M. W. Enkin, *Randomized Controlled Trials: Questions, Answers and Musings* (Wiley, 2008).

[4] D. Neuhauser, "Ernest Amory Codman, MD, and End Results of Medical Care," *International Journal of Technology Assessment in Health Care* 6, no. 02 (1990): pp. 307–325.

[5] J. A. Glover, "The Incidence of Tonsillectomy in School Children," *Indian Journal of Pediatrics* 5, no. 4 (1938): pp. 252–258.

[6] D. Sanders, A. Coulter and K. McPherson, *Variations in Hospital Admission Rates: A Review of the Literature* (King Edward's Hospital Fund for London, 1989).

[7] G. Marshall, et al., "Streptomycin Treatment of Pulmonary Tuberculosis: A Medical Research Council Investigation," *British Medical Journal* 2, no. 4582 (1948): pp. 769–782.

[8] "Controlled Trials from History," http://www.rcpe.ac.uk/controlled_trials/.

[9] A. L. Cochrane, *Effectiveness & Efficiency: Random Reflections on Health Services* (Taylor & Francis, 1999).

Cochrane identified both the paucity of evidence of effectiveness for much health care at the time, and also strongly advocated the RCT as its solution. The 1970s also saw *Limits to medicine*, in which the Austrian Ivan Illich described the medical establishment as a major threat to health;[10] and Thomas McKeown's *The role of medicine*, which challenged the idea that major improvements in the population's health were due to advances in medical care.[11] Health economics as a distinct academic specialty grew steadily from the mid-1970s; and in the 1980s, research on variations in health care, successors to Glover's work, became widespread.[12] A notable example was the work by Wennberg et al. in the USA, demonstrating large variations in the rates of prostatectomy for benign prostatic hyperplasia.[13] Those researchers suggested that the existence of such variations meant either under-provision in some places and/or over-provision (and possibly ineffective treatment) in others.[14]

These pioneering perspectives provided the tools for the assessment of both new and existing health care technologies: scepticism, the investigation of variations, RCTs and cost-utility analysis. The most recent addition to the toolkit—systematic reviews—has dramatically accelerated the development of robust HTA. The need for reviews to be systematic was clearly demonstrated by Mulrow in her scathing assessment of the narrative reviews that used to dominate the review article in the medical literature.[15] Responding to this and other challenges, The Cochrane Collaboration has provided a world-wide lead in helping "people make well-informed decisions about healthcare by preparing, maintaining and promoting the accessibility of systematic reviews of the effects of healthcare interventions."[16] At the time of writing, the Cochrane Database of Systematic Reviews in the Cochrane Library (2003, issue 1) had 2796 entries. As a result of all this hard work, the systematic review, complemented with analysis of cost-effectiveness, has become the centre-piece of health services' increasingly voracious appetite for accurate information on the value of health technologies.

Forces for HTA

That appetite has been driven by a number of forces. The first is the widespread realization that many medical interventions may be under-researched and may not do more good than harm. Many interventions are seen to be based on conventional wisdom rather than robust science, with perhaps only 50% of health care procedures based on good RCTs.[17] (Some have reported a figure as low as 15%,[18] although the meaning of such figures has also been disputed.[19]) The long-term follow-up of outcomes has also demonstrated that unproven

[10] I. Illich, *Limits to Medicine: Medical Nemesis: The Expropriation of Health* (M. Boyars, 1995).

[11] T. McKeown, *The Role of Medicine: Dream, Mirage, or Nemesis?* (Princeton University Press, 2014).

[12] Sanders, *Variations in Hospital Admission*.

[13] J. E. Wennberg, et al., "An Assessment of Prostatectomy for Benign Urinary Tract Obstruction: Geographic Variations and the Evaluation of Medical Care Outcomes," *Journal of the American Medical Association* 259, no. 20 (1988): pp. 3027–3030.

[14] J. Wennberg, J. Freeman and W. Culp, "Are Hospital Services Rationed in New Haven or over-Utilised in Boston?", *The Lancet* 329, no. 8543 (1987): pp. 1185–1189.

[15] C. D. Mulrow, "The Medical Review Article: State of the Science," *Annals of Internal Medicine* 106, no. 3 (1987): pp. 485–488.

[16] "The Cochrane Collection," http://www.cochrane.org/.

[17] D. Sackett, et al., "Inpatient General Medicine Is Evidence Based," *The Lancet* 346, no. 8972 (1995): pp. 407–410.

[18] R. Smith, "Where Is the Wisdom . . . ?", *British Medical Journal* 303, no. 6806 (1991): p. 798.

[19] T. Greenhalgh, "Is My Practice Evidence-Based?", *British Medical Journal* 313, no. 7063 (1996): pp. 957–958.

technologies may not have their intended benefits (radical mastectomy for breast cancer,[20] for instance)—or even worse, do more harm than good (as with, dramatically, the thalidomide disaster[21]).

In 1992, the Department of Health published a landmark report on *Assessing the effects of health technologies.*[22] This proposed a fourfold classification of the use of technologies that is still helpful today. First were widely used technologies ultimately shown to be ineffective or harmful, such as the freezing of peptic ulcers, and the use of prophylactic anti-arrhythmics in myocardial infarction. Second, the report highlighted the sometimes damaging delay in the introduction of valuable technologies, such as tamoxifen in early breast cancer and aspirin following myocardial infarction. Third were new technologies falsely promoted over existing ones, such as routine use of tissue plasminogen activator over streptokinase in acute myocardial infarction and chorion villous sampling over amniocentesis. Finally, the report pointed to uncertainty about the value of technologies as demonstrated by variations in their use, such as prostatectomy and caesarean section.

Not only was there clearly a shortage of evidence in many situations, but also sometimes where the evidence had amassed there was a costly (in terms of lives) delay in its being translated into accepted "knowledge." A retrospective cumulative meta-analysis of therapies for myocardial infarction demonstrated in 1992, for instance, that there had been a 10–15 year delay between the sufficient accumulated evidence of the value of streptokinase and its acknowledgement in standard medical texts (review articles and book chapters).[23]

The second principal driver for HTA has been, of course, cost. Cost-containment has been a concern of the NHS virtually since its inception and in practice almost no technologies (except perhaps immunization) have ever been cost reducing. Cost pressures on health services come from a number of elements: general inflation in the economy, growing demand as a result of population ageing and changing expectations, altered methods of working and, notably, the impact of new technologies.[24]

New technologies drive up costs in three main ways. First, there is the impact of the apparently exponential increase in numbers of new technologies. Over the last three decades, this has been particularly visible with expensive diagnostic technologies (CT scanning, MRI, digital imaging systems, teleimaging), but for the last 10 years (and for the foreseeable future) disease-modifying technologies have also come to the fore. Some have been treatments for previously untreatable conditions (although their value has at times been questioned), such as donepezil in Alzheimer's disease and beta-interferon in multiple sclerosis. Second, the unit cost of the new technologies has often been startlingly higher than the treatments they replace. Selective serotonin reuptake inhibitors, for example, cost six times as much as tricyclic antidepressants;[25] taxanes are several

[20] Early Breast Cancer Trialists' Collaborative Group, "Effects of Radiotherapy and Surgery in Early Breast Cancer; an Overview of the Randomized Trials," *New England Journal of Medicine* 333 (1995): pp. 1444–1455.

[21] The Sunday Times Insight Team, *Suffer the Children: The Story of Thalidomide* (London: Andre Deutsch, 1979).

[22] *Assessing the Effects of Health Technologies* (London: Department of Health, 1991).

[23] E. M. Antman, et al., "A Comparison of Results of Meta-Analyses of Randomized Control Trials and Recommendations of Clinical Experts: Treatments for Myocardial Infarction," *Journal of the American Medical Association* 268, no. 2 (1992): pp. 240–248.

[24] D. Wanless and G.B. Treasury, *Securing Our Future Health: Taking a Long-Term View: Final Report* (HM Treasury, 2002).

[25] J. Mason, N. Freemantle and P. Young, "Articles–the Effect of the Distribution of Effective Health Care Bulletins on Prescribing Selective Serotonin Reuptake Inhibitors in Primary Care," *Health Trends* 30, no. 4 (1998): pp. 120–122.

thousand pounds per patient treated more expensive than previous anti-cancer treatments;[26,27] and two new drugs for severe rheumatoid arthritis—etanercept and infliximab—can cost nearly £10 000 per patient for every year that they are treated.[28] Third, many new technologies are less unpleasant for patients than those they replace, so lowering clinicians' treatment thresholds and encouraging patients to seek treatment, and thus increasing the total number of patients treated. The rapid replacement of open by laparoscopic cholecystectomy in the early 1990s is an example.[29]

The third driver for HTA has been the rise in consumer expectations and demand. This has been important both indirectly (by increasing the use of health care and so fuelling the pressures described above) and directly (as consumers have become more demanding, one of the things they have demanded is better information, to help them make informed choices[30,31]). This consumer demand for HTA is fairly new but will surely be of great importance in the future.

. . .

The Future

We believe that HTA is here to stay. The need to contain costs and to reduce unjustified variations in clinical practice and health service provision will mean that decision-makers need more, not less, high-quality information on treatments' impacts. Developments specific to the NHS may mean an even greater need for HTA. The UK government's commitment to NHS modernization and sustained increases in health service spending leads to the need to increase investment in treatments and services likely to be of benefit to patients. HTA should be a central mechanism for ensuring that this modernization has its desired impact.

---

[26] *Guidance on the Use of Taxanes for Ovarian Cancer. Technology Appraisal Guidance No. 3* (London: National Institute for Clinical Excellence, 2000).

[27] *Guidance on the Use of Taxanes for Ovarian Cancer. Technology Appraisal Guidance No. 6* (London: National Institute for Clinical Excellence, 2000).

[28] *Guidance on the Use of Etanercept and Infliximab for the Treatment of Rheumatoid Arthritis. Technology Appraisal No. 36* (London: National Institute for Clinical Excellence, 2002).

[29] A. J. McMahon, et al., "Impact of Laparoscopic Cholecystectomy: A Population-Based Study," *The Lancet* 356, no. 9242 (2000): pp. 1632–1637.

[30] J. Irwig, L. Irwig and M. Sweet, *Smart Health Choices: How to Make Informed Health Decisions* (Allen & Unwin, 1999).

[31] M. Gray, *The Resourceful Patient* (eRosetta Press, 2002).

EXCERPT 3

Abridged text from:

D. Banta and E. Jonsson, "History of HTA: Introduction," *International Journal of Technology Assessment Health Care* 25, no. S1 (2009): pp. 1–6.

History of HTA: Introduction

David Banta and Egon Jonsson

. . .

The Beginnings of HTA

The field of HTA was developed in a systematic way beginning in the US Office of Technology Assessment (OTA), which published its first report on the subject in 1976.[1] HTA began to spread to the rest of the world in the late 1980s, with the formation of the Swedish Council on Technology Assessment in Health Care (SBU). During the two decades since that time, HTA has spread to nearly all European countries, then to some of the wealthier countries in Central Europe, Latin America, and Asia. This spread has been facilitated with help from international organizations such as the World Bank and, to a lesser extent, the WHO. Also of importance here are the membership associations in HTA, notably ISTAHC [the International Society for Technology Assessment in Health Care] and its successor organization, Health Technology Assessment International (HTAi), and the INAHTA [International Association for Health Technology Assessment, now known as International Network of Agencies for Health Technology Assessment]. . . .

[1] Office of Technology Assessment, *Development of Medical Technology, Opportunities for Assessment* (Washington, DC: US Government Printing Office, 1976).

The early products from OTA shaped the field of HTA. The OTA had the opportunity of examining possibilities for the new field, focusing on methods and concentrating on efficacy, safety, and cost-effectiveness.[2,3,4] The key method for HTA involved synthesizing available information, which has generally come to be called "systematic review" by the Cochrane Collaboration and others. In addition, these initial reports examined health policies that might be influenced by HTA, or that might use HTA results in their decisions. These two critical issues largely determined the general shape of HTA programs around the globe.

An early result of these reports on efficacy and safety was that they encouraged the US Congress to develop the National Center for Health Care Technology (NCHCT), which existed from 1980 to 1982. This was the first national agency in the world to deal with HTA (formally speaking, OTA existed to serve the US Congress, not the general public or the Executive Branch of the US government). In several ways NCHCT was a pioneer during its short life, especially in advising the US Medicare program on technologies to cover. Other pioneering actions of NCHCT were to carry out systematic reviews on selected technologies, to develop methods for setting priorities between health technologies, and to begin to identify new and emerging health technologies as candidates for assessment.

After NCHCT was abolished, the Institute of Medicine (IOM) of the National Academy of Sciences decided to develop a national

[2] Office of Technology Assessment, *Policy Implications of the Computed Tomography (CT) Scanner* (Washington, DC: US Government Printing Office, 1978).

[3] Office of Technology Assessment, *The Implications of Cost-Effectiveness Analysis of Medical Technology* (Washington, DC: US Government Printing Office, 1980).

[4] Office of Technology Assessment, *Assessing the Efficacy and Safety of Medical Technologies* (Washington, DC: US Government Printing Office, 1982).

Council on Health Care Technology to serve in its stead. The Council performed several important tasks. However, it eventually did not attract sufficient funding and was also dissolved. The IOM has supported the development of HTA in various ways. In addition to developing the Council, a notable move was to form the Committee for Evaluating Medical Technologies in Clinical Use. The main output of the Committee was the development of a rather definitive book on the field of HTA, *Assessing Medical Technologies*.[5] Since that time, HTA has not found a home in the US Federal government, especially after OTA was abolished in 1995. However, several public and private sector developments that followed these events kept the field alive. The recent significant attention to *comparative effectiveness* in health care in the United States by the Obama administration indicates a much broader support for HTA in the United States.[6]

Consensus development conferences, an important activity related to HTA, also developed first in the United States through the National Institutes of Health. These began in the United States in 1977, and such conferences have been held since that time at a rate of approximately 5 per year.[7] The goal is to bring together various concerned parties—physicians, researchers, economists, epidemiologists, consumers, ethicists, and so on—to seek consensus on the scientific basis of the safety, efficacy, and appropriate conditions for use of various healthcare technologies. A panel of experts listens to presentations by leading medical researchers addressing a specific set of questions. After 2 days of hearings, the panel is sequestered to write a consensus statement, which is read the next day and associated with a press conference. In the early years of HTA, consensus conferences were organized by public bodies in several countries, including Sweden, Denmark, Finland, France, the Netherlands, and the United Kingdom.

ISTAHC and HTAi

Those working in HTA realized early on that HTA had to become an international field. By the mid to late 1970s, informal meetings were held with those who identified with such work. The OTA health program received a steady stream of international visitors, as did the Swedish Planning and Rationalization Institute of the Health Services (Spri). Exchanges between the two organizations became frequent, and in 1979, Spri sponsored the first international conference on HTA in Stockholm, involving individuals from several European countries and the United States.[8]

The expansion in international contact prompted many of those working in HTA to attempt to form an international society or network of people interested in HTA. The first meeting was held in Copenhagen and attracted approximately sixty people from sixteen countries. The success of this meeting was unexpected by most, but was encouraging for the development of a society. ISTAHC was founded at the Copenhagen meeting with Seymour Perry as president. The new *International Journal for Technology Assessment in Health Care* was accepted a few years later as the official publication of ISTAHC. After 18 years, ISTAHC was liquidated for financial reasons in 2003. At its height ISTAHC included more than 1500 members. A new international society, HTAi, was formed in 2003, with Chris Henshall as president. HTAi presently has approximately 1000 individual members. It holds annual meetings and recognizes the journal as its official publication.

---

[5] Institute of Medicine, *Assessing Medical Technologies* (National Academies Press, 1985).

[6] H. D. Banta, "Considerations in Defining Evidence for Public Health," *International Journal of Technology Assessment in Health Care* 19, no. 03 (2003): pp. 559–572.

[7] Institute of Medicine, *Consensus Development at the NIH: Improving the Program* (National Academies Press, 1990).

[8] Spri, "International Workshop on Evaluation of Medical Technology, Swedish Planning and Rationalisation Institute of the Health Services," *Spri* 3089 (1979): p. 1.

INAHTA

As national programs began to appear, the need for communication and cooperation at the agency level was recognized. Several international meetings led to the formation of INAHTA in 1993. INAHTA presently has forty-six members from twenty-four countries who work mainly on issues related to coordination of assessment, including carrying out joint assessments on occasion. These agencies are generally similar in the priorities they identify, the methods they use (mainly systematic review), and their relation to national and regional policy making. As increasingly better information has become available on the "value for money" of health technology, countries have become more involved in attempting to ensure that decisions are made with at least the input of HTA findings. An important example is the use of HTA as part of health insurance coverage decisions, which is a priority in countries such as the Netherlands, France, Switzerland, Spain, the United Kingdom, and some non-European countries, notably Brazil, Argentina, and Uruguay in Latin America and Taiwan in Asia.

. . .

The Collaboration

The UK Cochrane Centre was established in 1992 to facilitate and coordinate systematic reviews of (mainly) randomized controlled trials. That Centre became the first Cochrane Centre in what would become the worldwide Cochrane Collaboration. The development and growth of the Cochrane Collaboration has been of great value to the field of HTA, for example, in terms of methodological improvements in searching and grading scientific studies, in access to systematic reviews and other important information, and in fostering a broader understanding of the need for evidence in clinical decision making and in health policy making. More details on the events of its development are available at http://www.cochrane.org/docs/cchronol.htm.

. . .

Future

HTA has strong political support in many countries where agencies in the field have been established. This may be due mainly to the fact that resources for health care are limited. Hence, choices must be made, and rational choices need to be informed by evidence. The use of evidence, whether one calls it HTA, EBM [Evidence Based Medicine], scientifically based health services, or something else, has become an essential element in modern health care at the policy, administrative, and clinical levels.

It is likely that HTAs of the future will move more closely toward the idea of *comparative effectiveness*.[9] Many HTA agencies have been doing comparative effectiveness analyses since their inception, so the concept offers nothing new for them. Others, who are doing assessments by focusing on one technology at a time, will eventually recognize the advantages of reviewing and assessing all options concerning a specific technology, including health promotion and other forms of prevention. For example, to some extent colorectal cancer is one of the few preventable forms of cancer, but most published HTAs on the technology of screening for this condition do not include the option of prevention.

A major challenge for HTA in the future concerns *impact*—to bridge the gap between evidence and health policy and practice. This may require some type of mechanism to hold decision makers accountable for making use of evidence.

. . .

---

[9] D. Hailey, P. Jacobs and E. Jonsson, *Comparative Effectiveness—A Review of Definitions* (Edmonton AB: Institute of Health Economics, 2009).

Further Resources

Relevant Organizations

Governmental

Medical Services Advisory Committee: Provides advice to the Minister for Health in Australia on the strength of evidence relating to comparative safety, clinical effectiveness, and cost-effectiveness of new or existing medical services or technology. Additional information can be found at http://www.msac.gov.au

Nongovernmental

Cochrane: A nonprofit, international organization that conducts systematic reviews of healthcare interventions and diagnostic tests. Additional information can be found at http://uk.cochrane.org/

International Network of Agencies for Health Technology Assessment: Aims to connect HTA agencies to each other to support knowledge sharing and the exchange of information. Additional information can be found at http://www.inahta.org

International Society for Pharmacoeconomics and Outcomes Research (ISPOR): A nonprofit professional membership society that focuses on health economics and outcomes research, in addition to policy and education. Additional information can be found at http://ispor.org/

Literature

Cotter, Dennis. "The National Center For Health Care Technology: Lessons Learned," *Health Affairs Blog*, January 22, 2009.

Fields, Robin. "God Help You. You're on Dialysis." *The Atlantic*, December, 2010.

Hofmann, Bjørn Morten. "Why Ethics Should Be Part of Health Technology Assessment." *International Journal of Technology Assessment in Health Care* 24, no. 04 (2008): 423–429.

Kolata, Gina. "Ideas & Trends: Increasingly, Life and Death Issues Become Money Matters," *New York Times*, March 20, 1988.

National Institute for Health and Care Excellence. "NICE Technology Appraisal Guidance." https://www.nice.org.uk/about/what-we-do/our-programmes/nice- guidance/nice-technology-appraisal-guidance.

RAND Europe. "Analysing the Economic Impact of the Health Technology Assessment Programme." https://www.rand.org/content/dam/rand/pubs/research_briefs/RB9800/RB9800/RAND_RB9800.pdf.

Sullivan, Sean D., John Watkins, Brian Sweet, and Scott D. Ramsey. "Health Technology Assessment in Health-Care Decisions in the United States." *Value in Health* 12: S39–S44.

Theories and Principles of Resource Allocation

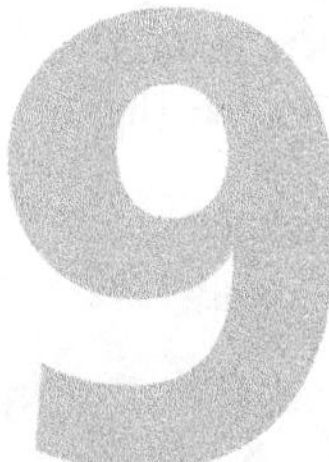

The concept of Universal Health Care (UHC) coverage was first endorsed by the World Health Organization in 2005, understood as requiring states to provide "access to [necessary] promotive, preventive, curative and rehabilitative health interventions for all at an affordable cost."[1] The health coverage cube, popularized by the World Health Organization (WHO), illustrates that coverage decisions require determinations in three interrelated dimensions: (1) how many people should be covered, (2) what services ought to be provided, and (3) what level of cost-sharing, if any, there should be (Figure 9.1). These three dimensions form the general background for resource allocation discussions and immediately raise the normative question of whether among the dimensions there is one that should have priority.

There is an increasingly broad consensus that the fundamental imperative is to prioritize leaving no one behind, and so discussions subsequently focus on the two other dimensions.[2] For example, the Lancet Commission on Investing in Health rejected expanding all three dimensions simultaneously and instead advocated progressive universalism by including "people who are poor from the beginning."[3] Similarly, half a century earlier, Aneurin Bevan, one of the architects of the British National Health Service (NHS) that was founded in 1948, observed in his book *In Place of Fear* that "no society can legitimately call itself civilized if a sick person is denied medical aid because of lack of means."[4] Currently, around 60 countries—just under one-third of the global total—have some

---

[1] World Health Organization, *57th World Health Assembly: Sustainable Health Financing, Universal Coverage and Social Health Insurance* (Geneva: 2005).

[2] K. Watkins, "Leaving No One Behind: An Agenda for Equity," *Lancet* 384, no. 9961 (2014): pp. 2248–2255.

[3] D. Gwatkin and A. Ergo, "Universal Health Coverage: Friend or Foe of Health Equity?", *Lancet* 377, no. 9784 (2011).

[4] A. Bevan, *In Place of Fear* (Ilkley: EP Publishing, 1976).

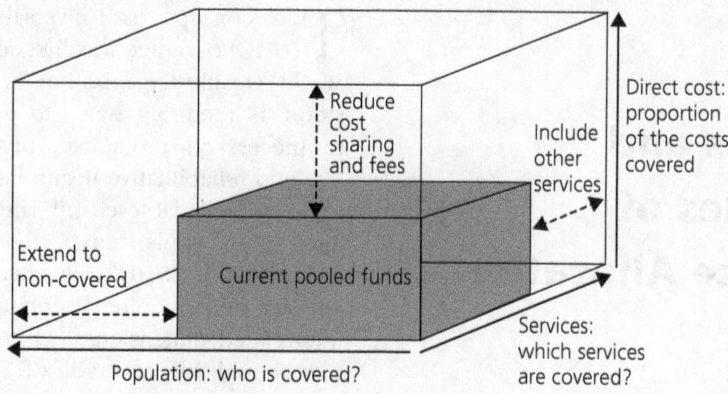

Figure 9.1 Three dimensions of health coverage.[5]

form of UHC.[6] The US Affordable Care Act of 2010 introduced an insurance mandate for all Americans along with structures to ensure affordable access for the first time. Following the inclusion of UHC as a target under the United Nation's Sustainable Development Goals[7] (successors to the influential Millennium Development Goals), increasing numbers of countries around the world are expected to move toward affordable healthcare for all.

With the moral imperative to "leave no one behind"[8] in place, the focus immediately shifts to the dimensions of service coverage and cost to users. In the words of Gro Harlem Brundtland, former director general of the WHO, "if services are to be provided for all, then not all services can be provided. The most cost-effective services should be provided first."[9] But what package of services would this comprise? And is cost-effectiveness really the right criterion to use for coverage decisions? These questions are of central relevance for countries striving for UHC, but determining value for money equally matters in settings where UHC is not recognized.

In the first excerpt of this chapter, Eddy advocates a cost-effectiveness calculation for determining essential health benefits.[10] "While few would debate the importance of benefits and harms [in determining essential care] some might object to including costs. But cost is the very problem that drives the concept of essential care. If costs were of no concern, there would be no problem; everyone could get everything that has benefit."[11] Eddy's approach produces the following formula: "Interventions that have great benefits, no harms, and low costs are essential. Interventions that have no benefits, or for which the benefits only slightly outweigh the harms, and that have high costs are not."[12] And the line between the two depends on value judgments. The value judgments, Eddy argues, should be

[5] World Health Organization, "The World Health Report 2013 – Research for Universal Health Coverage" (Geneva: World Health Organization, 2013). (First set out in: R. Busse, J. Schreyögg, and C. Gericke, "Analyzing Changes in Health Financing Arrangements in High-Income Countries: A Comprehensive Framework Approach" [2007].)

[6] Stuckler, David, et al. "The Political Economy of Universal Health Coverage." Background paper for the global symposium on health systems research. (Geneva: Health Organization, 2010).

[7] "Future We Want – Outcome Document," United Nations, 2012, https://sustainabledevelopment.un.org/futurewewant.html.

[8] Watkins, "Leaving No One Behind."

[9] World Health Organization, *World Health Report 1999: Making a Difference* (Geneva: The World Health Organization, 1999).

[10] D. M. Eddy, "What Care Is 'Essential'? What Services Are 'Basic'?", *JAMA* 265, no. 6 (1991): pp. 782–788.

[11] Ibid., p. 782.

[12] Ibid., p. 786.

based on patients' views on how to weigh benefits, harms, and cost. Eddy develops a critique for determining how to make these value judgments, taking the needs of average citizens, and based on the cost of care relative to median incomes:

> (1) [E]stimate the benefits and harms of the intervention, (2) estimate the costs in real dollars, (3) convert the costs into an equivalent wage, using the median wage as the reference point, (4) ask each judge if he or she is willing to pay that equivalent wage to receive the intervention, and (5) define as essential anything that the average Patient would want for himself or herself . . . if the average person would not choose an intervention for himself or herself, it need not be considered essential for others.[13]

Other approaches do not tie coverage as part of essential benefit packages to median incomes in the way that Eddy proposes but nonetheless seek to devise formulas that can quantify the balance of benefits and harms relative to cost. Cost-effectiveness analysis (CEA) is currently the dominant theoretical approach when formal assessments of the value of interventions are made. CEA is grounded in the utilitarian approach outlined in Chapter 3. Accordingly, the aim is to maximize overall utility. As Weinstein and Statson describe, utilities in cost-effectiveness analysis are typically measured in quality adjusted life years (QALYs) (Excerpt 2).[14] QALYs are a metric to value health outcomes; it is a composite measure that incorporates both quality and quantity of life. QALYs are expressed on a scale of 0–1, with 0 representing death and 1 perfect health.

The QALY approach has two main advantages. Regarding within-condition comparisons, it enables one to identify which of several interventions for a specific disease or condition, such as radiation or surgery for prostate cancer, generates the largest health gain relative to its cost. In addition, QALYs permit comparisons across conditions or health sector interventions, such as between cardiac, oncological, and mental health interventions, or between clinical and public health interventions.

Nevertheless, it is now also widely accepted that QALYs face methodological and value-based objections.[15] First, the metric treats an improvement from 0.1 to 0.2 as equivalent to an improvement from 0.9 to 1.0. But, from an ethical perspective, it is often argued that progress further down on the scale matters more and should be deemed more valuable, as Brock and Wikler discuss later in Excerpt 3.[16] Second, it is not clear whose preferences should be considered in quality-of-life assessments. Using the perspectives of patients, healthcare providers, or the general public can produce very different results. In particular, as Dan Brock highlights in discussing the concept of adaptation, people with disabilities or on dialysis often rank their quality of life significantly higher than nondisabled people who are asked to imagine living with the respective condition (Excerpt 4).[17] Third, QALYs and CEA more generally have been criticized because of their potentially discriminatory effect.[18] As Menzel and colleagues discuss, the focus on remaining years at a high quality of life can disadvantage the elderly, disabled, and chronically ill (Excerpt 5).[19] They illustrate this through the example of two groups of people who both require a life-saving treatment. One

---

[13] Ibid., p. 787.

[14] M. C. Weinstein, G. Torrance, and A. McGuire, "QALYs: The Basics," *Value in Health* 12 (2009): pp. S5–S9.

[15] M. R. Gold, *Cost-Effectiveness in Health and Medicine* (New York: Oxford University Press, 1996).

[16] D. W. Brock and D. Wikler, "Ethical Issues in Resource Allocation, Research, and New Product Development," in *Disease Control Priorities in Developing Countries, 2nd Edition*, edited by D. Jamison, et al. (Washington, DC: Oxford University Press and The World Bank, 2006), pp. 259–270.

[17] D. Brock, "Ethical Issues in the Use of Cost Effectiveness Analysis for the Prioritization of Health Resources," in *Handbook of Bioethics*, edited by G. Khushf (Springer Netherlands, 2004), pp. 353–380.

[18] Ibid.

[19] P. Menzel, et al., *Toward a Broader View of Values in Cost-Effectiveness Analysis of Health* (Hastings Center, 1999).

group was previously healthy, while the other was paraplegic (and will remain so if cured from the life-threatening condition). Both groups will not differ in their life expectancy if cured, yet, because of the lower base-line levels of health, conventional CEA would:

> recommend saving the first group, who can be returned to full health, before saving an equal number in the second group. It would recommend shifting priority to the paraplegia group only if the number of lives saved there at similar cost was at least 20 percent greater than the number of persons saved and returned to normal health.[20]

Perhaps most importantly, CEA and related approaches that seek to maximize total health are silent on how those gains in QALYs should be distributed. Specifically, CEA is neutral on whether a few people receive significant gains or many people receive modest gains. Weinstein and Statson[21] note:

> If the equitable distribution of benefits and costs across individuals or groups are of concern, a single cost-effectiveness measure will not do. However, as economists are wont to argue, over large numbers of programs and practices the inequities are likely to even themselves out and, with some exceptions, may reasonably be ignored.

John Harris[22] profoundly disagrees with this approach, arguing that maximizing health gains implies (Excerpt 6):

> the subordination of the health needs of individuals to something very abstract, and in some circumstances something very trivial indeed—namely, the improved health status of the whole community. For this could imply sacrificing the life of one person who was very ill and expensive to treat, if doing so would make even a tiny improvement to the aggregate health status, an improvement which no individual would even notice.

This observation is not merely a theoretical possibility but can arise directly as a result of specific applications of CEA, as Chapter 10 shows regarding the use of CEA in the real world to determine coverage decisions in Oregon. Harris is clear that CEA holds little potential, and he urges that health systems should instead "offer beneficial health care on the basis of individual need, so that each [person] has an equal chance of flourishing to the extent that their personal health status permits."[23] Menzel and colleagues focus on the special case of life-saving treatment in the face of death.[24] CEA typically would not favor costly interventions that only marginally extend life expectancy. Yet many peoples' intuitions support providing such treatment. Menzel and colleagues unfold several of the underlying assumptions that can be traced to the powerful concept of the rule of rescue, which is "rooted in the Kantian tradition of considering the individual to whom one is relating as an ultimate end-in-herself [and] resists the usual quantitative aggregation of economic analysis."[25]

Brock and Wikler contend that CEA can—and must—be combined with an equity approach.[26] They outline some of the central considerations in relation to prioritizing the worst-off because it is not straightforward to identify which groups of people should be considered worst-off and how much priority they should be given. They also highlight tensions arising from balancing fair chances and best

[20] Ibid., p. 10.

[21] M. C. Weinstein and W. B. Statson, "Foundations of Cost-Effectiveness Analysis for Health and Medical Practices," *New England Journal of Medicine* 296, no. 13 (1977): p. 718.

[22] J. Harris, "The Rationing Debate: Maximising the Health of the Whole Community. The Case Against: What the Principle Objective of the NHS Should Really Be," *BMJ* 314 (1997): p. 670.

[23] Ibid., p. 672.

[24] Menzel, *Toward a Broader View of Values.*

[25] Ibid., p. 9.

[26] Brock, "Ethical Issues in Resource Allocation."

outcomes in allocation decisions. CEA typically "ascribes a higher priority to those who can be helped more easily or cheaply. This thinking, in turn, implies that some patients will lose out simply because their needs are more difficult or expensive to meet."[27]

Clearly, the use of CEA is controversial, and there is no consensus on which approach should guide resource allocation decisions—or on the decisions themselves. Reasonable people can—and frequently do—disagree. One option would be to settle, once and for all, the question of what should be the right normative framework that serves as a foundation for allocation decisions. But, as noted in the discussion around political liberalism in Chapter 3, this has been an elusive goal in pluralist contemporary democracies. One influential response is to shift from substance to process by arguing that instead of seeking to achieve agreement on substantive ethical principles for resource allocation, the focus should move to agreement on fair procedures for decision-making.

Norman Daniels proposes the model of Accountability for Reasonableness (A4R) as a fair procedure to make allocation decisions (Excerpt 7).[28] A4R seeks to hold those limiting access to services accountable for the reasonableness of their decision. The idea is that justification for any allocation decision must meet four conditions. It must (1) be relevant to the decision, (2) be publicly accessible, (3) provide opportunities for appeals and revisions of policies, and (4) be enforced. Conditions 2 through 4—transparency, appeals, and enforcement—are relatively uncontroversial. Thus, the novel element—and the intellectual and ethical work—in A4R is Condition 1, the relevance condition. The relevance condition specifies that a rationale for limiting access to a health-care service "will be reasonable if it appeals to reasons and principles that are accepted as relevant by people who are disposed to finding terms of cooperation that are justifiable mutually."[29]

While A4R has been widely embraced, it has also been widely criticized. First, there is a concern that A4R provides no practical guidance, including a voting procedure.[30] Second, as Alex Friedman argues, the appeal to public reason and philosophically informed perspectives to resolve what weight to give to different ethical considerations seems too narrow (Excerpt 8).[31] A far wider range of views—including those of lay people—is plausibly relevant:

> [H]ow can a process that by virtue of its very nature excludes almost everyone from meaningful participation (from a very cynical point of view—everyone except the political philosophers who are proponents of such processes) confer democratic legitimacy on its outcomes? . . . many stakeholders in public policy debates might find reasons grounded in [Utilitarianism or Kantianism, etc.] not in the least bit compelling.[32]

Finally, while the approach may ensure legitimacy of decisions, it has been questioned whether it can be said to achieve fairness in any meaningful way. The very premise of the "presumption of undecidability" of allocation decisions has been challenged and criticized for prematurely relieving philosophers of their responsibilities to help solve difficult ethical choices.[33]

Despite these and further criticism, A4R has exerted considerable policy influence, not least because of the absence of an alternative. Accountability pressures in public

[27] Ibid., p. 264.

[28] N. Daniels, "Decisions About Access to Health Care and Accountability for Reasonableness," *Journal of Urban Health* 76, no. 2 (1999): pp. 176–191.

[29] Ibid., p. 179.

[30] A. Rid, "Justice and Procedure: How Does "Accountability for Reasonableness" Result in Fair Limit-Setting Decisions?", *Journal of Medical Ethics* 35, no. 1 (2009): pp. 12–16.

[31] A. Friedman, "Beyond Accountability for Reasonableness," *Bioethics* 22, no. 2 (2008): pp. 101–112.

[32] Ibid., p. 109.

[33] R. E. Ashcroft, "Fair Process and the Redundancy of Bioethics: A Polemic," *Public Health Ethics* 1, no. 1 (2008): pp. 3–9.

healthcare systems, such as the NHS, typically require decision-makers to be explicit about the normative foundations and operative principles that guide policy. But the criteria of private health systems, as found in numerous employer-sponsored health plans in the United States, are typically more implicit. While A4R's adequacy as a response to lacking transparency and accountability remains contested, its starting assumption—for better or worse—remains valid. To be ethical, coverage decisions of any kind require explicit justification of underlying criteria and, in particular, the use of CEA.

Questions for Discussion

1. Was Gro Harlem Brundtland, former director general of the WHO right in her observation that "if services are to be provided for all, then not all services can be provided. The most cost-effective services should be provided first?"
2. John Harris, a critic of CEA, argues in Excerpt 6 that health systems should instead "offer beneficial health care on the basis of individual need, so that each [person] has an equal chance of flourishing to the extent that their personal health status permits." Is this realistic?
3. In what ways does the QALY approach disadvantage the elderly, disabled, and chronically ill (give examples)?
4. The approach of Accountability for Reasonableness, discussed in Excerpts 7 and 8, has been criticized on a number of counts. Should it be abandoned? If so, what alternative approach would you put in place to guide resource allocation?
5. Menzel and colleagues (Excerpt 5) argue that the rule of rescue is rooted in Kantian philosophy and offers a powerful objection to CEA. Do you agree? How would you implement the rule of rescue in practice?

EXCERPTS

Note: The following excerpts have generally been edited for length, and omissions are indicated with ellipses. Editing includes footnotes and endnotes, which have also been renumbered. For citation and related purposes, the full original source texts should be used.

EXCERPT 1

Abridged text from:

D. M. Eddy, "What Care Is "Essential"? What Services Are "Basic"?", JAMA 265, no. 6 (1991): pp. 782–788.

What Care Is "Essential"? What Services Are "Basic"?

David M. Eddy

The concept is very appealing. It postulates that there is a minimum set of services to which everyone should have access, regardless of ability to pay. This set of services would form a floor for insurance policies, health plans, and government programs. People who want to receive more services could purchase them, either by buying more comprehensive (and expensive) insurance policies or plans, or by paying out-of-pocket. But everyone would at least receive this basic level of care. In the concept of essential care we find a compromise between the idealistic view that society should provide everyone with everything free of charge, and the practical fact that, as a society, we cannot pay the price of doing that. It strikes an ethical balance between society's obligation to the individual and the individual's obligation to society.

The concept is indeed appealing. Unfortunately, putting the concept into practice is far more difficult. Despite the fact that terms such as *essential care* and *basic services* come up in virtually every discussion of rationing, the uninsured poor, care for the aged, mandated benefits, and national health insurance, they have never been defined in truly operational terms.

The general principles have been well described. For example, Callahan[1] has written:

> *A "minimal level of adequate care" consists, first of full support for caring. . . ; second, of full support for those public health measures that promote general societal health as well as access to primary and emergency care; and, third, of access to more individualized forms of cure compatible with a sensible allocation of resources to the health sector in relationship to other societal requirements.*

General definitions of this type serve as useful guides, directing our attention, for example, to a balance between caring and prevention vs curing. But they leave unanswered the specific questions about just which interventions provide "full support" or are a "sensible allocation of resources."

Other definitions that do attempt to be operational usually end up defining broad categories of services. For example, the recent report of the Pepper Commission[2] defines the "recommended minimum benefit package" as:

> *hospital care, surgical care and other inpatient physician services, physician office visits, diagnostic tests, and limited mental health services (45 inpatient days and 25 outpatient visits), and preventive services including prenatal care, well-child care, mammograms, Pap smears, colorectal and prostate cancer screening procedures, and other preventive services that evidence shows are effective relative to costs.*

This type of definition *is* operational in the sense that a physician or administrator could determine whether an intervention was essential. But with the possible exception of the four cancer screening tests, which for unstated reasons are singled

[1] D. Callahan, *What Kind of Life?: The Limits of Medical Progress* (Georgetown University Press, 1995), p. 191.

[2] Pepper Commission, "A Call for Action. Final Report to the US. Bipartisan Commission on Comprehensive Health Care" (Washington, DC: US Government Printing Office, 1990), p. 61.

out for special mention, this definition is so broad that it is very unlikely to accurately sort out services that are truly essential in the usual sense of the word. Whether a service is essential appears to depend more on where it is provided, by whom and when, than on its actual value to patients. For example, an extremely expensive, very low-yield diagnostic test provided in a hospital would apparently be considered essential by this definition (because it is provided in a hospital), whereas a lifesaving antibiotic that could be taken at home would not. The definition does include a guiding principle for selecting preventive services ("that evidence shows are effective relative to costs"), but it leaves to others the task of determining what amount of effectiveness is worth what cost.

Defining Essential Care

. . .

The central problem that underlies the concept of essential care is that different interventions have different worths, determined by their benefits, harms, and costs. While few would debate the importance of benefits and harms, some might object to including costs. But cost is the very problem that drives the concept of essential care. If costs were of no concern, there would be no problem; everyone could get everything that has benefit, and the distinction between essential and "luxury" care would never arise. . . .

Whether an intervention is essential will depend on how the benefits, harms, and costs are weighed. Interventions that have great benefits, no harms, and low costs are essential. Interventions that have no benefits, or for which the benefits only slightly outweigh the harms, and that have high costs, are not. The central issue is where and how to draw the line.

This formulation of the problem has several implications. First, in order to determine if a service is essential, it is necessary to have some idea of its benefits, harms, and costs. . . .

The second implication is that the need for information about benefits, harms, and costs means that essential care must be defined at the level of particular interventions. "Hospital care," "surgical care," "diagnostic tests," and even "prenatal care" are far too broad to enable any useful estimates of benefits, harms, and costs. Furthermore, for many interventions it will be necessary to narrow the target to specific indications. Carotid endarterectomy might well be considered essential for a 65-year-old man with transient ischemic attacks, 80% stenosis, and history of stroke, but not for a 50-year-old asymptomatic man with 20% stenosis. For some interventions, it might even be necessary to identify a particular protocol. A Papanicolaou smear every 5 years is almost certainly essential; a Papanicolaou smear every 2 months is almost certainly not.

A third implication is that defining essential care will inevitably involve making value judgments. Sometime and somewhere, some group of people will have to compare benefits vs harms, and compare health outcomes vs costs. These three implications add up to the following: to determine what constitutes essential care, it is necessary to (1) identify specific interventions, patient indications, and protocols; (2) estimate their benefits, harms, and costs (compared with specified alternatives); and (3) weigh the benefits vs harms and costs.

Now let us assume that we have identified an intervention and have estimated its benefits, harms, and costs. . . . Suppose, for example, we are interested in a hypothetical drug that decreases the probability of dying of a myocardial infarction from 9% to 8% (an actual decrease of 1 percentage point, or 0.01), and that costs $10 000. The decision to cover the drug can also be viewed from the perspective of an insurance rider. A man or woman who has a five out of 1000 chance (0.005) of having a heart attack in the coming year would pay $50 (0.005 × $10 000) to buy coverage for the drug that would decrease his or her chance of dying of a heart attack by one in 20 000 (0.005 × 0.01). We now face the third step. Who should decide if this treatment is essential?

Who Should Decide?

Decisions about benefits, harms, and costs should be made by the people who will actually receive the benefits and harms and eventually bear the costs—that is, Patients. It is their lives and their money. The easiest way to appreciate that the choices should be made by Patients is to ask—who is in a better position to weigh the benefits, harms, and costs than the people who will have to live with the benefits and harms, and who will eventually have to pay the costs? Thus the general strategy is to identify some representative Patients (let us call them judges); present them with information on the benefits and harms of the intervention; tell them what it will cost them to receive those outcomes (being careful to construct settings in which the options, outcomes, and costs are realistic); and observe their choices.

This approach is clearly a good way to learn how people weigh benefits and harms. However, it faces a major problem in the evaluation of costs. Since costs are at the heart of any definition of essential care, this problem deserves careful thought. The problem is that the amounts of money that people are willing to pay to receive the outcomes of a health intervention depend critically on their financial status (eg, income and net worth). A poor person who makes, say, $5000 a year might well find $50 to be far too high a price to pay for a drug that reduces the probability he or she will die of a heart attack by one in 20,000. In contrast, a person making $300,000 a year might consider it a best buy to pay $50 a year to reduce the chance of a heart attack by one in 20,000. If we use the value judgments of the wealthiest people to define essential care, nearly everything will be essential—which is clearly not helpful (nobody except the wealthiest people will be able to afford it). If we use the judgment of the poorest people, very few interventions will be called essential—which fails to achieve our goal of providing an ethical floor for health services. What financial status should be used as a reference point?

To begin the discussion, let us suppose that we use the median financial status in the United States as the reference for defining essential services. . . . Thus, to be more specific, let us say that an intervention will be considered essential if Patients with median incomes find the health outcomes (benefits and harms) of the intervention to be worth its costs. Other cutoff points could obviously be chosen. For example, if a public debate reveals that we are inclined to be more generous, we can increase the level to say, 125% of the median income. . . . The median has a nice symmetry. It not only corresponds to the criterion we use for most other public decisions—majority vote—but it roughly defines the "average American."

. . .

One strategy is to index the perceived costs of the interventions to the income levels of the individual judges, using the median US income as the reference point. For example, costs could be presented in terms of daily wages. To keep the numbers round, suppose the median daily wage is $100. To a median-income person, coverage for the heart attack drug ($50) would cost a half-day's wage. This could be used to standardize the costs for people with different incomes. For example, a person who earned only $40 a day could be asked if he or she was willing to pay half a day's wage (which to him or her is $20). A person whose average daily income was $1000 would also be asked to pay a half a day's wage (which to him or her is $500). This strategy does not discriminate against gender, race, age, or any other factor that might be connected with income. In fact, it is designed to eliminate income discrimination. It is also important to understand that this strategy does *not* call for actually charging everyone a cost that is indexed to his or her income. Rather, this maneuver would be used only to learn the choices judges would make after adjustment for their incomes to make them "average."

To summarize, the steps for defining essential care that adjust for differences in income now become (1) estimate the benefits and harms of the intervention, (2) estimate the costs in real dollars, (3) convert the costs into an equivalent wage, using the median wage as the reference point, (4) ask each judge if he or she is willing to pay that equivalent wage to receive the intervention, and (5) define as essential anything that the average Patient would want for himself or herself. Others can no doubt improve on the details of this strategy; it is the principle I want to emphasize. The spirit of this proposal is much like the Golden Rule: Do unto others as you would have them do unto you. If the average person would choose the intervention for himself or herself, it should be considered essential for others. But if the average person would not choose an intervention for himself or herself, it need not be considered essential for others.

Design Issues

. . .

Most of these issues can be addressed using established principles from statistics. Two issues deserve special mention: (1) What if the judges are not unanimous? and (2) How do we deal with interventions whose outcomes affect different parties in conflicting ways? First, we can expect that the decisions of judges will rarely be unanimous. Suppose 37% of men at risk of heart attacks choose to buy coverage for the heart attack drug, while 63% decide that the coverage is not worth the cost. Clearly the degree of unanimity provides very useful information about the degree of "essentialness," as perceived by Patients. But some rule will still be needed to place this treatment on one side of the line or the other. The first step is to see if there are any identifiable factors that separate those who choose the intervention from those who do not. Perhaps there is some subgroup of people who have a different value system that must be respected. If that is the case, it might be possible and desirable to include those factors in the list of patient indications, and develop separate policies for the different groups of people. But assuming that no such factors can be identified or that it is not practical or ethical to separate people by that factor, an obvious strategy for resolving split decisions is to consider an intervention essential if it is chosen by a majority of judges. This not only is consistent with other public decisions, but maximizes the number of people who will be pleased with the results.

The other issue deals with judgments that affect different interest groups. Up to this point, I have tacitly assumed that the outcomes of interventions only affect the people who actually receive the intervention. In fact, many interventions affect several parties, in conflicting ways. A policy to isolate a person who has a highly infectious disease is an obvious example. From a purely selfish point of view, the patient who has the infection would say the harms and costs of isolation outweigh its benefits. But people who might be exposed to the infection would argue the other way. In problems of these types, both sides have reasonable and legitimate interests.

There are several ways to reconcile the interests of the different parties. One is to select a set of judges who are neutral in the sense that they do not represent either party. Preferably, they should be vulnerable to the possibility of eventually ending up in either party. These neutral judges would then be presented with information on the outcomes that affect each party *and* the probabilities that they (the neutral judges) might eventually end up in either party. Because the judges must face the possibility that they will be in either party, their interests will span both parties, and they will be forced to weigh the interests of both parties. This approach is a variation of the "original position" described by Rawls.[3]

When dealing with these or any other of the methodological issues, it is important to keep them in perspective. First, the definition of essential care is in its infancy. Our initial steps must be tentative, open to review, and eager for improvement. Second, it is quite likely that there is no single set of methods, much less a perfect set of methods, that will be applicable to all problems. Like experimental designs for clinical research, the appropriate methods will undoubtedly be different interventions, and will have to be tailored to fit particular problems. Also, like experimental designs, each method will undoubtedly have its strengths, weaknesses, and biases, and will require interpretation. Our immediate goal is not to be perfect, but to improve on what we are doing now. Given that, at present, there is no systematic approach at all to learning how Patients weigh benefits and harms, or how

---

[3] J. Rawls, *A Theory of Justice, Revised Edition* (Cambridge: Harvard University Press, 1999).

much they are willing to pay for health interventions, that goal should be easy to achieve.

Observations

First, this approach, which for convenience I will call "majority choice by average Patients," does not depend on or promote any particular mechanism for *financing* essential care. This approach could be applied in our current heterogeneous financing system to define a basic insurance policy, a basic managed care plan, or essential services for Medicaid and Medicare. Alternatively, it could be used to define a basic benefit package for a mandated employer-based program for the uninsured poor, or for a national health plan. This approach addresses the *content* of essential care, not its financing.

A second observation is that inherent in this approach, indeed inherent in the very idea of essential care, is that it is acceptable for different people to end up receiving different levels of care. The ethics of having multiple levels of care depends critically on where the levels are set. There is good agreement that it is unacceptable to have some people receive a very high level of care while other people receive virtually no care at all. However, there is also good agreement that it is acceptable to have some people receive a very high level of care while others receive less care, *provided* that the lower level of care covers everything that is essential. The majority choice of average Patients defines that lowest acceptable level of care to be that which an average American would want for himself or herself if he or she were paying the bill. By definition, if people with median financial stakes were offered a more comprehensive package (at a higher cost), they would turn it down. This is the basis for saying that this level satisfies essential needs. However, we *can* expect wealthier people to buy more comprehensive packages. No doubt several different levels of insurance and health plans would eventually be offered, and bought. It is even easy to imagine insurance companies and health plans competing by offering different levels of care, for different prices.

The third observation is at first thought startling. If this approach were to be used to define essential care, policies that will affect millions of people and billions of dollars would be based on the value judgments of a small group of judges, perhaps 50 to 2000 people. That seems like a very fragile basis for such a huge impact. Ironically, as fragile as that might seem, it is considerably more stable than what we do now. Currently, the great majority of policies are set with no explicit estimation at all of the benefits, harms, or costs of interventions, and no systematic exploration of how Patients weigh benefits, harms, and costs. Whatever the methodological flaws of defining essential care by the majority vote of average Patients, they are trivial compared with the methodological flaws of current methods used to set these policies.

Finally, this approach can be applied piecemeal—one intervention at a time—with very little investment, and without any major commitment to legislative change, financing, or even implementation. Whenever a new technology raises questions about benefits, harms, or costs, its outcomes could be estimated, a representative group of Patients could be identified, the questions could be asked, and the Patients' choices could be learned. Let's pick a few controversial interventions, try it out, and see what happens.

EXCERPT 2

Abridged text from:

M. C. Weinstein and W. B. Statson, "Foundations of Cost-Effectiveness Analysis for Health and Medical Practices," *New England Journal of Medicine* 296, no. 13 (1977): pp. 716–721.

Foundations of Cost-Effectiveness Analysis for Health and Medical Practices

M. C. Weinstein and W. B. Statson

. . .

General Analytic Approaches

Cost-effectiveness analysis and benefit-cost (or cost-benefit) analysis are two related, but quite different, approaches to the assessment of health practices. Confusion frequently exists between the two approaches, and many analyses that are technically cost-effectiveness analyses are often labeled "cost-benefit" analyses, and vice versa. The key distinction is that a benefit-cost analysis must value all outcomes in economic (e.g., dollar) terms, including lives or years of life and morbidity, whereas a cost-effectiveness analysis serves to place priorities on alternative expenditures without requiring that the dollar value of life and health be assessed.

The underlying premise of cost-effectiveness analysis in health problems[1,2,3] is that, for any given level of resources available, society (or the decision-making jurisdiction involved) wishes to maximize the total aggregate health benefits conferred. Alternatively, for a given health-benefit goal, the objective is to minimize the cost of achieving it. In either formulation, the analytical methodology is the same. First of all, health benefits and health-resource costs must each be expressed in terms of some common unit of measurement. Health-resource costs are inevitably measured in dollars. Health benefits, or health effectiveness, may be expressed in a variety of ways, the most common being either lives or life years, or some variant of them. The use of "quality-adjusted life years" has the advantage of incorporating changes in survival and morbidity in a single measure that reflects tradeoffs between them.

The ratio of costs to benefits, expressed as cost per year of life saved or cost per quality-adjusted year of life saved, becomes the cost-effectiveness measure. Alternative programs or services are then ranked, from the lowest value of this cost-per-effectiveness ratio to the highest, and selected from the top until available resources are exhausted. The point on the priority list at which the available resources are exhausted, or at which society is no longer willing to pay the price for the benefits achieved, becomes society's cutoff level of permissible cost per unit effectiveness. . . .

A limitation is that the benefits and costs to individual members of society need to be aggregated. If the equitable distribution benefits and costs across individuals or groups are of concern, a single cost-effectiveness measure will not do. However, as economists are wont to argue, over large numbers of programs and practices the inequities are likely to even themselves out and, with some exceptions, may reasonably be ignored.

The technics of decision analysis[4,5,6,7] are, in our opinion, essential adjuncts to either cost-effectiveness or benefit-cost analyses. Decision

[1] M. C. Weinstein and W. B. Stason, *Hypertension: A Policy Perspective* (Harvard University Press, 1976).

[2] J. P. Acton and Rand Corporation, *Evaluating Public Programs to Save Lives: The Case of Heart Attacks* (Rand, 1973).

[3] R. Zeckhauser, "Procedures for Valuing Lives," *Public Policy* 23, no. 4 (1975): pp. 419–464.

[4] H. Raiffa, *Decision Analysis: Introductory Lectures on Choices under Uncertainty* (Random House, 1986).

[5] W. B. Schwartz, et al., "Decision Analysis and Clinical Judgment," *The American Journal of Medicine* 55, no. 4 (1973): pp. 459–472.

[6] S. C. Schoenbaum, B. J. McNeil, and J. Kavet, "The Swine-Influenza Decision," *New England Journal of Medicine* 295, no. 14 (1976): pp. 759–765.

[7] S. G. Pauker, "Coronary Artery Surgery: The Use of Decision Analysis," *Annals of Internal Medicine* 85, no. 1 (1976): pp. 8–18.

analysis provides a cohesive framework for dealing with both uncertainty and complex value judgments, as well as the complex sequencing of decisions based on the current level of information. Since all these elements are usually present, the ensuing description of the elements of cost-effectiveness analysis includes many technics drawn from this field.

. . .

Cost-Effectiveness Ratio

The criterion for cost-effectiveness is the ratio of the net increase of health-care costs to the net effectiveness in terms of enhanced life expectancy and quality of life. The lower the value of this ratio, the higher the priority in terms of maximizing benefits derived from a given health expenditure.

The rationale for the division between the elements of the numerator (cost) and denominator (effectiveness) is straightforward. The former includes only resources drawn from the health-care budget: it describes the net change in the total number of dollars spent on health care as a result of the program or practice in question. The denominator, net health effectiveness, includes the life and other health benefits conferred, measured in lives, life years or quality-adjusted life years.

. . .

Discounting Future Costs and Health Benefits: Present-Value Analysis

Rarely do all costs and benefits occur at the same time. It is therefore necessary to combine present and future costs, as well as present and future benefits, in comparable units. One simple way would be to add up all dollar costs, regardless of when they are incurred, and all benefits, regardless of when they occur. This procedure, however, ignores the fact that a dollar in 1977 is worth more than it will be in 1978 or 2077. Present-value analysis is a widely accepted method of weighting future dollars by a discount factor to make them comparable' to present dollars. For consistency, the same discount factor should be applied to future health benefits (i.e., quality-adjusted life years) as well.

. . .

The reason is that a dollar not spent now can be invested productively to yield a larger number of real dollars in the future. Assuming an annual return of 5%, it follows that $X spent n years hence should be valued in present terms as $\$X/(1.05)^n$ because this quantity invested at 5% would yield $X in n years.

. . .

Currently, economists espouse discount rates, after correcting for inflation, of as high as 10% (the rate used by the United States Office of Management and Budget, subject to much criticism) or as low as 0 (or negative) per cent; most consensus lies between 4 and 6%. In any cost-effectiveness or benefit-cost analysis, a range of discount rates should be tested.

On the health-benefit side, the use of discounting requires more justification. For programs involving screening for disease, where the life years saved are far in the future, it matters a great deal whether expected benefits are discounted. Without discounting, a program that saves one quality-adjusted life year 40 years hence at a present-value cost of $10,000 would have a cost-effectiveness ratio of $10,000 per QALY. With discounting at 5% per year, the present value of that future QALY is reduced to $1/(1.05)^n$ or about 0.14, and the ratio becomes $70,000 per QALY, a remarkable difference in the implied priority of the program in the range of possible alternative uses of health resources.

The reason for discounting future life years saved is not that life years can, in any sense, be invested to yield more life years as dollars can be invested to yield more dollars. Nor is it necessary to assume that life years in the future, are less valuable than life years today in any absolute utilitarian sense. Rather, the reason for discounting future life years is precisely that they are being valued relative to dollars and, since a dollar in the future is discounted relative to a present dollar, so must a life year in the future be discounted relative to a present dollar. . . .

Conclusions on the Value and Application of Cost-Effectiveness Analysis in Health Care

The principal value of formal cost-effectiveness analysis in health care is that it forces one to be explicit about the beliefs and values that underlie allocation decisions. Opposing points of view can be clarified in terms of specific disagreements over assumptions, probability estimates or value tradeoffs.

Cost-effectiveness analysis often takes the societal point of view and is therefore directed at decision makers who act as agents for society as a whole. Nevertheless, the basic analytic framework should be useful to a variety of decision makers, who may include in the definitions of cost and benefit whatever elements they perceive to be within their domain. . . .

To facilitate such analyses, better data on the efficacy and costs of health practices are urgently needed. Application of the resource-allocation perspective, even with currently available data, can point to the kinds of data needed and the form in which they should be collected. The design of clinical trials and observational studies should take this perspective into account.

. . . Resource-allocation decisions do have to be made, and the choice is often between relying upon a responsible analysis, with all its imperfections, and no analysis at all. The former, in these times of increasingly complex decisions, difficult tradeoffs and limited resources, is by far the preferred choice.

EXCERPT 3

Abridged text from:
D. W. Brock and D. Wikler, "Ethical Issues in Resource Allocation, Research, and New Product Development," in *Disease Control Priorities in Developing Countries, 2nd Edition*, edited by D. Jamison, et al. (Washington, DC: Oxford University Press and The World Bank, 2006), pp. 259–270.

Ethical Issues in Resource Allocation, Research, and New Product Development

Dan W. Brock and Daniel Wikler

. . .

It is now widely recognized that CEA alone is not a satisfactory guide to resource allocation in all cases. CEA, as customarily formulated, measures the sum of costs and benefits and largely ignores the pattern of their distribution across the affected population. In some cases, the resulting allocation will strike most observers as unfair. Health resource allocators need to take distributional issues into account along with cost-effectiveness.

Priority to the Worst Off. Justice requires a special concern for the worst off, as is reflected in aphorisms such as "you can tell the justice of a society by how it treats its least well-off members," in the well-known Difference Principle in John Rawls's theory of justice, and by the special concern for the poor within many religious traditions.[1,2] This concern is often understood to reflect a concern for equality—in particular, equality in outcomes or welfare between people. . . .

A number of possible lines of reasoning support prioritarianism [that is, giving priority to the worst off or poorest members of society]. For example, the worse off that people are, the greater is the relative improvement that a given size of benefit will provide them, so the more the benefit may matter to them. Alternatively, the greater the undeserved health deprivation or need that an individual suffers, the greater is the moral claim to have it alleviated or met.

However priority to the worst off is justified, an important issue is who the worst off are. In the context of resource allocation in health care, the worst off might be those who are globally worst off, those with the worst overall well-being (such as the poor), or those with the worst health (that is, the sickest). General theories of justice usually focus on people's overall well-being, often allowing a lower level in one domain of well-being to be compensated for by a higher level in another domain. However, there are both moral and pragmatic reasons for what has been called a *separate spheres view*, according to which the worst off for the purpose of health resource allocation should be considered to be those with worse health. Morally, for example, Scanlon has argued that "for differences in level to affect the relative strength of people's claims to help, these differences have to be in an aspect of welfare that the help in question will contribute to."[3] Pragmatically, it may generally be too difficult, costly, intrusive, and controversial, as well as too subject to mistake and abuse, to have to inquire into all aspects of people's overall levels of well-being.

Even if health allocation to the worst off should be based on levels of health, other issues remain. For example, are those with worse health those who are sickest now, at the time a health intervention would be provided for them, or those with worse health over time, taking into account past and perhaps expected future health? The latter would give special weight to meeting the health needs of those with long-term chronic diseases and disabilities. Separate spheres would still include past and

---

[1] D. W. Brock, "Priority to the Worst Off in Health Care Prioritization," in *Medicine and Social Justice*, edited by M. Battin, R. Rhodes, and A. Silvers (New York: Oxford University Press, 2002).

[2] J. Rawls, *A Theory of Justice* (Cambridge: Harvard University Press, 1971).

[3] T. Scanlon, *What We Owe to Each Other* (Cambridge: Harvard University Press, 1997), p. 227.

future health. Should special priority also be given to those whose health is not worse now but is especially vulnerable to becoming worse?

Finally, how much priority should the worst off receive? Giving absolute priority to the worst off is implausible because it faces the bottomless pit problem—using very great amounts of resources to produce very limited or marginal gains in the health-related quality of life of the severely ill or disabled. However, there is no apparent principled basis for determining how much priority the worst off should receive.

. . .

Fair Chances and Best Outcomes. The thesis that resources should be targeted to interventions in which they will do the most good ascribes a higher priority to those who can be helped more easily or cheaply. This thinking, in turn, implies that some patients will lose out simply because their needs are more difficult or expensive to meet. Consider, for example, a ward with 100 patients, 50 of whom require one pill and 50 of whom require two pills to recover. The patients are otherwise similar. The clinic has 50 pills and must decide how to distribute them. To achieve the best outcome, all 50 pills should be given to the patients who need only one to recover. However, to give each patient an equal chance to recover, entitlement to treatment should be awarded randomly. Seventeen fewer cures would result.

Limited surveys indicate a sharp difference between health professionals and the general public in their responses to this conflict. Most health professionals favor distribution to one-pill patients only, and most members of the general public insist that people should not be penalized for needing two pills.[4] This division of opinion goes to the heart of CEA, which is precisely a guide to identifying the route to the best outcomes that can be hoped for with existing resources. It also creates a dilemma for those health professionals who maintain that health policy should be based on values most frequently endorsed by the population affected.

The conflict between fair chances and best outcomes arises not only from differences in the costs of treating otherwise similar groups of patients, but also when one group of patients will receive somewhat greater benefits than another at the same cost. The appeal of a fair-chances solution is greater when the difference in cost-effectiveness between the two programs is relatively small compared with the potential gain or loss to individual patients. Suppose that health program A will produce 5,000 QALYs while program B will produce 4,500 QALYs and that the effect on the health or life of each patient served is large—in the extreme, life saving. Patients who would be served by program B could complain that it is not fair that all the resources go to program A and none to B when they have nearly as pressing health needs and would be benefited by treatment nearly as much as the patients served by program A. If all cannot be treated, they might go on to argue, they deserve a fair chance to have their needs met rather than having no chance for treatment only because treating them would produce slightly less benefit than treating the patients served by program A. The small difference in benefits produced for the two groups—for example, a slightly greater life expectancy or more serious disability averted in program A—they argue, is too small to justify the tremendous difference in how the two groups are treated. In the extreme case, some live and others die. The better outcome is produced by funding program A rather than program B, but that additional good is insufficient to justify morally the huge difference in the way the two groups of patients are treated. The conflict between fair chances and best outcomes can arise in a variety of contexts.[5]

Preferring the most cost-effective program can also seem unfair because it compounds existing unfair inequalities. For example, screening slum-dwelling black men for hypertension targets the group with the highest incidence and greatest risk of premature death. However, it is more cost-effective to target

[4] E. Nord, *Cost-Value Analysis in Health Care: Making Sense out of QALYS* (Cambridge University Press, 1999).

[5] F. M. Kamm, *Morality, Mortality: Death and Whom to Save from It* (Oxford University Press, 1998).

well-to-do suburban white men, because they have more ordered lives, comply better, have personal doctors and the means to obtain medical services, are more educated, and are more likely to modify their lifestyles wisely. However, if the poor black men are not screened for this reason, it only compounds their existing unjust deprivation and, of course, is also in conflict with giving priority to the worst off.

If those who need a less cost-effective program deserve a fair chance to have their needs met, what would be a fair chance? Some argue that a fair chance is an equal chance, so some random method of selecting which program to fund should be used.[6] Others suggest proportional chances or a weighted lottery, in which the chance of each program being selected is proportional to the amount of health benefit each would produce, as a way of balancing fair chances against best outcomes.[7] Alternatively, some resources might go to each program (which is usually possible at the macro level), thereby benefiting some patients in each group—at least if their relative benefits are not strikingly dissimilar—instead of all going to the most cost-effective programs.

Another consideration supports spreading some resources to less cost-effective programs instead of devoting them all to the most cost-effective: to give all—or at least more—patients a reason to hope that their health needs will be met. This consideration may be especially important in developing countries where resource scarcity is more severe and adhering strictly to cost-effectiveness criteria could result in large numbers of patients with serious—or even life-threatening—health needs having no hope that their needs will be met.

. . .

[6] J. Broome. *Fairness*. In *Proceedings of the Aristotelian Society*. (JSTOR, 1990).

[7] D. W. Brock, "Ethical Issues in Recipient Selection for Organ Transplantation," in *Organ Substitution Technology: Ethical, Legal, and Public Policy Issues*, edited by D. Mathieu (Boulder and London: Westview Press, 1988).

EXCERPT 4

Abridged text from:

D. Brock, "Ethical Issues in the Use of Cost Effectiveness Analysis for the Prioritization of Health Resources," in *Handbook of Bioethics*, edited by G. Khushf (Springer Netherlands, 2004), pp. 353–380. Republished with kind permission of Springer Science + Business Media.

Ethical Issues in the Use of Cost-Effectiveness Analysis for the Prioritization of Health Care Resources

Dan W. Brock

. . .

First Issue: How Should States of Health and Disability Be Evaluated?

. . .

A central issue concerning whose evaluations of different states of disability or functional limitation should be used arises from the typical responses of individuals to becoming disabled: adaptation, that is improving one's functional performance through learning and skills development, coping, that is altering one's expectations for performance so as to reduce the self-perceived gap between them and one's actual performance; and adjustment, that is altering one's life plans to give greater importance to activities in which performance is not diminished by disability.[1] The result is that the disabled who have gone through these processes often report less distress and limitation of opportunity and a higher quality of life with their disability than the non disabled in evaluating the same condition. If the evaluations of disability states by the non disabled are used for ranking different states of health and disability, then disabilities will be ranked as more serious health needs, but these rankings are open to the charge that they are distorted by the ignorance of the evaluators of what it is like to live with the conditions in question. Moreover, those valuations will assign less value to extending the lives of persons with disabilities. If the evaluations of the disabled themselves are used, however, the rankings are open to the charge that they reflect a different distortion by unjustifiably underestimating the burden of the disability because of the process of adaptation, coping, and adjustment that the disabled person has undergone. Moreover, they will assign less value to prevention or rehabilitation for disability because of the results of this process. The problem here is to determine an appropriate evaluative standpoint for ranking the importance of different disabilities which avoids these potential distortions.[2]

Since the preferences for different states of disability or [Health Related Quality of Life] HRQL used to determine their relative values should be informed preferences, it is natural to think that the preferences of those who actually experience the disabilities should be used. Because they should have a more informed understanding of what it is actually like to live with the particular disability in question, we can hope to avoid uninformed evaluations. But this is to miss the deeper nature of the problem caused by adaptation, coping, and adjustment to disabilities.

Fundamental to understanding the difficulty posed by adaptation, coping, and adjustment to disabilities for preference evaluation of HRQL with various disabilities is that neither the non-disabled nor the disabled need have made any

[1] C. J. L. Murray, "Rethinking DALYS," in *The Global Burden of Disease: A Comprehensive Assessment of Mortality and Disability from Diseases, Injuries, and Risk Factors in 1990 and Projected to 2020*, edited by C. J. L. Murray and A. D. Lopez (Cambridge, MA: World Health Organization and Harvard University Press, 1996).

[2] D. W. Brock, "Justice and the Ada: Does Prioritizing and Rationing Health Care Discriminate against the Disabled?", *Social Philosophy and Policy* 12, no. 02 (1995): pp. 159–185.

mistake in their different evaluations of quality of life with that disability. They arrive at different evaluations of the quality of life with that disability because they use different evaluative standpoints as a result of the disabled person's adaptation, coping, and adjustment. Disabled persons who have undergone this process can look back and see that before they became disabled they too would have evaluated the quality of life with that disability as nondisabled people now do. But this provides no basis for concluding that their pre-disability evaluation of the quality of life with that disability was mistaken, and so in turn no basis for discounting or discarding it because mistaken. The problem that I call the perspectives problem is that the nondisabled and the disabled evaluate the quality of life with the disability from two different evaluative perspectives, neither of which is mistaken. It might seem tempting to use the non-disabled's preferences for assessing the importance of prevention or rehabilitation programs, but the disabled's preferences for assessing the importance of life-sustaining treatments for the disabled, but this ignores the necessity of a single unified perspective in order to compare the relative benefits from, and prioritize, the full range of different health interventions.

Moreover, what weight to give to the results of coping with one's condition may depend on the causes of that condition, for example disease or injury that are no one's fault as opposed to unjust social conditions. Most measures of HRQL include some measure of subjective satisfaction or distress, a factor that is importantly influenced by people's expectations. In a society which has long practiced systematic discrimination against women, for example, women may not be dissatisfied with their unjustly disadvantaged state, including the health differences that result from that discrimination. The fact that victims are sufficiently oppressed that they accept an injustice as natural and cope with it by reducing their expectations and adjusting their life plans should not make its effects less serious, as measures of HRQL with a subjective satisfaction or distress component would imply.

When measures like the [Health Utility Index] HUI or [Quality of Wellbeing] QWB are applied across different economic, ethnic, cultural, and social groups, the meaningful states of health and disability and their importance in different groups may vary greatly; for example, in a setting in which most work is manual labor limitations in physical functioning will have greater importance than it does in a setting in which most individuals are engaged in non physical, knowledge-based occupations, where certain cognitive disabilities are of greater importance. Different evaluations of health conditions and disabilities as seem to be necessary for groups with significantly different relative needs for different functional abilities, but then cross-group comparisons of health and disability, and of the relative value of health interventions, in those different groups will not be possible. The health program benefits will have been measured on two different and apparently incommensurable valuational scales. These differences will be magnified when summary measures of population health are employed for international comparisons across very disparate countries.

Some of this variability of perspective may be avoided by a focus on the evaluation of disability instead of handicap, as these are traditionally distinguished, such as in the 1980 International Classification of Impairments, Disabilities and Handicaps (ICIDH)[3], The ICIDH understands disabilities as "any restriction or lack (resulting from an impairment) of ability to perform an activity in the manner or within the range considered normal for a human being," whereas handicap is "a disadvantage for a given individual, resulting from an impairment or disability, that limits or prevents the fulfillment of a role that is normal (depending on age, sex, and social and cultural factors) for that individual." There will be greater variability between individuals, groups, and cultures in the relative importance of handicaps than of disabilities since handicaps take account of differences in individuals' roles and social conditions that disabilities do

[3] World Health Organization, "International Classification of Impairments, Disabilities, and Handicaps: A Manual of Classification Relating to the Consequences of Disease, Published in Accordance with Resolution WHA29. 35 of the Twenty-Ninth World Health Assembly, May 1976" (1980).

not. But it is problematic whether these differences should be ignored in prioritizing health resources for individuals, groups, and societies, that is, whether disabilities or handicaps are the correct focus for evaluation.

. . .

Conclusion

I have distinguished . . . issues about equity and justice that arise in the construction and use of cost effectiveness analysis to minimize the burdens of disease and to maximize health outcomes. . . . The concern for equity is in my view valid and warrants some constraints on a goal of unqualified maximization of health outcomes. [M]y point has been that there are important ethical and value choices to be made in constructing and using the measures; the choices are not merely technical, empirical, or economic, but moral and value choices as well. Each requires explicit attention by health policy makers using CEA. . . .

EXCERPT 5

Abridged text from:

P. Menzel, et al., *Toward a Broader View of Values in Cost-Effectiveness Analysis of Health* (Hastings Center, 1999).

Towards a Broader View of Values in Cost-Effectiveness Analysis of Health Care

Paul Menzel, Marthe R. Gold, Erik Nord, Jose-Luis Pinto Prades, Jeff Richardson, and Peter Ubel

. . .

[1]. *Lifesaving and Treatment in the Face of Death.* The most severe illnesses, of course, put people face to face with death. The propensity to regard situations where identifiable patients face great risk of avoidable death as holding a unique call on resources has been called the "Rule of Rescue."[1] Rooted in the Kantian tradition of considering the individual to whom one is relating as an ultimate end-in-herself, this "rule" resists the usual quantitative aggregation of economic analysis. Conventional CEA has conducted its business as if this propensity could be ignored—or at least, as if it was not the sort of factor that CEA could account for as part of the measurable value of different outcomes. This stance damages the credibility of health economics. Critics such as Hadorn, for example, have argued that "any plan to distribute health care services must take [this Rule of Rescue] . . . into account if the plan is to be acceptable to society."[2]

We are inclined to agree with Hadorn. Societal action provides ample evidence that we will expend great effort and large resources to avert death (the girl down the well, astronauts in space, sailors lost at sea, etc.). We also have examples from public life such as the state of Oregon, where all lifesaving services rose to a separate high priority category in the state Medicaid plan's eventual rationing list.[3] Several systematic studies provide corroborating evidence that people place a special value on care in the face of death that has a plausible prospect of success.[4]

A relatively simple thought experiment illustrates the intuitive power of lifesaving's value in the face of the contrary calculations of conventional CEA. Imagine two groups of patients stricken with a life threatening illness. The first group were previously in full health and can be returned to full health with treatment. The second group previously had paraplegia and, with treatment of their life threatening condition, will continue to have it. Both, if treated, will live the same number of additional years. Assume that the [Health Related Quality of Life] HRQoL of paraplegia is 0.8, as calculated from "time trade-off" responses in which persons with paraplegia themselves expressed a willingness to sacrifice 20% of their remaining life extension to obtain a complete cure of their condition. Conventional CEA would then recommend saving the first group, who can be returned to full health, before saving an equal number in the second group. It would recommend shifting priority to the paraplegia group only if the number of lives saved there at similar cost was at least 20% greater than the number of persons saved and returned to normal health. Yet few among us, reflecting seriously about the value of continuing to live, honestly believe that it is less important for society to save the lives of persons with paraplegia than the lives

[1] A. R. Jonsen, "Bentham in a Box: Technology Assessment and Health Care Allocation," *Law Medicine and Health Care* 14 (1986): p. 172.

[2] D. C. Hadorn, "Setting Health Care Priorities in Oregon: Cost-Effectiveness Meets the Rule of Rescue," *Journal of the American Medical Association* 265, no. 17 (1991): pp. 2218–2225.

[3] Ibid., note 10.

[4] E. Nord, J. Richardson and K. Macarounas-Kirchmann, "Social Evaluation of Health Care Versus Personal Evaluation of Health States: Evidence on the Validity of Four Health-State Scaling Instruments Using Norwegian and Australian Surveys," *International Journal of Technology Assessment in Health Care* 9, no. 04 (1993): pp. 463–478.

of others.[5] The value of lifesaving appears to overwhelm the influence of the differences in HRQoL on which conventional CEA focuses.

This example also reveals that lifesaving and treatment in the face of death pose particular concerns with respect to issues of discrimination against the disabled and the chronically ill.[6] In conventional economic analysis the value of saving lives can be influenced by whose lives, of what quality, they are. The disabled and the chronically ill will of course resist any such influence on valuations, and for good reason if we examine more carefully the implications of HRQoL judgments. Suppose, again, that the disabled person has ranked her individual quality of life at 0.8. This willingness to accept a 20% shorter remaining life in order to be cured from a permanent disability does not in any way indicate that she thought that her *life*, in relation to the prospect of *death*, was any less valuable and important to save than *another* fully healthy person's life.[7] While one number may have two meanings, we cannot take it for granted that it has; here, in fact, the 0.8 that expresses willingness to trade time within a life does not constitute a comparative judgment about the value of saving different persons' lives.

To be sure, this point about the potential for discrimination in the conventional model of CEA must not be overstated. The lifesaving interventions or programs being assessed in CEA rarely pertain selectively to a disabling condition such as paraplegia, so that discrimination against chronically ill and disabled people may be far less present in the actual use of CEA than one would surmise from its theoretical model.[8] Still, it is not a sufficient defense of conventional CEA to argue that, serendipitously, disabled patients rarely have life-threatening diseases or conditions requiring separate lifesaving treatments. First, such separate diseases and treatments can and do occur—an example would be HIV disease, for which there are HIV-specific medications. Second, rationing can indeed occur by medical categories of patients within the scope of a treatment, not just by an entire treatment. For example, chronic pulmonary disease patients might be poorer candidates for coronary artery bypass grafts than patients with normal lungs (and therefore, in carefully crafted practice guidelines, be excluded from such surgery).[9] Third, an allocation model's potential for discrimination against the disabled is hardly rendered irrelevant by probable pragmatic realities if conceptually the model's implications are sharply at odds with society's values about discrimination.[10]

---

[5] Few studies have investigated whether this claim is reflected in empirical preference data. One that found confirming data is E. Nord, "The Relevance of Health State After Treatment in Prioritising Between Different Patients," *Journal of Medical Ethics* 19, no. 1 (1993): pp. 37–42. For a philosophical discussion which concludes that quality of life differences are seldom relevant in trade-off lifesaving, see F. M. Kamm, *Morality, Mortality: Death and Whom to Save from It* (Oxford University Press, 1998), pp. 255–260.

[6] Such concerns receive extensive discussion by D. C. Hadorn, "The Problem of Discrimination in Health Care Priority Setting," *Journal of the American Medical Association* 268, no. 11 (1992): pp. 1454–1459, and P. G. Peters Jr., "Health Care Rationing and Disability Rights," *Indiana Law Journal* 70, no. 2 (1995): pp. 491–547.

[7] P. Menzel, *Strong Medicine* (New York: Oxford University Press, 1990).

[8] L. B. Russell, et al., "The Role of Cost-Effectiveness Analysis in Health and Medicine," *Journal of the American Medical Association* 276, no. 14 (1996): pp. 1172–1177.

[9] D. Orentlicher, "Rationing and the Americans with Disabilities Act," *Journal of the American Medical Association* 271, no. 4 (1994): pp. 308–314.

[10] In two companion papers, we explain how a two-stage model of CEA that separates HRQoL assessments at the level of individual utility from societal value judgments avoids precisely this problem of discrimination about lifesaving. One paper, written primarily for health economists, describes in some detail an actual model of a reformed CEA. The other, for a more general audience, integrates the former paper's description of an economic model with the current paper's ethical focus. The former is E. Nord, et al., "Incorporating Societal Concerns for Fairness in Numerical Valuations of Health Programmes," *Health Economics* 8, no. 1 (1999): pp. 25–39. The latter is P. A. Ubel, et al., "Improving Value

In any case, consideration for the special value of treatment in the face of death pertains to more than lifesaving services. Widespread attitudes toward hospice and other non-lifesaving terminal care also suggest the same special value of care in the face of death. Putting up with severe pain for a six-month period when one expects to live for many years is one thing; having to put up with it at the end of one's life is another. People generally, not just patients facing death, have a special concern that life not end in pain. Thus, palliative measures for patients with terminal conditions produce an extra value than what palliative measures of nominally equal effectiveness produce for other patients.[11]

In claiming that conventional CEA is deficient in its treatment of the value of care in the face of death, we are by no means agreeing with those who would inflate the value of life to an absolute. People are, in fact, perfectly and knowledgeably willing to trade some lifesaving for other health services. Yet at the same time, the value that a wide range of public opinion puts on care in the face of death appears to be inadequately captured by conventional economic analysis.

[2]. ***Level of Health Potential.*** The societal value of priority for more severe illnesses focuses independently on a patient's start point, as distinct from the size of treatment effect. Analogously, the end point may have independent relevance which is not accounted for in the calculation of the size of the treatment effect. We shall call this the "level of potential" factor, which is directly related to people's reluctance to disadvantage patients who are already burdened with lower potential for overall health.

This value has been operative in the paraplegia lifesaving example discussed above, but it speaks to many more cases than the lifesaving at issue there. To take the broader, non-lifesaving case, suppose that on a utility scale, treatment can improve one group of people from 0.6 to 0.8 and another from 0.6 to 1.0, and that the first group's end point of 0.8 represents its members' maximum prospective health potential. Should we really regard the second group's treatment effect as having twice the value of the first's? Treatment can, after all, "fully cure" even those in the first group within the perspective of each of their lives. That health potential defines, in significant part, the lives they can lead, and since a life with that potential is the only life that they in any case will have, it is plausible to think that reaching their 0.8 level counts as notably more than half the value of other people's improvement from 0.6 to full health.

The essential ethical claim here is that where people are "located" in life in relation to their maximum realistic potential is an important factor to take into account in the context of resource allocation. In part this may be a function of aversion to inequality: the gap between the 1.0 for one person and the 0.6 for another that is likely to result from giving priority to treatment for illness B over A is larger than the gap between 0.8 and 0.6 that is likely to result from treating A before B. With more empirical research, other moral elements besides aversion to inequality may come to light as involved in the societal preference for compensating for the downward pressure of low end-state potential in net "effectiveness."

The same study of Norwegian politicians that has previously been mentioned in connection with severity of illness also provides suggestive empirical support for the level of potential factor.[12] The respondents were given

---

Measurement in Cost-Effectiveness Analysis," *Medical Care* 38, no. 9 (2000): pp. 892–901. On the larger context for proposing a two-stage model, see E. Nord and J. Richardson, *Cost-Value Analysis in Health Care* (Cambridge: Cambridge University Press, 1999).

[11] The general point here has been made by J. Harris, "QALYfying the Value of Life," *Journal of Medical Ethics* 13, no. 3 (1987): pp. 117–123.

[12] E. Nord, "Health Politicians Do Not Wish to Maximize Health Benefits," *Journal of the Norwegian Medical Association* 113 (1993): note 6. See also data in E. Nord, "The Relevance of Health State," note 13, and in E. Nord, "Health Status Index Models for Use in Resource Allocation Decisions: A Critical Review in the

another dilemma. Two illnesses, both equally common and involving the same degree of suffering, have treatments that are equally costly. The best treatment of illness A helps patients a little, and the best treatment of illness B helps a lot. With an increase in funding that can cover treatment of only the patients with one of these illnesses, not both groups, respondents were asked to choose between two different allocations: (1) Most of the increase should be allocated to treatments for illness B, since the effects are greater. (2) The increase should be divided evenly between the two groups, on the grounds that they are equally entitled to treatment. Almost half (48%) chose the second (egalitarian) view, while 24% chose the first.

Admittedly, the currently available public preference data are less clear in confirming consideration for limited level of health potential as an important societal value than in confirming the importance of severity of illness. They still, however, appear to conflict with the way that health potential is considered in conventional CEA.[13] Moreover, the ethical relevance of special consideration for level of long-term health potential can be powerfully articulated.

. . .

Light of Observed Preferences for Social Choice," *International Journal of Technology Assessment in Health Care* 12, no. 01 (1996): pp. 31–44.

[13] In addition to the previous reference, see E. Nord, et al., "Maximizing Health Benefits Vs Egalitarianism: An Australian Survey of Health Issues," *Social Science and Medicine* 41, no. 10 (1995): note 5.

EXCERPT 6

Abridged text from:

J. Harris, "The Rationing Debate: Maximising the Health of the Whole Community. The Case Against: What the Principle Objective of the NHS Should Really Be", *BMJ* 314 (1997): pp. 669–672.

The Rationing Debate: Maximising the Health of the Whole Community. The Case Against: What the Principal Objective of the NHS Should Really Be

John Harris

. . .

Means and Ends

It is common ground I suppose that we have to think about the ethics both of means and of ends. Even if it were to be accepted that the healthcare system ought principally to aim at maximising aggregate health gain, it does not follow that the most effective ways of achieving this are legitimate. If all seriously ill people were to be allowed to die this might dramatically improve the aggregate health of the community at large. I hope such a policy would not seem ethically defensible. Yet this is precisely what measures which use quality adjusted life years, or similar mechanisms, do: they systematically accord preference to those who have better health prospects, and, by selecting against those with worse prospects, tend to improve the aggregate health status of the whole community at the expense of the life chances of those with poorer prognosis.

We should notice that to make aggregate improvements a principal objective, even if not the only objective, is to imply the subordination of the health needs of individuals to something very abstract, and in some circumstances something very trivial indeed—namely, the improved health status of the whole community. For this could imply sacrificing the life of one person who was very ill and expensive to treat, if doing so would make even a tiny improvement to the aggregate health status, an improvement which no individual would even notice.

Distributive Justice

Distributive justice must be built into any articulation of principal objectives for the NHS, but it cannot be enough to define the relevant principle of distributive justice in terms of a more equal distribution of health across populations, because such an objective could be achieved as much by levelling down as by levelling up. One method of allocating a scarce resource which apparently satisfies the requirements of justice is, of course, not to allocate that resource to anyone. All are then treated equally.

The fallacy of such a supposition is easily illustrated. The principles of justice, and indeed the principles of equality, are moral principles, principles that are designed to be more than impartial, that are designed among other things to respect and to do justice to people. In some sense this must involve some benevolent attitude to people which is often abbreviated as "respect for persons." Such an attitude to others is as different as it is possible to be to that of simply showing an equality of lack of respect or an equal indifference to their fate.

So, neither the failure to allocate resources that would save lives or protect individuals nor the simple attempt to move towards a more equal distribution of health could be part of a claim to satisfy the requirements of equality or justice conceived of as moral principles (and how else are we to think of them?). This is because equality or distributive justice has at its heart the claim that people's lives and fundamental interests are of value, that they matter. Anyone who denied resources which would protect life and other fundamental interests is not valuing the lives of those to whom she denies these protections. Although she might be treating people equally in the sense of treating them all the same, she is not treating them as equals, as people who matter and hence matter equally.

Now this brings us close to the positive part of my account, because I believe it to be an integral part of any principle of distributive justice that people's moral claims to resources are not diminished by who they are; how old they are; how rich or poor, powerful or weak, they are; or by the quality of their lives. A principle of justice worth its salt covers young and old, healthy and sick, weak and strong, regardless of race, creed, colour, sex, quality of life, and life expectancy.

. . .

NHS Is There to Protect Life and Liberty

Imagine an industrialised state that has big conurbations where millions of citizens are concentrated, many smaller towns, and thousands of tiny villages. It has vast sparsely populated tracts of agricultural land and vaster mountainous areas and wilderness where few people live. How should it distribute its access to health care? Probably it will place the major hospitals and medical schools in the centres of population, but smaller hospitals and medical centres will serve the smaller towns and isolated villages. For the remotest areas there will probably be an air rescue service or even a flying doctor or flying hospital service.

For geographical reasons if for no other, those in the most remote regions will be generally more expensive to treat. To fly the remote farmer and backwoodsman to the major centres of excellence for specialised treatment will be naturally more costly and hence less cost effective than to bus suburban commuters downtown. We will assume, what is probably true, that the funds devoted to servicing the health needs of citizens who are geographically remote from major centres would have treated more people had they been allocated to urban populations. Why do societies divert resources available for health care away from the more numerous city dwellers in a way which must adversely affect their ability to maximise aggregate improvements in health status or indeed to maximise numbers treated?

I believe the ends subserved by public healthcare systems are broadly the same as those which justify the high priority given to national defence. All governments and would be governments boast the strongest commitment to national defence. The question that is seldom asked is what is national defence for, what justifies its prominent place in national priorities? The simplistic answer is, of course, that without national defence there might be no nation and hence no national priorities. But pressed further it is reasonable to ask for the underlying values and interests it subserves.

Equal Protection

Arguably protecting citizens against threats to their lives, liberties, and fundamental interests is the first priority for any state. When in 1651 Thomas Hobbes wrote "The obligation of subjects to the sovereign, is understood to last as long, and no longer, than the power lasteth, by which he is able to protect them" he was providing an answer to this question. On this view, any citizen's obligation to the state and to obey its laws is conditional on the state for its part protecting that citizen against threats to her life and liberty. If we reflect on what citizens today want and need in the way of protection I believe we will find that in most contemporary societies the most important threats to life and liberty come not in the form of soldiers with snow on their boots but from illness, accident, and poverty. This is why it is arguable that the obligation to provide health care, and in particular life saving health care, to each and every citizen, regardless of its effect on the aggregate health status of the community, takes precedence over the obligation to provide defence forces against external (and often mythical) enemies.

There is a good principle which states that real and present dangers should be met before future and speculative ones. If this is right the healthcare system should have first claim on the national defence budget. I should make clear that no part of my argument assumes a given budget for health care; rather I argue that the budget could and should be larger, that the health budget has first call on the defence budget, but that whatever the budget is, there are ways of distributing the budget which are to be avoided because they are unjust.

Another feature of the state's obligation to defend its citizens which is often overlooked is its egalitarian nature. Just as each citizen owes his or her obligation to obey the law regardless of such features as race, religion, sex or age, quality of life, or prognosis, so the state must discharge its obligation of protection with the same impartiality. If we expect people to obey the law even though their life expectancy is short and the quality of their life poor, we must not deny them the equal protection that is an essential part of the social contract. I have suggested that the protection of the healthcare system is one of the principal elements of the state's side of this contract and that discrimination against those with poor quality of life or shorter life expectancy in the allocation of such resources is a betrayal, not only of those citizens, but of the social contract. Where all cannot be treated and priorities must be set the basis of prioritisation should not be the effect on the aggregate health of the whole community, for this will tend to discriminate against those arguably most in need of health care.

The principal objective of the NHS should be to protect the life and health of each citizen impartially and to offer beneficial health care on the basis of individual need, so that each has an equal chance of flourishing to the extent that their personal health status permits.

EXCERPT 7

Abridged text from:

N. Daniels, "Decisions About Access to Health Care and Accountability for Reasonableness," *Journal of Urban Health* 76, no. 2 (1999): pp. 176–191.

Decisions About Access to Health Care and Accountability for Reasonableness

Norman Daniels

. . .

In our system, private, generally for-profit employers and health plans make decisions about access to medical care that have the potential to affect our health and welfare in fundamental ways. Some of these decisions are "direct" ways of limiting access to services, such as coverage decisions for new technologies and decisions about the contents and design of a [drug] formulary. Other decisions "indirectly" limit access by implementing novel forms of risk-sharing incentives with physician groups; the incentives induce physicians to limit access to care. Ideally, setting limits in the appropriate ways can improve the quality of outcomes of a covered population by eliminating unnecessary care, implementing outcomes-based clinical guidelines, ensuring improved continuity and integration of care, and setting fair priorities under resource constraints. In practice, however, limit setting is greeted with suspicion and distrust, for many fear that it is only the costs to powerful stakeholders that drive decisions, not a commitment to meeting health needs fairly in a covered population. As a result, an increasing number of Americans fear that a treatment they need will not be covered by their insurer.[1]

In what follows, I argue that we cannot ensure the fairness or legitimacy of direct or indirect limit setting unless we implement forms of public accountability not now in place.[2] Specifically, we must go beyond demanding *market accountability,* the simple demand for clear information about options and performance, and must instead implement measures that establish *accountability for reasonableness.*[3] Accountability for reasonableness demands public access to rationales for limit-setting decisions. It also requires that these rationales be ones that "fair-minded" people can agree are relevant to meeting population health needs fairly under resource constraints. In effect, this is a call for the transformation of the corporate culture in which these decisions are made. I try to be quite practical in suggesting how this accountability can be established in key areas of direct and indirect limit setting.

. . .

Legitimacy and Accountability for Reasonableness

Elsewhere, I have argued (with James Sabin) that the direct and indirect limit-setting decisions made by health plans and other insurers pose a "legitimacy problem."[4,5] Specifically, why should moral authority for such important and morally controversial decisions be lodged with these institutions? More constructively, under what conditions should we come to view the exercise of such authority as legitimate and fair?

---

[1] Kaiser Family Foundation/Harvard, "Kaiser Family Foundation/Harvard National Survey of Americans," Views on Consumer Protection in Managed Care, 1998, http://www.kff.org/kff/library.html.

[2] N. Daniels and J. Sabin, "Limits to Health Care: Fair Procedures, Democratic Deliberation, and the Legitimacy Problem for Insurers," *Philosophy & Public Affairs* 26, no. 4 (1997): pp. 303–350.

[3] N. Daniels and J. Sabin, "The Ethics of Accountability in Managed Care Reform," *Health Affairs* 17, no. 5 (1998): pp. 50–64.

[4] Daniels, "Limits to Health Care."

[5] N. Daniels and J. Sabin, "Closure, Fair Procedures, and Setting Limits within Managed Care Organizations," *Journal of the American Geriatrics Society* 46, no. 3 (1998): pp. 351–354.

A standard reply to this question is that when consumers exercise informed choices about their insurance options, then their choice of plan counts as "informed consent" to the limits it imposes. According to this view, consumers do not need to know why plans set the limits they do any more than they need to know why car or computer manufacturers make the design decisions they make. It is sufficient that the limits are clear so that clear choices can be made. Questions about legitimacy are dissolved by the consent involved in the purchase of a plan—or car or computer—at a given price.

The facts that legitimacy requires consent and consent comes through actual informed choice show the key limits of this view. First, nearly half of American workers have no choice of plans: their employers choose for them. In addition, many of us become aware of what limits mean for us only in the context of treatment, when it is too late to make another choice of health plan. Second, the enormous uncertainty that surrounds health care is different from that involved in the purchase of other goods.[6] We have better information about our computer or automobile "needs" and how to match them to appropriate computers or cars than we do about our health needs and how to match them to appropriate plans, clinicians, or treatments. (This information problem makes our ongoing, interactive relationship with clinicians we can trust crucial to health care delivery, but not car buying.) In addition, if we buy a car or computer that no longer meets our needs, we can sell it and buy one that does, perhaps with some inconvenience and cost, but without serious impact on our well-being. When a plan turns out not to meet our newly discovered health care needs, we may not be welcome in another one, or we may be too urgently ill to shop around.

Perhaps most important, if the computer market fails to provide us with machines that meet all our information-managing needs, that is too bad, but no injustice is done. But, if health plans fail to meet our needs fairly under necessary resource constraints, we violate a societal obligation to provide appropriate care for those needs. . . .[7] That means an injustice is done. There is simply no way to hold plans accountable for their role in meeting that societal obligation if we do not insist on accountability for making reasonable decisions. There is simply no way to guarantee that even an ideal market will provide people with reasonable coverage and treatment options without holding players in that market explicitly accountable for reasonableness.

To implement accountability for reasonableness, four conditions must be met (they are necessary, but probably not sufficient, conditions).[8]

1. *Publicity:* Decisions regarding coverage for new technologies (and other limit-setting decisions) and their rationales must be accessible publicly.
2. *Reasonableness:* The rationales for coverage decisions should aim to provide a reasonable construal of how the organization should provide "value for money" in meeting the varied health needs of a defined population under reasonable resource constraints. Specifically, a construal will be reasonable if it appeals to reasons and principles that are accepted as relevant by people who are disposed to finding terms of cooperation that are justifiable mutually.
3. *Appeals:* There is a mechanism for challenge and dispute resolution regarding limit-setting decisions, including the opportunity for revising decisions in light of further evidence or arguments.
4. *Enforcement:* There is either voluntary or public regulation of the process to ensure that conditions 1–3 are met.

Condition 1 requires openness or publicity, that is, transparency with regard to reasons for decisions. If it is implemented, for example, in decisions about coverage for new technologies or

[6] K. J. Arrow, "Uncertainty and the Welfare Economics of Medical Care," *The American Economic Review* (1963): pp. 941–973.

[7] N. Daniels, *Just Health Care* (Cambridge University Press, 1985).

[8] Daniels, "Limits to Health Care."

in decisions about the design of a formulary, then a kind of "case law" is established. Plans reveal their commitment to appropriate reasons for limiting care through the demand that these constitute a coherent, defensible body of decisions over time.

Condition 2 requires the most explanation since it involves some constraints on the kinds of reasons that can play a role in the rationale. At its core, it recognizes the fundamental interest all parties in a cooperative scheme for delivering health care have in finding a justification all can accept as reasonable. We can think of Condition 2 as requiring that we limit ourselves to reasons that fair-minded people can agree are relevant to pursuing appropriate patient care under necessary resource constraints.

Fair-minded people are those who seek terms of cooperation that are mutually justifiable. In sports, we consider people fair minded if they play by accepted rules of the game. Indeed, fair-minded people want the rules of the game to promote its essential skills and the excitement their use produces. For example, they want rules that permit blocking in football, but not clipping or grabbing face masks, because they want to encourage teamwork and skill and not the mere advantage that comes from imposing injuries. Of course, having rules of a game that fair-minded people accept does not eliminate all controversy about their application, but it does narrow the scope of controversy and methods for adjudicating them.

Similarly, if the "game" is delivering health care, whether in public or private insurance schemes, then fair-minded people will seek reasons all can accept as relevant to meeting people's needs fairly under resource constraints. As in sporting games, the rules shape a conception of the common good that is the goal of cooperation (or competition). In both games, people who seek "mere advantage" by ignoring the rules, or by seeking rules that give advantage only to them, are not fair minded. There still will be disagreement about how to apply the rules, but seeking mutually acceptable rules, as fair-minded people do, narrows the scope of disagreement and the grounds on which disputes can be adjudicated.

Conditions 3 and 4 provide mechanisms for connecting deliberation and decisions within managed-care organizations (MCOs) to a broader deliberative process, that is, for making them accountable to the results of a wider deliberation about fairness requirements in health care. The kind of appeals process required by Condition 3, for example, establishes a form of due process and helps open discussion about contested decisions to broader scrutiny. At the same time, if properly designed, these appeals should diminish adversarial confrontation in the courts.[9] Condition 4 recognizes that public regulation may be necessary if self-regulation proves inadequate, but the combined intention behind the four conditions is to focus regulation on process rather than on "organ-by-organ" mandates in health plans. Current reform efforts contain elements of accountability for reasonableness, but they have not focused clearly on that as a central goal.[10]

. . .

[9] N. Daniels and J. E. Sabin, "Last Chance Therapies and Managed Care Pluralism, Fair Procedures, and Legitimacy," *Hastings Center Report* 28, no. 2 (1998): pp. 27–42.

[10] Daniels, "The Ethics of Accountability."

EXCERPT 8

Abridged text from:
A. Friedman, "Beyond Accountability for Reasonableness," *Bioethics* 22, no. 2 (2008): pp. 101–112.

Beyond Accountability for Reasonableness

Alex Friedman

. . .

It is [a] regrettable but equally inescapable fact that no society has been able to reach anything resembling a consensus on how much should be spent on health care, or how the allocated resources should be distributed. Faced with these difficulties, Norman Daniels and James Sabin suggest that we give up on attempts to resolve our differences by finding principles or values that will yield the "right" answers, and instead focus on putting in place procedures that will ensure fairness and legitimacy of whatever outcomes they generate.[1] If we cannot agree on views regarding the key issues underlying disputes about health care resource allocation, they argue, we should at least be able to agree on fair ways of making the unavoidable decisions that even those who disagree with the outcome should, and hopefully will, accept as reasonable and legitimate.[2]

Daniels and Sabin offer four criteria that a decision-making process for allocation of health care resources must meet in order to be (and be perceived as) legitimate, regardless of whether it occurs within a private organization or a government institution:

1. *Publicity Condition*: Decisions regarding both direct and indirect limits to care and their rationales must be publicly accessible.
2. *Relevance Condition*: The rationales for limit-setting decisions should aim to provide a *reasonable* explanation of how the organization seeks to provide "value for money" in meeting the varied health needs of a defined population under reasonable resource constraints. Specifically, a rationale will be reasonable if it appeals to evidence, reasons, and principles that are accepted as relevant by fair-minded people who are disposed to finding mutually justifiable terms of cooperation.
3. *Revision and Appeals Condition*: There must be mechanisms for challenge and dispute resolution regarding limit-setting decisions, and, more broadly, opportunities for revision and improvement of policies in the light of new evidence or arguments.
4. *Enforcement*[3] *Condition*: There is either voluntary or public regulation of the

[1] Since the problem under consideration is, at least in part, practical, Daniels and Sabin rightly worry not only about actual legitimacy and fairness, but also about perceptions of legitimacy and fairness. A legitimate and fair procedure (or outcome) that is not considered either fair or legitimate by the public will not solve the problem of distrust or eliminate its more unpleasant manifestations, such as endless litigation. A consequence of that is that we need to be concerned with both what people *do*, in fact, accept as legitimate (reasonable, fair, etc.) and with what they *should* regard as such. Of course, the two do not always coincide; and of the two, actual legitimacy should, almost certainly, take precedence—while a legitimate procedure that is not viewed as such is "merely" impractical, an illegitimate procedure that is accepted as legitimate may constitute (and be a source of) injustice that is extremely difficult to remedy.

[2] N. Daniels and J. Sabin, *Setting Limits Fairly: Can We Learn to Share Medical Resources?* (Oxford University Press, 2002), ch. 1–4. Regarding the scope and intractability of our moral disagreements about resource allocation, see especially pp. 30–39. On the subject of giving priority to questions of actual, as opposed to perceived, legitimacy, see, for instance, p. 10.

[3] The condition is referred to as *"Regulative"* in Daniels and Sabin, *Setting Limits Fairly,* but I will follow much of the literature in opting for the more intuitive *"Enforcement"* label from N. Daniels and J. Sabin, "The Ethics of Accountability in Managed Care Reform," *Health Affairs* 17, no. 5 (1998): pp. 50–64.

process to ensure that conditions 1–3 are met.[4]

Together, these four conditions comprise the Accountability for Reasonableness framework, which has been gaining increasing acceptance worldwide over the last decade,[5] arguably to the point of becoming the dominant paradigm in the field of health policy. But is the Accountability for Reasonableness approach the decisive breakthrough that it is widely believed to be?

. . .

The big question, is whether or not the Relevance Condition can be justified. The Relevance Condition follows a Rawlsian tradition of considerable pedigree.[5] Its practical motivation is to limit disagreement to "reasonable" disagreement—by excluding the kinds of reasons that cannot be expected to motivate others if they do not already share certain extremely controversial and empirically unverifiable assumptions, e.g. a particular type of religious belief.[6] Excluding such "non-public" reasons[7] is supposed to narrow the range of disagreement and to make the disagreements that remain more tractable. Such exclusion is also argued to be just, as free and equal citizens should not be bound by laws grounded only in a system of beliefs that they have no reason to accept.[8] . . .

Despite its initial appeal, the Relevance Condition is unnecessary for ensuring a legitimate decision-making process and would, in fact, be detrimental to such a process, both procedurally and substantively. . . .

As Daniels and Sabin suggest, once we have agreed on which considerations matter, should it not be a relatively easy "practical matter" to negotiate (or settle by vote) the weights that should be attached to each of the considerations?[9] And would not even the "losers" in such a process accept the outcome as reasonable and fair because "the preference of the majority rests on the kind of reason that even the minority must acknowledge appropriately plays a role in the deliberation"?[10] Unfortunately, this would only be the case on the assumption that the truly intractable value-laden disputes are limited to the "which considerations matter" level, whereas the "assignment of weights" level is somehow more technical and pragmatic, and less fundamental. And there is no reason to accept this correlation.

---

[4] Daniels and Sabin, *Setting Limits Fairly,* p. 45.

[5] See, for instance, J. Rawls, "The Idea of Public Reason," in *Political Liberalism* (New York: Columbia University Press, 1993). For one of the more recent expositions of a Rawls-inspired view that incorporates a similar condition, see A. Gutmann and D. Thompson, *Democracy and Disagreement* (Harvard University Press, 2009).

[6] In fact, Daniels and Sabin may have something even stronger in mind, as their formulation of the Relevance Condition talks about reasons that fair-minded people *do not* find relevant, as opposed to reasons that fair-minded people *can not* or *should not* find relevant. If taken entirely at face value, that would imply that all that matters is whether people are, in fact, motivated by certain reasons, not whether or not they can or should be so motivated. It is not clear to what extent Daniels and Sabin are committed to this view, which is more controversial but much easier to apply on a practical level. Other quotes from Daniels & Sabin, *op. cit.* note 2, for instance: ". . . the preference of the majority rests on the kind of reason that even the minority *must* acknowledge appropriately plays a role in the deliberation" (p. 36) and ". . . these reasons must be ones that "fair-minded" people *can* agree are relevant . . ." (p. 44) [italics added for emphasis], suggest that the commitment is, at the very least, not absolute; but difficulties with the Relevance Condition abound either way. Since the practical problem of how to overcome disagreement must be addressed in any case, in what follows I will mostly, but not exclusively, focus on what people are likely to find *actually* relevant. Thanks to Henry Richardson for pointing out the need to address this issue.

[7] The term is borrowed from Rawls, "The Idea of Public Reason," note 14.

[8] Daniels and Sabin, *Setting Limits Fairly*, p. 45.

[9] "Suppose that a deliberation appeals only to reasons that all can recognize as acceptable or relevant, but that consensus about an outcome is still not achieved. To settle the *practical* matter, we rely on a majority vote." [italics added for emphasis] Daniels, *Setting Limits Fairly.*

[10] Daniels, *Setting Limits Fairly,* p. 36.

Perhaps what motivates the idea that there is a sharp divide between the two types of disagreement is the illusion that disputes over weights would take the form of "now that we have all agreed that utility, freedom of choice, and equality of access are the only considerations relevant to making this particular decision, do we count utility for 60%, equality for 30%, and freedom of choice for 10%, or do we count utility for 55%, equality for 32% and freedom of choice for 13%?" If that were the case, the dispute would certainly appear to be minor and much more pragmatic than a disagreement about whether Utilitarianism or Kantianism (or some other alternative) is the correct comprehensive approach to ethics, or about whether opinions with regard to revealed truth are relevant, or even about whether or not self-responsibility for medical conditions is a factor that should be taken into account when making resource allocation decisions.

Would even the "losers" in such a dispute over weights accept the reasonableness of the outcome with relative ease, since their own view will have been so close, both philosophically and pragmatically, to the view that eventually triumphed? Perhaps they would, but only on the crucial assumption that the resource allocation decisions in question will not be of the all-or-nothing variety. Otherwise, for instance, a group of elderly patients facing kidney failure and denied access to dialysis would hardly find the decision any more acceptable simply because a tiny change in how considerations were weighted—say, if utility had counted for 2% less and equality of access for 2% more—would have resulted in them having access to dialysis.[11] If anything, such knowledge could infuriate the "losers" by making what for them are life-or-death decisions seem arbitrary despite all the thinking and reasoning that had gone into them. In the end, if the stakes at the level of policy are substantial, they are likely to be better predictors of how obstinately the stakeholders with the most to lose will fight for their positions than the magnitude of the underlying theoretical differences. But, in any case, most (if not all) disagreements about weights—in health care, or in ethical debates more generally—will not be of such a "trifling" sort.[12]

For instance, while I am not a utilitarian, I believe that utility is very relevant in ethics generally, and in health care resource allocation in particular. So, I agree with the utilitarians that utility considerations matter. Is our disagreement about the extent to which utility considerations matter "merely" technical or pragmatic? Would the scope and severity of the disagreement be reduced if my utilitarian opponent was willing to concede that all the other factors, which I believe should be taken into account when making the decision in question, can sometimes matter—for instance, as tiebreakers if utility calculations come out even or nearly even—so that we had agreement on a list of relevant considerations?[13] The answer is clearly "No".

For example, suppose that the utilitarian insists that organs for transplantation should be distributed on the basis of medical prognosis (with and without a transplant) so as to achieve

[11] Nor does there seem to be a good reason why they *should* accept the outcome as reasonable and legitimate simply because the theoretical differences underlying the disagreement were so small and revolved entirely around weights.

[12] In addition, an assignment of numerical weights is only one possible way of dealing with a plurality of values. An example of an alternative would be some sort of a lexical priority principle. Clearly, it would be, if anything, even harder to claim that a conflict between alternative priority principles is less problematic than a disagreement about which values matter in the first place. Thanks to Alan Wertheimer for calling my attention to this point.

[13] An even more extreme situation would arise if the utilitarian assigned weights of 0 to all considerations other than utility in all circumstances. Clearly, reclassifying a disagreement about moral significance ("relevance" in Daniels' and Sabin's terminology) as a disagreement over whether to assign a certain factor a weight of 0, does not in any way change the nature or severity of the disagreement. This may already cast some doubt on the plausibility of a radical distinction between disagreements about relevance and disagreements about weights.

the best consequences possible—i.e. what really matter are the degree of urgency, the likelihood of severe complications or death if a transplant is attempted, how healthy the person would be if the transplant is successful, and how long he/she is likely to live after the transplant. Other factors, such as equality of access or overall prior quality of life, can be considered in cases of ties. Such an approach would, on balance, probably result in the youngest and (otherwise) healthiest candidates receiving the needed organs. And suppose I object that while medical prognosis is certainly a morally significant factor, it would be unfair to deny older patients, for instance, any chance at life-saving treatment just because they have (on average) fewer years left if cured; or that it may be unjust to deny organs to someone solely because of comorbidities, especially if they are of a kind largely beyond a person's control and strongly correlated with lower socioeconomic status. Therefore, utility, equality of access, and prior quality of life should all be taken into account, without utility being accorded the status of a trump.

The disagreement here is, in a sense, "just" a matter of weights. But it is no more technical, pragmatic, or insignificant than my disagreement with utilitarianism was to begin with. What is at stake is not "merely" a slight numerical variation, but radically and fundamentally different approaches that arrive at very different conclusions (with life-or-death implications) because of entirely different conceptions of persons, morality, justice, etc.[14] Such disagreements about weights, which the Relevance Condition cannot help us avoid, are no less fundamental, significant, or intractable than any disagreement that it could ever hope to preclude.[15]

To sum up my discussion of assumptions 1 and 2: we should not expect the Relevance Condition to reduce all of our moral disagreements to "merely" disagreements about weights. And even if that were possible, the gains, contrary to what Daniels and Sabin appear to envision, would, even in the best case scenario, be slight gains in degree as opposed to large gains in kind. . . .

Section 4: Is the Relevance Condition Just?

Why might the Relevance Condition be unjust and/or unfair? The most obvious concern is that the kind of reasoning and deliberation about one's own views that Daniels and Sabin, as well as most other political philosophers, would like to see, is hard to find in real life. . . .

Many stakeholders in public policy debates might find reasons grounded in one of these ethical theories not in the least bit compelling, and be no more interested in learning more about the theory in question and examining it in detail than they would be in learning the particulars of someone else's religious views. Someone convinced that the main purpose of allocating resources for organ transplantation must be to achieve the best possible aggregate outcome, need not react to an objection that a

[14] Daniels and Sabin seem to come at least partway towards acknowledging as much in Daniels, *Setting Limits Fairly*, p. 321 ("The weightings that different people give to different moral concerns, such as helping the worst off versus not sacrificing achievable medical benefits, probably depend on how these moral concerns fit within wider moral conceptions people hold. If so, there is good reason to think these disagreements will be a persistent feature of the situation . . .") but do not appear to have found the concern particularly disturbing.

[15] It should also be noted that there is sometimes a tendency, when searching for common moral ground, to reclassify disagreements over the moral significance of a certain consideration as agreement on a very broad and vague principle with the interpretation, scope, and weight of the principle remaining to be specified (see, for example, Daniels' and Sabin's discussion of the principle of protection of opportunity in Daniels, *Setting Limits Fairly,* note 2, p. 54). It is important to remember that such reclassification, in itself, does absolutely nothing to change the nature or scope of the disagreement—exactly the same questions need to be settled in order for the dispute to be resolved.

policy based on that assumption would not necessarily benefit those who are worst off (or that it would restrict the liberty of some "merely" in order to produce more beneficial results for others) any differently from the way he would react to an objection that such a policy would contradict some important religious text. And if our utilitarian does end up taking any one of these criticisms seriously, it would hopefully be not because of the objection's genealogy but because of its substantive merits in pointing out the moral shortcomings of a purely consequentialist approach to organ transplantation.

The point here is certainly not that we should never appeal to comprehensive ethical theories, or that they should not, in some cases, be seriously considered in the course of policy deliberations. The point is that there is no clear and non-controversial way to draw the line demarcating "bad" (non-public) religious reasons from "good" (public) philosophical ones. In fact, many stakeholders in policy deliberations who do not share the assumptions from the realm of political philosophy that underlie the Relevance Condition, are very likely to find Daniels' and Sabin's reasons for drawing that line unconvincing in the first place and to claim that the difference between faith-based and ethical-theory-based (or even political-philosophy-based) reasons is of no relevance. If they have a case, then the a priori exclusion of faith-based perspectives would be arbitrary, unfair, and unjust. This is not to say that there are no differences at all between religious reasons and philosophical ones—a religious reason is, for instance, somewhat more likely to have nothing to recommend it other than the belief of some that it represents revealed truth. The differences, however, are a matter of degree, not of kind, and so do not justify a wholesale prohibition on the use of faith-based reasons in public deliberation.[16]

. . .

[16] Rawls disagrees with the position that reasons that are not purely political can ever be public—see Rawls, "The Idea of Public Reason" note 14; as well as S. Freeman, "Public Reason and Political Justifications," *Fordham Law Review* 72 (2003): p. 2021. According to his view, reasonable comprehensive doctrines like Utilitarianism and Kantianism can be distilled into "inoffensive" political conceptions of justice that may be appealed to in public deliberation. Everything that is not part of the distilled version must be left out of public debate. But this does not suffice to vindicate an exclusion criterion like the Relevance Condition as a pragmatic stepping stone towards avoiding or resolving disagreement in public deliberation. While a detailed discussion of the Rawlsian approach is far outside the scope of this paper, it should be noted that the distinction between political conceptions of justice and comprehensive doctrines is itself extremely controversial and difficult to draw, especially in a manner which will leave enough substance intact in the distilled political version of the doctrines to ground normative conclusions. The difficulties discussed above merely get shifted from the task of distinguishing between religion-based (and similar) comprehensive doctrines and other comprehensive ethical doctrines to the task of distinguishing between political and comprehensive conceptions of justice.

Further Resources

Relevant Organizations

Governmental

Division for Sustainable Development: Promotes and coordinates implementation of the sustainable development agenda for the United Nations. Additional information can be found at https://sustainabledevelopment.un.org/

The National Institute for Health and Care Excellence (NICE): An executive, nondepartmental public body of the Department of Health in the United Kingdom, providing guidance and advice to improve health and social care in the UK. Additional information can be found at www.nice.org.uk

The Pharmaceutical Benefits Scheme (PBS): Makes recommendations to the Minister for Health and Ageing regarding drugs which should be made available to Australians as pharmaceutical benefits. Additional information can be found at http://www.pbs.gov.au/pbs/home

Literature

Ashcroft, Richard. "Fair Process and the Redundancy of Bioethics: A Polemic." *Public Health Ethics* 1, no. 1 (April 1, 2008): 3–9.

Daniels, Norman. *Just Health: Meeting Health Needs Fairly* (New York: Cambridge University Press, 2008).

National Institute for Health and Clinical Excellence, Citizens Council. "Quality Adjusted Life Years (QALYs) and the Severity of Illness." https://www.nice.org.uk/Media/Default/Get-involved/Citizens-Council/Reports/CCReport10QALYSeverity.pdf.

White, Stuart, "Social Minimum," The Stanford Encyclopedia of Philosophy (Winter 2015 Edition), Edward N. Zalta (ed.), http://plato.stanford.edu/archives/win2015/entries/social-minimum/.

Williams, Alan. "QALYS and Ethics: A Health Economist's Perspective." *Social Science & Medicine* 43, no. 12 (12/ 1996): 1795–1804.

Other Media

"How Much Would You Pay For A Year of Life?" Narrated by Molly Webster. *Radiolab,* 2014. http://www.radiolab.org/story/what-year-life-worth/. Host and guest discuss the value of a life year in regard to healthcare decisions.

Snowden, Edward. *Citizenfour*. Directed by Laura Poitras. New York City: HBO Films: The film documents Edward Snowden, who publicized a secret government program, raising issues related to transparency in governance of priority setting.

Implementing Principles in Policy and Practice

10

Evidence-based medicine (EBM), comparative effectiveness research (CER), and health technology assessment (HTA) all have decisive roles to play in resource allocation decisions. Each in its own way links ethical and economic concepts to actual healthcare decisions. Unfortunately, these different concepts are not always clearly distinguished. Luce and colleagues helpfully clear up much of the confusion (Excerpt 1).[1] They characterize EBM chiefly as an evidence synthesis and decision process aimed at assisting patients' and/or physicians' decisions. EBM also includes the development of clinical guidelines. CER comprises both evidence generation and synthesis and focuses on assessments in routine practice settings. CER does not generally include economic evaluations and thus needs to be distinguished from cost-effectiveness analysis which is explicitly an economic analysis. However, outputs of CER inform clinical guideline development, as well as EBM and HTA. HTA is centered on appraisals of clinical effectiveness and broader social and economic evaluations. It typically includes cost-effectiveness analysis (CEA) or other economic evaluations, as well as associated implicit and explicit ethical values (see also Table 10.1). While EBM centrally focuses on how best to improve health for individual patients, CER and HTA focus on the population and societal levels.

Chapter 9 addressed central ethical issues arising from economic evaluations that are carried out as part of HTA. But salient ethical issues also arise in EBM and CER. First, the empirical facts resulting from research, as well as their interpretations, are not value-free. Judgments need to be made regarding what kind of study designs are regarded as sufficiently robust, what study endpoints are adequate, and how the balance of benefits and harms should be struck in recommending for or against an intervention.[2,3]

---

[1] B. R. Luce, et al., "EBM, HTA, and CER: Clearing the Confusion," *Milbank Quarterly* 88, no. 2 (2010): pp. 256–276.

[2] D. Strech and J. Tilburt, "Value Judgments in the Analysis and Synthesis of Evidence," *J Clin Epidemiol* 61, no. 6 (2008): pp. 521–524.

[3] P. A. Ubel, "Medical Facts Versus Value Judgments: Toward Preference-Sensitive

Empirical facts alone provide no guidance here. Furthermore, values also come into play in process terms, regarding who should be involved in what role in allocation policy and concrete decisions. Decisions are not simply made between patients and their physicians, but also require determinations of the respective roles of healthcare professionals, healthcare payers such as insurers or governments covering services, and sometimes politicians and the broader public through different types of engagement processes.

Countries differ considerably in how they organize EBM, CER, and HTA. Kalipso Chalkidou and colleagues note in a comparison of Australian, French, German, and British government-initiated institutions concerned with synthesizing and appraising evidence of healthcare interventions that all except the British began with CER narrowly construed (Excerpt 2).[4] But "in each case the lack of economic assessment was found to limit these organizations' ability to complete their assessments" and was subsequently added, broadening out to the HTA scope.[5] Economic and ethical evaluations in different forms have become indispensable beyond these three countries.[6] At the same time, there remains a lack of consensus on how best to incorporate them into resource allocation decisions. For instance, different countries have adopted very different approaches on using QALYs and cost thresholds (see overview in Table 10.1).[7]

Table 10.1
Differences in Four Countries Regarding the Implementation of Central Economic and Ethical Concepts in Heath Technology Assessment and Coverage Decisions at the National Level

	QALYs	Economic Evaluation	Cost Threshold	Rule of Rescue[a]
UK	Yes	Yes	Yes	No
Australia	Yes	Yes	No	Yes
Germany	No	No	No	Yes
USA	No	No	No	Yes

[a] See Chapter 9

The UK's National Institute for Health and Care Excellence (NICE)[8] develops clinical guidelines and advises the National Health Service (NHS) on which interventions to cover within the publicly funded healthcare system that is accessible to all residents at minimal cost burden. As Rawlins and Culyer describe (Excerpt 3),[9] NICE has probably attracted most interest and controversy for its explicit use of QALYs in combination with a somewhat flexible cost threshold of approximately £30,000 per QALY gained[10] (further context is provided by Corinna Sorenson and Adam Oliver in Excerpt 4).[11]

In addition, NICE has made an explicit policy decision against the so-called rule of rescue, which demands genuine resource commitments "when an identified person's life is visibly threatened if effective rescue measures are available."[12] The rule of rescue is addressed

Guidelines," *New England Journal of Medicine* 372, no. 26 (2015): pp. 2475–2477.

[4] K. Chalkidou, et al., "Comparative Effectiveness Research and Evidence-Based Health Policy: Experience from Four Countries," *Milbank Quarterly* 87, no. 2 (2009): pp. 339–367.

[5] Ibid., p. 353.

[6] A. Gerber-Grote and J. Windeler, "Welchen Beitrag Leisten Kosten-Nutzen-Bewertungen Bei Entscheidungen Im Gesundheitswesen: Erfahrungen Aus 7 Ausgewählten Ländern," *Zeitschrift fuer Evidenz, Fortbildung und Qualitaet im Gesundheitswesen* 7, no. 108 (2014): pp. 355–357.

[7] Ibid.

[8] National Institute for Clinical Excellence, accessed June 16, 2015, https://www.nice.org.uk/.

[9] M. D. Rawlins and A. J. Culyer, "National Institute for Clinical Excellence and Its Value Judgments," *BMJ* 329, no. 7459 (2004): pp. 224–227.

[10] National Institute for Health and Care Excellence, *Social Value Judgements—Principles for the Development of NICE Guidance (2nd Ed)* (London: National Institute for Health and Care Excellence, 2008).

[11] A. Oliver and C. Sorenson, "The Limits and Challenges to the Economic Evaluation of Health Technologies," edited by J. Costa-Font, C. Courbage, and A. McGuire (Oxford University Press, 2009), pp. 212–214.

[12] D. C. Hadorn, "Setting Health Care Priorities in Oregon: Cost Effectiveness Meets the Rule of Rescue," *JAMA* 265, no. 17 (1991): p. 2219.

directly in the Social Value Judgments (SVJs), a guidance document containing eight principles for use by NICE's staff, those conducting specific appraisals of interventions, and external stakeholders, including the public.[13] The SVJs are issued by NICE's board and also draw on input from a 30-strong Citizens Council comprised of lay members of the public. While the Citizen's Council had sympathy for an adoption of the rule of rescue,[14] the SVJ then argues:

> NICE recognises that when it is making its decisions it should consider the needs of present and future patients of the NHS who are anonymous and who do not necessarily have people to argue their case on their behalf. NICE considers that the principles provided in this document are appropriate to resolve the tension between the needs of an individual patient and the needs of present and future users of the NHS. The Institute has not therefore adopted an additional "rule of rescue."[15]

While NICE uses an explicit procedure to determine value for money, as Rawlins and Pearson outline in Excerpt 5:

> It is important to note that NICE does not take the budget impact of a new technology into account. For example, although a new drug might have a favorable cost-effectiveness ratio of $30,000 per QALY, the overall impact might be too great for the NHS budget if very large numbers of patients were to be eligible for treatment. Affordability is not the responsibility of NICE; the government remains accountable for the overall NHS budget and must therefore judge a particular intervention unaffordable for the NHS even though NICE might have judged it cost-effective. Such a situation has not yet arisen.

[13] NICE, *Social Value Judgements*.

[14] NICE Citizens Council, *NICE Citizens Council Report: Rule of Rescue* (2006).

[15] NICE, *Social Value Judgements*, pp. 20–21.

Australia's Pharmaceutical Benefits Scheme (PBS),[16] which broadly serves very similar policy objectives as NICE, has adopted a different approach on these issues. As Bulfone, Younie, and Carter describe, the PBS evaluations are also based on QALYs but avoid using a cost threshold (Excerpt 6).[17] In part this is because "HTA was not introduced into Australia with a main objective of cost containment but rather as a means of ensuring that funding of interventions was evidence-based and represented value-for-money."[18] This does not mean that the budgetary impact of interventions is ignored. Economic evaluations do come into play regarding the coverage of high-cost interventions that can pose large questions of affordability. The authors point out that government becomes involved when covering an intervention will raise costs substantially:

> new drugs with a budgetary impact greater than $5 million [need to] be considered by the Department of Treasury and Finance and . . . new drugs with a budgetary impact greater than $10 million [require] approval from Cabinet . . . before any recommendation to make a drug available is implemented.[19]

This requirement explicitly acknowledges that allocation decisions in publicly funded healthcare systems can quickly move beyond the realm of scientific evidence, technical economic evaluations, and basic ethical principles, to become the subject of political processes. The requirement also matters in view of the fact that the rule of rescue is explicitly accepted in Australia. The authors note that for the rule to be invoked, three conditions must be fulfilled: (1) a severe illness that considerably

[16] The Pharmaceutical Benefits Scheme (PBS), accessed June 16, 2015, http://www.pbs.gov.au/pbs/home.

[17] L. Bulfone, S. Younie, and R. Carter, "Health Technology Assessment: Reflection from the Antipodes," *Value Health* 12, no. 2 (2009): pp. S28–S39.

[18] Ibid., p. S31.

[19] Ibid., p. S32.

shortens life, (2) an illness that affects only a small number of people, and (3) an illness for which there is no alternative treatment in Australia.

Germany has taken a different approach to incorporating economic considerations into resource allocation decisions. First, Germany has two separate bodies that engage with CER and coverage decisions. The Federal Joint Commission (Gemeinsamer Bundesausschuss, G-BA) is the central body that makes decisions on which services will be covered by public health insurance.[20] The G-BA brings together representatives from payers and providers of healthcare as well as patient groups. As a major input to its decision making, the G-BA requests advice on efficacy, effectiveness, and efficiency from the Institute for Quality and Efficiency in Healthcare (Institut für Qualität und Wirtschaftlichkeit im Gesundheitswesen, IQWiG).[21] Regarding economic evaluations, as Caro and colleagues outline, IQWiG reviewed internationally used approaches but found that none was "universally accepted" (Excerpt 7).[22] In looking for alternatives, the Institute "insisted on a method that does not address the broader issue of prioritizing across the health-care system."[23] Thus, the IQWiG does not use QALYs.[24] Instead, IQWiG draws on an efficiency frontier that uses existing interventions as benchmarks and then compares the relative benefits of other interventions in terms of life expectancy, side effects, and health-related quality of life. Thus, unlike NICE in England and PBS in Australia, Germany does not use QALYs nor does it have a cost-effectiveness threshold, whether fixed or flexible.

Germany also differs considerably on the rule of rescue. Normally, the rule of rescue seems reasonable only if there is an effective (albeit expensive) intervention. But in Germany, the highest court affirmed that it is valid even when evidence of an intervention's efficacy is lacking. In the so-called St. Nicholas case, a 19-year-old muscular dystrophy patient requested bio-resonance therapy, an unproved treatment using electrical stimulation. The Bundesverfassungsgericht ruled that for life-threatening conditions, interventions that lack a solid scientific basis but have a "not entirely remote chance of healing or recovery" must be covered.[25]

The United States differs from the other countries in how it approaches economic and ethical considerations in coverage decisions. In the United States, the healthcare system is fragmented and there is no central body making coverage decisions. Different payers make different use of CER data in their coverage and benefit design decisions. Around half of the population is covered by employer-based healthcare; approximately a third is covered by government programs—Medicare, Medicaid, and CHIP—for children, elderly or low-income populations; a small but significant proportion of the population purchase insurance privately; and 3% are covered as active or former military service personnel.[26] The Affordable Care Act (ACA) established the Patient-Centered Outcomes Research Institute (PCORI)[27] to fund and coordinate CER. PCORI does not make coverage decisions and has

[20] "The Federal Joint Committee: About Us," 2010, accessed June 16, 2015, https://www.g-ba.de/downloads/17-98-2804/2010-01-01-Faltblatt-GBA_engl.pdf.

[21] Institut Für Qualität Und Wirtschaftlichkeit Im Gesundheitswesen, accessed June 16, 2015, https://www.iqwig.de/de/startseite.2724.html.

[22] J. J. Caro, et al., "The Efficiency Frontier Approach to Economic Evaluation of Health-Care Interventions," *Health Economics* 19 (2010): p. 1119.

[23] Ibid.

[24] Gerber-Grote, "Welchen Beitrag Leisten."

[25] R. Hess, "Alternative Behandlungsmethoden Bei Lebensbedrohlichen Erkrankungen: Auseinandersetzung Mit Dem Beschluss Des Bundesverfassungsgerichts Vom 6.; Dezember 2005," *Gesundheit und Gesellschaft: G + G* Vol. 6, No. 4, p. 7–14 (2006).

[26] "Health Insurance Coverage of the Total Population," accessed June 16, 2015, http://kff.org/other/state-indicator/total-population/

[27] "Patient-Centered Outcomes Research Institute: About Us," accessed June 16, 2015, http://www.pcori.org/about-us.

no enforcement mechanisms to encourage or require either public or private payers to use its findings. Just as other government payers of healthcare, PCORI is legally prohibited from using QALYs and a threshold of any kind in its evaluations. The ACA explicitly noted in establishing PCORI that it

> shall not develop or employ a dollars-per-quality adjusted life year (or similar measure that discounts the value of a life because of an individual's disability) as a threshold to establish what type of health care is cost effective or recommended. The Secretary [of Health] shall not utilize such an adjusted life year (or such a similar measure) as a threshold to determine coverage, reimbursement, or incentive programs under title XVIII [the public Medicare program].[28]

While there is no formal legal or other endorsement of the rule of rescue, by implication, the US's explicit objection to considering cost places it closer to the German approach. Still, it has been suggested that payers, hospitals, and others increasingly demand cost-effectiveness data,[29] introducing economic evaluations in a decentralized manner. This situation raises equity issues in that it is possible that three people who are neighbors all have different entitlements to health care, if, for example, one has employer-based insurance, one has coverage through Medicare, and one through the Veterans Health Administration (providing for former military personnel). Similar variation in coverage, albeit at the level of postal codes, was one of the reasons that led to the establishment of the UK's NICE in 1999.[30]

As was highlighted in Chapters 8 and 9, historically and currently, CER and HTA centrally focus on identifying effectiveness, which is a necessary albeit not sufficient condition for decisions about an intervention's efficiency. In this regard, the fact that the United States is the most hostile to centralized economic considerations also needs to be seen in the context of its relationship between spending and health outcomes in comparison to other countries. The ethical significance lies in the entailed opportunity cost: high cost with no significant health gains due to interventions with unduly limited effectiveness constitute waste and typically deplete funding for more effective healthcare services. Moreover, waste in not just undesirable in an abstract sense, but has direct implications for healthcare users. It increases costs and therefore insurance premiums or taxation, as well as out-of-pocket costs such as co-payments and other user fees. In addition, where government resources are the main funding source, budgets of other non–healthcare services, such as education, are typically affected negatively. As Figure 10.1 shows, the US situation warrants closer examination because private and public spending individually exceed the median of the combined private and public spending of all member countries of the Organization for Economic Cooperation and Development (OECD) as a percentage of gross domestic product (GDP).

The US's high spending—at around $9,000 per capita total healthcare costs currently account for a little over a sixth of the economy[31]—does not, however, translate into better care or better outcomes, as an annually updated comparison of the US system in international comparisons consistently shows (Figure 10.2).

In this context, a major report by the nonpartisan Institute of Medicine (IOM) to advise on defining essential health benefits (EHBs) is of particular relevance. Excerpt 8 delineates the

---

28 *Patient Protection and Affordable Care Act,* H.R. 3590, Section 1182.

29 J. C. Robinson, "Biomedical Innovation in the Era of Health Care Spending Constraints," *Health Affairs* 34, no. 2 (2015): pp. 203–209.

30 R. R. Faden and K. Chalkidou, "Determining the Value of Drugs: The Evolving British Experience," *New England Journal of Medicine* 364, no. 14 (2011): p. 1290.

31 Peter G. Peterson Foundation, "Americans Spend over Twice as Much Per Capita on Healthcare as the Average Developed Country Does," 2014, accessed May 2015, http://pgpf.org/Chart-Archive/0006_health-care-oecd.

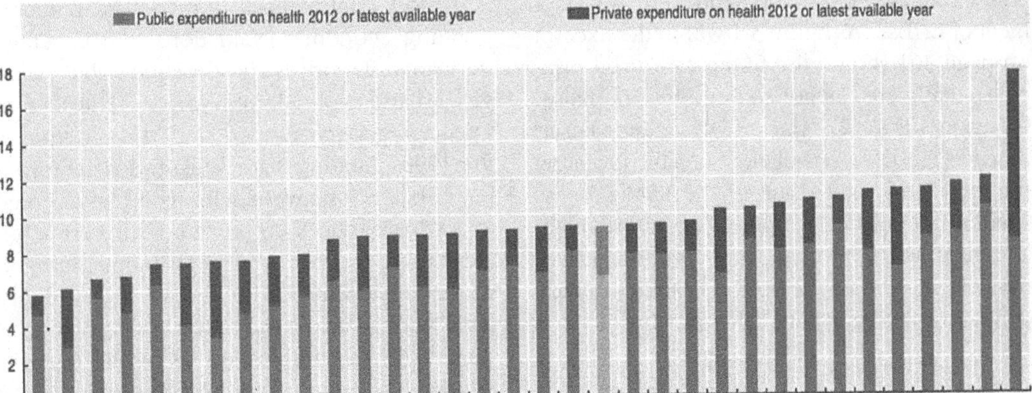

Figure 10.1 Public and private expenditure on health as a percentage of gross domestic product (GDP), 2011.

Organization for Economic Co-operation and Development.

COUNTRY RANKINGS

Top 2+
Middle
Bottom 2+

	AUS	CAN	FRA	GER	NETH	NZ	NDR	SWE	SWIZ	UK	US
OVERALL RANKING (2013)	4	10	9	5	5	7	7	3	2	1	11
Quality Care	2	9	8	7	5	4	11	10	3	1	5
Effective Care	4	7	9	6	5	2	11	10	8	1	3
Safe Care	3	10	2	6	7	9	11	5	4	1	7
Coordinated Care	4	8	9	10	5	2	7	11	3	1	6
Patient Centered Care	5	8	10	7	3	6	11	9	2	1	4
Access	8	9	11	2	4	7	6	4	2	1	9
Cost-Related Problem	9	5	10	4	8	6	3	1	7	1	11
Timelines of Care	6	11	10	4	2	7	8	9	1	3	5
Efficiency	4	10	8	9	7	3	4	2	6	1	11
Equity	5	9	7	4	8	10	6	1	2	2	11
Healthy Lines	4	8	1	7	5	9	6	2	3	10	11
Healthy Expenditures/Capita, 2011**	$3,800	$4,522	$4,118	$4,495	$5,099	$3,182	$5,669	$3,925	$5,643	$3,405	$8,508

Figure 10.2 Quality rankings of 11 member countries of the Organization for Economic Cooperation and Development (OECD) by five key criteria (2013 or nearest year).[a]

[a] Includes ties. ** Expenditures shown in $US PPP (purchasing power parity); Australian $ data are from 2010.

Calculated by the Commonwealth Fund based on 2011 International Health Policy Survey of Sicker Adults; 2012 International Health Policy Survey of Primary Care Physicians; 2013 International Health.

IOM's framework to help guide the development of EHBs.[32] As figure 3-1 within the Excerpt on page 361 shows, the framework used principles that were categorized into four domains: (1) economics, (2) ethics, (3) evidence-based practice, and (4) population health. Probably the most important result of the IOM process was an unequivocal emphasis on affordability and maximizing coverage over comprehensiveness of benefits. As the IOM's "Criteria to guide content of the aggregate EHBs states:

> In the aggregate, the EHB must:
>
> 1) Be affordable for consumers, employers, and taxpayers.
> 2) Maximize the number of people with insurance coverage.
> 3) Protect the most vulnerable by addressing the particular needs of those patients and populations.[33]

The criteria go on to emphasize advancing "stewardship of resources," "addressing the medical concerns of greatest importance," and "protecting against the greatest financial risks." And, finally, it suggests that individual services should "be cost effective, so that the health gain for individual and population health is sufficient to justify the additional cost to taxpayers and consumers."[34]

Thus, the IOM strongly endorsed emphasizing cost and minimizing cost for maximal health benefits. After robust conversations, the IOM "ultimately decided that costs were a critical component of the definition" of EHBs.[35]

Ultimately, however, none of this mattered. In December 2011, the Secretary avoided defining a uniform package of EHBs that all Americans would be entitled to and instead granted each state authority to define its EHBs by determining covered services in reference to existing benefits.[36]

Despite the general aversion to consideration of cost in healthcare in the United States, it has also been the site of one of the boldest and most controversial approaches to incorporating economic evaluations into coverage decisions. David Eddy describes the background and evolution of reforms of the state of Oregon's publicly funded Medicaid program in the 1990s, lauding it for seeking to "achieve a better balance between who receives coverage and what services are covered" (Excerpt 9).[37] Despite severe budgetary constraints, Oregon wanted to extend Medicaid coverage to all eligible people below the federal poverty level.[38]

Initially, a combination of public engagement and a very direct application of CEA was used to rank services that would be covered. One of the consequences was that comparatively minor benefits that accrued to a very large number of patients were prioritized over very significant benefits for a smaller number of people. For example, tooth capping for a large number of people was ranked higher than life-saving appendectomies for far fewer. David Hadorn argues that the policy represents a fundamental and irreconcilable conflict between CEA and the rule of rescue (Excerpt 10).[39] He describes how the initial list, based on CEA, was subsequently revised by ordering a set of 17 categories that concern varying types or degrees of expected health benefit from treatments according to three criteria: (1) perceived value to the individual, (2) value to society, and (3) necessity. Norman Daniels focuses on whether Oregon's policy makes disadvantaged groups better or worse off, whether entailed inequalities are justifiable, and whether the procedure for determining the basic level of healthcare is a just or fair one (Excerpt 11).[40]

---

[32] Institute of Medicine, *Essential Health Benefits: Balancing Coverage and Cost* (Washington, DC: The National Academies Press, 2012).

[33] Ibid., p. 55.

[34] Ibid., p. 55.

[35] Ibid., p. 82.

[36] Center for Consumer Information and Insurance Oversight, "Essential Health Benefits Bulletin," 2011.

[37] D. M. Eddy, "What's Going on in Oregon?", *JAMA* 266, no. 3 (1991): p. 419.

[38] Ibid.

[39] D. C. Hadorn, "Setting Health Care Priorities in Oregon: Cost Effectiveness Meets the Rule of Rescue," *JAMA* 265, no. 17 (1991): pp. 2218–2225.

[40] N. Daniels, "Is the Oregon Rationing Plan Fair?", *JAMA* 265, no. 17 (1991): pp. 2232–2235.

To some extent, the variations in approach to considering CEA as part of HTA reflect different cultural traditions or the force of particularly strong budgetary pressures. However, such constraints aside, if health systems are to prioritize higher value interventions, then there has to be some way to compare interventions across diseases. Many oppose rigid QALY thresholds alone for complex resource allocation questions. But, as the Australian example showed, QALYs need not be linked to thresholds. Rather, QALYs can provide crucial baseline orientation, elucidating society's willingness to pay by providing a common currency, thus enabling comparisons of the relative capacity of different interventions to improve length and quality of life. To address shortcomings such as those highlighted in Chapter 9, economic evaluations can furthermore be balanced with other moral values, as Johri and Norheim show (Excerpt 12).[41] Their systematic review examined formal mechanisms for integrating equity considerations in the context of CEA and identified 51 studies that offered feasible suggestions. These can be grouped into three clusters: more than half integrated distributional concerns through equity weights and social welfare functions, and around 20% each used mathematical programming and multicriteria decision analysis.

While policy-makers and politicians centrally shape the framework that determines which scientific considerations and value judgments affect resource allocation, their voices are not the only ones that influence coverage decisions. Increasingly, there is an acknowledgment that the lay perspective matters and should be included in some way. The US's PCORI requires public engagement "from topic selection through design and conduct of research to dissemination of results [as] such engagement can influence research to be more patient-centered, useful, and trustworthy."[42] Julia Kreis and Harald Schmidt analyzed engagement processes in HTA and coverage decisions in the UK, Germany, and France (Excerpt 13).[43] They found that, despite similar policy objectives, there is no consensus about which members of the public should be involved in which processes, what weight their views should have in influencing decisions, how they should be recruited and supported, and how potential conflicts of interests should be addressed. Equally, there appears to be lack of clarity about which of several commonly cited rationales for public engagement should be guiding: contributing facts, values, improving the legitimacy or acceptability of policy, and disseminating knowledge about decisions and processes.

Whether CEA is applied crudely, in a more nuanced way, or, as in the German case, it plays no role at all, an entirely separate question in policy terms is how to implement the relative value that an intervention is deemed to have in coverage decision, benefit design, and clinical practice. The starkest choice is clearly between coverage and noncoverage. But there is a wide range of further levers that can be used to affect the behavior of different actors in the health system toward more high-value care.[44] Table 10.2 provides an overview of some of the more prominent options. Their occurrence, feasibility, and impact differs

---

[41] M. Johri and O. F. Norheim, "Can Cost-Effectiveness Analysis Integrate Concerns for Equity? Systematic Review," *International Journal of Technology Assessment Health Care* 28, no. 2 (2012): pp. 125–132. See also World Health Organization (WHO), *Making Fair Choices on the Path to Universal Health Coverage: Final Report of the WHO Consultative Group on Equity and Universal Health Coverage* (Geneva: WHO).

[42] Patient-Centered Outcomes Research Institute (PCORI), "What We Mean by Engagement," http://www.pcori.org/funding-opportunities/what-we-mean-engagement.

[43] J. Kreis and H. Schmidt, "Public Engagement in Health Technology Assessment and Coverage Decisions: A Study of Experiences in France, Germany, and the United Kingdom," *Journal of Health Politics, Policy and Law* 38, no. 1 (2013): pp. 89–122.

[44] D. J. Morgan, et al., "Understanding Overdiagnosis, Overtreatment and Medical Overuse: A Consensus-Derived Research Agenda," *BMJ* 351, no. h4534 (2015).

Table 10.2
Policy Options for Encouraging High-Value Care by Changing Behavior of Different Agents*

Policy Type	Initiated by	Primary Target Audience
Compulsory review:[a] Require that any safe and efficacious interventions submitted for use by the health care system undergoes effectiveness and efficiency evaluations.	Government, policy-makers	Industry
Coverage refusal or removal:[b] Payers do not, or cease to, cover interventions judged to have poor value (for all patient populations that an intervention is intended for, or for patients with specific characteristics such as health status, genetic or other factors, that significantly affect an intervention"s value)	Public and private payers	Industry, healthcare providers, healthcare professionals
Conditional coverage:[c] Interventions are covered "only in research" or as "coverage with evidence development": payers receive a rebate if performance falls behind the producers" claims.	Policy-makers, Public and private payers	Industry
Reference pricing:[d,e] All safe and effective interventions or procedures are made available, but reimbursement rates are tied to the lowest cost options among equally effective interventions or procedures	Policy-makers, Public and private payers	Industry, healthcare providers
Guideline adherence:[f] Reimbursement is tied to compliance with evidence-based guidelines regarding best practice or "do-not-do" guidelines.[g]	Policy-makers, Public and private payers	Industry, healthcare providers, healthcare professionals
Value-based insurance design (VBID):[h,i] Copayments or other out-of-pocket cost are waived for lower cost options among equally effective interventions	Policy-makers, Public and private payers	Patients
Shared Decision Making:[j,k] Provide patients with evidence-based decision aids[l,m] and other evidence-based means to empower their standing in genuinely shared decisions with healthcare provider	Public and private payers, Healthcare professionals,	Healthcare professionals, patients
Ban direct-to-consumer advertising:[n] Provide information on treatment options through the health care system and curb supply-induced-demand for low-value services	Government, policy-makers	The public, patients

*Adapted from: Elshaug, A.G., Rosenthal, M.B., Lavis, J.N., Brownlee, S., Schmidt, H., Nagpal, S., Littlejohns, P., Srivastava, D., Tunis, S. and Saini, V., 2017. Levers for addressing medical underuse and overuse: achieving high-value health care. *The Lancet.*

[a] Chalkidou, "Comparative Effectiveness Research."

[b] G. MacKean, et al., "Health Technology Reassessment: The Art of the Possible," *Int J Technol Assess Health Care* 29, no. 4 (2013): pp. 418–423.

[c] S. R. Tunis and K. Chalkidou, "Coverage with Evidence Development: A Very Good Beginning, but Much to Be Done. Commentary to Hutton Et Al," *Int J Technol Assess Health Care* 23, no. 4 (2007): pp. 432–435.

[d] P. Kanavos and U. E. Reinhardt, "Reference Pricing for Drugs: Is It Compatible with US Health Care?", *Health Affairs* 22, no. 3 (2003): pp. 16–30.

[e] J. C. Robinson and K. MacPherson, "Payers Test Reference Pricing and Centers of Excellence to Steer Patients to Low-Price and High-Quality Providers," *Health Aff (Millwood)* 31, no. 9 (2012): pp. 2028–2036.

[f] J. N. Lavis, et al., "Evidence-Informed Health Policy 1 – Synthesis of Findings from a Multi-Method Study of Organizations that Support the Use of Research Evidence," *Implementation Science: IS* 3 (2008): pp. 53–53.

[g] S. Garner, et al., "Reducing Ineffective Practice: Challenges in Identifying Low-Value Health Care Using Cochrane Systematic Reviews," *J Health Serv Res Policy* 18, no. 1 (2013): pp. 6–12.

[h] T. B. Gibson, et al., "Value-Based Insurance Design: Benefits Beyond Cost and Utilization," *Am J Manag Care* 21, no. 1 (2015): pp. 32–35.

[i] M. E. Chernew, A. B. Rosen, and A. M. Fendrick, "Value-Based Insurance Design," *Health Affairs* 26, no. 2 (2007): pp. w195–w203.

[j] A. G. Mulley, C. Trimble, and G. Elwyn, *Stop the Silent Misdiagnosis: Patients" Preferences Matter* (2012).

[k] E. Oshima Lee and E. J. Emanuel, "Shared Decision Making to Improve Care and Reduce Costs," *New England Journal of Medicine* 368, no. 1 (2013): pp. 6–8.

[l] Ottawa Hospital Research Institute, "Patient Decision Aids," 2014, accessed June 16, 2015, http://decisionaid.ohri.ca/.

[m] J. Hersch, et al., "Use of a Decision Aid Including Information on Overdetection to Support Informed Choice About Breast Cancer Screening: A Randomised Controlled Trial," *The Lancet* 385, no. 9978): pp. 1642–1652.

[n] B. A. Liang and T. Mackey, "Reforming Direct-to-Consumer Advertising," *Nat Biotech* 29, no. 5 (2011): pp. 397–400.

across countries, in no small part because the structural background conditions of health systems favor some approaches over others (for example, varying co-payments is only meaningful where there are co-payments).

Whether principles of resource allocation are declared explicitly in transparent processes or can only be reconstructed implicitly, by analyzing how access to services in situations of relative scarcity is structured, ethical values are at the heart of any healthcare system. Both explicit and implicit approaches require justification—there is no value-free space in either policy or practice.

Questions for Discussion

1. What is the difference between EBM, CER, and HTA?
2. Consider the British use of QALYs: What do you see as the most significant ethical benefit and what as the most significant harm?
3. Is the Australian approach to the rule of rescue fair?
4. The United States has the highest health spending of all OECD countries, yet no superior health outcomes. Although CEA is not used centrally, it is suggested that payers, hospitals, and others increasingly demand it. Why might this be so?
5. Julia Kreis and Harald Schmidt found in a review of public engagement activities in HTA and coverage decisions in the UK, Germany, and France that there was no agreement on which of five fundamental rationales for engagement should be the most important: contributing facts, values, improving the legitimacy or acceptability of policy, and disseminating knowledge about decisions and processes (Excerpt 13). Which do you consider most important and why?

EXCERPTS

Note: The following excerpts have generally been edited for length, and omissions are indicated with ellipses. Editing includes footnotes and endnotes, which have also been renumbered. For citation and related purposes, the full original source texts should be used.

EXCERPT 1

Abridged text from:

B. R. Luce, et al., "EBM, HTA, and CER: Clearing the Confusion," *Milbank Quarterly* 88, no. 2 (2010): pp. 256–276.

EBM, HTA, and CER: Clearing the Confusion

Bryan R. Luce, Michael Drummond, Bengt Jönsson, Peter J. Neumann, J. Sanford Schwartz, Uwe Seibert, and Sean D. Sullivan

The International Working Group for HTA Advancement; United BioSource Corporation; University of York; Stockholm School of Economics; Tufts Medical Center; University of Pennsylvania; University for Health Sciences, Medical Informatics and Technology; University of Washington

. . .

Redefining EBM, HTA, and CER

[W]e propose clarifying the typology, nomenclature, and interrelationships of the evidence terms. . . . Figure [10.3] depicts EBM, HTA, and CER again as rectangles. The key related concepts are in circles and ovals, and the most important decision-making processes are shown as diamonds. The arrows illustrate the principal relationships among the various concepts. The dotted lines labeled A through C indicate relationships about which there is considerable dispute. . . .

Considering first the column headed "Can it work?" we can see that evidence generated from traditional efficacy RCTs is used for decisions about the market approval of new interventions. These RCTs are also currently the major input to systematic reviews of trials. SRTs include, too, pragmatic clinical trials that are becoming more common, and they also are inputs to clinical guidelines, which we view as straddling the first two columns in the diagram.

Comparative-effectiveness research is firmly situated in the column "Does it work?" covering both evidence generation and evidence synthesis. That is, we expect a two-way link between CER and pragmatic clinical trials, and we expect a similar link between CER and SREs. In turn, SREs (systematic reviews of evidence) consider evidence from RCTs, PCTs, and observational studies. We also depict the outputs of CER activities as influencing EBM either directly or indirectly through clinical guidelines, whose development we consider to be one activity of EBM. The outputs of CER activities also are an important input to HTA activities (e.g., the results of nationally funded CER studies may be an important input to HTAs conducted by different payers). One important aspect of this definition of CER is that it has no direct link to any decision process, although its purpose is to do so and thus it ideally influences patients' and physicians' decisions through EBM, or coverage decisions including those through HTA.

EBM is characterized as a decision process, focusing on decisions by individual patients and physicians, but it does cross into the "evidence synthesis" space. In our representation, EBM focuses mainly on the question "Does it work?" although it also contains an element of the question "Is it worth it?" specifically from the patient's perspective. As mentioned previously, we acknowledge that the development of clinical guidelines is an important aspect of EBM, but we think of it from a patient's perspective rather than a societal perspective. We regard the production of guidelines from a societal perspective as being closer to HTA.

Health technology assessment straddles the last two columns in the figure, and is viewed as a method of evidence synthesis that receives inputs from CER, economic evaluation, and the consideration of social, ethical, and legal

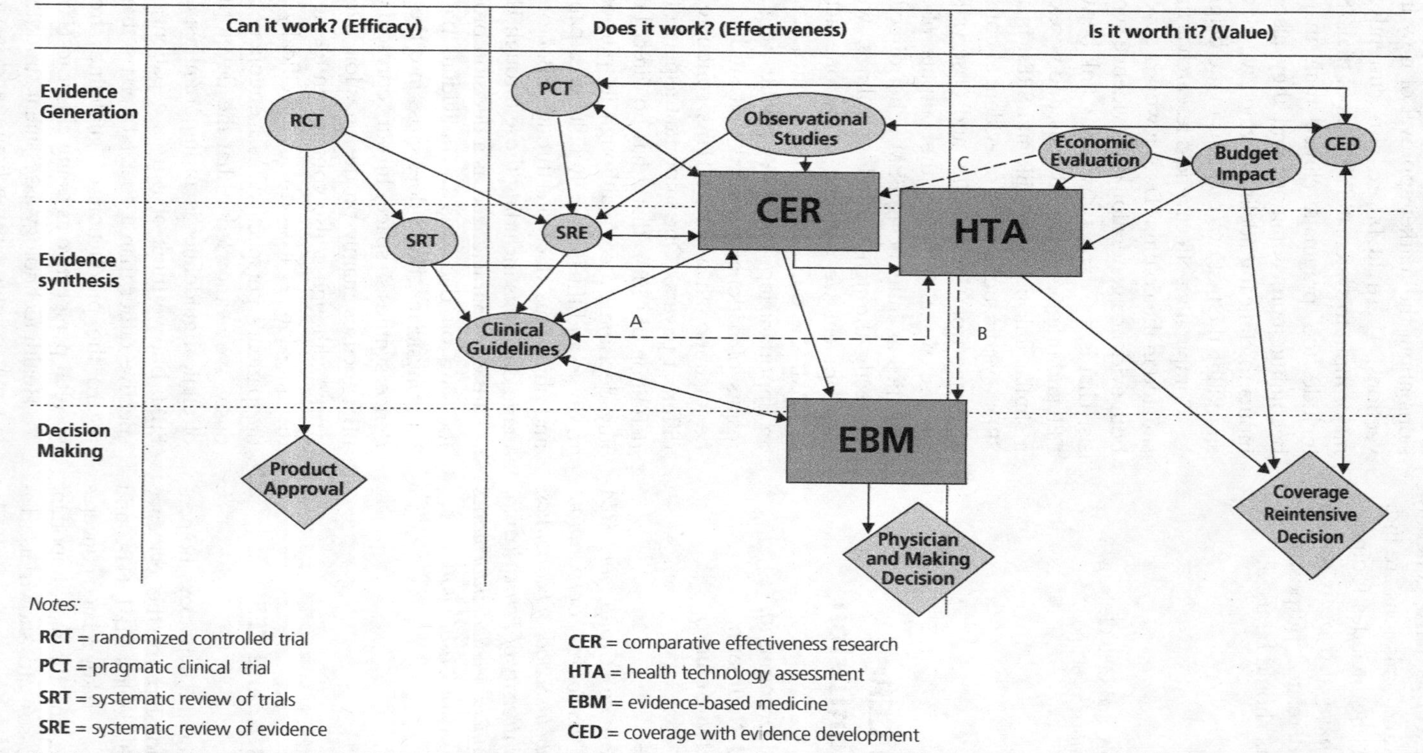

Figure [10.3] Redefined relationships of evidence processes.

RCT, randomized controlled trial; *PCT*, pragmatic clinical trial; *SRT*, systematic review of trials; *SRE*, systematic review of evidence; *CER*, comparative effectiveness research; *HTA*, health technology assessment; *EBM*, evidence-based medicine; *CED*, coverage with evidence development.

Solid lines indicate clear relationships and dotted lines indicate disputed relationships. Diamonds represent decision on processes; circles and ovals represent all other evidence activities, except for the rectangles, which are reserved for EBM, HTA, and CER.

aspects. As we depict it, HTA is a main input to coverage decisions, which may also be influenced by budget implications.

Finally, conditional coverage (depicted in the diagram as CED) is represented as both a decision and an evidence generation process involving the commissioning and use of observational studies and, occasionally, pragmatic RCTs.

Although we believe that our organizing framework and accompanying definitions do help distinguish concepts and depict relationships of EBM, HTA, and CER (and other related terms), some relationships remain the subject of debate. These are identified by the broken lines in the figure. Line A indicates that there could be a link between clinical guidelines and HTA, opening up the possibility that clinical guidelines may—and sometimes do—explicitly include a consideration of cost-effectiveness and, through HTA, be linked to coverage decisions. We consider this to be entirely appropriate, and it is the approach followed by NICE in the United Kingdom and other countries.[1] Our diagram reflects the current majority view that clinical guidelines, as practiced through EBM, are primarily concerned with improving the quality of care for the patient rather than increasing value for money for the payer or society.

Line B suggests that there could be a link between EBM and HTA. First, as we acknowledged earlier, some health technology assessments may focus on the clinical effectiveness and quality of care, rather than on value for money. Second, as we argued earlier, some of the objectives of quality of care and value for money are closely aligned. For example, removing interventions that contribute only little to improving patients' outcomes and are inconvenient to the patient, are expensive, or are risky will increase the quality of care and save resources. Nevertheless, we still feel that it is preferable to distinguish between activities that concentrate primarily on benefits to the patient (EBM) and those that concentrate primarily on benefits to society at large (HTA).

Line C, going directly from Economic Evaluation to CER, is probably the most controversial of all. This relationship implies that CER studies should include consideration of cost-effectiveness, a suggestion that has led to considerable debate in the United States.[2,3] At the time of this writing, however, US legislation, for instance, that associated with health care reform, does not include cost-effectiveness.[4] We can see the merits of both sets of arguments. But our basic diagram, without line C, has balance, in that CER studies are viewed as an important source of information for those conducting both EBM and HTA.

Those who believe that cost-effectiveness should be routinely incorporated into CER make two arguments. First, CER studies represent an important opportunity for collecting data on resource use and cost, which in turn are useful for subsequent HTAs. Second, if cost-effectiveness is not part of CER, subsequent HTAs may not be fully informed. For example, individual health plans may not have the expertise, time, resources, or even inclination to conduct proper cost-effectiveness analysis. In such cases, the argument is that coverage decisions tend to focus on the acquisition cost of a new technology, rather than to consider fully its economic value.

The counterargument is that the direct inclusion of cost-effectiveness considerations in CER studies changes the overall balance in the emphasis and use of these studies, concentrating on their use in HTA and possibly disregarding their use in EBM. This may lead to objections that would hamper the overall CER movement. We firmly believe, though, that because all decisions have resource implications, cost-effectiveness considerations should play a role in coverage

[1] "Special Issue: Health Technology Assessment in Evidence-Based Health Care Reimbursement Decisions around the World: Lessons Learned," *Value in Health* 12, no. s2 (2009).

[2] American College of Physicians, "Information on Cost-Effectiveness: An Essential Product of a National Comparative Effectiveness Program," *Annals of Internal Medicine* 148, no. 12 (2008): pp. 956–961.

[3] G. R. Wilensky, "Cost-Effectiveness Information: Yes, It's Important, but Keep It Separate, Please!", *Annals of Internal Medicine* 148, no. 12 (2008): pp. 967–968.

[4] US Congress, Senate. 2009. *The Patient Protection and Affordable Care Act.* 111th Cong., 1st sess., H.R. 3590.

decisions, through either inclusion in CER studies directly or adequately conducted HTAs.

Finally, we note the potential for inherent conflicts that inevitably resides in some, if not all, the concepts that we have tried to clarify and distinguish from one another in this article. For example, consider EBM and HTA. If we take as given that the proper and full expression of EBM includes individual patients' values, which itself can include patients' out-of-pocket costs, the societal aggregate of these values would quickly conflict with societal HTA. This is because the former assumes that individual patients are to be satisfied one by one, whereas HTA may take a societal approach, often within budget constraints, meaning that not everyone may get everything he or she desires. Thus, although we seek to differentiate, bind, and relate EBM-HTA-CER (plus other related evidence-based processes) within one holistic graphic, we are not contending that they all have a central unifying aspect.

Bearing all this in mind, the following are our preferred definitions of the three key terms:

1. Evidence-based medicine (EBM) is an evidence synthesis and decision process used to assist patients' and/or physicians' decisions. It considers evidence regarding the effectiveness of interventions and patients' values and is mainly concerned with individual patients' decisions, but is also useful for developing clinical guidelines as they pertain to individual patients.
2. Comparative effectiveness research (CER) includes both evidence generation and evidence synthesis. It is concerned with the comparative assessment of interventions in routine practice settings. The outputs of CER activities are useful for clinical guideline development, evidence-based medicine, and the broader social and economic assessment of health technologies (i.e., HTA).
3. Health technology assessment (HTA) is a method of evidence synthesis that considers evidence regarding clinical effectiveness, safety, cost-effectiveness and, when broadly applied, includes social, ethical, and legal aspects of the use of health technologies. The precise balance of these inputs depends on the purpose of each individual HTA. A major use of HTAs is in informing reimbursement and coverage decisions, in which case HTAs should include benefit-harm assessment and economic evaluation.

Conclusions

[We offered] more precise definitions of key terms based on an organizing framework that clarifies the differences and relationships among EBM, HTA, CER, and related concepts. All three terms address the "Does it work?" question, but none asks the "Can it work?" question. Health technology assessment is the primary activity that considers "Is it worth it?" although as we point out, EBM should also address the more limited question "Is it worth it to the patient?" taking into account the costs to the patient. Of the three concepts, only EBM is a decision process, although both HTA and CER are applied specifically to feed into decision making.

Acknowledgments: The International Working Group for HTA Advancement was established in July 2007 with unrestricted funding from the Schering Plough Corporation (now Merck & Co). The Working Group's mission is to provide scientifically based leadership to facilitate significant continuous improvement in the development and implementation of practical, rigorous methods into formal health technology assessment (HTA) systems and processes, by facilitating the development and adoption of high-quality, scientifically driven, objective, and trusted HTA to improve patient outcomes, the health of the public, and the overall quality and efficiency of health care. We are grateful to Emily Sargent for her outstanding graphics work, formatting, and general manuscript preparation and for the many helpful comments by several anonymous reviewers as well as Bradford Gray. The views expressed in this article are those of the authors and do not necessarily reflect the opinions of any of these individuals.

EXCERPT 2

Abridged text from:

K. Chalkidou, et al., "Comparative Effectiveness Research and Evidence-Based Health Policy: Experience from Four Countries," *Milbank Quarterly* 87, no. 2 (2009): pp. 339–367.

Comparative Effectiveness Research and Evidence-Based Health Policy: Experience from Four Countries

Kalipso Chalkidou, Sean Tunis, Ruth Lopert, Lise Rochaix, Peter T. Sawicki, Mona Nasser, and Bertrand Xerri

National Institute for Health and Clinical Excellence (UK); Center for Medical Technology Policy (USA); Department of Health and Ageing (Australia); Haute Autorit'e de Sant'e (France); Institut für Qualität und Wirtschaftlichkeit im Gesundheitswesen (Germany)

8296->1685

. . .

This article builds a matrix of features identified from the international models studied that offer insights into near-term decisions about the location, design, and function of a US-based CER entity. While each country has developed a CER capacity unique to its health system, elements such as the inclusiveness of relevant stakeholders, transparency in operation, independence of the central government and other interests, and adaptability to a changing environment are prerequisites for these entities' successful operation. . . .

. . . (See Table [10.3])

Relationship to health care system: The relationship of each CER entity to the health care system in which it operates ranges from an integrated model in the case of [the UK's] NICE, which forms part of and issues its advice directly to the NHS, to an arm's-length relationship in the case of [Germany's] IQWiG, which advises the Federal Joint Committee (FJC). The responsibility for developing and implementing health policy in light of IQWiG's advice lies with FJC, which includes representatives from the providers (hospitals and professional associations) and the payers (insurance funds). France's HAS also is at arm's length from insurers and government and other stakeholders, even though these stakeholders help determine its annual work program. In Australia, the Pharmaceutical Benefits Advisory Committee (PBAC) makes recommendations to the minister for health and ageing, who must have a positive recommendation in order to list a drug on the PBS formulary. Any decisions whose net cost to the program is expected to exceed AUS$10 million per year must be endorsed by the cabinet.

. . .

Consideration of costs: All four entities explicitly consider costs and cost-effectiveness when making decisions or recommendations. PBS was the first to include costs in the 1990s, followed by NICE, when it was established in 1999. HAS and IQWiG added or enhanced cost considerations as part of their remit by law, in 2008 and 2007, respectively. With the exception of NICE, the original focus of CER entities was to conduct comparative clinical effectiveness reviews without considering costs, but in each case the lack of economic assessment was found to limit these organizations' ability to complete their assessments.

. . .

Dissemination and Implementation

. . .

Interestingly, the implementation of CER decisions in the health care system originally was outside the remit of all the four CER entities reviewed. Traditionally, separate bodies were responsible for ensuring that providers and payers adhered to CER-based guidance through monitoring, regulation, and pay-for-performance schemes. NICE and HAS are the two examples of agencies for which implementation is now becoming an important

Table [10.3]
Key Attributes Across CER Entities

Attributes	NICE [UK]	HAS [France]	IQWiG [Germany]	PBS [Australia]
1. State objective and purpose	Reduce variation in practice; accelerate uptake of new technologies; set quality standards and improve efficiency.	Improve the quality of health care services through hospital accreditation, best care standards, and continuous professional development; evaluation of medical effectiveness, public health impact, and health technology assessments (new and within the existing formulary).	(1) Search for, assessment, and presentation of current scientific evidence on diagnostic and therapeutic procedures for specific diseases; (2) Preparation of scientific reports and expert opinions on quality and efficiency issues of Statutory Health Insurance fund, taking age, gender, and personal circumstances into account; (3) Appraisal of evidence-based clinical practice guidelines on epidemiologically most important diseases; (4) Development of recommendations on disease management programs; (5) Provision of understandable evidence-based information for patients and public.	(To support) timely access to the medicines that Australians need, at a cost that individuals and the community can afford.
2. Subject and scope of assessment (e.g., drugs, technologies, management strategies)	Medical technologies including drugs, devices, and diagnostic tests; clinical guidelines for disease management; public health guidance on disease prevention; information for patients and the public.	Medical technologies including drugs, devices, procedures, and diagnostic tests; clinical guidelines for disease management; public health guidance on disease prevention and health care system organization.	Pharmaceuticals (drugs), medical devices, quality control interventions, surgical procedures, diagnostic tests, clinical practice guidelines and aspects of disease management programs, and evidence-based information for patients.	Limited to assessment of prescription medicines for subsidy; the Pharmaceutical Benefits Advisory Committee (PBAC) also evaluates vaccines for inclusion on the National Immunization Program.
. . .	. . .	. . .	. . .	. . .
4. Type of research evidence used (prospective trials, claims data analysis, systematic reviews, and decision analysis)	Mostly evidence synthesis of existing experimental and observational studies; economic modeling; small number of prospective trials funded by public sources.	Synthesis of existing experimental and observational studies; increasing use of economic modeling and public health analyses; analysis of postmarketing and postlisting studies data when available.	Mostly evidence synthesis of existing experimental studies, economic modeling, guidelines, and, occasionally, method studies. For patient information, high-quality systematic reviews.	Applicant identifies, synthesizes, and presents evidence. PBAC prefers evidence from meta-analyses of well-conducted head-to-head RCTs of proposed drug and main comparator but has no minimum standard. Economic modeling is generally required.

...	...	...	...	...
6. Structure and relationship to health care system	Part of NHS; independent of central government, issues guidance directly to health service and broader public sector (local authorities, transport, and education boards).	Independent of central government, health ministry, or insurance funds. Accountable to the French parliament	Established by the Federal Joint Committee, independent from government, private foundation, receives commissions from Federal Joint Committee and Ministry of Health and advises FJC who issue their directives to Statutory Health Insurance funds.	Policy and program management is responsibility of the Pharmaceutical Evaluation Branch (PEB) of Pharmaceutical Benefits Division of Department of Health and Ageing; the PEB supports the PBAC and its subcommittees and manages evaluation process, pricing negotiations and arrangements, public dissemination of decisions, and liaison with pharmaceutical
7. Budget and source of funding	£35 million per year: funded by Department of Health.	In 2006, € 70 million funded by the following sources: 34% through earmarked taxes levied on drug companies spending on advertising, 15% from hospitals' accreditation fees, 7% from fees from manufacturers, 32% by NHI, 10% by government, 2% by investment income.	€ 15 million; 50% from a levy on every hospital case to be invoiced and 50% from an increase in reimbursement rate of medical and dental outpatient services paid by the health insurance funds. Details determined by the Federal Joint Committee.	The PBS is a demand-driven program with an uncapped appropriation. Management of the PBS listing process is part of Department of Health and Ageing portfolio funding and is approximately AUD $ 14 million per year.
8. Consideration of costs (e.g., budget impact analysis, CEA, other)	Comparative cost-effectiveness analysis part of its remit since establishment in 1999. Budget impact analysis to inform implementation but not as a decision input.	Since January 2008, consideration of economic and other social dimensions as part of remit to inform decisions about sustainability and feasibility.	Since 2007, description of relationships between costs and benefits along with an efficiency frontier and a budget impact analysis to provide a decision basis for ceiling prices of drugs (currently under development).	Comparative cost-effectiveness analysis since 1988 (mandatory since 1993); budget impact analysis (mandatory and considered as part of recommendation, and by government for final decision).

(continued)

Table [10.3] (Continued)

Attributes	NICE [UK]	HAS [France]	IQWiG [Germany]	PBS [Australia]
9. Status of guidance (e.g., mandatory, advisory) and relationship with coverage and reimbursement decisions	Guidance on use of medical technologies mandatory (funds must be made available to cover recommended technologies). Public health and clinical guideline recommendations have advisory status.	Guidance on drugs and devices mandatory since 1999. Recommendations on use of procedures and other public health and clinical guideline recommendations have advisory status.	Advisory to the Federal Joint Committee. After approval by the Ministry of Health, the directives by Federal Joint Committee based on IQWiG reports are mandatory.	As part of listing recommendations, PBAC may recommend specific circumstances in which medicines should be subsidized; positive advice is subject to ministerial/ parliamentary approval. Negative advice is mandatory.
10. Dissemination and implementation/ enforcement strategies (e.g., audit, educational tools, academic detailing, financial incentives – P4P)	Responsibility for supporting implementation since 2004: audit and educational tools, field consultants, budget impact analysis, continuous medical education. Financial and regulatory performance schemes to encourage uptake.	Implementation is fostered by integration of recommendation within various dimensions of HAS's remit, from hospitals' accreditation to continuous professional development and patient information.	Implemented through directives of the Federal Joint Committee, which considers equipment and training needed for implementation by the insurance funds. Insurance funds can use different health plan strategies within directives' frame.	National Prescribing Service (NPS), established in 1998, is an independent organization funded by government that promotes quality use of medicines (QUM) through professional education, academic detailing, training in rational prescribing, clinical audits, conferences, the national Therapeutic Advisory and Information Service, and a range of publications for prescribers. Prescriber audit is the responsibility of Medicare Australia.

priority. Since 2004, NICE has included "supporting implementation" in its remit and its implementation team is the fastest growing in the institute. This may be the result of the realization that merely making information available is insufficient for its effective and timely adoption, especially advisory standards for non-pharmacological interventions. Financial and regulatory incentives are increasingly used to promote the adoption of NICE guidance and reduce inappropriate variation and wasteful practice through (1) a stronger system of incentives, directly linking NICE guidance to monetary rewards for primary care physicians (Quality and Outcomes Framework) and secondary care providers (through regular adjustments of DRG prices to reflect NICE guidance and a move to normative CER-based DRGs, whose "price tag" reflects the cost of best practices, like not paying for an extended stay or high rates of caesarean sections); (2) a new accreditation scheme for providers linking their accreditation with, among other things, adherence to NICE standards; and (3) an NHS constitution, making access to NICE-recommended treatment regimes a right for every NHS patient. For HAS, implementation is facilitated by the fact that its purview is very wide, thereby allowing its guidance to be translated into various HAS functions, from hospital accreditation to professional guidelines and continuous professional development programs. No direct incentives or sanctions are associated with guidance follow-up, however. In Germany, implementation is part of the responsibilities of FJC, not IQWiG. FJC takes into consideration the benefit of the medical services along with the applicability and feasibility of implementing these services through mandatory directives issued by the health insurance funds, which cover health care expenses for 90% of the population.

Acknowledgments: The authors would like to thank the Commonwealth Fund for funding this analysis and the London workshop and Steve Pearson, Tony Culyer, Gail Wilensky, and Michael Rawlins for participating in the workshop and sharing their views with us. We are grateful to Andrew Dillon from NICE; Klaus Koch, Anna-Sabine Ernst, Stefan Lange, Hilda Bastian, and Thomas Kaiser from IQWiG; Lloyd Sansom from PBAC; and Laurent Degos, François Meyer, and Margaret Galbraith from HAS for their comments on the draft. We also thank Reetan Patel for managing the international group of authors and coordinating the London workshop. Our views expressed in this article are those of the authors and do not reflect those of their employers or of the Commonwealth Fund, its directors, officers, or staff.

EXCERPT 3

Abridged text from:

M. D. Rawlins and A. J. Culyer, "National Institute for Clinical Excellence and Its Value Judgments," *BMJ* 329 (2004): pp. 224–227.

National Institute for Clinical Excellence and Its Value Judgments

Michael D. Rawlins and Anthony J. Culyer

. . .

NICE's Approach to Economic Evaluation

On its own, clinical effectiveness is insufficient for maintaining or introducing any clinical procedure or process. Cost must also be taken into account. When good evidence exists of the therapeutic equivalence between two or more clinical management strategies, the cheaper option is preferred. . . .

Incremental Cost Effectiveness Ratio

However, in most instances NICE is confronted with a clinical management strategy that is better than current standard practice but which costs more. NICE must then decide what increase in health (compared with standard practice) is likely to accrue from the increase in expenditure. This is the incremental cost effectiveness ratio. Such ratios can be expressed in many ways. NICE's preferred measure is the cost per quality adjusted life year (QALY), but if appropriate data on quality of life are not available, it uses alternatives such as the cost per life year gained.

NICE rejects the use of an absolute threshold for judging the level of acceptability of a technology in the NHS for four reasons:

- There is no empirical basis for deciding at what value a threshold should be set
- There may be circumstances in which NICE would want to ignore a threshold
- To set a threshold would imply that efficiency has absolute priority over other objectives (particularly fairness)
- Many of the technology supply industries are monopolies, and a threshold would discourage price competition.

Rather than apply an arbitrary threshold, NICE makes its decisions on a case by case basis, as shown stylistically in the figure (see Figure [10.4]). As the incremental cost effectiveness ratio increases, the likelihood of rejection on grounds of cost ineffectiveness rises. The critical issues are the values of incremental cost effectiveness ratios at inflexions A and B.[1,2,3] Clinical management pathways with ratios to the left of A would generally be regarded as cost effective. Those with ratios to the right of B would, if adopted, be likely to deny other patients (with different conditions) access to more cost effective treatments.

There is no empirical basis for assigning particular values to A or B,[4] but NICE and

---

[1] M. L. Weinstein, "From Cost Effectiveness Ratios to Resource Allocation: Where to Draw the Line," in *Valuing Health*, edited by F. A. Sloan (Cambridge: Cambridge University Press, 1995).

[2] A. Towse, C. Pritchard and N. Devlin, eds., *Cost Effectiveness Thesholds: Economic and Ethical Issues* (London: Office of Health Economics, Kings Fund, 2002).

[3] A. Laupacis, et al., "How Attractive Does a New Technology Have to Be to Warrant Adoption and Utilization? Tentative Guidelines for Using Clinical and Economic Evaluations," *Canadian Medical Association Journal* 146, no. 4 (1992): pp. 473–481.

[4] A. J. Culyer, "The Rationing Debate: Maximising the Health of the Whole Community. The Case For," *British Medical Journal* 314, no. 7081 (1997): p. 667.

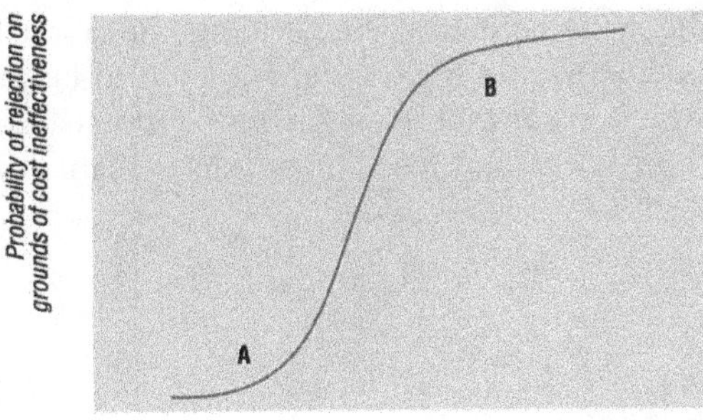

Figure [10.4] Relation between likelihood of a technology being considered as cost-ineffective plotted against the log of the incremental cost-effectiveness ratio.

its advisory bodies have taken the view that inflexion A occurs at around £5000–£15,000/QALY and inflexion B at around £25,000–£35,000/QALY. NICE would be unlikely to reject a technology with a ratio in the range of £5000–£15,000/QALY solely on the grounds of cost ineffectiveness but would need special reasons for accepting technologies with ratios over £25,000–£35,000/QALY as cost effective. The main considerations in making judgments about cost effectiveness for ratios of £25,000–£35,000/QALY are:

- The degree of uncertainty surrounding the estimate
- The particular features of the condition and population using the technology
- The innovative nature of the technology
- When appropriate, the wider societal costs and benefits
- When appropriate, reference to previous appraisals.

The phrase "particular features of the condition and the population using the technology" incorporates matters that include the availability and clinical effectiveness of other interventions for the condition, particular public health issues (such as communicable diseases), and special considerations of equity. Boxes [10.1] and [10.2] show examples of the application of some of these principles.

Box [10.1] Cost Ineffectiveness

Anakinra for Rheumatoid Arthritis

Anakinra seems to be less effective than etanercept or infliximab for rheumatoid arthritis.[i] It costs £7450/year for each patient. The incremental cost effectiveness ratio for anakinra is estimated to be

£69,000/QALY for rheumatoid arthritis, which is an unacceptable opportunity cost.

Interferon beta and glatiramer acetate for multiple sclerosis

Interferon beta and glatiramer acetate reduce the frequency and severity of relapse in relapsing-remitting multiple sclerosis.[ii] The mid-range estimates of the incremental cost effectiveness ratios (£/QALY) depend on the time horizon examined:

- 5 years = £580,000
- 10 years = £308,000
- 20 years = £70,000

The opportunity costs for each of these scenarios are unacceptable.

[i] National Institute for Clinical Excellence, *Anakinra for Rheumatoid Arthritis* (London: NICE, 2003).

[ii] National Institute for Clinical Excellence, *Beta Interferon and Glatiramer Acetate for the Treatment of Multiple Sclerosis* (London: NICE, 2002).

Judgments about whether incremental cost effectiveness ratios can be considered "reasonable" are made by the independent members of NICE's advisory committees (particularly the appraisal committee) and the guideline development groups. Membership is drawn from clinicians and health managers working in the NHS, technical experts (statisticians and health economists), and patients or patient advocates.

Box [10.2] Cost Effectiveness

Imatinib is licensed for the treatment of chronic myeloid leukaemia in the chronic phase (after failure of interferon alfa)[10] and in the accelerated and blast crisis phases (for those not treated earlier with imatinib). The mid range estimates of the incremental cost effectiveness ratios (£/QALY) are:

- 37,000 for the chronic phase
- 38,400 for the accelerated phase
- 49,000 for the blast crisis phase.

In the absence of any effective alternative treatment (apart from bone marrow transplantation) imatinib was considered to be cost effective in the chronic phase after interferon alfa. Denial of imatinib in the accelerated phase was considered to be inconsistent because the ratio was similar to that for the chronic phase

Denial of imatinib to patients in the blast cell phase was considered unfair. Patients at this advanced stage could reasonably have expected, in view of the decisions made already, to have had the opportunity of treatment with imatinib at an earlier stage of their condition. The fact that they were not given this chance would have been due to failings in the healthcare system. On grounds of equity, therefore, it was considered that imatinib should be available to patients in the blast cell phase of chronic myeloid leukaemia who had not previously been treated with the drug.

Affordability

NICE does not take affordability into account when making judgments about cost effectiveness. The term is not a technical one, but we use it to mean that a particular activity should be funded by increasing the total funds available for health care rather than from existing resources. This would imply increasing taxation, borrowing on the markets, or diversion of funds from another publicly funded activity. Affordability, in this sense, is a matter for the government when deciding the annual budget for the NHS. It is NICE's job to judge whether something ought to be purchased from within the resources made available to the NHS.

. . .

Social Value Judgments

Social value judgments have a critical role if resources are to be distributed with efficiency and equity. NICE and its advisory bodies, however, have no particular legitimacy to determine the social values of those served by the NHS. To ensure that these values resonate broadly with the public, NICE has formed a Citizens Council.[5,6]

. . .

Equity

Equity lies at the heart of the NHS. Lack of equity (in the form of so-called postcode prescribing) was one of the reasons why NICE was established. Much of the philosophical literature on equity is far from being applicable to the real world.[7,8] NICE has therefore had to make its own judgments. For NICE, equity also refers to fairness in the ways in which the costs and benefits of available care are distributed

[5] NICE Citizens Council, *Report of the First Meeting: Determining Clinical Need* (London: NICE, 2003).

[6] NICE Citizens Council, *Report on Age* (London: NICE, 2003).

[7] A. J. Culyer and A. Wagstaff, "Equity and Equality in Health and Health Care," *Journal of Health Economics* 12, no. 4 (1993): pp. 431–457.

[8] A. J. Culyer, "Economics and Ethics in Health Care," *Journal of Medical Ethics* 27, no. 4 (2001): pp. 217–222.

among all those who use the NHS.[9,10,11] NICE's recommendations are intended to apply across the whole of England and Wales, regardless of where people live or work. Thus, NICE has made the social value judgment that local variations in cost ought not to result in variations in availability of health care.[12]

Value judgments about equity are often implicit within both clinical and cost effectiveness analyses. An assumption that underlies most of NICE's technology appraisals has been that "a QALY is a QALY is a QALY." By this NICE means that a QALY gained or lost in respect of one disease is equivalent to a QALY gained or lost in respect of another. It also means that the weight given to the gain of a QALY is the same, regardless of how many QALYs have already been enjoyed, how many are in prospect, the age or sex of the beneficiaries, their deservedness, and the extent to which the recipients are deprived in other respects than health. The decision to give no differential weight is the result of a social value judgment that an additional adjusted life year is of equal importance for each person.[13]

. . .

[9] Culyer, "Economics and Ethics in Health Care."

[10] A. J. Culyer, "Equity – Some Theory and Its Policy Implications," *Journal of Medical Ethics* 27, no. 4 (2001): pp. 275–283.

[11] A. J. Culyer, "Need: The Idea Won't Do—but We Still Need It," *Social Science & Medicine* 40, no. 6 (1995): pp. 727–730.

[12] NICE Citizens Council, *Report of the First Meeting*.

[13] NICE Citizens Council, *Report on Age*.

EXCERPT 4

Abridged text from:

A. Oliver and C. Sorenson, "The Limits and Challenges to the Economic Evaluation of Health Technologies," edited by J. Costa-Font, C. Courbage, and A. McGuire (Oxford University Press, 2009), pp. 212–214.

The Limits and Challenges to the Economic Evaluation of Health Technologies

Adam Oliver and Corinna Sorenson

. . .

[T]he cost-effectiveness threshold employed by the [National Institute for Health and Care Excellence, NICE] for has been a source of contention. The threshold at which NICE deems interventions to be cost-effective, although implicit, appears to be somewhere between £20,000 and £30,000 per QALY gained,[1] with the more generous end of this range being employed when an intervention has particular positive characteristics; for example, if the intervention is especially innovative.[2] This threshold has been criticised as being too generous, arbitrary, and out of line with NHS products and services not assessed by NICE,[3] and Williams[4] argued that the NHS should pay no more than the average per capita GDP of about £18,000 for each QALY gained. However, NICE faces significant media-driven public pressure when it rules against the provision of interventions, emphasised by past decisions vis-à-vis drug therapy for multiple sclerosis. Indeed, given the political difficulties of recommending against the use of treatments, NICE guidance often only goes so far as to advocate restricted use in certain patient categories.[5] This . . . can upset physicians, many of whom believe that broad brush guidance, even when applied in relation to specific patient categories, tends to overlook the unique situation of many patients, including the presence of co-morbidities, particular socio-economic circumstances, etc. NICE seems almost destined to be damned for going "too high" or "too low" in its choice of a cost-effectiveness threshold, depending on the perspective of the particular critic. Regardless of the actual threshold, however, it is generally agreed that the rationale and method of its determination should be much more transparent.

Further concerns have been cited. For instance, some have written that NICE has insufficient capacity to assess a meaningful number of interventions, and that it has traditionally focused too heavily on new interventions, overlooking a potentially large number of cost-ineffective interventions in the NHS. . . . In a recent study, Linden et al[6] looked at 159 technologies reviewed from 88 appraisals between March 2000 and June 2006, and found that 84 (53%) were new technologies and 75 (47%) were existing technologies, from which they argued that this did not indicate a bias (p. 213) towards new technologies. It is worth bearing in mind, however, that the number of existing technologies far outnumbers the number of new interventions, and therefore an approximately 50–50 split may still represent a significant bias towards assessing the newer products and services. The

---

[1] I. Williams, S. Bryan and S. McIver, "How Should Cost-Effectiveness Analysis Be Used in Health Technology Coverage Decisions? Evidence from the National Institute for Health and Clinical Excellence Approach," *Journal of Health Services Research & Policy* 12, no. 2 (2007): pp. 73–79.

[2] S. Birch and A. Gafni, "Economists" Dream or Nightmare? Maximizing Health Gains from Available Resources Using the NICE Guidelines," *Health Economics Policy and Law* 2, no. 2 (2007): p. 193.

[3] J. Appleby, N. Devlin and D. Parkin, "NICE's Cost Effectiveness Threshold," *British Medical Journal* 335, no. 7616 (2007): p. 358.

[4] A. Williams, *What Could Be Nicer Than NICE?* (Office for Health Economics, 2004).

[5] Williams, "How Should Cost-Effectiveness Analysis Be Used."

[6] L. Linden, et al., "Does the National Institute for Health and Clinical Excellence Only Appraise New Pharmaceuticals?", *International Journal of Technology Assessment in Health Care* 23, no. 03 (2007): pp. 349–353.

limited capacity of NICE may create legitimate cause for concern that its impact will inevitably be limited, although one could counter this concern by arguing that the producers of medical interventions face the risk that their products *may* be assessed and thus have an incentive to make their products more cost-effective than they would be otherwise.

Despite the transparency of many aspects of NICE, with its processes and assessment reports published in detail and available for expert and—in theory—public scrutiny, the level of technical sophistication now applied in measurements of costs and outcomes somewhat undermines any claim that HTA-based decision making affords greater transparency to the public.[7] This is particularly worrying when one keeps in mind that the methods of economic evaluation are far from perfect.

Another key concern regards the slow and variable implementation of NICE guidance to date.[8] To address this issue, NICE guidance to the NHS was made mandatory in 2001,[9] and primary care trusts (PCTs), the local purchasers of health care, must not deny funds for treatments that have been recommended for use by NICE when more than 3 months have passed since the guidance was issued.[10] Unfortunately, this may steer the NHS towards a sub-optimal focus upon those interventions that NICE assesses, and away from other possibly higher priority investments or cutbacks in other activities.[11,12] Moreover, there is little evidence that these efforts have adequately improved the implementation of guidance and, therefore, remedied the "post-code" prescribing that NICE was intended to rectify.

As a result of poor implementation, some have pondered whether NICE itself is cost-effective.[13] One could argue that it is an inefficient use of NHS resources to support an appraisal system that is not fully implemented or prioritized by local purchasers. It appears that NICE guidance is more likely to be effectively adopted and implemented when it runs parallel to the support of opinion leaders, professional bodies, and marketing efforts by pharmaceutical companies,[14] and when NHS organizations have established structures and processes to manage implementation.[15]

NICE can, however, be seen in a more positive light. Many of the problems discussed above are methodological or process-orientated, and it may be possible to address these adequately with time. Moreover, one has to consider NICE with respect to the pre-NICE era, when general practitioner and hospital prescribing were influenced heavily by pharmaceutical companies and powerful hospital consultants and interest groups.[16],[17] The political path of least resistance is to say "yes" to powerful lobbies and "no" to weaker ones, irrespective of the products and services on offer. NICE has thus far offered a more systematic, transparent, and evidence-based approach to ascertaining the value of health technologies and (p.214) making subsequent recommendations. Moreover, while there are existing limitations to economic evaluation, the Institute has made efforts towards improving its methods

[7] J. Coast, "Is Economic Evaluation in Touch with Society's Health Values?", *British Medical Journal* 329, no. 7476 (2004): p. 1233.

[8] T. A. Sheldon, et al., "What's the Evidence That NICE Guidance Has Been Implemented? Results from a National Evaluation Using Time Series Analysis, Audit of Patients' Notes, and Interviews," *British Medical Journal* 329, no. 7473 (2004): p. 999.

[9] The mandate does not apply to clinical guidelines.

[10] A. Stevens and R. Milne, "Health Technology Assessment in England and Wales," *International Journal of Technology Assessment in Health Care* 20, no. 1 (2004): pp. 11–24.

[11] Ibid.

[12] Birch, "Economists" Dream or Nightmare?'

[13] N. Freemantle, "Is NICE Delivering the Goods?", *British Medical Journal* 329, no. 7473 (2004): pp. 1003–1004.

[14] Sheldon, "What's the Evidence That NICE Guidance Has Been Implemented?"

[15] The Audit Commission, "Managing the Financial Implications of NICE Guidance," 2005.

[16] Stevens, "Health Technology Assessment in England and Wales."

[17] M. Drummond, "NICE: A Nightmare Worth Having?", *Health Economics, Policy and Law* 2, no. 02 (2007): pp. 203–208.

and procedures. For instance, it has offered funding for methods development and attempts to address stakeholder concerns surrounding social judgements and the estimation of costs. To that end, the Institute is probably the one HTA body that formally involves a wide range of stakeholders in its process, such as its use of a Citizens Council;[18] although, there has been much debate regarding the influence of stakeholder input. Overall, although NICE is beset with challenges, its underlying motivation is largely honourable and, although the jury is still out, it may, with time and with the appropriate developments, positively benefit the populations of England and Wales.

. . .

[18] The Citizens Council, open to participation of the wider public, assists NICE decision making by offering views from the public on key issues informing the development of guidance, especially regarding social values and judgments in relation to equity and need.

EXCERPT 5

Abridged text from:

S. D. Pearson and M. D. Rawlins, "Quality, Innovation, and Value for Money: NICE and the British National Health Service," *JAMA* 294, no. 20 (2005): pp. 2618–2622.

Quality, Innovation, and Value for Money: NICE and the British National Health Service

Steven D. Pearson and Michael D. Rawlins

The interplay among quality of care, technological innovation, and cost control creates a policy challenge for all health care systems. Improvements in the quality of care can reduce health care costs; for example, better management of chronic conditions may lessen the chance of hospitalization, and new drugs and medical devices might improve the quality and efficiency of care. Often, however, innovation comes with a significant additional cost. Even the most affluent health care systems must consider the benefits of medical innovation compared with other efforts to improve the quality of care. This article describes how this policy challenge is being addressed in Britain through the activities of the National Institute for Health and Clinical Excellence (NICE).

NICE was established in 1999. . . .

NICE Guidance

The institute . . . appraises individual or classes of health technologies (eg, pharmaceuticals, devices, procedures, diagnostic methods), taking account of both their clinical effectiveness and cost-effectiveness. . . .

Economic Evaluation. Of all the elements of NICE guidance, the most distinctive, from a US perspective, is its use of economic evaluation to help judge the value of technologies that provide additional benefit but at an increased cost. The key measure used by NICE to assess the marginal value of a technology for different patient groups is the additional cost per quality-adjusted life-year (QALY) gained. If appropriate data on quality of life are unavailable, cost-effectiveness is estimated using alternatives such as cost per life-year gained.

Whether to recommend the use of a technology for certain patients and indications depends in part on the point at which the incremental cost per QALY is judged to no longer be cost-effective. Recognizing this central feature of economic evaluation, NICE has carefully described its approach and expects its advisory bodies to use estimates of cost-effectiveness to inform, but not determine, their decisions.[1] In other words, NICE does not have a specific cost per QALY threshold above which a technology is rejected. Although research is continuing in this area, there is currently no empirical basis for assigning a specific cost per QALY threshold within the NHS; even if there were an empirical guide, an explicit threshold would suggest that health utility as measured by QALYs has absolute priority over other objectives, including various forms of equity. Nevertheless, NICE has arrived operationally at a band of approximately $30,600 to $45,900 per QALY (based on purchasing power parity of US $1 = £0.65) as the threshold above which it would be increasingly likely to reject a technology on grounds of cost-ineffectiveness. For example, the institute has approved the use of etanercept and infliximab, both with incremental cost-effectiveness ratios of $47,430 per QALY, in the treatment of rheumatoid arthritis, but it has rejected anakinra, with an incremental ratio of $102,510 per QALY.[2]

---

[1] M. D. Rawlins and A. J. Culyer, "National Institute for Clinical Excellence and Its Value Judgments," *British Medical Journal* 329 (2004): pp. 224–227.

[2] National Institute for Clinical Excellence, "Guidance on the Use of Etanercept and Infliximab for the Treatment of Rheumatoid Arthritis," accessed 2005, http://www.nice.org.uk/pdf/RA-PDF.pdf.

Adopting this range of $30,600 to $45,900 per QALY as a benchmark for cost-effectiveness maintains consistency across the many different types of health care technologies that NICE appraises and, at the same time, provides NICE's advisory bodies with latitude to consider the degree of uncertainty surrounding the estimate, the particular features of the condition, the innovative nature of the technology, and, where appropriate, the wider societal costs and benefits.[3]

It is important to note that NICE does not take the budget impact of a new technology into account. For example, although a new drug might have a favorable cost-effectiveness ratio of $30,000 per QALY, the overall impact might be too great for the NHS budget if very large numbers of patients were to be eligible for treatment. Affordability is not the responsibility of NICE; the government remains accountable for the overall NHS budget and must therefore judge a particular intervention unaffordable for the NHS even though NICE might have judged it cost-effective. Such a situation has not yet arisen.

Implementation. Not all of NICE's guidance is mandatory for the NHS. For technology appraisals, however, every local health care body within the NHS is legally required to provide funding from its overall government allocation within 3 months to support care for all patients who meet NICE-approved indications for treatment. This has raised concerns that local health care organizations will be forced to displace other, allegedly more cost-effective interventions.[4] Without a mandatory feature, however, it is likely that expensive new technologies would remain subject to continued postcode prescribing. From a policy perspective, the mandatory funding of NICE technology appraisals also serves the important purpose of fostering innovation. If NICE guidance is acted on consistently, manufacturers producing novel cost-effective technologies have an explicit mechanism to gain funding for their products, and patients have security of access to new technologies wherever they live in the United Kingdom.

. . .

Criticisms of NICE

Not surprising for an organization at the fulcrum of decisions that can have far-reaching implications for patients, clinicians, and manufacturers, NICE and its guidance have received much attention in the United Kingdom, and not all of it has been favorable. . . .

Some critics have pointed out that NICE's approach to using cost-effectiveness, although touted as a mechanism for making difficult decisions to limit the approval of new technologies, has in fact led to the approval for funding, at least for some indications, of most new drugs and devices. NICE has thus been called a "golden goose" for the pharmaceutical industry and has been blamed for NHS inflation and the creation of a constant stream of new budgetary requirements for local health care authorities struggling to support local spending priorities of higher value.[5,6,7]

NICE in fact has operated during the halcyon days of an unprecedented period of sustained growth in the overall NHS budget, a rate of growth (7.3% annually since 2000) that cannot continue indefinitely.[8] When budgets cease to grow, a new day will dawn for NICE and the NHS as they manage the delicate balance between cost-effective new technologies

---

[3] Rawlins, "NICE and Its Value Judgments."

[4] R. Cookson, D. McDaid and A. Maynard, "Wrong Sign, NICE Mess: Is National Guidance Distorting Allocation of Resources?", *British Medical Journal* 323, no. 7315 (2001): pp. 743–745.

[5] Ibid.

[6] A. Maynard, K. Bloor and N. Freemantle, "Challenges for the National Institute for Clinical Excellence," *British Medical Jouranl* 329, no. 7459 (2004): pp. 227–229.

[7] A. Gafni and S. Birch, "NICE Methodological Guidelines and Decision Making in the National Health Service in England and Wales," *Pharmacoeconomics* 21, no. 3 (2003): pp. 149–157.

[8] S. Stevens, "Reform Strategies for the English NHS," *Health Affairs* 23, no. 3 (2004): pp. 37–44.

and local health authority budgets. Critics foreseeing this funding squeeze often suggest that NICE should become engaged more directly in the true trade-off budgetary decisions within the NHS. This could occur by adjusting its cost-effectiveness threshold downward to reflect the preferences of local authorities, by shifting its work program to identify a greater number of "obsolete" technologies whose funding should be eliminated, or by having a yearly fixed budget itself, out of which all funding for new innovations would have to come.[9]

From the other end of the spectrum, drug and device manufacturers have a mixed view of NICE. Some are eager to have their products appraised by NICE to gain rapid entry into the UK market. Others claim publicly that economic modeling based on QALYs is unreliable and inappropriate to use as the standard for early evaluations of many new products.[10] Many of those opposed to NICE's approach probably have the chief concern that a negative appraisal would have adverse consequences on global sales. Manufacturers of all views, however, continue to appeal many of NICE's decisions when the guidance is viewed as too restrictive or when the guidance declines to promote one product over another in appraisals of several drugs in the same class.

. . .

NICE in the United States?

. . . NICE was able to neutralize much of the early concern about its role by taking great efforts to produce guidance of the highest possible quality and ethical legitimacy. The rigor and independence of NICE's scientific review process brings an objectivity to NICE guidance that is widely respected.[11] Through scrupulous adherence to its principles of stakeholder involvement and procedural transparency, the positive effects of scientific rigor and independence are strengthened and help to underscore the legitimacy of all of NICE's guidance.

An important point for the United States is that NICE has also demonstrated that cost-effectiveness analysis can work at the core of a national guidance program, and the institute has made strong claims for its ethical and practical benefits. A key to this success lies in the balance between NICE's use of cost-effectiveness to set limits and the institute's explicit role in facilitating the funding of innovative new technologies. Manufacturers have benefited not only from the funding mandate that comes with NICE approval but also from clarification of the rules of the game. Manufacturers now know what data they will need from clinical trials to provide acceptable evidence of the clinical effectiveness and cost-effectiveness of their products; they can therefore see and engage in a clear process.

NICE's arm's-length structure within the NHS and use of independent advisory groups also holds important policy lessons related to its success. Much like the US Federal Reserve Board, NICE is able to operate with a sense of security from any direct political influence. This independence was recently tested when NICE produced draft guidance proposing the elimination of funding for drug therapies for Alzheimer disease because of cost-ineffectiveness. Public pressure mounted against this draft decision, with the media trumpeting NICE's "attack" on the elderly. The issue reached the floor of the House of Commons, where the prime minister reasserted that NICE was an independent body whose judgments should be respected and not open to political pressure. He faced no opposition to this statement. Structural independence is necessary to build this kind of durable support. . . .

---

9 Maynard, "Challenges for NICE."

10 F. Schubert, "Health Technology Assessment. The Pharmaceutical Industry Perspective," *International Journal of Technology Assessment in Health Care* 18, no. 2 (2002): pp. 184–191.

11 S. Hill, et al., "Technology Appraisal Programme of the National Institute for Clinical Excellence: A Review by WHO" (2003).

EXCERPT 6

Abridged text from:
L. Bulfone, S. Younie, and R. Carter, "Health Technology Assessment: Reflection from the Antipodes," *Value Health* 12, no. 2 (2009): pp. S28–S39.

Health Technology Assessment: Reflections from the Antipodes

Liliana Bulfone, Sandra Younie, and Rob Carter

. . .

As the predominant use of HTA (including economic evaluation) is within the [Pharmaceutical Benefits Advisory Committee,] PBAC and [the Medical Services Advisory Committee,] MSAC processes in Australia, much of the discussion that follows is primarily in the context of these settings.

Australia has found that a process involving the formal use of HTA (including economic evaluation) to inform reimbursement decision-making for health technologies is both feasible and able to be effectively implemented. While acceptance of an evidence-based and cost-effectiveness process in health-care decision-making has been a little slower than advocates might have liked, it has gradually gained acceptance across the health sector. Nevertheless, there has been some resistance to the use of evidence-based medicine to guide availability of interventions especially if it conflicts with clinical freedom or reduces income to the healthcare provider.[1] For cost-effectiveness evaluation to be an accepted part of the decision-making process, the use and acceptance of comparative clinical efficacy as a basis for decision-making needs to be well established. That is, there needs to be a culture of reliance on evidence-based medicine to guide medical practice. This can then be used as a foundation on which to build an HTA process.

Decision-makers in Australia aim to focus on the relative therapeutic value (i.e., the value of the health technology as compared with best current practice) rather than simply efficacy relative to control (often placebo) as may be demonstrated in a trial. As discussed in the guidelines published by PBAC and MSAC, the positioning of the proposed intervention in the management algorithm for the condition of interest is required to be explicit and the incremental effects of changing the algorithm from current practice to practice including the intervention is of paramount interest to the committees.

The use of HTA is now generally well accepted for the evaluation of pharmaceuticals but is less so for medical technologies (particularly for prosthesis and devices). This is partly because of the lack of availability of high-quality evidence as this sector does not have the same history of designing trials that correspond to the highest levels of evidence. Also, adoption of new technologies in the medical services areas can follow a different pathway to that for pharmaceuticals, i.e., new technologies can be adopted by clinicians in the absence of high-quality evidence demonstrating efficacy and safety.

Relationship Between Decision-Making Agencies Using HTA and Government

[A]ustralia has a universal health insurance scheme, Medicare, based on a philosophy that medical services should be delivered on the basis of ability to benefit rather than ability to pay. Like elsewhere, Australia has budget constraints on public health expenditure, and HTA has proven a useful measure to inform government, policymakers, and clinicians about the

[1] A. Harris and L. Bulfone, "Getting Value for Money: The Australian Experience," in *Health Care Coverage Determinations: International Comparative Study*, edited by T. S. Jost (Maidenhead: Open University Press, 2005).

relative value of technologies. Nevertheless, the successful integration of HTA into a healthcare system requires policymakers and HTA bodies, who are typically independent of each other in their decisions, to share a mutual set of principles underlying their decision-making. It needs to be recognized, for example, that pursuing "value-for-money" and pursuing "cost containment" are two quite different objectives, although often confused and conflated. HTA was not introduced into Australia with a main objective of cost containment but rather as a means of ensuring that funding of interventions was evidence-based and represented value-for-money.

This being said, it needs to be acknowledged that the Australian system is prone to affordability issues that generate ongoing tensions. This reflects the absence of any specified decision rule to define "acceptable cost-effectiveness," the key role of fee-for-service in our health insurance payment arrangements, and the absence of any explicit expenditure caps on the MBS and PBS schemes. The increasing availability of effective but expensive drugs and new technologies is likely to continue in the future. Accepting that a tension exists between the availability of cost-effective technologies and affordability, the key Australian HTA arrangements (as operated by PBAC and MSAC) does nonetheless provide a mechanism whereby the government can justify decisions in relation to health expenditure. To ensure that affordability is considered and to ensure that the system remains sustainable, the decision-making role of the PBAC is supplemented with a requirement that new drugs with a budgetary impact greater than $5 million be considered by the Department of Treasury and Finance and that new drugs with a budgetary impact greater than $10 million obtain approval from Cabinet (the decision-makers within the elected government) before any recommendation to make a drug available is implemented. If necessary, additional mechanisms to limit access can be introduced, policy advice may be issued, or an increase in public contributions through copayments or taxes can be arranged.

Transparency in Assessment and Decision-Making

Pharmaceutical companies and manufacturers of some other health technologies have been reluctant to have their submissions to the TGA, PBAC, and MSAC released in the public domain on the grounds that they contain commercially sensitive information. Sponsors requesting registration or subsidy of health technologies through these agencies are permitted to provide information on a commercial-in-confidence basis as part of their submissions. The TGA, unlike the Food and Drug Administration in the United States and the European Medicines Evaluation Agency, does not release any details of its evaluations.

In the past, the PBAC has accepted submissions on a commercial-in-confidence basis and the reasoning behind PBAC decisions was not publicly disclosed. Nevertheless, the recent Free Trade Agreement between Australia and the United States has influenced the PBAC to release their reasons for decisions publicly over the Internet, although much information (particularly details of economic analyses) is not disclosed. Generally, only summary clinical and economic information is released.

MSAC on the other hand, a more recent HTA initiative, releases its complete evaluation report, with censoring of information deemed commercial-in-confidence. . . . The release of the whole evaluation report by MSAC was in response to criticisms[2] that MSAC decisions were not clear and often at odds with the recommendations included in the evaluation reports. Therefore, recommendations arrived at by MSAC, and their reasoning, are publicly available documents along with copies of the evaluation report. Included with the reasoning is an indication as to whether

---

[2] "Report of the Review of the Medical Services Advisory Committee: May 2005," http://www.msac.gov.au/internet/msac/publishing.nsf/Content/review-1.

commercial-in-confidence information was relied upon in coming to a decision.

In our view, there is a strong argument that data submitted to support a request for public subsidy should be open to public scrutiny as public funds will be used to pay for the technologies. Furthermore, we contend that evaluations of these data conducted by government agencies should also be made available to health professionals and consumers. The successful operation of the system is contingent on health professionals complying with restrictions applied to a technology and their cooperation is more likely if they can understand the reasons behind a decision to restrict the availability of a technology.

There have now been many calls for transparency in regulatory and reimbursement decisions in Australia and internationally. For example, there have been calls for an international register of clinical trials so that unfavorable results cannot be hidden.[3,4] The Australian HTA experience has been one of increasing transparency, in response to greater public demands for more information about the basis on which the PBAC and MSAC make their decisions, together with the impact of the Australia–United States Free Trade Agreement.

Factors Influencing Decisions

Some may consider it desirable for decision-makers to designate an explicit decision threshold (e.g., in terms of incremental cost per additional quality-adjusted life-year [QALY] gained) as constituting acceptable cost-effectiveness. Others argue that the nomination of a decision threshold is problematic as it may encourage "gaming" of the system (where interventions are priced at the maximum price that results in an incremental cost-effectiveness ratio (ICER) below the threshold) and because such formulae-driven approaches ignore other factors that influence whether a particular estimate of incremental cost-effectiveness is considered acceptable or not. These broader considerations include: 1) the degree of uncertainty around the point estimate of incremental cost-effectiveness; 2) the burden and severity of the disease or condition; 3) the prevalence of the disease or condition; 4) the availability of alternative treatments; and 5) the net financial implications of making the therapy available (including the potential for widespread use of the intervention outside any proposed restrictions).

In Australia, neither the PBAC nor the MSAC have nominated any decision threshold as representing acceptable cost-effectiveness and nomination of thresholds indicating that acceptable cost-effectiveness is unlikely to occur. The role of economic evaluation in decision-making in Australia remains as a part of the whole and not the "end game." Results of an analysis conducted by Harris et al.[5] of the relative influence of factors in decisions for public insurance coverage of new drugs in Australia found that "there is no evidence of a fixed public threshold value of life years or QALYs, but willingness-to-pay is clearly related to the characteristics of the clinical condition, perceived confidence in the evidence of effectiveness and its relevance, as well as total cost to government." No similar analysis has been reported in relation to MSAC decisions; Nevertheless, similar considerations underlie their decision-making.

As listed above, other factors, apart from economic considerations, can also be considered in deciding whether a particular estimate of incremental cost-effectiveness is "acceptable" or not. The potential for use of an intervention

---

[3] C. DeAngelis, et al., "Clinical Trial Registration: A Statement from the International Committee of Medical Journal Editors," *Medical Journal of Australiat* 181, no. 6 (2004): pp. 293–294.

[4] C. D. De Angelis, et al., "Is This Clinical Trial Fully Registered?: A Statement from the International Committee of Medical Journal Editors," *New England Journal of Medicine* 352, no. 23 (2005): pp. 2436–2438.

[5] A. H. Harris, et al., "The Role of Value for Money in Public Insurance Coverage Decisions for Drugs in Australia: A Retrospective Analysis 1994-2004," *Medical Decision Making* 28, no. 5 (2008): pp. 713–722.

beyond any restriction that might apply (also known as "leakage") is one of these considerations. For example, where a drug that is listed on the PBS for one reason may also be used for another purpose, needs to be considered, particularly where the market authorization (through TGA in Australia) is broader than the subsidy decision. Examples of use beyond a restriction (leakage) include use of therapy in patients with the same disease as those for whom the intervention is available but in whom cost-effectiveness has not been demonstrated (e.g., where the listing is restricted to a specific subgroup of patients with a disease, but evidence of cost-effectiveness is not available in other subgroups). . . .

Another factor that the PBAC identifies as a special circumstance affecting its decisions is known as "rule of rescue," which applies in exceptional circumstances and is particularly influential in favor of listing. The following three factors need to apply concurrently for the "rule of rescue" to be satisfied:

1. No alternative exists in Australia to treat patients with the medical condition meeting the criteria of the requested restriction. This is an absolute requirement.
2. The medical condition defined by the requested restriction is severe, progressive, and expected to lead to premature death. The more severe the condition, or the younger the age at which a person with the condition might die, or the closer a person with the condition is to death, the more influential the rule of rescue consideration is.
3. The medical condition defined by the requested restriction applies to only a very small number of patients. Again, the fewer the patients, the more influential the rule of rescue might be. Nevertheless, the PBAC is also mindful that the PBS is a community-based scheme and cannot cater for individual circumstances.

As with all considerations in the "other relevant information" category, the rule of rescue supplements, rather than substitutes for, the evidence-based consideration of comparative cost-effectiveness. A decision on whether the rule of rescue is relevant is only necessary if the PBAC would be inclined to reject a submission based on its assessment of comparative cost-effectiveness (and any other relevant factors).

. . .

EXCERPT 7

Abridged text from:

J. J. Caro, et al., "The Efficiency Frontier Approach to Economic Evaluation of Health-Care Interventions," *Health Economics* 19 (2010): pp. 1117–1127.

The Efficiency Frontier Approach to Economic Evaluation of Health-Care Interventions

Jaime Caro, Erik Nord, Uwe Seibert, Alistair McGuire, Maurice McGregor, David Henry, Gérard de Pouvourville, Vincenzo Atella, and Peter Kolominsky-Rabas

. . .

The initial legislation specified that [the Institute for Quality and Efficiency in Healthcare, German: Institut für Qualität und Wirtschaftlichkeit im Gesundheitswesen,] IQWiG should assess the clinical effects of health technologies according to "internationally recognized standards of evidence-based medicine" (EBM). In early 2007, the German parliament passed additional legislation, which expanded IQWiG's responsibilities to include the "cost-benefit" assessments of pharmaceuticals or medical procedures according to "accepted international standards of health economics." Although *Nutzen* was translated from the German into "benefit," it is clear that Parliament did not intend to mandate a specific methodology (i.e. cost-benefit analysis). Instead, the idea was that IQWiG would develop the methods it would use for economic evaluation, consistent with the legal requirements.[1] These requirements were made operational by IQWiG and reaffirmed by the German Federal Ministry of Health, which is legally responsible,[2] and this defined the context for the Panel's development of the methods.

. . .

The basis for these evaluations, as defined by the Ministry and IQWiG, is not the same as in many other health-care systems: it does not involve establishing funding priorities across the German health-care system. Instead, it envisions the narrower goal of establishing a maximum reimbursement amount for "patented innovations as well as pharmaceuticals of importance"[3] in a given disease area. The process of setting this amount is informed (but not determined) by estimating the additional benefit and incremental costs beyond those of currently available interventions in the disease area in question. This was a logical extension of the current IQWiG practice of establishing relative health benefit at the therapeutic level. It is also in line with common application of economic analysis as an aid to decision making, as opposed to determining decisions. Thus, any additional expenditure need not be weighed formally against what could be achieved in other therapeutic areas, nor by investments in other sectors of the economy, such as education or the military. As these comparisons would require judgments about the societal value of treating one disease versus another and no universally accepted method for doing this has been identified by IQWiG (including the cost-per-quality-adjusted life year [QALY] approach[4,5]; IQWIG insisted on a method that does not address the broader issue of

[1] SGB, *Gesetz Zur Stärkung Des Wettbewerbs in Der Gesetzlichen Krankenversicherung* (Bundesgesetzblatt, 2007).

[2] Bundesministerium für Gesundheit, "Stellungnahme Zur Methodik Der Kosten-Nutzen-Bewertung Von Arzneimittel," 2008, http://www.bmg.bund.de/cln_117/nn_1168258/SharedDocs/Standardartikel/DE/AZ/K/Glossar-Kosten-Nutzen-Bewertung/Stellungnahme.html.

[3] SGB, *Gesetz Zur Stärkung Des Wettbewerbs.*

[4] E. Nord, N. Daniels and M. Kamlet, "QALYs: Some Challenges," *Value in Health* 12 (2009): pp. S10–S15.

[5] M. D. Smith, M. Drummond and D. Brixner, "Moving the QALY Forward: Rationale for Change," *Value in Health* 12 (2009): pp. S1–S4.

prioritizing across the health-care system. That application of citizens' values was to be left to the decision-making bodies designated by law.

According to the legal framework (SGB V, § 35b), a second constraint is that the economic evaluations should only address those interventions that have been judged to be superior (presumably to existing ones) and that the health benefits to be considered in the economic assessment are those which have been estimated by IQWiG following its published Methods grounded in the principles of EBM.[6] This has several implications. It means that new inferior therapies have no place in the system, even if they are considerably less expensive than existing ones. It also means that the effectiveness component must reflect the review carried out by IQWiG beforehand—no additional benefits, even if indirectly implied by the EBM measures, are to be included.

A third requirement imposed in Germany is that the costs be assessed primarily from the perspective of the community of the citizens insured by [Statutory Health Insurance,] SHI. This implies that it is the costs which citizens bear that should be included. This means that some costs that might be excluded from evaluations (e.g. personal health-care costs) should be incorporated in this case.

A fourth requirement was that patients not be excluded from therapeutic benefits on cost grounds alone.

3. The Proposed Method

The approach recommended by the Panel takes as its point of departure that the efficiency of an intervention relative to others in the same disease area is relevant to decision makers—that is, that an important input (though not the only one) to setting the maximum reimbursement is the health value obtained for a given expenditure and that, accordingly, newer interventions should not provide less value without strong justification. Thus, the efficiency frontier, for a particular disease area, is defined by the most efficient interventions at increasing levels of benefit. The efficiency frontier presents the trade-off between costs and benefits and identifies the interventions that provide the most value for any given level of investment. It can be displayed graphically (see Figure [10.5]) by plotting the interventions at their estimated net cost (horizontal axis) and benefits (vertical axis) and drawing line segments linking the options that are not dominated by any other (further explanation below). Although the axes could be inverted (as is common in the "cost-effectiveness plane" of pharmacoeconomics[7]), it is preferable to do it as proposed because the resulting slopes have a ready interpretation in terms of efficiency and this accords better with the format used in other fields. The slopes of the line segments give the "going rate" (how much is gained per unit of cost).

The efficiency frontier represents the best that the system can do with available agents

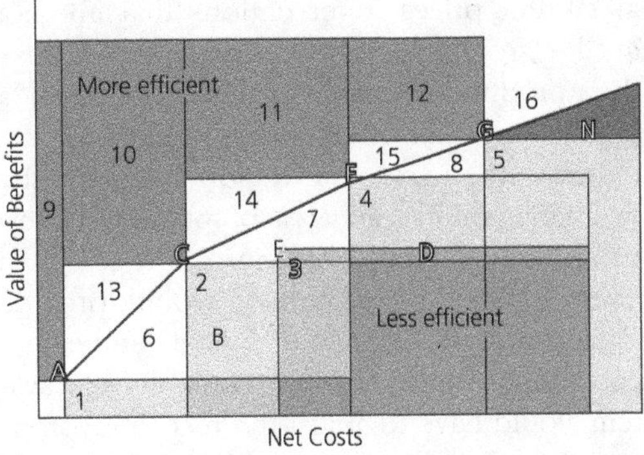

Figure [10.5] Plot of the efficiency frontier dividing the space into more or less efficient interventions and various guidance zones.

[6] "IQWiG Methoden 3.0," 2009, http://www.iqwig.de/download/IQWiG_General_methods_V-3-0.pdf.

[7] W. C. Black, "The CE Plane: A Graphic Representation of Cost-Effectiveness," *MedicalDecision Making* 10, no. 3 (1990): pp. 212–214.

at current prices. Interventions that are not at the frontier are less desirable because they produce the same or less benefits at a higher cost than other existing interventions; by the same token, the region "beyond" the frontier identifies an area of potential interventions that would be more efficient than existing ones because they would provide equal or more benefits at less or equivalent cost. Should they become available, the system would have to adjust the mix to incorporate them because the resulting combination would deliver more with available resources. The general approach is compatible with the use of economic analysis to support decisions rather than make them (Gold et al., 1996), as well as being compatible with theoretical underpinnings.[8,9]

. . .

Using Relative Efficiency to Provide Guidance

In Germany, the efficiency frontier will be used to provide guidance to the G-BA for setting the maximum reimbursement amount. This guidance is not intended to be an appraisal conveying the decision itself but rather information that can be used by the decision makers—together with other inputs—to arrive at such an amount. Relative efficiency is only one piece of information; its components (value of the benefits and total net costs) are also important, as are the estimated budget impact and the uncertainty around all the estimates.

Guidance will be provided to G-BA by plotting the efficiency frontier and using it to assess the position of the intervention at issue relative to what already existed in the market. In Germany, unlike many other countries, the evaluations take place ex post—that is, the intervention being assessed is already on the market and has an established price. Thus, there is no need to project the frontier into unknown space but rather to consider the efficiency of the intervention at issue in comparison with the efficiency of other interventions on the market in that therapeutic area.

As seen in the figure, plotting of the frontier (interventions A, C, F, G) delineates three guidance zones. Any interventions that would plot in the areas below and to the right of the frontier would be considered inefficient as they cost more and provide less value than existing ones (those falling in the shaded rectangles labeled 1-5, such as B and D) or they are in a position where there is a lower price that would place them on the frontier (those plotting inside a triangle labeled 6–8, such as E). It is not expected—at least initially—that any evaluations in Germany will find newer interventions falling in this zone because of the two-stage process of determining benefit first and only if it is judged to be superior, going on to the economic assessment.

A second guidance zone is given by the area above and to the left of the frontier. This zone indicates positions where a newer intervention would dominate an existing frontier intervention because it would provide benefits of greater value and at less cost (shaded rectangles 9–12) or would be in a position of "extended dominance" by providing benefits more efficiently than the neighboring segment of the frontier (triangles 13–16). Indeed, any intervention falling in these areas would redefine the frontier. Most of this frontier-redefining area will also not be used in Germany because of the requirement for superiority of benefits before economic evaluation is undertaken (the exception is the portion above the next best available intervention, indicating a newer, superior intervention that has been priced very attractively and redefined the frontier).

The third guidance zone is the triangle (labeled N) that indicates superior benefits but a lower efficiency than the next best intervention on the frontier. In this third case, decision

---

[8] S. Birch and A. Gafni, "Cost Effectiveness/Utility Analyses: Do Current Decision Rules Lead Us to Where We Want to Be?", *Journal of Health Economics* 11, no. 3 (1992): pp. 279–296.

[9] While open to the criticism of being a "partial analysis," the efficiency frontier approach is broadly compatible with the integer programming approach.

makers would need to consider how much lower the efficiency is and whether there is justification for the decrease. A small decrement could still be viewed as reasonable, whereas large ones would be more problematic.

The slope of the efficiency frontier tends to decrease as benefits increase, reflecting, in many cases, diminishing marginal returns (i.e. the fact that even in the subset of "most efficient therapies," increases in costs of research and development and of production provide less and less additional value[10]). If there are sufficient points on the frontier, then further analysis can be carried out to determine the rate at which efficiency has been decreasing as a function of increasing value. This estimate of the rate of decline indicates "what is to be expected" in terms of cost increases for new interventions that provide more value than earlier ones. This would provide a basis for assessing how reasonable the last decrease in efficiency is.

Additional criteria, such as the citizens' willingness to pay for additional benefits in that therapeutic area, could be applied in principle. Obtaining these valuations is quite challenging, however.[11]

. . .

[10] K. Murphy and R. Topel, "Diminishing Returns? The Costs and Benefits of Improving Health," *Perspectives on Biology and Medicine* 46, no. 3 Suppl (2003): pp. S108–S128.

[11] M. Ryan, et al., "Eliciting Public Preferences for Healthcare: A Systematic Review of Techniques," *Health Technology Assessment* 5, no. 5 (2001): pp. 1–186.

EXCERPT 8

Abridged text from:
Institute of Medicine, *Essential Health Benefits: Balancing Coverage and Cost* (Washington, DC: The National Academies Press, 2012), pp. 47–58, 79-102.

Essential Health Benefits: Balancing Coverage and Cost

. . .

3. Policy Foundations and Criteria for the Essential Health Benefits

. . .

The Secretary asked the Institute of Medicine (IOM) committee to develop an explicit framework for considering the Essential Health Benefits (EHB) package that would serve the Department of Health and Human Services (HHS) now and in the future.[1]

POLICY FOUNDATIONS

The committee finds that no single policy lens is sufficient or comprehensive enough for explicitly framing decisions about the EHB. Figure [10.6] graphically illustrates the four domains and principles associated with those domains. Each of these distinct perspectives—complementary in some cases, overlapping in others, conflicting at times—influences how we think about what health insurance should cover and how it should be implemented.

Economics

A benefit design framework rooted in economics primarily conceives of coverage as *insurance*—protecting individuals and their families against the risk of unforeseen health care needs, particularly those associated with large expenses.[2] An economics approach uses markets to promote value and efficiency, relying heavily on these markets to find the equilibrium between price and demand. With respect to the ACA, new markets are being developed for health insurance products that will include the EHB.

. . .

Ethics

An ethical framework requires consideration of stewardship of shared population-wide resources and, at the same time, fidelity to the needs of the individual.[3,4] Stewardship is not just a matter of living within a budget, but of having a broader obligation for the judicious use of resources so that they are available when people who contribute to the resource pool most need them.

The American Medical Association's (AMA's) Ethical Force Program proposed five content areas directly related to the fairness of a health benefits design and subsequent administration, stating that health care coverage decisions should be (1) transparent, (2) participatory, (3) equitable and consistent, (4) sensitive to value, and (5) compassionate (Box 3.1).

The five areas suggested are to be advocated for because

4. **Transparency** is necessary for market accountability;

[1] S. Glied, "Testimony to the IOM Committee on the Determination of Essential Health Benefits by Sherry Glied, Assistant Secretary for Planning and Evaluation," 2011.

[2] R. E. Santerre and S. P. Neun, "The Demand for Medical Insurance: Traditional and Managed Care Coverage," in *Health Economics: Theory, Insights, and Industry Studies*, edited by R. E. Santerre and S. P. Neun (Mason, OH: South-Western, Cengage Learning, 2010).

[3] N. Daniels and J. Sabin, "Limits to Health Care: Fair Procedures, Democratic Deliberation, and the Legitimacy Problem for Insurers," *Philosophy & Public Affairs* 26, no. 4 (1997): pp. 303–350.

[4] N. Daniels and J. Sabin, *Setting Limits,* 2nd ed (Oxford University Press, 2002).

Economics	Ethics
• Insurance must protect against the risk of unforeseen large health care expenses. • Competition can be used to promote quality and efficiency. • Government should address market failures that result in incomplete or excessively costly insurance options. • Incentives may be useful to promote high-value services.	• Decisions about the distribution of societal resources must be done fairly and transparently. • There is a duty to protect society's most vulnerable. • The stewardship of limited resources requires at tention to maximizing health benefits. • Shared responsibility for improving health should be promoted among consumers, employers, insurers, providers, and government.
Evidence-Based Practice	**Population Health**
• EBP provides a systematic way to apply the best scientific evidence to clinical decision making. • EBP clarifies the contribution of scientific evidence to value-based decisions. • EBP integrates clinical expertise, patient values, and best research evidence into patient care decision making.	• Insurance should facilitate efforts to improve population health. • Primary, secondary, and tertiary prevention need attention. • Access for the vulnerable must be assured. • Disparities should be eliminated.

Figure [10.6] Four policy domains with associated foundational principles for thinking about essential health benefits development and implementation.

5. **Participatory** processes ensure that public concerns are understood and considered, foster a heightened sense of fairness and legitimacy among stakeholders, and additionally promote quality improvement by drawing attention to grievances;
6. **Equity and consistency** safeguard against inappropriate discrimination (both for legal reasons in setting and enforcing precedents and for promoting public acceptability of a system);
7. **Sensitivity to value** is rooted in the consequentialist approach of promoting the greatest good; and
8. **Compassion** is consistent with the health insurance function of protecting against an imbalance in individual risk, requiring that health care resource allocation transcend the formulaic by incorporating flexibility and responsiveness to extraordinary individual circumstances and informing itself on such individual variations.[5]

. . .

Population Health

. . . Population health focuses on improving the *overall* health status of a community, thus departing from the predominant late 20th century medical care model of focusing interventions only on the individual.[6] The function of health insurance, in this framework, is to encourage access to health-promoting

[5] AMA, *Ensuring Fairness in Health Care Coverage*.

[6] D. A. Kindig, "Understanding Population Health Terminology," *Milbank Quarterly* 85, no. 1 (2007): pp. 139–161.

care services, through primary and secondary prevention (e.g., immunizations to reduce transmission of communicable diseases; screenings for conditions such as high blood pressure, type 2 diabetes mellitus, or certain cancers, in which a delay in the initiation of treatment is associated with increased mortality).

. . .

CRITERIA

. . .

. . .

Insurance is a method of pooling the risk of financial loss across a group or a population. This prompts the question, "Which medical services should be paid for using a limited pool of shared funds?" Insurance policies exclude certain benefits; HHS will certainly have to exclude benefits that might be important to certain stakeholders, and these may even be services that have an evidence base that shows at some level they are effective. Most of us will be paying into insurance pools, directly through purchasing insurance and/or indirectly through taxes. Thus, we all depend on the possibility of spending from these shared pools and should want financial protection against catastrophic illnesses and conditions and assurances that care paid for out of shared resources is medically necessary. In contrast to other policy foundations, an insurance/economic frame emphasizes mitigation of short-term risk. Thus, relying on this frame alone is insufficient for establishing the EHB; coverage of prevention services, which are often relatively low cost and whose use can be anticipated, would tend not to be covered under an insurance frame solely.

The ACA puts an emphasis on prevention, and it will be necessary to invest in effective prevention and treatment practices for leading causes of morbidity and mortality to advance population health. In setting that as a goal, however, there must always be, as the ACA requires, attention to diverse segments of society and a spectrum of needs throughout the lifecycle and across a variety of conditions to prevent discrimination in the choice of benefits.

. . .

5. Defining the EHB

. . .

Applying Committee Criteria

. . .

The committee recommends a set of criteria for evaluating both the specific elements for inclusion and the overall package, as well as criteria to guide the process by which the overall package and its elements are defined (see Figure [10.7]). Specifically, in considering whether particular categories or services are included, the committee recommends evaluating each to determine whether it is safe, effective, likely to enhance patient outcomes when compared with available alternatives, and that the cost is justified by the health gain. Included elements should perform acceptably on all of these criteria. The committee also recommends evaluating the overall set of benefits to determine whether the package is affordable, likely to maximize the number of people with insurance, able to protect the most vulnerable, likely to encourage best practices, consistent with the principle of advancing stewardship of finite resources, likely to protect people against the greatest financial risks, and addresses the medical concerns of greatest importance for the eligible populations.

. . .

STEP 2: INCORPORATE COST INTO THE DEVELOPMENT OF THE INITIAL EHB

Early in its deliberations, the committee concluded that the costs associated with offering

Criteria to Guide Content of the Aggregate EHB Package
In the aggregate, the EHB must: • **Be affordable** for consumers, employers, and taxpayers. • **Maximize the number of people with insurance coverage.** • **Protect the most vulnerable** by addressing the particular needs of those patients and populations. • **Encourage better care practices** by promoting the right care to the right patient in the right setting at the right time. • **Advance stewardship of resources** by focusing on high value services and reducing use of low value services. Value is defined as outcomes relative to cost. • **Address the medical concerns of greatest importance** to enrollees in EHB-related plans, as identified through a public deliberative process. • **Protect against the greatest financial risks** due to catastrophic events or illnesses.
Criteria to Guide EHB Content on Specific Components
The individual service, device, or drug for the EHB must: • **Be safe**—expected benefits should be greater than expected harms. • **Be medically effective** and supported by a sufficient evidence base, or in the absence of evidence on effectiveness, a credible standard of care is used. • **Demonstrate meaningful improvement** in outcomes over current effective services/treatments. • **Be a medical service**, not serving primarily a social or educational function. • **Be cost effective**, so that the health gain for individual and population health is sufficient to justify the additional cost to taxpayers and consumers.
Caveats:
Failure to meet any of the criteria should result in exclusion or significant limits on coverage. Each component would shall be subject to the criteria for assembling the aggregate EHB package. Inclusion does not mean that it is appropriate for every person to receive every component.

Figure [10.7] Criteria for assessing content of essential health benefits (EHB) as a whole and for specific components.

the EHB would materially affect the likelihood that the ACA would achieve its goal of significantly reducing the number of people without health insurance. The committee, therefore, incorporates into its recommended process, consideration of overall costs to frame choices about what would ultimately be included in the EHB package. . . .

Rationale for Incorporating Costs into the Definition of Essential Health Benefits

. . .

First, and most importantly, cost provides a useful mechanism to help frame tradeoffs between competing options for inclusion in a benefit package. In fact, the law makes clear that the essential health benefits should reflect the scope of a typical employer plan, and typical employers commonly use premiums as a key element in deciding on the benefit package they will offer employees. For employers, establishing a budget creates one way to explicitly consider benefit package tradeoffs when resources are limited.

Second, in examining the legislative history of the ACA and in testimony received from congressional staff involved in the development of the law, it is clear that improving access to care by expanding the number of people with health insurance was the primary goal of the legislation. Because one important determinant of the number of people who have health insurance is the cost of obtaining coverage[7], the price of the EHB package will influence the ability to achieve the law's goal.

Third, the committee observed that the cost estimates developed by the Congressional Budget Office (CBO) for the ACA were a key element in its ultimate passage. Those cost projections incorporated an estimate of the average premium price of health insurance to be purchased on the exchanges, which in turn affected the total cost of the subsidy and the cost of the federal portion of Medicaid.

Fourth, the committee reflected on the current concern around the deficit and the impact of existing open-ended entitlements, such as Medicare, on the manageability of the federal budget. From a pragmatic viewpoint, requiring a benefit package that was more expensive than typical packages was not regarded by the committee as consistent with today's fiscal realities.

Fifth, the idea of having an explicit budget has been recognized as both an ethical and practical precondition for expanding access to care in medicine.[8] The committee recommends three cost-related criteria—affordability of insurance, stewardship of resources and maximizing access to care—for the Secretary to use to assess the overall EHB package.

For all of these reasons, the committee concluded that the Secretary must use cost to provide guidance in developing the essential health benefits package.

. . .

STEP 3: RECONCILE INITIAL LIST TO THE PREMIUM TARGET

The central debate in constructing the EHB package has been balancing the comprehensiveness of benefits with their costs so as to promote value. This is not an academic exercise but one that has real repercussions for how many people will be able to afford the premium—because the essential health benefits apply to individual and small group policies both inside and outside the exchanges. Furthermore, it will have an impact on state and federal budgets through subsidies and whether people are able to obtain commercial insurance or need to remain fully on public programs. The committee envisions that the Secretary will be able to calculate the estimated national average premium, as well as obtain the actuarial estimates for the categories and services that comprise the list of potential benefits. These may then be compared to reconcile the list to ensure that the incremental cost of all of the proposed benefits will fit within the premium target.

The use of a public deliberative process for setting priorities provides an effective method for meeting many of these requirements. Thus, the committee recommends, in this stage of the process, that structured, public deliberation sessions be conducted to set

[7] J. M. Abraham and R. Feldman, "Taking up or Turning Down: New Estimates of Household Demand for Employer-Sponsored Health Insurance," *INQUIRY: The Journal of Health Care Organization, Provision, and Financing* 47, no. 1 (2010): pp. 17–32.

[8] M. A. Levine, et al., "Improving Access to Health Care: A Consensus Ethical Framework to Guide Proposals for Reform," *Hastings Center Report* 37, no. 5 (2007): pp. 14–19.

priorities within the concept of a budgetary constraint. . . .

Required Elements for Consideration

. . . (See Box [10.3].)

Balance Across Categories and Diverse Segments

. . .

The EHB should incorporate a spectrum of care that meets the evidence-based needs of the varied medical conditions and services that a diverse population of patients requires.

In response to the committee's online query about balance and diversity, various approaches to assessing performance on these dimensions were suggested. Both employers and insurers tended to support having balance across categories defined by a marketplace norm of typical employer plans. The committee believes this is a reasonable approach at the outset, and any information the Secretary has obtained that describes such norms regarding limits and cost-sharing practices would likely be informational not regulatory. Another suggestion, provided by both WellPoint and the American Medical Association[9], was that the goal of balance should be to ensure parity in access to health care services—for example, by having "equal access to providers in each of the 10 categories, as determined by network adequacy standards".[10]

Utilization patterns were most often offered as a way to measure and set norms of practice and identify diverse patient needs.[11,12,13] This information may be helpful in actuarial estimation, but there are limits to the utility of this approach given the ACA's addition of new service categories to the standard benefit package. Consumers and providers that provided input to the committee were often wary of depending solely on existing utilization and coverage patterns to assess balance.[14,15] They argued that current utilization data or even the experience in typical employer plans cannot identify previously unaddressed needs related to some of the 10 categories of care, such as habilitation, mental health and substance abuse parity, and expanded access to preventive services. Others raised the problem of using utilization patterns to identify appropriate multidisciplinary or specialized care.[16]

---

[9] M. A. Maves, "Online Questionnaire Responses Submitted by Michael Maves, CEO and Executive Vice President, American Medical Association, to the IOM Committee on the Determination of Essential Health Benefits, December 20," 2010.

[10] A. Walter-Dumm, "Online Questionnaire Responses Submitted by Ashley Walter-Dumm, Health Policy Director, Wellpoint, Inc. To the IOM Committee on the Determination of Essential Health Benefits, December 6," 2010.

[11] R. Sacco, "Online Questionnaire Responses Submitted by Ralph Sacco, President, American Heart Association to the IOM Committee on the Determination of Essential Health Benefits, December 21," 2010.

[12] R. Sandstrom, "Online Questionnaire Responses Submitted by Robert Sandstrom, Associate Professor, Department of Physical Therapy, Creighton University to the IOM Committee on the Determination of Essential Health Benefits, December 6," 2010.

[13] S. Wojcik, "Online Questionnaire Responses Submitted by Steve Wojcik, Vice President, Public Policy, National Business Group on Health to the IOM Committee on the Determination of Essential Health Benefits, December 6," 2010.

[14] J. Kotch, "Online Questionnaire Responses Submitted by Jonathan Kotch, Professor, Unc Gillings School of Global Public Health to the IOM Committee on the Determination of Essential Health Benefits, November 29," 2010.

[15] J. Touschner, "Online Questionnaire Responses Submitted by Joe Touschner, State Health Policy Analyst, Georgetown Center for Children and Families to the IOM Committee on the Determination of Essential Health Benefits, December 6," 2010.

[16] M. Rice, "Online Questionnaire Responses Submitted by Michelle Rice, Regional Director of Chapter Services, National Hemophilia Foundation to the IOM Committee on the Determination of Essential Health Benefits, December 6," 2010.

Box [10.3] Selected Required Elements for Consideration

Section 1302 (b) (4) REQUIRED ELEMENTS FOR CONSIDERATION.–In defining the essential health benefits under paragraph (1), the Secretary shall –

(A) ensure that such essential health benefits reflect an appropriate balance among the categories described in such subsection, so that benefits are not unduly weighted toward any category;

(B) not make coverage decisions, determine reimbursement rates, establish incentive programs, or design benefits in ways that discriminate against individuals because of their age, disability, or expected length of life;

. . .

Arguments were also presented against traditional "utilization" determinants for pediatric populations, pointing out that this population typically has consumed fewer resources than adults and that investing in preventive services for children presents an opportunity for life-long impact.[17] Nevertheless, the committee supports measures of use as one approach to guide and assess balance considerations. For example, if enrollees of a given plan were systemically not using services considered high value (e.g., not managing their chronic disease adequately), the Secretary might examine the benefit offerings or design for evidence of inappropriate "imbalance."

. . .

[17] A. Racine, "Testimony to the IOM Committee on the Determination of Essential Health Benefits by Andrew Racine, American Academy of Pediatrics, Washington, DC, January 14," 2011.

EXCERPT 9

Abridged text from:

D. M. Eddy, "What's Going on in Oregon", *JAMA* 266, no. 3 (1991): pp. 417–420.

What's Going on in Oregon?

David Eddy

. . .

In July 1989 the Oregon legislature passed the Oregon Basic Health Services Act, a three-part program designed to ensure that every person in Oregon would be covered for at least basic health care. The three components are to expand Medicaid to include all citizens with a family income below the federal poverty level, to require that employers offer workplace-based coverage for employees and their dependents through a small-business insurance pool, and to establish an all-payers' high-risk pool. Thus, the public sector would be responsible for everyone below the federal poverty level, while the private sector would be responsible for those above it. The act also stipulates that providers should be fully reimbursed for the cost of their services.

A central feature of the program is to set priorities for health services. The act created the Oregon Health Services Commission and charged it with producing a ranked list of services that could be used to define a basic care package for coverage by Medicaid. The same package would also define the minimum set of services to be covered by the private sector insurance pools. The commission defined *services* as pairs of conditions (defined by the *International Classification of Diseases, Ninth Revision [ICD-9]* codes) and treatments (defined by *Current Procedural Terminology, Fourth Edition [CPT-4]* codes) and proceeded to analyze more than 1600 condition-treatment pairs. The initial method used a benefit-cost formula that incorporated the health outcomes that could be expected from the condition with and without the treatment, the duration of benefit, the values Oregon residents place on the outcomes, and the cost of the treatment.

When the initial draft of the priority list was released in May 1990, several problems were apparent. The major ones were (1) that some condition-treatment pairs were defined too broadly (eg, minor esophageal strictures that require only medical treatment were grouped with extreme strictures that require resection); (2) there was inadequate differentiation of the durations of the benefit of different treatments (eg, the same "lifetime benefit" was assigned to treatments for self-limited measles, chronic diabetes mellitus, and life-threatening appendicitis); (3) the cost data were incomplete or inaccurate; and (4) there were questions about whether the cost-benefit calculations captured social values accurately, especially values relating to lifesaving treatments. In response to these problems, the commission regrouped and narrowed the definitions of condition-treatment pairs, refined the calculations of duration of benefit, and reviewed the cost assumptions. The commission also loosened the method for ranking the services to incorporate subjective judgments about the types of services and outcomes, along with the objective estimates of benefits and cost.

A revised priority list was published February 20, 1991, and received wider acceptance. Actuaries then estimated the cost of each service and the budget necessary to cover different packages of services. A final priority list and actuary report were submitted to the governor and legislature May 1, 1991. In June, the legislature voted on the reports and a specific funding level. This funding level defines the basic health care package—services covered in order of their ranking in the priority list until the allocated funds are exhausted. Services that rank below the cutoff point are not covered from public funds.

Implementation of the program will require a waiver of the federal law, which can be granted administratively by the Health Care Financing Administration (HCFA) or statutorially by Congress. Two components in particular require a waiver: Oregon needs permission to modify the types, amounts, and scopes of services and to add new groups who have incomes below the federal poverty level but who do not currently qualify. Oregon will apply to both the HCFA and Congress for the waiver. If the waiver is approved by either the HCFA or Congress, Oregon will implement the Basic Health Services Program in the summer of 1992.

The Current Program

Evaluating the impact and merits of the proposed program requires an understanding of Oregon's current Medicaid program. Oregon's program today is the result of a collection of laws, built up over the years by both federal and state governments, that define who is eligible and what they are eligible for. Six main building blocks define who is eligible: the presence of children in a family, the ages of the children, whether a woman is pregnant, whether someone is aged, the presence of a major disability, and income. Using criteria based on these building blocks, federal law defines certain groups of people who must be covered, other groups of people for whom coverage is optional, and still other groups of people for whom coverage is forbidden. The result truly justifies the adjective *patchwork*. . . .

The program covers virtually every medical service for a subset of poor people but covers nothing for a far larger number of people who are poor or nearly poor. Approximately 200,000 people fit the criteria for Medicaid eligibility in Oregon. However, more than twice that number—approximately 450,000 people, or 18% of the state's population—do not have any health insurance. Approximately 120,000 of the 450,000 have incomes below the federal poverty level, but they are not poor enough (eg, incomes below 50% of the federal poverty level) or they do not have the right family status (eg, no children, not pregnant, or children too old) to qualify for Medicaid. A family of four with an income of $541 a month is "too rich" to qualify, even though private insurance would cost them about $204 a month.

The financial cost of the program is high, approximately $230 million in 1990. This cost is shared by the federal government (63%) and the state (37%). But more alarming and frustrating is that, under current laws, the costs grow without control. The budget for physical medical services alone (excluding mental health and chemical dependency services and long-term care) has risen at an annual rate exceeding 18% since 1984, more than twice the rate for other goods and services in the economy. The next biennial budget for medical services will be up 30% over the previous budget. Part of this increase reflects the inexorable inflation of medical care that affects both private and public sectors. But another cause is the propensity of the federal government to add patches to the Medicaid quilt. For example, the Omnibus Budget Reconciliation Act of 1990 added coverage for children born after September 30, 1983 (currently 8 years old) whose families have incomes below 100% of the federal poverty level. This will gradually expand the age limit for children until the year 2004, when the limit will be capped at 21 years.

. . .

The current program covers approximately 60% of the poor (those below the federal poverty line) for virtually every service, including services of relatively low or even unknown value but leaves approximately 40% of the poor with no coverage, even for services that are well documented to have high value. It also leaves uncovered approximately 330,000 other people whose incomes exceed the federal poverty level. The proposed program would offer coverage for all 450,000 Oregon residents who currently have no coverage, but only for services that pass a priority threshold. The shift in balance between who and what is well symbolized by the two main components of the program that require waivers—one would permit Oregon to be more selective in determining what services are covered, allowing the state to cut coverage for low-priority services, and the other would give Oregon more freedom to define who is covered, allowing it to expand the criteria to everyone below the federal poverty level.

The objective of the Oregon plan is not to save money, nor will it have that effect. The proposed program is estimated to cost at least 25% more than the current program. Rather, the objectives of the Oregon plan are to provide better coverage, better incentives, a better balance between health services and other social services, and, most important, better health.

Contributions

In taking these steps, Oregon has made major contributions to the national debate on the cost, access, and quality of health care.

First, Oregon has focused national attention on important problems with the current Medicaid system.[1] One problem is that the current Medicaid system rations people (or for those who dislike the word *ration,* the current system "prioritizes" people). A 6-year-old child is in, a 7-year-old child is out; a woman who is pregnant is in, but if she is not pregnant, she is out; a single adult with a child is in, but single adults without children and two-parent families and childless couples are out. The current system is an excellent example of rationing by meat ax.[2] A second problem is that the current system does not recognize that different medical services have different degrees of effectiveness. It is willing to place different values on different people but not on different services. A third problem is that the current system does not curb Medicaid's appetite for resources that belong to other social programs, even programs that are important to health. Keeping a child healthy requires more than periodic physical examinations and vaccinations; it requires good playgrounds, schools, parents with jobs, crime-free neighborhoods, and counseling about drugs, tobacco, and reproduction. A fourth problem is that the current system fails to address the conflict between the individual and society.[3,4] It has no mechanism for shifting hundreds of thousands of dollars from supportive care for one brain-dead accident victim to basic prevention or medical care for thousands of people.

A second contribution from Oregon is that the state and its leaders have demonstrated the political courage to take action. . . .

Third, Oregon has created an open and explicit social process for addressing the state's health care needs. . . .

A fourth contribution is the initial focus on principles and the subsequent derivation of methods from principles and results from methods. . . .

Fifth, Oregon has used explicit outcomes-based and preference-based methods to set its priorities.[5] . . .

Finally, Oregon included costs and cost-effectiveness as important factors in setting priorities for services. This is political dynamite but is the only way to achieve the desired balance between value and cost.[6]

. . .

[1] J. Kitzhaber, "A Healthier Approach to Health Care," *Issues in Science and Technology* (1991): p. 7

[2] D. M. Eddy, "Rationing by Patient Choice," *Journal of the American Medical Association* 265, no. 1 (1991): pp. 105–108.

[3] D. M. Eddy, "The Individual Vs Society: Is There a Conflict?", *Journal of the American Medical Association* 265, no. 11 (1991): pp. 1446–1450.

[4] D. M. Eddy, "The Individual Vs Society: Resolving the Conflict," *Journal of the American Medical Association* 265, no. 18 (1991): pp. 2399–2406.

[5] D. M. Eddy, "Practice Policies: Guidelines for Methods," *Journal of the American Medical Association* 263 (1990): pp. 1839–1841.

[6] D. M. Eddy, "Connecting Value and Costs: Whom Do We Ask, and What Do We Ask Them?", *Journal of the American Medical Association* 264, no. 13 (1990): pp. 1737–1739.

EXCERPT 10

Abridged text from:
D. C. Hadorn, "Setting Health Care Priorities in Oregon: Cost Effectiveness Meets the Rule of Rescue," *JAMA* 265, no. 17 (1991): pp. 2218–2225.

Setting Health Care Priorities in Oregon: Cost Effectiveness Meets the Rule of Rescue

David C. Hadorn

. . .

Cost-Effectiveness Analysis

Traditional cost-effectiveness theory dictates that in developing a priority list of services the cost of each service should be divided by some measure of the health benefit that is expected from treatment. Benefit is often defined in terms of "quality-adjusted life years" in order to integrate the expected longevity benefit or harm of a treatment with its overall impact on quality of life.[1]

. . .

OHSC followed this prescription exactly in generating its draft priority list.

. . .

Table [10.4] depicts the factors that were combined to produce the priority ratings for the four treatments [tooth capping, surgery for ectopic pregnancy, splints for temporomandibular joint disorder, and appendectomy]; similar line items were generated for each of the more than 1600 condition and treatment pairs (eg, appendectomy for appendicitis) contained in the list. Three factors were estimated for each line item: (1) the expected net benefit from treatment, (2) the expected duration of this benefit, and (3) the direct costs of providing the treatment. Priority ratings were then obtained using the following formula: Priority Rating = Cost of Treatment/(Net Expected Benefit x Duration of Benefit). This formula is a faithful reflection of classic cost-effectiveness theory, including the calculation of quality-adjusted life years in the denominator.

While a description of the procedures used to arrive at the various estimates of cost and outcomes is beyond the scope of this article,[2] the estimates in Table [10.4] appear reasonable. Dental caps, for example, were estimated to produce an average quality-of-life improvement of about 8% vs nontreatment, whereas an appendectomy was expected to produce a 97% improvement (virtually the difference between being alive and being dead).

. . .

The Rule of Rescue

What's wrong with the priority order of Oregon's initial list? After all, in an economic or utilitarian sense it may be true, as implied by the relative location of services on the draft list, that the overall value to society of treating 50 to 100 patients who have temporomandibular joint disorders or dental pulp exposures is comparable to the value of a single life. Treating many patients for a painful condition could, in theory, be considered equivalent to saving one life.

However, any plan to distribute health care services must take human nature into account if the plan is to be acceptable to society. In this regard, there is a fact about the human psyche that will inevitably trump the utilitarian rationality that is implicit in cost-effectiveness analysis: people cannot stand idly by when an identified person's life is visibly threatened

[1] G. Loomes and L. McKenzie, "The Use of QALYs in Health Care Decision Making," *Social Science & Medicine* 28, no. 4 (1989): pp. 299–308.

[2] D. C. Hadorn, "The Oregon Priority-Setting Exercise: Quality of Life and Public Policy," *Hastings Center Reports* 21, no. 3 (1991): pp. S11-S16.

Table [10.4]
Factors Producing the Priority Scores of Four Treatments in Oregon's Draft List

Treatment	Expected Net Benefit From Treatment[a]	Expected Duration of Benefit, y	Cost, $	Priority Rating[b]	Priority Ranking
Tooth capping	.08	4	38.10	117.6	371
Surgery for ectopic pregnancy	.71[c]	48	4015	117.8	372
Splints for temporomandibular joint disorder	.16	5	98.51	122.2	376
Appendectomy	.97	48	5733	122.5	377

[a]Maximum achievable benefit = 1.0.
[b]Priority ratings were obtained using the following formula: Priority rating = Cost of Treatment/(Net Expected Benefit X Duration of Benefit). Ratings ranged from 1.45 (highest priority) to 999.998 (lowest priority).
[c] The net benefit is relatively low because Oregon's consultant physicians estimated that (only) 70% of patients with ectopic pregnancy would die if not operated on. Increasing the estimated net benefit from surgery to 1.0 would move this treatment to 326 on the draft priority list.

if effective rescue measures are available. This strong proclivity has been dubbed the "Rule of Rescue" by Jonsen,[3] who recognized the difficulties posed by the Rule for resource allocation planning:

> *Many of the technologies under assessment relieve illness or pain or disability, but do not directly save life, do not rescue people from imminent death. Those technologies that do stave off death pose a particularly daunting problem [for resource allocation planners] . . . a barrier difficult to climb, a chasm difficult to leap: namely, the imperative to rescue endangered life.*[4]

This duty-based imperative, Jonsen believes, cannot be "expunged from our collective moral conscience," even by the "most evangelical utilitarian." Moreover, although the Rule of Rescue clearly is most compelling in the context of life-saving interventions, it is also a factor whenever an identified patient is in need of treatment (eg, for a fractured arm).

[3] A. R. Jonsen, "Bentham in a Box: Technology Assessment and Health Care Allocation," *Law, Medicine, and Health Care* 14, no. 3-4 (1986): pp. 172–174.

[4] Ibid.

. . .

Is the Rule of Rescue justified or simply an emotional reaction of some kind? Very likely, it is both. Depending on one's conception of distributive justice (ie, what we owe each other), the Rule might be seen as facilitating a sense of fairness in providing for the needs of others—a sense that might be poorly developed otherwise. Clearly, however, as noted above, there is also an emotional component to the Rule of Rescue that can interfere with the development and implementation of fair allocation systems. Society cannot afford to provide every possible beneficial service to every patient—identified or not—as Oregon's planners realized when they embarked on their priority-setting mission. Yielding to the Rule of Rescue in every case of apparent need would lead to an impossibly expensive system.

How then should we cope with the Rule of Rescue when setting health care priorities, as we surely must do if equitable and rational systems of resource allocation are to be developed?[5]

[5] D. C. Hadorn, "The Role of Public Values in Setting Health Care Priorities," *Social Science & Medicine* 32, no. 7 (1991): pp. 773–781.

To answer this question, let's look at how OHSC proceeded following the release of its draft priority list.

Development of the Final Priority List

Stung by public criticism of its initial list, and themselves dismayed by the intuitive unacceptability of the draft list's priority order, OHSC moved swiftly to adopt a different method for purposes of developing its final priority list. . . .

After trimming the Alternative Methodology Subcommittee's draft set of 26 categories [depicting varying types or degrees of expected health benefit from treatments] to 17, OHSC ranked the final set of categories (Table [10.5]) in order of importance, based on three criteria: (1) the category's perceived value to the individual, (2) its value to society, and (3) the "necessity" of the category. Next, OHSC assigned each line item (eg, appendectomy for appendicitis) to one specific category. Several runs were made through the categories by different commissioners in an attempt to achieve consensus and relative consistency in category assignments.

Encouraged by the results of these exercises, OHSC voted on September 5, 1990, to adopt the categorization approach as an alternative to cost-effectiveness analysis for preparing its final list. The next 5 months were spent adjusting category descriptions and definitions, assigning and reassigning line items to the various categories, and continuing to make line item data corrections. Final adjustments in category ranking and line item assignments were made by OHSC on February 2, 1991.

The final priority list was prepared by "stacking" categories on top of each other in rank order so that all the line items in the top-ranked category were deemed to be of higher priority than all the items in the second-ranked category, and so on. Services were ordered within each category according to the net benefit component of the cost-effectiveness ratio. This criterion was selected because in earlier test runs it had seemed to generate the most sensible priority order. Thus, cost was eliminated as a systematic factor in the ordering of services on the final priority list.

To a very minor extent, cost was reintroduced in the concluding step of the process, during which OHSC rearranged line items "by hand." Between February 13 and February 20 (the date of OHSC's meeting, at which time the final priority list was released), the commissioners of OHSC moved individual line items higher or lower on the priority list based on their collective judgment concerning the overall importance of each item in relation to the others. These judgments were guided informally by several factors (as articulated by the commissioners during their discussion and debate), including the number of people who were expected to benefit from a treatment, the value placed on the treatment by society (eg, higher weights on prevention and maternal and child care), and on the item's cost-effectiveness ratio (ie, priority rating Table [10.4]). Thus, service costs were factored into Oregon's final priority list to a minor extent; the influence of cost on the final ordering of services was negligible, however, in comparison with the effect of the categories and the initial within-category ranking of services by net benefit.

Approximately 33% to 50% of the line items contained in the final list were rearranged, although only about 5% to 10% were moved more than 50 positions from the locations arrived at by the prioritization method just described. This rearrangement rate seems reasonable in view of the tremendous complexity of the prioritization task. Surely far more "list jockeying" (as the commissioners sometimes called the process) would have been necessary had the original cost-effectiveness formula been retained, since the Rule of Rescue would still have been a factor. Because service costs were essentially eliminated from Oregon's final priority list, however, the Rule of Rescue was quiescent; as a result, the priority order of the final list generally appears to be far more sensible than the initial list. For example, surgery for appendicitis and for ectopic pregnancy are now both ranked in the top 10 services, while splints for temporomandibular joint disorder dropped near the bottom of the list and dental caps were eliminated entirely as a separate line item.

Events in Oregon continue to evolve. An actuarial analysis of the final priority list will be completed by May 1, which will furnish estimates of the costs required for the state to provide the various services on the priority list—based on historical conjunctions of the various diagnosis and treatment codes used by OHSC to define each line item. These codes were taken from the *International Classification of Diseases, Ninth Revision (ICD-9)* and *Current Procedural Terminology, Fourth Edition (CPT-4)* manuals. Multiple copies of these manuals were always present (and heavily used) during OHSC's meetings.

After estimating the costs of line items, actuaries will calculate the total cost of providing services down to each of several possible "cut points" in the final list. The Oregon Legislative Assembly will then review the final list and decide, by late spring 1991, whether to accept it as the basis for changing the Oregon Medicaid program. If the list is accepted, legislators will "draw a line" somewhere on the list to divide the services that will be covered under Oregon's Medicaid program (those "above the line") from services that will not to be covered (those "below the line"). Legislators are not authorized to change the order of the priority list.

In its final report, scheduled for release May 1, 1991, OHSC will issue a series of findings and recommendations, including the finding that "essential health care" consists of almost all of the services in categories 1 through 9 (Table [10.5]) and most of the services in categories 10 through 13. Services in categories 14 through 17 are deemed nonessential. Based on the location of services on the final list (a total of 714 items), a line drawn somewhere between item 450 (removal of an ovary or fallopian tube for benign conditions) and item 500 (lobectomy for benign pulmonary neoplasm) would appear to fulfill OHSC's definition of essential care.

Finally, if Oregon's Legislative Assembly accepts the priority list and specifies a funding cutoff point, Oregon's leaders will petition both the US Congress and the Health Care Financing Administration for a Medicaid waiver—required for the restructuring of Oregon's Medicaid program to proceed. Prospects for a waiver will be dim if the Legislative Assembly fails to find services in accordance with OHSC's definition of essential care.

. . .

Modified Cost-Effectiveness Analysis

[W]e have seen how Oregon's final priority list was generated primarily by reference to category assignment, which in turn was based on the expected health benefit of treatment. Moreover, services were arranged within categories (prior to hand-rearranging) according to the net benefit component of the cost-effectiveness formula. Thus, service costs were effectively eliminated in generating the final priority list. It was also noted that the Oregon legislature will specify a cutoff point for funding under Medicaid (assuming the final priority list is deemed acceptable). The cutoff point would determine the balance between the range of services covered under Oregon's Medicaid program and the cost of that program.

This two-stage process represents a modification rather than an abandonment of traditional cost-effectiveness theory, since services are still ranked and "selected from the top until resources are exhausted."[6] The key difference, of course, is that Oregon's final list was not

[6] M. C. Weinstein and W. B. Stason, "Foundations of Cost-Effectiveness Analysis for Health and Medical Practices," *New England Journal of Medicine* 296, no. 13 (1977): pp. 716–721.

Table [10.5]
Oregon Health Services Commission's Service Category Definitions (in Rank Order of Deemed Importance)*

1. Treatment of acute life-threatening conditionst where treatment prevents imminent deaths with a full recovery[§] and return to previous health state[§]
   Examples: Appendectomy for appendicitis
   Repair of deep, open wound of neck
2. Maternity care, including disorders of newborn
   Examples: Obstetrical care for pregnancy
   Medical therapy for low-birth-weight babies
3. Treatment of acute life-threatening conditions[†] where treatment prevents imminent death) without a full recovery! or return to previous health state[§]
   Examples: Surgical treatment for head injury with prolonged loss of consciousness
   Medical therapy for acute bacterial meningitis
4. Prevention care for children (includes well-child care)[||]
   Examples: Immunizations
   Screening for vision or hearing problems
5. Treatment of a fatal, chronic condition where, with treatment, one would have improvement in life span[††] and
   QWB[¶]
   Examples: Medical therapy for type I diabetes mellitus Medical therapy for asthma
6. Reproductive services (excluding maternity and infertility)[*]
   Examples: Contraceptive management, vasectomy, tubal ligation
7. Comfort care[**]
8. Preventive dental care
   Example: Cleaning and fluoride
9. Preventive (A, B, C), adults[||]
   Examples: Mammograms, blood pressure screening
10. Treatment of acute,[§] nonfatal[†††] non-self-limited[§] conditions with return to previous health state[§]
    Examples: Medical therapy for acute thyroiditis
    Medical therapy for vaginitis
11. One-time treatment of nonfatal,[†††] chronic[§] conditions with improvement in
    QWB[¶]
    Examples: Hip replacement
    Laser surgery for diabetic retinopathy
12. Treatment of acute,[§] nonfatal[†††] conditions where treatment will improve QWB[¶] without return to prior health state[§]
    Examples: Relocation of dislocated elbow
    Arthroscopic repair of internal derangement of knee
13. Repetitive treatment[§] of nonfatal,[†††] chronic[§] (with recurrent or continuous symptoms) conditions with improvement in QWB[¶] with short-term benefit[§]
    Examples: Medical therapy for chronic sinusitis
    Medical therapy for migraine headache
14. Treatment of acute,[§] nonfatal,[†††] self-limited[§] condition where treatment will expedite return to prior health state[§]
    Examples: Medical therapy for diaper rash
    Medical therapy for acute conjunctivitis
15. Infertility services
    Examples: Medical therapy for anovulation Microsurgery for tubal disease
16. Preventive (D, E), adults[||]
    Examples: Dipstick urinalysis for hematuria in adults who are younger than 60 years
    Sigmoidoscopy for persons who are younger than 40 years

Table [10.5]
Continued

17. Treatment of fatal† or nonfatal††† conditions with minimal or no improvement in QWB¶ or life span§ *Examples:* Medical therapy for gallstones without cholecystitis Medical therapy for viral warts

*OHSC refers to Oregon Health Services Commission. Category descriptions are verbatim from working documents used by the OHSC. Examples are taken from material released by OHSC for its press conference on February 20,1991, at which the final list was announced.
†Five-year mortality rate estimated at 1% or greater.
†† Reduces expected 5-year mortality rate by 25% or more.
§Not defined, left to the judgment of commissioners.
||Defined by reference to the US Preventive Services Task Force Report, except that well-child care is defined using American Academy of Pediatrics guidelines.
¶QWB refers to quality of well-being, the Commission's term for quality of life; derived from the QWB Index of Robert Kaplan and colleagues[9]
*Also includes abortion for "unwanted pregnancy." OHSC will issue a separate disclaimer stating that it advises no change in current Oregon Medicaid policy with respect to abortion.
†††Five-year mortality rate <1%.

constructed using cost-effectiveness ratios as the initial criterion of priority, as posited by traditional theory.

In my view, this two-stage, modified approach represents a significant advance over traditional cost-effectiveness analysis for purposes of setting health care priorities. Setting priorities first on the basis of net expected health benefit, followed by a determination of the degree of benefit required before services are deemed necessary (eg, how close to the top of the list they must be for coverage), provides a reasonable compromise between a public-good, utilitarian framework and the need to accommodate the Rule of Rescue.

. . .

EXCERPT 11

Abridged text from:

N. Daniels, "Is the Oregon Rationing Plan Fair?", *JAMA* 265, no. 17 (1991): pp. 2232–2235.

Is the Oregon Rationing Plan Fair?

Norman Daniels

. . .

What Does the Oregon Plan Do to the Worse-Off Groups?

Critics of Oregon's plan appeal to widely held egalitarian concerns when they argue that it makes the poor bear the burden of this effort to close the insurance gap. The strongest sense of "bear the burden" is "being made worse off." Does the plan, as the critics charge, make the poor worse off instead of giving priority to improving their well-being?[1,2]

Consider the simplest case first, a zero sum game with resources. For example, if extrarenal transplants are removed from coverage and no higher-priority services, unavailable before the plan, are added, then current Medicaid recipients will lose some services and the health benefits they produce. They will no doubt then make this complaint: "We bear the burden of the plan. Since we are already the most indigent group, or close to it, we should not have to give up lifesaving or other important medical services so that the currently uninsured can get basic level health care."

It is important to grasp the moral force of this complaint. Notice that *aggregate* health status for *all* the poor, including current Medicaid recipients and the uninsured, can be improved by the plan, even though current Medicaid recipients are made worse off. The loss of less important services by current recipients is more than counterbalanced by the gains of the uninsured. As a result, the plan reduces overall inequality between the poor and the rest of society, albeit at the expense of current Medicaid recipients. Therefore, the complaint cannot be that the plan makes society less equal; instead, it is that even greater reductions in inequality are possible if other groups sacrifice instead of Medicaid recipients. It is unfair for current Medicaid recipients to bear a burden that others could bear much better, especially since inequality would then be even further reduced.

How stringent is the priority owed the poorest groups when we seek to improve aggregate well-being? Three positions are possible: (1) help the poor as much as possible *(strict priority);* (2) make sure the poor get some benefit *(modified priority);* or (3) allow only modest harms to the poor in return for significant gains to others who are not well off *(weak priority)*. Critics of the Oregon plan insist that we should not settle for weak priority, especially since feasible alternatives help the poor more. The Oregon plan leaves the bulk of the health care system intact. By eliminating the inefficiencies it contains, eg, by establishing a low-overhead public insurance scheme (as in Canada), or by developing treatment protocols that eliminate unnecessary services, we might be able to avoid making current Medicaid recipients any worse off. Alternatively, by broadening rationing to cover most of society, as in Canada or Great Britain, we could avoid the criticism that only the poor are being made to bear the burden of improving access.

. . .

If the current Medicaid recipients are made worse off, there is a serious, though not necessarily fatal, objection to the Oregon plan. If we hold only a weak version of the requirement that we give priority to the worse off, we might still think the plan acceptable even though some of the poor bear the burden of reducing overall inequality. In any case, the Oregon planners hope that rationing will yield a result

[1] N. Daniels, *Just Health Care* (Cambridge University Press, 1985).

[2] J. Rawls, *A Theory of Justice* (Cambridge: Harvard University Press, 1971).

in which all the poor are better off than now. Political judgments differ about the likelihood of this preferred outcome.

Are the Inequalities the Oregon Plan Accepts Justifiable?

By rationing lower-priority services to the poor, rather than excluding whole groups of the poor and near-poor from insurance, the Oregon plan reduces inequality in our society, even if current Medicaid recipients are, to some extent, worse off than they are now. Somewhat paradoxically, even under the scenario in which no one is worse off, there is still a sense in which the poor bear the burden of the plan, since the plan accepts as official policy an unjustifiable inequality in the health care system.

. . .

To see why one structure of inequality seems worse than the other, consider how the poor would feel under both. Under the Oregon plan, the poor can complain that society as a whole is content not only to leave them economically badly off, but also to deny them medical services that would protect the range of opportunities that are open to them.[3] There is a basis here for reasonable regrets or resentment, for society as a whole seems content to shut the poor out of mainstream opportunities. They may reasonably feel that the majority is too willing to leave them behind, under terms in which the benefits of social cooperation do not reflect their moral status as free and equal agents.[4,5] Alternatively, if health care protects opportunity in a way that is roughly equal for all, except that the most advantaged group has some extra advantages, then this may seem somewhat unfair, but no one group is then singled out for special disadvantages that are viewed as "acceptable" by the economically and medically advantaged majority. Consequently, no group would have a basis for the strong and reasonable regrets that the poor have under the Oregon plan, despite their improvement relative to the current situation.

. . .

[3] Daniels, *Just Health Care*.

[4] J. Cohen, "Democratic Equality," *Ethics* (1989): pp. 727–751.

[5] T. M. Scanlon, "Contractualism and Utilitarianism," in *Utilitarianism and Beyond*, edited by A. K. Sen and B. Williams (New York: Cambridge University Press, 1982), pp. 103–128.

Is the Public Process for Deciding What Is "Basic Care" Fair?

The Oregon plan involves public, explicit rationing; it disavows rationing hidden by the covert workings of a market, or buried in the quiet, professional decisions of providers. Its rationing decisions are the result of a two-step process involving separate, publicly accountable bodies. First (step 1), OHSC, which is charged with taking "community values" into consideration, determines priorities among services in a possible benefit package. Second (step 2), the legislature decides how much to spend on Medicaid, given competing demands on state funds. Some lower-priority services may thus not be covered, but the resulting Medicaid benefit package must still be approved by the Department of Health and Human Services. Assessing the fairness of the rationing process requires examining both steps.

Oregon's insistence on publicity is controversial. Calabresi and Bobbit[6] argue that "tragic choices" are best made out of the public view in order to preserve important symbolic values, such as the sanctity of life. Despite the importance of such symbols, however, justice requires publicity. People who view themselves as free and equal moral agents must have available to them the grounds for all decisions that affect their lives in fundamental ways, as rationing decisions do. Only with publicity can they resolve disputes about whether the decisions

[6] G. Calabresi and P. Bobbitt, *Tragic Choices* (Norton, 1978).

conform to the more basic principles of justice that are the accepted basis of their social cooperation.[7]

Actually, going beyond a concern for publicity, Oregon calls for broad public participation in the development of priorities. Public participation is desirable because it may yield agreement about how to resolve disputes among winners and losers in a fair way. It also makes it more likely that outcomes reflect the consent of those individuals who are affected and, since there may not be one uniquely fair or just way to ration services, participation allows the shared values of a community to shape the result. Is the public participation process itself fair, and does it have a real effect on outcomes?

OHSC held public hearings on health services and asked Oregon Health Decisions to hold community meetings throughout the state "to build consensus on the values to be used to guide health resource allocation decisions."[8] At 47 meetings that were held during the early part of 1990, citizens were asked to rank the importance of various categories of treatment and were asked, "Why is this health care service *important to us?*" From these discussions, an unranked list of 13 "values" was distilled. A tally was kept of how often each value was discussed, but we cannot rank the importance of the values on that basis.

. . .

OHSC is well aware of this limitation and views the list of values only as a "qualitative check" on the process of ranking services (Paige Sipes-Metzler, personal communication, June and July 1990). Thus, it believes the community concern for equity is met because the system guarantees universal access to basic care. Community concerns about mental health and chemical dependency, or prevention, are met by making sure that these services are included in the ranking process. Although no weights were assigned to values such as quality of life or cost-effectiveness, they are included as factors in the formal ranking process. The only direct community input into the first attempt at ranking services, however, came from a telephone survey aimed at finding how Oregonians ranked particular health outcomes that affect their quality of life. By combining this information with expert judgments about the likely outcomes of using particular procedures to treat certain conditions, as well as with information about the costs of treating a population with those procedures, OHSC generated a preliminary cost-benefit ranking of services. Because this ranking drew extensive criticism (*New York Times*. July 9, 1990; sect A: 17) and failed to match its own expectations about priorities, OHSC modified its procedure for ranking services. As a result, the OHSC commissioners themselves ranked general categories of services according to their importance to the individual, to society, and to the health plan and "adjusted" other items.[9] It remains unclear how this process reflects community values, and until we know just how the final rankings were "adjusted," we cannot know what influence public participation has had.

The rationing process involves two decisions, not one. Suppose that we have a fair procedure and a perfect outcome at step 1: the ranking of services captures relevant facts about costs and benefits and represents community values fairly. Unfortunately, fairness at step 1 does not assure it at step 2, because the voting power of the poor is negated in a political process that generally underrepresents them, judging from past voting patterns and outcomes. Therefore, even if there is a consensus at step 1 about what the basic, minimum package should be, there may be well-founded worries that the legislature will not fund it. Indeed, the situation is somewhat worse because OHSC only ranks services, it does not decide what is basic. The funding decision of the legislature determines what basic care is provided.

---

[7] J. Rawls, "Kantian Constructivism in Moral Theory," *The Journal of Philosophy* (1980): pp. 515–572.

[8] R. Hasnain and M. Garland, *Health Care in Common: Report of the Oregon Health Decisions Community Meetings Process* (Portland: Oregon Health Decisions, 1990).

[9] J. Kitzhaber, *Summary: The Health Services Prioritization Process* (Salem: Oregon State Senate, 1990).

Clearly, political judgments diverge on how much we can trust the legislature. The crucial issue from the point of view of process, however, is this: because the Oregon plan explicitly involves rationing primarily for the poor and near-poor, funding decisions face constant political pressure from more powerful groups who want to put public resources to other uses. In contrast, if the legislature were deciding how to fund a rationing plan that applied to themselves and to all their constituents, then we might expect a careful and honest weighing of the importance of health care against other goods. The legislature would then have stronger reasons not to concede to political pressures to divert resources, and other groups would be less likely to apply such pressure. If the plan is expanded to include other groups, then the poor may find important allies.

Worries about fairness in the Oregon rationing process thus come from the plan's being aimed at the poor rather than at the population as a whole. Concerns about fairness in the process thus converge with concerns about the kinds of inequality the system tolerates. This does not mean that the Oregon experiment should not be tried; it may produce less overall inequality in health status than we now have. But we should recognize from the start that a system that rations only to the poor is less equitable and less fair than alternative systems that ration for the great majority of people. To the extent that the inequality ends up troubling many participants in the system, including physicians who will be able to do only certain things for some children and more for others, the strains of commitment to abiding by the rationing will be greater, and rationing may get a worse name than it deserves.

. . .

This work was generously supported by grant RH-20917 from the National Endowment for the Humanities and grant 1RO1LM05005 from the National Library of Medicine, Washington, DC.

Helpful information, materials, or comments were provided by Dan Brock, PhD, Arthur Caplan, PhD, Michael Garland, PhD, John Golenski, SJ, Bruce Jennings, PhD, Sen John Kitzhaber, and Paige Sipes-Metzler, DPA.

EXCERPT 12

Abridged text from:

M. Johri and O. F. Norheim, "Can Cost-Effectiveness Analysis Integrate Concerns for Equity? Systematic Review," *International Journal of Technology Assessment Health Care* 28, no. 2 (2012): pp. 125–132.

Can Cost-Effectiveness Analysis Integrate Concerns for Equity? Systematic Review

Mira Johri and Ole Frithjof Norheim

The aim of this study was to promote approaches to health technology assessment (HTA) that are both evidence-based and values-based. We conducted a systematic review of published studies describing formal methods to consider equity in the context of cost-effectiveness analysis (CEA). . . .

The fifty-one studies took three broad approaches to facilitate quantitative consideration of equity concerns in CEA (Table 1): integration of distributional concerns through equity weights and social welfare functions (33 of 51; 65%), exploration of the opportunity costs of alternative policy options through mathematical programming (9 of 51; 18%), and multi-criteria decision analysis (9 of 51; 18%). We critically review their main features.

. . .

Discussion

This review has identified three formal mechanisms to consider equity in the context of CEA, all of which are technically feasible. Yet, despite sustained methodological work spanning 2 decades, consideration of equity issues remains peripheral to CEA.[1,2] A central problem relates to the fact that equity is understood in multiple ways, each demarcating a distinct set of intuitions concerning fairness. Each method takes a distinct approach to how values should articulate with cost-effectiveness evidence. We synthesize the major findings below. An important limitation of this review concerns the failure to assess the quality of studies with respect to conceptualization and empirical implementation.

Equity Weights and Social Welfare Functions

Authors advocating these approaches have usually envisioned a definitive amendment to the QALY model incorporating specific values for equity weights, or identification and parameterization of a correct form of the SWF.

To justify specification of weights or parameters, several studies looked to empirical surveys of stated preferences of members of the general public or decision makers. At least six problems arise from this approach, reflecting difficulties in eliciting true and stable preferences,[3] and questions about the normative role public opinion is being called upon to play: (i) The manner in which questions are asked is known to influence

---

[1] F. Sassi, L. Archard, and J. Le Grand, "Equity and the Economic Evaluation of Healthcare," *Health Technology Assessment (Winchester, England)* 5, no. 3 (2001): p. 1.

[2] H. Weatherly, et al., "Methods for Assessing the Cost-Effectiveness of Public Health Interventions: Key Challenges and Recommendations," *Health Policy* 93, no. 2 (2009): pp. 85–92.

[3] A. J. Lloyd, "Threats to the Estimation of Benefit: Are Preference Elicitation Methods Accurate?", *Health Economics* 12, no. 5 (2003): pp. 393–402.

responses;[4] (ii) Large-scale surveys elicit opinions rather than considered judgments; (iii) Questions are posed in isolation; however, we require information on the joint effects of equity dimensions;[5] (iv) The average value is a statistical compromise imposed on a wide distribution of opinion;[6] (v) Even where a clear consensus exists, majority opinion can simply be wrong;[7] (vi) The public may not have well-considered judgments about complex distributive issues. Public consultation is clearly important in democratic societies and improved techniques are being developed.[8] However, public opinion by itself offers insufficient normative grounds to justify the choice of specific values for equity weights or functional forms.

SWF studies have also sought guidance from theories of fair distribution from welfare economics or moral and political philosophy. These theories offer coherent and sophisticated normative frameworks that can be used as analytic lenses. However, they are developed at a high level of generality and their application to concrete problems of health policy is challenging.

To summarize, surveys reveal no consensus on specific values for weights, parameter values or functional forms, and studies offer no strong theoretical basis to establish such values. We, therefore, believe that exploratory use of these techniques, for example in sensitivity analyses, is most promising.

[4] P. A. Ubel, "How Stable Are People's Preferences for Giving Priority to Severely Ill Patients?", *Social Science & Medicine* 49, no. 7 (1999): pp. 895–903.

[5] Sassi et al., "Equity and the Economic Evaluation of Healthcare."

[6] M. Johri, et al., "The Importance of Age in Allocating Health Care Resources: Does Intervention-Type Matter?", *Health Economics* 14, no. 7 (2005): pp. 669–678.

[7] D. W. Brock, "Empirical Ethics, Moral Philosophy, and the Democracy Problem," in *Summary Measures of Population Health*, edited by C. Murray, et al. (Geneva: World Health Organization, 2003).

[8] J. S. Fishkin, *Democracy and Deliberation: New Directions for Democratic Reform* (Yale University Press, 1991).

Mathematical Programming and the Exploration of Opportunity Costs

Developed primarily by researchers engaged in cost-effectiveness modeling, MP shares many features of the SWF approach. Specifically, maximization and health equity are presented in a unified framework, and equity is conceived as a constraint on an optimization problem with a quantifiable cost. MP studies trace the opportunity costs of alternative policy options leaving the choice of which option to pursue to decision makers. Accordingly, pure efficiency results are presented separately from equity-based scenarios.

To support normative claims, MP studies advocate general principles such as equality or proportionality in health benefits or financial investment between groups, defined in terms of clinical characteristics, risk factors, socio-demographically or geographically.[9,10,11,12,13,14,15] Horizontal equity, or the

[9] S. Cleary, G. Mooney, and D. McIntyre, "Equity and Efficiency in HIV-Treatment in South Africa: The Contribution of Mathematical Programming to Priority Setting," *Health Economics* 19, no. 10 (2010): pp. 1166–1180.

[10] S. R. Earnshaw, et al., "Optimal Allocation of Resources Across Four Interventions for Type 2 Diabetes," *Medical Decision Making* 22, no. suppl 1 (2002): pp. s80–s91.

[11] D. M. Epstein, et al., "Efficiency, Equity, and Budgetary Policies Informing Decisions Using Mathematical Programming," *Medical Decision Making* 27, no. 2 (2007): pp. 128–137.

[12] E. H. Kaplan and M. H. Merson, "Allocating HIV-Prevention Resources: Balancing Efficiency and Equity," *American Journal of Public Health* 92, no. 12 (2002): pp. 1905–1907.

[13] A. A. Stinnett and A. D. Paltiel, "Mathematical Programming for the Efficient Allocation of Health Care Resources," *Journal of Health Economics* 15, no. 5 (1996): pp. 641–653.

[14] G. S. Zaric and M. L. Brandeau, "Optimal Investment in a Portfolio of HIV Prevention Programs," *Medical Decision Making* 21, no. 5 (2001): pp. 391–408.

[15] S. A. Zenios, L. M. Wein and G. M. Chertow, "Evidence-Based Organ Allocation," *The American Journal of Medicine* 107, no. 1 (1999): pp. 52–61.

principle of equal treatment for equal need, has also been invoked.[16] Zenios and colleagues discuss a compelling case where heterogeneity between patient subgroups results in kidney transplantation being less cost-effective for black than for white Americans. While the logic of efficiency would suggest defining subgroup-specific cost-effectiveness ratios and potentially restricting transplantation to those with more favorable cost-effectiveness, equity is addressed through a constraint preventing race from influencing access to treatment.[17]

In the kidney transplantation example, the criterion for defining groups is intuitively morally important. However, for the majority of analyses, the definition of what constitutes a group often seems ad hoc or of questionable moral relevance.

Several studies attempt to address equity by giving all stake-holder groups a slice of the pie, without asking why these groups should have special fairness claims. With a notable exception,[18,19] MP papers are not clearly linked to the theoretical literatures on equity. Their main focus to date has been to explore and advance technical methods that can be used to address fairness concerns in CEA. Despite considerable strengths in modeling and methods, the lack of a clear normative basis is currently a limiting factor to their utility.

Multi-Criteria Decision Analysis

In MCDA, equity and efficiency figure among several priority-setting concerns that contribute to define a ranking of health interventions.[20] To identify relevant concerns, MCDA draws on the values of a small group of stakeholders. The exercise to identify and weigh criteria contributes to procedural fairness by encouraging clarity, transparency, and discussion among stake-holders, as well as appropriate use of scientific evidence. Studies have generally recruited individuals with an elected or managerial responsibility for the public's health to ensure that use of their values to inform health priorities is legitimate.[21,22,23] Through recognition of the plurality of relevant concerns and its pragmatism, MCDA has made a substantial contribution to priority setting. It has modest data and modeling requirements and can be done relatively quickly in a variety of settings.

MCDA is an empirical and context-specific approach about which several important questions can be posed. One might be worried that selection of criteria is somewhat arbitrary in that it depends on a small group of individuals. Moreover, criteria selected to date have sometimes been defined in overlapping terms, reflecting the lack of a clear theoretical relationship between these criteria and a broader theory of justice. The stability of econometric results is also at issue, as it is unclear to what extent rankings are sensitive to the composition of the respondent group. A fractional factorial design allows for estimation of all main effects, but not of interactions. The design of

[16] Epstein, "Efficiency, Equity, and Budgetary Policies."

[17] Zenios, "Evidence-Based Organ Allocation."

[18] P. Anand, "QALYs and the Integration of Claims in Health-Care Rationing," *Health Care Analysis* 7, no. 3 (1999): pp. 239–253.

[19] P. Anand, "The Integration of Claims to Health-Care: A Programming Approach," *Journal of Health Economics* 22, no. 5 (2003): pp. 731–745.

[20] R. Baltussen and L. Niessen, "Priority Setting of Health Interventions: The Need for Multi-Criteria Decision Analysis," *Cost Effectiveness and Resource Allocation* 4, no. 1 (2006): p. 14.

[21] R. Baltussen, et al., "Towards a Multi-Criteria Approach for Priority Setting: An Application to Ghana," *Health Economics* 15, no. 7 (2006): pp. 689–696.

[22] R. Baltussen, et al., "Priority Setting Using Multiple Criteria: Should a Lung Health Programme Be Implemented in Nepal?", *Health Policy and Planning* 22, no. 3 (2007): pp. 178–185.

[23] C. Jehu-Appiah, et al., "Balancing Equity and Efficiency in Health Priorities in Ghana: The Use of Multicriteria Decision Analysis," *Value in Health* 11, no. 7 (2008): pp. 1081–1087.

the experiments published thus far has been orthogonal, without correlations between the attributes. Nonorthogonal designs could be considered in future to model situations of dependence between attributes and those for which the choice probabilities are dependent on the attribute levels. Informational loss related to the aggregation process may result in lack of transparency in final rankings. Perhaps most importantly, one might be concerned that the aggregation function used to construct the final ranking is empirically and statistically driven rather than being based on cultivation of judgment. It combines on an equal footing the best-known scientific evidence and opinions of uncertain validity. Deliberative approaches to MCDA merit exploration, as do methods integrating qualitative dimensions.[24]

Concluding Remarks

Viable techniques now exist to facilitate consideration of equity in CEA. These range from descriptive approaches[25] to the quantitative methods studied in this review. In our view, the principal obstacles impeding their use now lie at the normative rather than the technical level. We conclude with two recommendations for HTA bodies seeking to strengthen consideration of equity in decision making.

The term "equity" is used to refer to a multiplicity of concepts and values. Talking at cross-purposes has often hindered understanding. As a practical tool to focus discussion, HTA bodies require a comprehensive map of the principle equity concerns. Based on this review, Table 2 provides a synthesis of additional normative criteria relevant to CEA. Achieving greater clarity at the conceptual level will facilitate effective data gathering on the equity effects of interventions and the tradeoffs between maximizing overall health benefits and equity considerations. Greater conceptual clarity will also help to ensure that such data are reliable, valid, and contribute to the cumulative growth of knowledge on interventions to promote health equity.

Value pluralism is a universal feature of democratic societies, and there is no widely accepted normative source on which to ground normative choices. Cost-effectiveness rankings provide extremely important and useful information for resource allocation choices. However, many additional criteria related to the many dimensions of equity, and other goals such as feasibility and affordability are also relevant to HTA decisions. To foster the best overall decision under specific circumstances, we recommend that HTA bodies use techniques for explicit consideration of equity such as those reviewed in this study as part of a deliberative process that emphasizes procedural fairness through accountability, transparency, consistency, and the proper use of scientific evidence.[26] While we value the insights they can provide, we eschew using quantitative techniques for consideration of equity to provide a definitive ranking of priorities. These techniques can do most when used in an open-ended manner as part of a fair decision-making process.

. . .

[24] E. Makundi, L. Kapiriri and O. F. Norheim, "Combining Evidence and Values in Priority Setting: Testing the Balance Sheet Method in a Low-Income Country," *BMC Health Services Research* 7, no. 1 (2007): p. 152.

[25] R. Cookson, M. Drummond and H. Weatherly, "Explicit Incorporation of Equity Considerations into Economic Evaluation of Public Health Interventions," *Health Economics, Policy and Law* 4, no. 02 (2009): pp. 231–245.

[26] N. Daniels, *Just Health Care* (Cambridge University Press, 1985).

EXCERPT 13

Abridged text from:

J. Kreis and H. Schmidt, "Public Engagement in Health Technology Assessment and Coverage Decisions: A Study of Experiences in France, Germany, and the United Kingdom," *Journal of Health Politics, Policy and Law* 38, no. 1 (2013): pp. 89–122.

Public Engagement in Health Technology Assessment and Coverage Decisions: A Study of Experiences in France, Germany, and the United Kingdom

Julia Kreis and Harald Schmidt

. . .

We explore operational processes and underlying rationales of public engagement at HTA agencies in France, Germany, and the United Kingdom. The analysis is based on website information, legal framework documents, published and gray literature, and semi-structured, in-depth interviews with officials at Chief Executive or Chairperson level at these agencies.

We use the term *public* as the broadest generic term to include engagement of individual citizens, patients, consumers (or users), laypeople, or formal or informal representatives of groups of these.[1]

Engagement processes differ across agencies, particularly regarding the areas in which the public is involved, which groups of the public are involved, what weight they have in influencing decisions, how they are recruited and supported, and how potential conflicts of interests are addressed (see Table [10.6].) . . .

. . .

Interviewees were asked to rate the importance of five hypothetical rationales that we identified from the literature.

. . .

. . .

Why Engage in the First Place? The Relevance of Different Rationales

There was noteworthy variation in the implied and declared rationales of carrying out engagement activities, with the least disagreement about the importance of legitimacy and value mining, which also received the highest average ranks across the key informants (see Table [10.7].). . .

Fact Mining and Incorporating the "Knowledge Privilege." On the public's ability to contribute factual knowledge, NICE's key informant assigned the highest marks, G-BA's the lowest, and HAS's an in-between score. However, it should be noted that in Germany, key tasks in generating evidence reports are carried out by IQWiG, which in turn involves patient groups in determining study endpoints. Still, there appear to be varying perceptions, in that NICE's key informant also judged input on facts to be the most important of all rationales. In what might be termed patients' "knowledge privilege," having a direct first-person perspective on all aspects of living with a particular condition was valued as an opportunity to complement data from the scientific literature that often draws on abstract standardized instruments to measure patients' quality of life. Given that NICE has the most extensive experience with engagement (of the organizations reviewed here as well as in general, considering other similar bodies), this could warrant further exploration to ascertain whether this form of engagement is a particularly effective and unique way of incorporating patients' perspectives. However, it is not clear that personal testimony is the only way this outcome could be achieved. The assumption would need to be ascertained in formal evaluations, which would need to compare personal testimony to other methods of capturing patients' views and taking into account their perspectives, such as from survey or interview work.[2] . . .

---

[1] F. -P. Gauvin, et al., ""It All Depends": Conceptualizing Public Involvement in the Context of Health Technology Assessment Agencies," *Social Science and Medicine* 70, no. 10 (2010): pp. 1518–1526.

[2] K. Facey, et al., "Patients" Perspectives in Health Technology Assessment: A Route to Robust Evidence and Fair Deliberation', *International Journal of Technology Assessment in Health Care* 26, no. 03 (2010): pp. 334–340.

Table [10.6]
Selected Aspects of Scope and Type of Public Engagement at NICE, G-BA, and HAS

	NICE [UK]	G-BA [Germany]	HAS [France]
Public engagement at board level	Yes	Yes	No
Main recruitment mechanism	Open advertising/ individuals	Nominated by organizations/ representatives	Not Applicable
Voting rights	Full voting rights	None (but the right to propose agenda items and request a vote)	Not applicable
Public engagement in appraisal committees	Yes	Yes	Depends on type of committee
Main recruitment mechanism	Open advertising/ individuals	Nominated by organizations/ representatives	Nominated by organizations/ representatives
Voting rights	Full voting rights	None (but the right to propose agenda items and request a vote)	Full voting rights where they are represented
Final guidance/decision by	NICE[a]	G-BA[b]	Department of Health
Assessing the general public's value judgments	Citizens Council elicits societal values (feed into codified document that appraisal committees are expected to consider in decisions)	Values implicitly taken into consideration in appraisals (via patient representatives)	Focus groups and public debates carried out for sensitive and controversial topics
Conflicts of interest of individuals	To be declared, published	To be declared internally, not published	To be declared, published
Legal requirement for industry to declare funding of patient groups	None	None	Funding to be declared to HAS, published
Remuneration of members of the public	Yes	Yes	Yes
Training opportunities for individuals	Yes, in-house	Yes, in-house	No

NICE, National Institute for Health and Clinical Excellence; *G-BA*, Gemeinsamer Bundesausschuss; *HAS*, Haute Autorité de Santé.

[a]Generally, the NHS is obliged to provide approved interventions within three months, although the Department of Health may decide that in specific cases longer periods may be appropriate.

[b]The Ministry of Health may formally object to the G-BA's decisions within a two-month period before their entry into force.

Value Mining. There was broad agreement among informants that when it comes to values, the public has much to contribute, and it is important for the organizations to obtain a good understanding of the public's views. HAS's and G-BA's key informants emphasized that values are relevant, particularly when evidence alone is highly inconclusive but coverage decisions still need to be made or when topics are addressed that go beyond the more

Table [10.7]
Key Informants' Views on Different Rationales for Public Engagement

Rationale[a]	Key informants' institution		
	NICE	G-BA	HAS
Facts Engagement may generate new knowledge about people's views or medical preferences, such as endpoints	5	2	3
Values Engagement may generate insights into people's normative preferences and values, regarding, for example, prioritization in treatment	3–4	3–3.5	4
Legitimacy Engagement may strengthen an agency's moral and legal authority in decision making through openness and transparency, either by identifying new facts or values, or simply by carrying out engagement processes	3–4	3.5–4	4
Acceptability Engagement may help increase awareness of HTA processes and improve understanding that difficult decisions need to be made when not all needs can be met	1	5	3
Dissemination Engagement may help spread knowledge about particular decisions	2–3	3	4

NICE, National Institute for Health and Clinical Excellence; *GBA*, Gemeinsamer Bundesausschuss; *HAS*, Haute Autorité de Santé.

Interviewees (one key informant at chief executive or chairperson level per agency) were asked to rate on a scale of 1–5, with 5 signifying the greatest importance. In some cases, intermediate rankings were assigned (e.g., 3.5). Note that the views are those expressed by the interviewees and must not be taken to be official position statements of the respective organizations.

narrowly defined medical context. Values play a role in all forms of engagement, but, as observed above, only NICE has a dedicated forum for eliciting value judgments in its Citizens Council, largely due to its specific function and objectives. Culturally, institutions such as citizens' juries are also more salient in the United Kingdom, and NICE's key informant alluded to their presence in describing what led to the council's establishment. In the legal context, too, technical and complex matters often need to be resolved. But trust is placed in the belief that a group of reasonable people, each with individual sets of facts and values, can provide valuable scrutiny that is more appropriate than that of representatives of a particular interest group. Such a permanent forum is absent in the German context and in the case of HAS is given only in ad hoc focus groups or public hearings.

As with fact mining, it is not clear that there is a "right" way of gathering the general public's values. Again, the appropriateness of specific initiatives needs to be seen and evaluated in light of alternatives such as surveys, focus groups, or deliberative polling.[3]

Legitimacy, Representation, and Relevant Reasons. Across all three organizations, there is also broad agreement about the importance of the rationale of legitimacy. However, as is true for terms such as *fairness* or *justice*, there

[3] C. Davies, M. Wetherell and E. Barnett, "Opening the Box: Evaluating the Citizens Council of NICE. Report Prepared for the National Coordinating Centre for Research Methodology, NHS Research and Development Programme," March. (Milton Keynes, UK: Open University, 2005).

is no single canonical understanding of *legitimacy* in philosophy and political science.[4] Here we focus on two specific dimensions of legitimacy that are of central relevance to virtually all normative accounts. These dimensions concern issues around representation and the identification and analysis of relevant reasons, both of which the key informants appealed to.

The concept of representativeness features in many engagement activities and in comments such as that the public has a right to be heard since the NHS is publicly owned. Yet the shortcomings of such claims are obvious and generally recognized. Consultations are in principle open to everyone and can be a useful tool to ascertain the relevance of issues that come up in appraisal processes, but factors such as self-selection require care in interpreting results. In addition, while NICE's Citizens Council tries to reflect the diversity of the British public as closely as possible, there are clear limits resulting, in particular, from the size of the group. Even doubling or quadrupling numbers will fail to fully represent actual diversity. The forum is therefore best viewed not as exhaustively representing the public's view but as providing some insights into the thoughts of a group of ordinary people that constitutes a (weighted) sample of the wider population.[5,6] Furthermore, council members have no formal mandate from the public to represent it, and the same is true for lay members of NICE's appraisal committees, who participate as individuals and may vote in actual decisions. In the case of G-BA and HAS, there are formal criteria that govern the involvement of patient group representatives. This decentralized arrangement may be appealing in the sense that participating groups can cascade information through their networks and determine internally which person is best suited to participate. But as the G-BA discussions on voting rights illustrated, while in the best case representatives reflect the interests of all their members, they have no monopoly over the respective patient population, not least because many patients do not engage with the organizations' work and may in fact disagree with their policies. Much care is therefore required in interpreting any results of engagement processes as genuinely representative of the public or particular patient groups.

However, key informants also touched on another aspect of legitimacy in highlighting the importance of explicit justification of their decisions. In this sense legitimacy is a function of the extent to which organizations provide fair opportunities to the public (and other stakeholders) to submit relevant reasons in open, transparent, and lawful processes where their views are likely to make a difference.[7] We noted two ways in which this could be achieved. First, in a somewhat passive but nonetheless important sense, lay presence on committees can encourage experts to argue their case more explicitly and comprehensibly. Second, when members of the public can provide their own facts or values they may identify new or different reasons that might otherwise have been ignored. For this input to have an effect, appropriate mechanisms (at relevant stages throughout the appraisal process) need to be instituted to allow for analysis of views submitted and, where adequate, response. Such arrangements can help ensure that the organizations provide more thorough and comprehensive justification based on a broader and better set of relevant reasons than might otherwise have been the case.

---

[4] F. Peter, "Political Legitimacy," in *The Stanford Encyclopedia of Philosophy*, edited by E. N. Zalta (2010).

[5] N. Daniels, "Accountability for Reasonableness and the Citizens Council," in *Patients, the Public, and Priorities in Healthcare*, edited by P. Littlejohns and M. Rawlins (Oxford: Radcliffe, 2009).

[6] J. Parkinson, "Legitimacy Problems in Deliberative Democracy," *Political Studies* 51, no. 1 (2003): pp. 180–196.

[7] N. Daniels and J. Sabin, *Setting Limits Fairly: Can We Learn to Share Medical Resources?* (Oxford University Press, 2002).

It is interesting to note that G-BA is legally required to organize training for patient representatives and to provide dedicated manpower to this end. In France patient representatives are by law entitled to training in order to facilitate the exercise of their mandate. A plausible rationale for this stipulation is that for engagement to be meaningful and for those engaged to be able to act at the same level as experts, required skills cannot be taken for granted and must be supported and developed.

Acceptability. The acceptability of decisions might be seen as depending exclusively on the extent to which they are legitimate. But decisions may well be legitimate and nonetheless not be accepted by all. Organizations may also want to use engagement more directly to improve acceptance. Key informants differed considerably in their grading of legitimacy and acceptability, with those for the latter showing the greatest variation: G-BA's informant assigned the highest rank (overall and across the three organizations) and NICE's informant the lowest (again, overall and across the three organizations). This finding needs to be seen in the context of the three organizations' public profiles: NICE has the highest, whereas G-BA is known mainly in stakeholder circles (the public generally presumes that the G-BA's work is done by the Ministry of Health). As noted, the G-BA applies the same structure that is used to bring together representatives from the payer and provider community to patient representatives, whose organizations may send delegates. The high ranking of the G-BA's key informant can perhaps be understood against this legal background, which likewise could be driven by the desire to increase acceptability by drawing on established patient and consumer groups.

G-BA's and HAS's observations that engagement signals that the organizations are not merely faceless administrative machines can perhaps be seen as explanations of why engagement can matter in improving acceptability, independent of the criterion of legitimacy. If it should emerge that acceptability can be improved on these grounds, such a finding could also have implications for conclusions one might draw from assessing the extent to which other rationales have been achieved. For example, even if evaluations demonstrate that the knowledge privilege can be obtained through other means, engagement may still be used to signal in a symbolic way that the respective body listens. Insofar as achieving this outcome means that the population is more willing to accept often controversial decisions, a nontrivial and in fact potentially quite substantial benefit will have been achieved.

Whether engagement has in fact been successful in improving acceptability, whether the opportunity for providing input is ranked as highly by the public as it is by the interviewees who made this point, and what the relationship is between acceptability and legitimacy in the public's eye are matters of opinion and empirical research, as carried out in related contexts. . . . Robust evidence from such research would help assess the perceived and real weight of carrying out engagement for the purpose of improving acceptability and could help guide investments (or disinvestments) in different forms of engagement.

Disseminating Information. There is also some variation regarding the use of engagement as a form of disseminating information, which, however, again needs to be seen in the context of the bodies' different functions. The rankings broadly reflect this, with HAS playing a more active role in informing patients, whereas in Germany this is shouldered by organizations other than the G-BA such as IQWiG, the sickness funds, or the Federal Center for Health Education, and in the United Kingdom by the NHS more broadly. Besides spreading information about particular decisions, members of the public could also disseminate information about how the particular decision was reached and why. In that sense, members of the public could become ambassadors of decisions, which might in turn again increase their acceptability. . . .

For each of the five rationales we have explored, three main questions are of central relevance in evaluations. First, what has the engagement activity contributed in terms of achieving the rationale? Second, could the results of engagement have been obtained in other ways? Third, has the contribution led to better processes or decisions than in the counterfactual case where no engagement took place? Evaluations should extend to assessing both the quality of the products of engagement (such as written or oral testimony or opinions) and the response mechanisms that organizations have in place to analyze and, where relevant, incorporate or reject input, with justification given as appropriate. . . .

Further Resources

Relevant Organizations

Governmental

Medical Services Advisory Committee: Provides advice to the Minister for Health in Australia on the strength of evidence relating to comparative safety, clinical effectiveness, and cost-effectiveness of new or existing medical services or technology. Additional information can be found at http://www.msac.gov.au

NICE Citizens Council: Provides public perspective on overarching moral and ethical issues that NICE has to take into account when producing guidance for UK health decisions. Additional information can be found at https://www.nice.org.uk/get-involved/citizens-council

Oregon Health Plan: State Medicaid program aiming to provide basic health care needs to low-income individuals and families. Additional information can be found at http://www.oregon.gov/oha/healthplan/pages/index.aspx

The Commonwealth Treasury: Establishes Australian policy in areas such as public service pay and conditions, welfare payments, and is also involved in the collection of statistics. Additional information can be found at http://www.treasury.gov.au/

The Federal Joint Committee (G-BA): Specifies which medical care services are reimbursed by the statutory health insurance funds in Germany. Additional information can be found at http://www.english.g-ba.de/

The Pharmaceutical Benefits Advisory Committee: Assesses applications for listing of medicines on the Pharmaceutical Benefits Scheme in Australia. Additional information can be found at pbac.pbs.gov.au/

Therapeutic Goods Administration: Australia's regulatory authority for therapeutic goods, carrying out assessment and monitoring activities to ensure quality and access of therapeutic goods. Additional information can be found at https://www.tga.gov.au/

Nongovernmental

Health Technology Assessment international (HTAi): A global professional society for those who produce, use, or encounter HTA. Additional information can be found at http://www.htai.org/

International Network of Agencies for Health Technology Assessment: Aims to connect HTA agencies to each other to support knowledge sharing and the exchange of information. Additional information can be found at http://www.inahta.org/

Institute for Quality and Efficiency in Health Care: Examines the benefits and harms of medical interventions for patients in Germany. Additional information can be found at https://www.iqwig.de/en/home.2724.html

Patient-Centered Outcomes Research Institute (PCORI): Provides data to improve health decisions. Additional information can be found at www.pcori.org

Literature

Carroll, Aaron E. "Forbidden Topic in Health Policy Debate: Cost Effectiveness," *New York Times*, December 15, 2014.

Dillon, Andrew. "Blog: Carrying NICE over the Threshold," *National Institute for Health and Clinical Excellence,* February 19, 2015.

Dovi, Suzanne, "Political Representation," The Stanford Encyclopedia of Philosophy (Spring 2014 Edition), Edward N. Zalta (ed.), http://plato.stanford.edu/archives/spr2014/entries/political-representation/.

Millman, Jason. "Price Transparency Stinks in Health Care. Here's How the Industry Wants to Change That," *The Washington Post*, April 16, 2014.

Oberlander, Jonathan, Theodore Marmor, and Lawrence Jacobs. "Rationing Medical Care: Rhetoric and Reality in the Oregon Health Plan." *CMAJ: Canadian Medical Association Journal* 164, no. 11 (2001): 1583–1587.

Oregon Health Plan. "The Prioritized List." http://www.oregon.gov/oha/healthplan/Pages/priorlist.aspx.

Pharmaceutical Benefits Advisory Committee. "Other Relevant Factors." https://pbac.pbs.gov.au/section-f/f3-other-relevant-factors.html.

Protheroe, Joanne, Don Nutbeam, and Gill Rowlands. "Health Literacy: A Necessity for Increasing Participation in Health Care." *The British Journal of General Practice* 59, no. 567 (2009): 721–723.

Other Media

"The Price of Life." Television Movie. Directed by Adam Wishart, BBC, June 17, 2009: Documentary about NICE drug appraisal process.

11

Four Illustrative Cases

Colon Cancer, Prostate Cancer, Gaucher's Disease, and Antiretroviral Treatments (ARTs)

Drug Formulary Exclusions as a Means for Cost Containment in Cancer Care

Memorial Sloan Kettering's Decision to Reject Zaltrap from its Colorectal Cancer Formulary

The Treatment Landscape for Advanced-Stage Colorectal Cancer

Colon cancer is the third most commonly diagnosed form of cancer and the fourth leading cause of cancer death worldwide.[1] There are roughly 1.4 million new diagnoses and 700,000 deaths annually.[2] When detected and treated in its earliest stages while tumors are localized, the 5-year survival rate of colon cancer is generally good—above 90%. But once it has spread to the nearby lymph nodes, the disease is far more deadly. And if it reaches other vital organs, such as the liver, it is incurable.[3]

For advanced-stage colorectal cancers, most patients undergo surgery to remove the segment of the colon containing the tumor. If the cancer is found to have spread to other tissues, chemotherapy typically follows.

The most common chemotherapy regimens for colon cancers center around a drug called 5-florouracil (5-FU), which was developed in 1957. In the decades since, pharmaceutical companies have attempted to generate new therapies in hopes of supplanting 5-FU. They have not yet succeeded. They have, however, introduced a host of new drugs that, when combined with 5-FU or other existing therapies, have been shown to extend survival by varying amounts of

---

[1] World Cancer Research Fund International, "Cancer Facts and Figures: Worldwide Data," 2014, accessed October 12, 2015, http://www.wcrf.org/int/cancer-facts-figures/worldwide-data.

[2] Ibid.

[3] American Cancer Society, *Colorectal Cancer Facts & Figures 2011–2013* (Atlanta, GA: American Cancer Society, 2011).

time. And because the US Food and Drug Administration (FDA) approves drugs solely on the basis of their safety and efficacy—and not according to their cost-effectiveness—pharmaceutical companies have successfully brought numerous drugs to market even if their exorbitant costs are offset by relatively small health benefits.

In 1996, Pfizer won FDA approval for a drug called Camptosar, which was found to extend median overall survival by 3 months for a cost of $5,300 per month of treatment. In 2004, ImClone, a biotech company, won approval for Erbitux, which was found to extend median overall survival by 4 months. Bristol-Myers Squibb and Eli Lilly acquired ImClone and now market Erbitux for $8,400 per month of treatment. Also in 2004, Genentech introduced Avastin (bevacizumab), which was approved after it was shown to extend average survival by nearly 5 months as a first-line therapy and by 1.5 months as a second-line therapy (after a first-line therapy has not worked adequately). Avastin today costs roughly $5,000 per month of treatment.[4]

Introduction of Zaltrap

On August 3, 2012, the FDA approved yet another chemotherapy agent for colorectal cancer, called Zaltrap (ziv-aflibercept), manufactured by Sanofi-Aventis. In a randomized clinical study of 1,226 patients with metastatic colorectal cancer, patients who received Zaltrap were shown to live 1.5 months longer compared to those who only received the standard FOLFIRI regimen (folinic acid, 5-FU and irinotecan). Tumors also reduced in size for 20% of the patients who received FOLFIRI with Zaltrap, compared to 11% of those who received FOLFIRI without it. The common side effects of Zaltrap included decreased white blood cell count, diarrhea, mouth ulcers, fatigue, high blood pressure, and weight loss.[5]

While the effectiveness and side effects of Zaltrap were similar to those of other drugs already on the market, including Avastin, it was the price of the drug that set it apart. Under US law, pharmaceutical manufacturers are granted periods of patent exclusivity during which competitors are barred from developing and marketing generic alternatives. This affords manufacturers monopoly-like conditions in which to set the initial price of new drugs when bringing them to market.

When Zaltrap came to market in August of 2012, the price was set at roughly $11,000 per month of treatment. Avastin, which was shown to prolong survival for exactly the same number of days in clinical trials, was priced at $5,000 per month.[6]

Reaction Among Providers

Exorbitantly high prices for chemotherapy agents under patent protection are not at all uncommon. Prices for cancer drugs have been rising exponentially over the past five decades. The median monthly price for cancer drugs at the time of FDA approval in the period from 1965 to 1970 was roughly $100 (in 2014 USD). It was roughly $10,000 per month in 2014 (Figure 11.1).[7]

In the United States, providers of medical care have been relatively slow to push back against rising chemotherapy prices, mostly because expensive drugs can be a major boon

[4] S. S. Hall, "The Cost of Living," *New York Magazine*, October 20, 2013.

[5] P. A. Tang and M. J. Moore, "Aflibercept in the Treatment of Patients with Metastatic Colorectal Cancer: Latest Findings and Interpretations," *Therapeutic Advances in Gastroenterology* 6, no. 6 (2013): p. 467.

[6] Hall, "The Cost of Living."

[7] P. B. Bach, "Price & Value of Cancer Drug," Memorial Sloan Kettering Cancer Center, 2015, accessed November 17, 2015, https://www.mskcc.org/research-areas/programs-centers/health-policy-outcomes/cost-drugs.

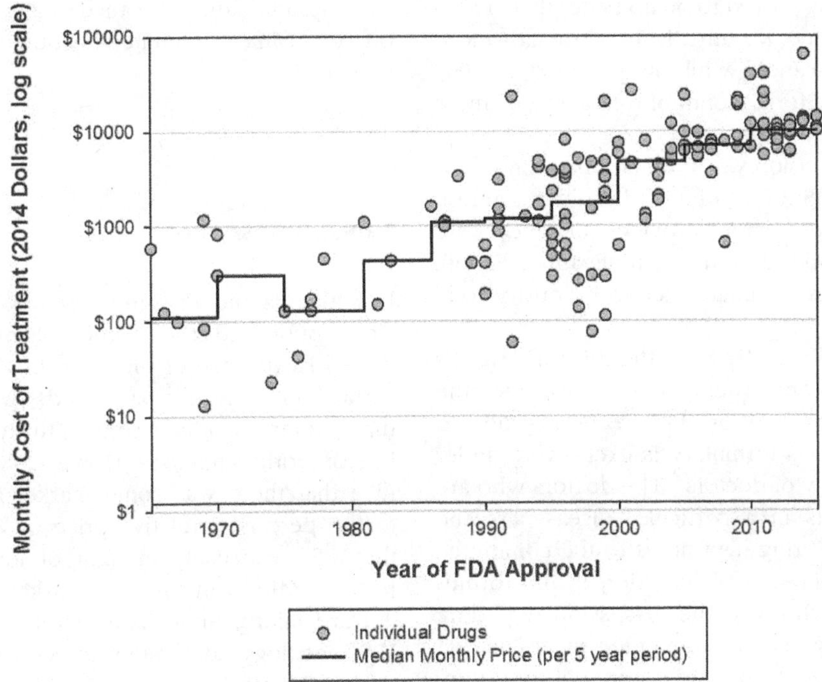

Figure 11.1 Monthly and median costs of cancer drugs at the time of FDA approval (1965–2015).[8]
Source: Memorial Sloan Kettering Cancer Center.

for doctors' and hospitals' revenue and profitability. For example, Medicare and many payers reimburse oncologists the average sales prices of chemotherapy drugs plus a 6% markup for practice cost.[9] This creates perverse incentives: an oncologist prescribing a $1,000 drug receives a $60 markup, while one who prescribes a $10,000 drug gets $600. Thus, providers have developed a preference for using higher priced drugs, even when less expensive, equally effective options are available because higher prices mean higher profits to physicians and hospitals.[10]

The Physicians of Memorial Sloan Kettering Cancer Center Decide to Buck the Trend

In October 2012, Peter B. Bach, Leonard B. Saltz, and Robert E. Wittes—three physicians at Memorial Sloan Kettering Cancer Center (MSKCC)—published an op-ed in the *New York Times* announcing a decision that "should have been a no brainer."[11] Drs. Bach, Saltz, and Wittes explained that physicians at MSKCC had decided to not "give a phenomenally expensive new cancer drug to [their] patients" because, they argued "The drug,

[8] Ibid.

[9] S. Glied and K. Haninger, "Medicare Part B Reimbursement of Prescription Drugs," 2014, accessed October 12, 2015, http://aspe.hhs.gov/report/medicare-part-b-reimbursement-prescription-drugs.

[10] H. Schmidt and E. J. Emanuel, "Lowering Medical Costs Through the Sharing of Savings by Physicians and Patients: Inclusive Shared Savings," *JAMA Internal Medicine* 174, no. 12 (2014): pp. 2009–2013.

[11] P. B. Bach, L. B. Saltz, and R. E. Wittes, "In Cancer Care, Cost Matters," *New York Times*, October 14, 2012.

Zaltrap, has proved to be no better than a similar medicine we already have for advanced colorectal cancer, while its price—at $11,063 on average for a month of treatment—is more than twice as high."

The decision was the first of its kind. And because MSKCC is one of the oldest, largest, and most prestigious providers of cancer care in the world, Zaltrap's manufacturer, Sanofi, and the rest of pharmaceutical industry took notice.

According to Dr. Saltz, the chair of MSKCC's Pharmacy and Therapeutic Committee, the decision to add or remove new drugs to the hospital's formulary is exclusively under the purview of doctors. "The doctors who are the experts in a particular disease are the ones who bring new drugs to the committee for consideration of inclusion in the formulary and who lead the discussion regarding those drugs at the committee meetings." At present, Dr. Saltz said, "none of our doctors who treat this disease have been able to identify a situation in which we would feel that the use of this drug might be appropriate. If new data emerge and that changes, we will certainly review those data and act accordingly."[12]

In their op-ed, the physicians argued, "ignoring the cost of care is no longer tenable." As healthcare costs have risen over the decades, the financial burdens on patients—both directly, through higher out-of-pocket spending and insurance premiums, as well as indirectly, through greater budget deficits and spending cuts—have risen, too. "When choosing treatments for a patient," they argued, "we have to consider the financial strains they may cause alongside the benefits they might deliver." And since the FDA, Medicare, and the major insurers seem to be too afraid to confront this issue for fear of charges of "rationing," the authors argue that physicians and hospitals should assume the responsibility. "The future of our health care system, and of cancer care, depends on our using our limited resources wisely," they said.[13]

Sanofi's Response

Less than a month after the MSKCC physicians published their op-ed, Sanofi abandoned its defense of the price of Zaltrap. In a statement, the company said, "We believe that Zaltrap is priced competitively as used in real-world situations. However, we recognize that there was some market resistance to the perceived relative price of Zaltrap in the U.S.—especially in light of low awareness of Zaltrap in the U.S. market. As such, we are taking immediate action across the U.S. oncology community to reduce the net cost of Zaltrap."[14]

The action Sanofi took was to offer 50% rebates to doctors and hospitals that offered Zaltrap. The rebates, however, did not change the official list price for the drug, which meant that insurance companies' and patients' out-of-pocket costs associated with the drug would remain pegged to the $11,000 original price. For Medicare patients without a supplementary insurance policy, many of whom are responsible for as much as 20% of the cost of chemotherapeutics, the out-of-pocket costs may be prohibitive—which, for Zaltrap, may be as high as $2,200 a month.[15] High out-of-pocket expenses like these are a large reason why 38% of patients with colorectal cancer experience severe financial hardship (defined as accruing debt, borrowing money from friends or family, selling/refinancing their

[12] L. B. Saltz, "The Cost of Cancer Care and Formulary Decisions—the Zaltrap Story," Practice Update, 2012.

[13] Bach, "In Cancer Care, Cost Matters."

[14] A. Pollack, "Sanofi Halves Price of Cancer Drug Zaltrap after Sloan-Kettering Rejection," *New York Times*, November 8, 2012.

[15] S. Ramsey and V. Shankaran, "Managing the Financial Impact of Cancer Treatment: The Role of Clinical Practice Guidelines," *Journal of the National Comprehensive Cancer Network* 10, no. 8 (2012): pp. 1037–1042.

primary home, or a 20% or greater decline in income).[16]

Sanofi's response did little to move MSKCC's Pharmacy and Therapeutic Committee to reconsider allowing Zaltrap on its formulary. The drug is still not used at MSKCC.

In the aftermath of the decision, Dr. Bach said, "We didn't set out to make an example of the drug. This was an instance where we thought things were particularly indefensible. We decided that what we felt was in the best interest of patients."[17]

[16] K. R. Yabroff, et al., "Economic Burden of Cancer in the United States: Estimates, Projections, and Future Research," *Cancer Epidemiology Biomarkers & Prevention* 20, no. 10 (2011): pp. 2006–2014.

[17] M. Dalzell, "Pushback on Zaltrap's Price Highlights Sensitive End-of-Life Issue," *Managed Care* 21, no. 12 (2012): p. 40.

Questions for Discussion

1. What are the advantages and disadvantages of having physician-led committees decide what drugs are included or excluded from hospital formularies?
2. In your opinion, should these decisions rest with doctors or other actors in the healthcare system—like patients, payers, or the government? Why?
3. Should the MSKCC Pharmacy and Therapeutics Committee include Zaltrap after Sanofi reduced the "effective" price but not the list price by 50%?
4. If Zaltrap was priced only 20% higher than Avastin, rather than 100%, would that have made a difference to you if you were a member of MSKCC Pharmacy and Therapeutics Committee?
5. Should MSKCC make these types of decisions for other medical equipment and procedures, in addition to costly cancer drugs?
6. Should MSKCC exclude certain types of wheelchairs, pacemakers, or surgeries because there are other more cost-effective alternatives? Why or why not?

EXCERPTS

Note: The following excerpts have generally been edited for length, and omissions are indicated with ellipses. Editing includes footnotes and endnotes, which have also been renumbered. For citation and related purposes, the full original source texts should be used.

EXCERPT 1

Choosing Among Treatment Options for Prostate Cancer: What Role Should Cost Play?

Prostate Cancer: Prevalence and Mortality Risk

Excluding skin cancers, there is no form of cancer more common among men in the United States than prostate cancer. According to the National Cancer Institute, approximately 15.3% of American men will be diagnosed with prostate cancer at some point in their lifetimes. An even greater number—perhaps as high as 40% of men over the age of 50—harbor an early as yet undetectable form of the disease.[1] Yet, due to slow progression and other tumor-specific characteristics, more men die with it than from it.[2]

Prostate cancer has always been a relatively common form of cancer. In 1975, there were approximately 95 new cases of prostate cancer for every 100,000 men. By 1992, there were more than 237 new cases for every 100,000 men.[3] (See Figure [11.2]) The dramatic increase in incidence was not due to any change in the disease or new vulnerability among American men. Rather, the advent of prostate-specific antigen (PSA) screening and greater awareness of the condition led to much more frequent detection of the disease—usually in its earlier, low-risk stages, before patients begin to show symptoms.[4] The number of new cases per year has since decreased consistently.

The mortality risk of prostate cancer varies substantially depending on the stage at which the disease is discovered. If the disease is discovered in its later stages, after it has spread to distant organs, there is a high mortality risk. The 5-year relative survival rate of prostate cancer that has metastasized beyond the regional lymph nodes is 28%. These cases, however, comprise only a small minority of new prostate cancer diagnoses. Just 4% of the prostate cancers discovered between 2004 and 2010 were found to have spread beyond the immediate region.[5]

The vast majority of new cases, by contrast, carry much lower mortality risk: 80% of new prostate cancer cases are diagnosed as localized, low-risk tumors. Another 12% are diagnosed as regional (i.e., the cancer has spread to the nearby lymph nodes but without any evidence of distant metastases). In these localized and regional diagnoses, the 5-year relative survival rate is nearly 100%.[6] When assessed as a whole, even factoring in the advanced-stage diagnoses, the long-term survival rate for new prostate cancer patients is still fairly good. The relative 10- and 15-year survival rates are 99% and 94%, respectively.[7] Compared to the survival rates of other forms of cancer, these numbers paint a much rosier picture.

---

[1] D. Ollendorf, et al., *Management Options for Low-Risk Prostate Cancer: A Report on Comparative Effectiveness and Value* (Boston, MA: Institute for Clinical and Economic Review, 2010).

[2] T. Wilt, et al., "Comparative Effectiveness of Therapies for Clinically Localized Prostate Cancer," *AHRQ Comparative Effectiveness Reviews* (2008): p. 1.

[3] National Cancer Institute, "SEER Stat Fact Sheets: Prostate Cancer," 2015, accessed November 17, 2015, http://seer.cancer.gov/statfacts/html/prost.html.

[4] R. A. Stephenson, "Prostate Cancer Trends in the Era of Prostate-Specific Antigen," *Urologic Clinics* 29, no. 1 (2002): pp. 173–181.

[5] Ibid.

[6] Ibid.

[7] American Cancer Society, "Survival Rates for Prostate Cancer," 2015, accessed October 13, 2015, http://www.cancer.org/cancer/prostatecancer/detailedguide/prostate-cancer-survival-rates.

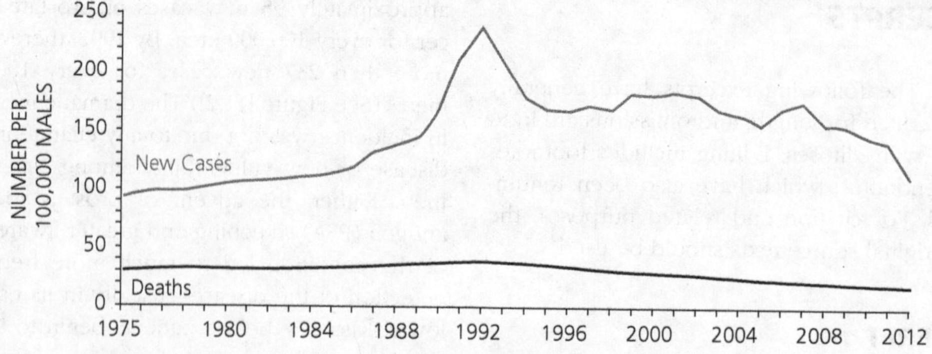

Figure [11.2] Prostate cancer new cases and deaths per 100,000 males, United States.[8]

Source: National Cancer Institute: Surveillance, Epidemiology, and End Results Program.

Options for Managing Low-Risk Prostate Cancer

Determining a course of treatment for low-risk prostate cancer, with localized disease confined to the prostate and without lymph node involvement, can be difficult. Patients and clinicians have numerous factors and options to weigh, but very little objective data to inform their decision. And while most prostate cancer treatment plans have roughly the same cure and disease recurrence rates, the side effects and the financial costs of each option differ substantially.

The Institute for Clinical and Economic Review (ICER) published a report in 2010 summarizing previous appraisals of five of the leading treatment options for low-risk prostate cancer.[9] The treatment options included (1) radical prostatectomy, (2) brachytherapy, (3) intensity-modulated radiation therapy, (4) proton beam therapy, and (5) active surveillance, also known as *watchful waiting* (the dominance in the US of the former term can be seen as a subtle yet revealing reflection of the professional and cultural reluctance to refrain from interventions) (See Figure [11.3].)

Radical Prostatectomy

Radical prostatectomy is a surgical procedure that removes the prostate gland and some of the surrounding tissue in hopes of extracting all the cancerous cells in and around the prostate. It can be performed as open surgery, most commonly through an incision in the lower abdomen, or as minimally invasive laparoscopic surgery, either by hand or with the assistance of robotic arms. The typical inpatient hospital stay associated with the treatment is 1–4 days. There are a number of potential risks and side effects from the surgery. Although surgeons have introduced "nerve-sparing" techniques, erectile dysfunction is a fairly common side effect, affecting roughly 40% of men between 1 and 2 years after surgery. Urinary incontinence is also common, affecting 40% of men within 90 days after the procedure and 14% of men at 1 year and beyond.[10]

Surgical treatment has grown in popularity in recent years due to a couple of factors. First, detection of the disease is now more common in younger and otherwise healthier men. Men who are younger and healthier are generally better able to recover fully from surgery. Additionally, men who discover the low-risk form of the disease later in life are more likely to die of causes other than the disease itself. By contrast, men who plan to live with the disease for 30 or

[8] National Cancer Institute, "SEER Stat Fact Sheets."

[9] Ollendorf, "Management Options for Low-Risk Prostate Cancer."

[10] Ibid.

	Active Surveillance	Radical Prostatectomy	Brachytherapy	IMRT
Potential Comparative Advantages	~40% never show clinical progression requiring active treatment Risk of "missed" aggressive tumors or tumor progression	Single procedure Low risk of bowel side effects Surgical complications	Single procedure Minimally invasive Lower risks of short-term incontinence or impotence than surgery	Noninvasive Lower risks of short-term incontinence or impotence than surgery Higher (~45) number of visits for treatment
Potential Comparative Disadvantages	Monitoring and biopsies required Extended life expectancy (>20 yrs)	Higher rates of short-term incontinence and impotence Higher surgical risks	Risk of short-term urinary obstruction Large prostate	Higher risk of bowel side effects (proctitis) Higher concern for normal bowel function
May Not Be Best For	High anxiety High potential for failure to follow-up	Higher concern for sexual function and urinary continence	History of urinary obstruction	High concern for normal bowel function
Relative Cost to Insurers	↓	↔	↔	↑

Figure [11.3] Low-risk prostate cancer management decision guide.[11]

40 years have a greater risk of progression if the cancerous cells are not removed. Younger men are often counseled to take curative action when prostate cancer is discovered. Second, the advent of robot-assisted surgery has further propelled the popularity of this option. Despite a lack of conclusive data that prove robot-assisted surgery leads to less risk or better outcomes, the availability of the technique has seemingly driven a precipitous rise in laparoscopic prostatectomy procedures due to successful marketing campaigns and a widespread belief that the new technology will reduce recovery times.[12,13]

The lifetime costs associated with surgery vary, but typically fall between $30,000 and $40,000, depending on the age at diagnosis.[14] Robot-assisted surgery is considerably more expensive due to the substantial institutional costs of acquiring and maintaining the technology, which is covered by the hospital. A new robotic surgical system, for example, can cost upward of $1.6 million, with annual maintenance costs of $100,000–$200,000.[15] Most insurance companies, including Medicare, will cover all types of radical prostatectomy, but they will not provide separate or additional reimbursement for the more expensive robot-assisted procedures.[16]

11 Ibid., p. 7.

12 J. C. Hu, et al., "Comparative Effectiveness of Minimally Invasive vs Open Radical Prostatectomy," *Journal of the American Medical Association* 302, no. 14 (2009): pp. 1557–1564.

13 M. L. Blute, "Radical Prostatectomy by Open or Laparoscopic/Robotic Techniques: An Issue of Surgical Device or Surgical Expertise?," *Journal of Clinical Oncology* 26, no. 14 (2008): pp. 2248–2249.

14 Ollendorf, "Management Options for Low-Risk Prostate Cancer," p. 50.

15 Ibid., p. 45.

16 Ibid., p. 27.

Brachytherapy

Brachytherapy involves the implantation of radioactive "seeds" into the prostate near the cancerous cells. The seeds are small pellets of radioactive material that emit radiation as they break down to become more stable isotopes. The aim is for the energy emitted to kill the cancerous cells. Placement of the seeds requires a short operation that typically necessitates an overnight hospital stay.

Like all radiation, the danger of brachytherapy is that normal, noncancerous tissue is also exposed to the radiation emitted from the seeds. This produces a risk of damage to the bladder and intestines, which can lead to incontinence, urgency, and other problems with urinary and bowel function, or treatment-related secondary malignancy. There is also risk that the seeds fall out of the prostate gland and migrate to other parts of the body.

Lifetime brachytherapy treatment costs roughly the same amount as surgery—between $30,000 and $38,000—with a large percentage of the expense devoted to procuring the radioactive isotope seed and the image guidance systems used to implant them.[17] The treatment is covered by Medicare and the major commercial insurers.[18]

Intensity-Modulated Radiation Therapy (IMRT) and Proton Beam Therapy (PBT)

IMRT and PBT are both forms of external beam radiation therapy. In both, a machine sends high-energy radiation to a specific part of the body through multiple beam angles and targets it using computer-guided imaging in hopes of maximizing the dose to the cancerous tissue and sparing adjacent noncancerous tissue. IMRT and PBT are typically conducted as outpatient procedures over the course of roughly 40 daily treatment visits. IMRT, which was developed in the mid-1990s, uses small radiation beams with varying intensities to shape the radiation beam to the cancerous target. PBT, developed more recently, draws its radiation energy from heavier proton particles, which—its proponents argue—can be controlled even more precisely than IMRT radiation. The depth to which protons penetrate the body can be fine-tuned to match the location of a tumor, which in theory would reduce the radiation dose to uninvolved, surrounding tissue.[19]

The short- and long-term risks of external beam radiation therapies for prostate cancer have been studied to a much lesser degree than they have for other courses of treatment. There is roughly a 1% risk of a radiation-associated secondary malignancy with IMRT and PBT due to radiation affecting surrounding tissue. As of 2014, there is no conclusive proof that PBT lowers this risk compared to IMRT. There is also risk of both short- and long-term gastrointestinal, urinary, and sexual side effects. Compared to other possible treatments, IMRT carries a greater risk of bowel side effects and perhaps a lower risk of impotence or incontinence.[20] More study of PBT is needed to assess the comparative risks and benefits, though initial research suggests similar rates to IMRT.

Where the external beam radiation therapies set themselves apart is in the realm of cost. IMRT and PBT are the most expensive courses of treatment for low-risk prostate cancer. The average lifetime costs for IMRT are between $43,000 and $51,000, while the average lifetime costs for PBT are between $60,000 and $69,000.[21] When compared to a radical prostatectomy, the incremental cost effectiveness ratio—that is, the cost per number of added quality-adjusted life years (QALY)—was $35,233 for IMRT and $169,867 for PBT, according to the ICER report.[22]

Despite the high costs, most major commercial insurers will cover external beam radiation, though many will do so only if certain conditions

[17] Ibid., p. 50.

[18] Ibid., pp. 27–28.

[19] Ibid., p. 18.

[20] Ibid., p. 6.

[21] Ibid., p. 50.

[22] Ibid., p. 51.

are met. For example, United Healthcare will cover IMRT, but only for cases in which "irregularly shaped tumors are in close proximity to vital structures or sensitive normal tissue AND one of the following criteria: non-metastatic prostate cancer for dose escalation >75Gy or equivalent hypofractionated regimen," meaning only in cases where the tumor would be hard to reach with other treatments and a high dose of radiation would be needed.[23] For PBT, insurers range from covering it unconditionally to not covering it at all. Humana's policy simply states, "Proton beam therapy is considered a covered benefit for the treatment of prostate cancer."[24] PriorityHealth's policy, by contrast, states, "Proton beam therapy for prostate cancer is not covered, because 'alternate equally effective forms of therapy which are more cost-effective exist.'"[25] Still other insurers, like Cigna and United, will cover PBT, but do not consider it "medically superior" to IMRT and will therefore only reimburse to cover the costs of the less expensive form of radiation treatment.[26]

Active Surveillance or Watchful Waiting

Localized, low-risk prostate cancer is considered a fairly nonaggressive form of cancer. Many men can harbor an early form of the disease with no symptoms and no pathological progression. With the advent of new screening techniques, including PSA testing, more newly diagnosed prostate cancer cases are detected in this early stage. In fact, estimates are that PSA screening detects prostate cancers an average of 9 years before clinical diagnosis or presentation of symptoms.[27]

Active surveillance entails no medication, radiation, or surgery—at least at the outset. It is a treatment protocol that calls for frequent and careful monitoring to assess the risk posed by an early-stage prostate tumor at any given time. If PSA levels rise beyond a certain level, a change in the course of treatment is triggered and a new definitive procedure—like surgery or radiation—is chosen. Roughly 40% of patients aged 65 and older who begin active surveillance will never require definitive treatment because they die of other causes before their cancer progresses to a dangerous degree (see Table [11.1]).[28]

The main risk of active surveillance is allowing the disease to progress for too long before beginning definitive treatment. There is also a risk that the uncertainty of cancer progression can increase patient anxiety. Patients who are younger (and who are likely to live long enough to require definitive treatment eventually), as well as those who are likely to fail to follow-up to be retested frequently are less ideal candidates for active surveillance. But, in the limited data that exist, symptom progression within 4 years of beginning active surveillance is rare.[29]

Unsurprisingly, the cost of active surveillance within the first year of treatment is relatively modest compared to other options. Whereas the first-year costs of radical prostatectomy and IMRT are roughly $14,000 and $24,000, respectively, active surveillance will cost just $4,000 annually to cover the cost of physician visits, screenings, and biopsies. Lifetime costs, however, are more comparable to other courses of treatment, since the cases that do progress will eventually require definitive intervention. Importantly, any side effects of treatment, if it is needed, are postponed for years or even decades. Lifetime costs for active surveillance are estimated between $39,000 and $47,000, dependent on the age of beginning surveillance.[30]

23 Ibid., p. 28.
24 Ibid., p. 29.
25 Ibid., p. 29.
26 Ibid., p. 29.
27 Ibid., p. 15.

28 Ibid., p. 5.
29 Ibid., p. 43.
30 Ibid., p. 50.

Table [11.1]
Lifetime Quality-Adjusted Life Expectancy and Costs for 65-Year-Old Men with Clinically Localized, Low-Risk Prostate Cancer, by Treatment Type[31]

Strategy	QALYs	Incremental QALYs	Cost	Incremental	Cost/QALY
AS	8.97	1.15	$30,422	$2,074	$1,803
Brachytherapy	8.12	0.30	$25,484	($2,864)	N/A[b]
IMRT	8.09	0.27	$37,861	$9,513	$35,233[a]
Proton Beam	7.97	0.15	$53,828	$25,480	$169,867[a]
RP	7.82	Reference	$28,348	Reference	

All incremental values relative to radical prostatectomy; strategies appear in alphabetical order.
RP, radical prostatectomy; *AS*, active surveillance; *IMRT*, intensity-modulated radiation therapy; *QALY*, quality-adjusted life years.
[a]Incremental cost-effectiveness ratios presented for purposes of transparency; findings of the Institute for Clinical and Economic Review (ICER) systematic review do *not* support substantial differences in overall effectiveness.
[b]Strategy is less costly and more effective than reference strategy.
Source: Institute for Clinical and Economic Review.

Decision-Making

Choosing a course of treatment for early-stage, low-risk prostate cancer is a highly individualized process. It must factor in tumor size and location, age, concerns for various side effects, and potential for metastases. In countries such as the US, it must also factor in insurance status and other financial considerations. The relative value of the available courses of treatment can vary widely.

Government and third-party payers, however, tend to try not to influence patient decision-making. By covering most, if not all, of the treatment options available, payers allow patients and physicians maximal flexibility in decision-making, even if this results in more patients choosing a treatment that costs considerably more while promising little added benefit compared to alternatives. The context in which such choices are made matters crucially. Given the complexity of the tradeoffs, evidence-based shared decision-making is vital. Prostate cancer is a prime example of a disease with a wide variety of treatment options that pose challenging ethical dilemmas of medical resource allocation.

[31] Ibid., p. 51.

Questions for Discussion

1. If you were a 65-year-old man suffering from early-stage prostate cancer, which treatment pathway would you prefer? How would you decide?
2. If you were an executive of a major commercial health insurance company, what would your policy toward prostate cancer treatments be? How would you decide?
3. If you were a senior administrator at the Center for Medicare and Medicaid Services, which prostate cancer treatment plans would you cover and why? Would your rationale be any different than if you were running a private, commercial insurance company? Why or why not?

Solving the Gaucher's Disease Dilemma: Connecting Patients with Exorbitantly Priced Drugs to Treat a Rare but Controllable Illness

Gaucher's Disease

Gaucher's disease is an inherited metabolic disorder. It arises from a genetic abnormality that causes a deficiency in glucocerebrosidase—an enzyme that helps break down fat in the body. The disease manifests differently in each patient, but, in its most common form, the enzyme deficiency causes fat to build up around the liver, spleen, and bone marrow, leading to symptoms of varying severity, including anemia, fatigue, osteoporosis, swelling in the abdomen, and organ damage. In more serious forms of the disease, the build-up of metabolic waste can damage the brain and spinal cord, which can cause severe neurological disability or death.[1]

Gaucher's disease is exceedingly rare. It occurs in roughly 1 in 40,000 individuals—though it is significantly more common in certain populations, particularly Jews of Eastern European ancestry.[2] As of today, there are only about 2,000 cases Gaucher's disease in the United States and fewer than 10,000 worldwide.[3]

While the disease is generally quite serious, most cases are manageable with proper treatment. In the 1990s, pharmaceutical companies began developing enzyme replacement therapy (ERT), which can augment enzyme activity and mitigate the danger of surplus metabolic waste. ERT drugs like Genzyme's Cerezyme have been proved highly effective at halting or even reversing the progression of Gaucher's disease.[4] There is, however, a major downside: for patients in the United States, ERT with Cerezyme can cost upward of $300,000 per year.[5]

The Orphan Drug Problem

Exorbitant prices for drugs designed to treat rare diseases like Gaucher's are not at all uncommon because of what is known as the "orphan drug problem." Most drugs are not orphan drugs—they treat diseases that affect large numbers of people, and, consequently, the universe of customers who might buy the drug is large. This possibility for high-volume sales is enough to entice pharmaceutical companies to foot the cost of research and development and to enter the market.

For rare diseases and the drugs that treat them, however, the calculus is different. Drugs that are developed to treat rare diseases—those that affect fewer than 200,000 individuals in the United States—have a much smaller market potential. For pharmaceutical companies, this creates a powerful incentive to forego investment in rare disease drug development and skip the market altogether. In fact, prior to the 1980s, most pharmaceutical companies did just that. From 1973 to 1983, fewer than

[1] WebMD, "Guacher's Disease," accessed October 13, 2015, http://www.webmd.com/a-to-z-guides/gauchers-disease-symptoms-causes-treatments.

[2] A. Mehta, "Epidemiology and Natural History of Gaucher's Disease," *European Journal of Internal Medicine* 17 (2006): pp. S2–S5.

[3] R. Weisman, "New Genzyme Pill Will Cost Patients $310,250 a Year," *Boston Globe*, September 2, 2014.

[4] N. J. Weinreb, et al., "Effectiveness of Enzyme Replacement Therapy in 1028 Patients with Type 1 Gaucher Disease After 2 to 5 Years of Treatment: A Report from the Gaucher Registry," *The American Journal of Medicine* 113, no. 2 (2002): pp. 112–119.

[5] Weisman, "New Genzyme pill will cost patients $310,250 a year."

10 pharmaceutical products were developed to treat rare diseases.[6]

In 1983, however, the United States Congress attempted to counter these strong disincentives by passing the Orphan Drug Act. The Act offered pharmaceutical companies a longer period of patent exclusivity, tax credits and grants for research and development, waivers for FDA approval fees, and a number of other financial incentives.[7] The European Union, Japan, Singapore, and Australia have since enacted similar policy initiatives. Today, by most measures, these initiatives have been successful in generating more treatments for rare diseases. But while availability has been improved, affordability often remains a major barrier.

Tania's Story

Tania Gonzalez grew up in Barranca de Puntarenas, a village near the Pacific coast in Costa Rica.[8] At age 8, she was diagnosed with Gaucher's disease. Her father, Jose, a beer deliveryman who earned about $800 a month, did not know to whom he could turn. Over 4 years, he had watched his daughter endure a "strange and frightening decline" which left her "[struggling] on frail limbs to carry her swollen abdomen."[9] Tania's doctors at the national children's hospital informed her family that, without treatment, she would die.

There was hope, however. If Tania could be treated with Genzyme's Cerezyme, she would be able to manage her Gaucher's disease and lead a full, normal life. As Costa Rican citizens, the Gonzalez family was insured through the Costa Rican Department of Social Security—so lack of coverage wasn't the issue. The problem was that, at the time, the drug cost more than $160,000 a year, and the government didn't cover it.

Luckily for Tania and her family, Genzyme was eager to provide Tania with the drug. Since Gaucher's is such a rare disease with so few patients, Genzyme's business strategy centered on finding as many patients as possible globally and keeping the per unit price of Cerezyme extraordinarily high. Thus, Genzyme would seek out desperate patients like Tania, help them get treatment, and then insist on being fully reimbursed despite the patients' inability to pay. Usually this entailed pressuring their governments to cover the cost.

Genzyme decided when it released the drug in the 1990s that it would not provide discounts no matter the circumstances. The policy was "full price or free."[10] As Alison Taunton-Rigby, a former Genzyme executive, put it, "If you're going to give on the price someplace, everyone's going to ask for a deal, and then you've got a massive mess—so from day one, it was one price."[11] The strategy proved enormously successful. In 2009, drug companies like Genzyme brought in more the $1.8 billion on Cerezyme while only serving 6,000 patients worldwide.[12]

In Tania's case, Genzyme provided the first few months of treatment free and then hired a consultant to determine how to secure coverage from that point onward by the Costa Rican government. This posed a vexing resource allocation dilemma. While the health budget was sufficient to cover Tania's treatment, doing so would deplete funds used for other priorities, like caring for the 600,000 Costa Ricans with

---

[6] US Food and Drug Administration, "Developing Products for Rare Diseases & Conditions," 2015, accessed October 13, 2015, http://www.fda.gov/ForIndustry/DevelopingProductsforRareDiseasesConditions/default.htm.

[7] M. M. Braun, et al., "Emergence of Orphan Drugs in the United States: A Quantitative Assessment of the First 25 Years," *Nature Reviews Drug Discoveries* 9, no. 7 (2010): pp. 519–522.

[8] Ibid.

[9] Ibid.

[10] Ibid.

[11] Ibid.

[12] P. B. Deegan and T. M. Cox, "Imiglucerase in the Treatment of Gaucher Disease: A History and Perspective," *Drug Design, Development and Therapy* 6 (2012): p. 81.

hypertension or the 120,000 Costa Ricans with diabetes.

Ultimately, the Costa Rican Health Ministry refused to cover the cost. In response, Genzyme's consultant directed the Gonzalez family to press the case in the Costa Rican courts. After an onslaught of media attention and an emotionally charged hearing in front of the Costa Rica's high court, the government agreed to cover the cost of Tania' s Cerezyme.

Today, Tania is able to lead a normal life. Every 2 weeks she travels to San Jose to receive her Cerezyme infusion, and she will continue to do so indefinitely. The Costa Rican government continues to pay for her treatment, but many officials worry about the precedent that has been set. Other drug companies have developed similar therapies for rare diseases and have modeled their pricing strategy off Genzyme's. Governments like Costa Rica's, consequently, remain concerned about their ability to continue to cover the exorbitant cost of these drugs while meeting the health needs of their broader population.

Alternative Pricing Models

Of course, the "full price or free" model isn't the only way expensive drugs for rare diseases can be marketed in developing countries. As Tania's battle for Cerezyme moved toward resolution, Dr. Albin Chaves, an official in the Costa Rican government, began advocating for an international agreement that would compel pharmaceutical companies to tie drug prices to a country's gross domestic product (GDP).[13] Under such a system, in future cases like Tania's, the Costa Rican government might pay more than its impoverished neighbor Nicaragua, but far less than wealthy countries like the United States. A tiered or scaled pricing system like the one Dr. Chaves supported might alleviate the burden that the "full price or free" model places on governments like Costa Rica's, but it would require a concerted effort by governments around the world to get pharmaceutical companies to comply. As of today, the consensus needed to build a tiered or scaled pricing system remains elusive.

Other countries have attempted to impose restrictions on public reimbursement for drugs like Cerezyme through advisory panels within their governments. In countries like Belgium, Canada, Australia, and Israel, public coverage decisions for orphan drugs are made by groups of officials who are directed to consider factors such as therapeutic value, the listed price from the manufacturer, the price available in other countries, clinical importance, and the budgetary impact of the drug.[14] Such factors, however, are malleable, which creates potential for uncertainty and inconsistency.

The economic and ethical dilemmas posed by conditions like Gaucher's disease remain unsolved. While governments have made great progress in encouraging pharmaceutical companies to manufacture drugs for rare diseases, the lack of effective price control mechanisms continues to pose harsh resource allocation dilemmas for both governments and private payers.

---

[13] Heuser, "One Girl's Hope."

[14] E. Picavet, D. Cassiman, and S. Simoens, "Reimbursement of Orphan Drugs in Belgium: What (Else) Matters?," *Orphanet Journal of Rare Diseases* 9, no. 1 (2014): pp. 1–9.

Questions for Discussion

1. In your view, was the Costa Rican Health Ministry ethically justified in denying Tania Gonzalez Cerezyme treatment for her Gaucher disease?
2. Should a court be the proper place to decide medical resource allocation decisions?
3. Would you support Albin Chaves's campaign for an international agreement that would compel drug companies to scale their prices to a country's GDP? Would it work? Why or why not?
4. Genzyme's business model allows the company to provide the drug to 300 patients in developing countries completely free of charge. If forcing Genzyme to lower the price of Cerezyme in Costa Rica for Tania's case meant discontinuing the provision of free doses to two other patients in another country, how would you advise Genzyme to proceed?
5. How would you optimize the pricing and reimbursement system for orphan drugs?

Distributing Antiretroviral Treatments for HIV/AIDS: Who Should get Treatment and Where Should Additional Health Assistance Funding Go?

According to UNAIDS, a joint United Nations Programme established in 1994 to reduce death and disability from HIV/AIDS, in 2015, there were approximately 37 million people living with HIV/AIDS. While new cases of HIV infection have fallen 35% since 2000, about 2 million people became newly infected in 2014. About 1.2 million people die of HIV/AIDS each year.[1]

In 2013, the World Health Organization (WHO) issued new standards for antiretroviral treatment (ART), recommending that all HIV infected individuals with CD4 counts (CD4 T lymphocytes within a sample of blood, used as a strong predictor of immune system strength and HIV progression) below 500 cells per microliter should be treated with highly active anti-retroviral treatment (HAART), a three-drug antiretroviral regimen.[2] According to this standard, approximately 28.6 million people globally should receive HAART. The Strategic Timing of AntiRetroviral Treatment (START) study recently showed that all 37 million HIV infected patients, regardless of CD4 count, could clinically benefit from HAART.[3] In 2015, only 41% of adults with HIV/AIDS were accessing treatment. That is, only 15 million people worldwide were on HAART.[4] Thus, there is a gap of 13 million HIV-infected people who are eligible for HAART according to WHO standards who are not receiving treatment. (And, according to the START data, a full 22 million HIV-infected people who could benefit are not receiving HAART.)

In 2015, approximately $20 billion was spent on HIV/AIDS in low- and middle-income countries.[5] Rich countries, foundations, nongovernmental organizations (NGOs), and others donate approximately $11 billion per year for HIV/AIDS care and treatment.[6] According to the Institute for Health Metrics and Evaluation, this amount has remained relatively flat since 2010.[7] According to UNAIDS, 44 low- and middle-income countries relied on international donors for 75% or more of the financial resources to combat HIV/AIDS.[8] UNAIDS (whose annual operating budget for fostering and supporting partnerships at global, regional, and country levels is $485 million[9]) estimates that, by 2020, $31.9 billion will be needed for the response to HIV/AIDS.[10]

This situation raises two fundamental ethical concerns. The first is a question of rationing. If not all HIV/AIDS patients can be treated

---

[1] UNAIDS, "Fact Sheet: 2014 Statistics," 2015, accessed November 19, 2015, http://www.unaids.org/en/resources/documents/2015/20150714_factsheet.

[2] World Health Organization, *Consolidated Guidelines on the Use of Antiretroviral Drugs for Treating and Preventing HIV Infection: Recommendations for a Public Health Approach* (Geneva, Switzerland: WHO, 2013), p. 28.

[3] National Institutes of Health, "Starting Antiretroviral Treatment Early Improves Outcomes for HIV-Infected Individuals: NIH-Funded Trial Results Likely Will Impact Global Treatment Guidelines," NIH, 2015, accessed November 19, 2015, http://www.nih.gov/news-events/news-releases/starting-antiretroviral-treatment-early-improves-outcomes-hiv-infected-individuals.

[4] UNAIDS, "Fact Sheet."

[5] Ibid.

[6] Institute for Health Metrics and Evaluation, Financing Global Health 2014: Shifts in Funding as the MDG Era Closes (Seattle, WA: IHME, 2015), p. 53.

[7] Ibid.

[8] UNAIDS, "Fact Sheet."

[9] UNAIDS, "Budget for 2014–2015," 2013, accessed November 19, 2015, http://www.unaids.org/sites/default/files/sub_landing/files/20131405GMAfinal_UBRAF_BUDGET%202014-2015.pdf.

[10] UNAIDS, "Fact Sheet."

Table [11.2]
Health Impacts in Low-Income Countries

Disease or Condition	Deaths in Low Income Countries (per 100,000 population)[a]	DALYs in Low-Income Countries (per 100,000 population)[b]	Current Global Funding Level (millions USD)[c]
Pneumonia	91	5,507	$640
HIV/AIDS	65	4,089	$11,000
Diarrhea	53	3,963	***
Stroke	52	1,277	$610
Ischemic heart disease	39	1,064	***
Malaria	35	3,114	$2,400
Pre-term birth complications	33	987	$3,000
TB	31	1,544	$1,400
Birth asphyxia	29	2,820	***
Malnutrition	27	1,649	***

[a] World Health Organization, "The Top 10 Causes of Death: 2012," 2014, accessed October 31, 2015, http://www.who.int/mediacentre/factsheets/fs310/en/index1.html.
[b] World Health Organization, "Estimates for 2000–2012: Disease Burden," WHO, accessed November 20, 2015, http://www.who.int/healthinfo/global_burden_disease/estimates/en/index2.html.
[c] Institute for Health Metrics and Evaluation, *Financing Global Health 2014: Shifts in Funding as the MDG Era Closes* (Seattle, WA: IHME, 2015).

with HAART, who should receive treatment? How should we select those people to receive treatment? Because of facilities, travel, distribution infrastructure, trained personnel, and other factors, it is more cost-effective to treat HIV-infected people in urban areas. Is it ethical to focus treatment on urban areas, or would this discriminate against those people who happen to live in rural communities? Does focusing on urban areas use a morally irrelevant factor in deciding who should receive treatment? Should those who are sickest receive treatment first? Should it be the young or those who are more economically productive?

There is a different resource allocation question: If global health assistance increases, should the additional funds be directed toward HIV/AIDS, or should other health problems be addressed instead? Should funding for tuberculosis, malaria, safe births, or diarrhea take priority over HIV/AIDS? Table [11.2] shows the health impacts of various diseases and conditions in the low-income countries and approximate levels of health assistance.

Norman Daniels's "Fair Process"

Norman Daniels, a political philosopher and bioethicist at Harvard University, recognized the essential difficulty at the heart of this question. Allocation decisions in situations of relative scarcity are never purely technical; they necessarily entail value judgments. And among the key stakeholders in healthcare—patients, doctors, governments, pharmaceutical companies, and others—there is, and will always be, reasonable moral disagreement regarding which principle or mix of principles should govern resource distribution. In Daniels's view, it is impossible to resolve such disagreement by appeal to substantive ethical principles.[11]

[11] N. Daniels, "Decisions About Access to Health Care and Accountability for Reasonableness," *Journal of Urban Health* 76, no. 2 (1999): pp. 176–191.

Given this unavoidable disagreement, endless debate over intractable ethical questions is unlikely to generate a widely acceptable and actionable policy. Rather, Daniels argues, healthcare decision-makers need to focus on constructing a "fair process" that will cultivate consensus around what is legitimate and fair.[12] As Daniels claims, central to this fair process, termed *accountability for reasonableness*, are four requirements: (1) a publicity condition, (2) a relevancy condition, (3) a revisability and appeals condition, and (4) an enforcement or regulation condition.[13]

"Fair Process" and Global Health Assistance

In a 2004 report written for the WHO, Daniels applied his "fair process" framework to HIV/AIDS and, by implication, to wider global health assistance issues.[14] Daniels contended that any policy aimed at resolving these issues must be derived from a fair process, whereby even those who disagree with the ultimate strategy can respect the final decision.

The Publicity Condition

In Daniels's view, the first requirement of a "fair process" is publicity—a degree of transparency and accessibility that imposes public scrutiny and democratic control on decision-makers. In many countries, in both the developed and the developing world, allocation decisions are made behind closed doors by insulated bureaucratic organizations. The public is thus shut out from the conversation and often entirely uninformed about the rationale behind allocation policies, which can breed resentment and a sense of illegitimacy. If, instead, decision-makers are open about the grounds for their decisions, the public can become more informed about the countervailing ethical considerations surrounding a problem and, hopefully, more accepting of an eventual solution. With publicity comes a degree of transparency that can raise the standards of argument and evidence that officials must meet to justify their decisions.

Daniels argues any resource allocation decisions should be accompanied by detailed explanations of the ethical grounds on which those decisions were made. If the policy was motivated by efficiency, officials should be expected to explain, in an accessible manner, why the efficiency gains outweigh the concerns of equity and access. Such explanations will certainly not win over every segment of the public, but it will leave everyone more informed and more engaged.

The Relevance Condition

The second requirement, relevance, limits the universe of acceptable policy justifications to only those that are rationally connected to meeting the needs of beneficiaries in a fair way. This requirement serves to exclude justifications based on irrelevant considerations that have no bearing on needs: for example, exclusions based on race.

In the global health context, Daniels argues that the arbiters of relevance are the primary populations that are affected by allocation decisions—namely, health providers, health planners, people with HIV and other diseases, and their family members. In order to harness the power of deliberative decision-making, the universe of policy rationales should not be limited to majority viewpoints. Minority views must be included as well. Possible relevant considerations might include equity of access, prognosis-based efficiency, ensuring some fair chance of treatment to all, giving priority to health workers, or maximizing sustainable delivery.

---

[12] N. Daniels, "Accountability for Reasonableness," *British Medical Journal* 321 (2000): pp. 1300–1301.

[13] Daniels, "Decisions About Access to Health Care," p. 179.

[14] N. Daniels, *How to Achieve Fair Distribution of ARTs in 3 by 5: Fair Process and Legitimacy in Patient Selection* (Geneva: World Health Organization, 2004).

The Revisability Condition

Daniels's third requirement is revisability, an assurance that stakeholders will have at least some ability to amend decisions should they have unfair consequences. Of course, not every challenge to a decision can yield a changed outcome. But, at the very least, Daniels contends, appeals can force policy-makers to fully articulate their rationale in their defense of their decisions, promoting understanding and broader social deliberation.

Daniels argues that any international agency administering global health aid should invite feedback from national and subnational level decision-makers. Policies should be revisited periodically with an eye toward remedying these complaints. When new evidence and arguments arise, they should be welcomed as a chance to improve quality.

The Regulation and Enforcement Condition

Finally, the fourth requirement is regulatory compliance. The details of any enforcement strategy, Daniels notes, will necessarily vary country-by-country according to the legal and regulatory infrastructure available. In the developing countries, enforcement often poses a significant challenge. Many countries have little transparency, little means of aggregating and synthesizing stakeholder views, and weak civic institutions to allow individuals to challenge policy decisions. Daniels has acknowledged that the enforcement condition "may be the soft under-belly of the problem of fair process, and that may be true because enforcement in this context is part of a much larger problem of assuring enforcement in the governance of the health sector more generally."[15] However, international agencies like the WHO, World Bank, and USAID can support this effort and gradually improve the efficacy of local regulation.

"Fair Process" Application in "3 by 5" and Beyond

While the WHO endorsed Daniels's "fair process" and its underlying rationale, it ultimately was not operationalized. The administrative and logistical challenges of implementing and scaling-up fair process infrastructure have proved daunting, and, to date, there is still a dearth of robust empirical data supporting the efficacy and feasibility of widespread fair process implementation. Daniels, however, remains optimistic about his approach and its ability to solve thorny allocation questions in the medical context. While he does not see it as a "magic bullet," in the right context and with the right leadership, Daniels believes fair process can help decision-makers build consensus and build solid solutions.[16]

---

[15] N. Daniels and J. Sabin, "Response to Commentaries: Further Thoughts on Implementing Accountability for Reasonableness," in *The Future of Bioethics: International Dialogues*, edited by A. Akabayashi (New York: Oxford University Press, 2014), pp. 590–592.

[16] Ibid., p. 590.

Questions for Discussion

1. Do you agree with Daniels's emphasis on process over substantive ethical decision as the means of cultivating greater consensus and legitimacy around contentious allocation decisions? What are the advantages and drawbacks?
2. If you were a WHO official, how would you respond to Daniels's fair process proposal? Would you support it? If no, what alternative process would you use to arrive at allocation decisions and why? If yes, what steps would you take to address the challenges of fair process implementation?
3. UNAIDS was established in 1994 to reduce death and disability from HIV/AIDS—but there is not a similar body for any other individual health issue. Dr. Peter Piot, then Executive Director UNAIDS, argued that an "agenda for a response commensurate with the challenges posed by the epidemic cannot be realised if we do not maintain the exceptionality of HIV."[1] There are no UN programmes for any other single conditions with similar or higher mortality and morbidity rates than HIV/AIDS. Explain whether you see the exceptional status of UNAIDS as helpful and justified from a resource allocation standpoint, or whether you see any problems.

---

[1] P. Piot, "Aids: From Crisis Management to Sustained Strategic Response," *The Lancet* 368, no. 9534): pp. 526–530.

Further Resources

Relevant Organizations

Governmental

The Joint United Nations Programme on HIV and AIDS (UNAIDS): Aims to prevent transmission of HIV, provide care and support to those living with the virus, and alleviate the impact of the epidemic. Additional information can be found at http://www.unaids.org/

Nongovernmental

Institute for Clinical and Economic Review (ICER): A nonprofit organization, located in Boston, Massachusetts, that evaluates evidence on the value of medical test, treatment, and delivery systems. Additional information can be found at http://icer-review.org/

Institute for Health Metric and Evaluation (IHME): A health research center at the University of Washington that aims to provide information on population health, its determinants, and the performance of health systems. Additional information can be found at http://www.healthdata.org/

Literature

Committee on Gynecologic Practice, Society of Gynecologic Surgeons. "Robotic Surgery in Gynecology." http://www.acog.org/-/media/Committee-Opinions/Committee-on-Gynecologic-Practice/co628.pdf?dmc=1&ts=20150819T1805215068.

European Commission. "Inventory of Union and Member State Incentives to Support Research into, and the Development and Availability of, Orphan Medicinal Products." http://ec.europa.eu/health/files/orphanmp/doc/orphan_inv_report_20160126.pdf.

Gericke, C., A. Riesberg, and R. Busse. "Ethical Issues in Funding Orphan Drug Research and Development." *Journal of Medical Ethics* 31, no. 3 (2005): 164–168.

Jacobs, B. L., Y. Zhang, F. R. Schroeck, et al. "Use of Advanced Treatment Technologies among Men at Low Risk of Dying from Prostate Cancer." *JAMA* 309, no. 24 (2013): 2587–2595.

Okulicz, J. F., T. D. Le, B. K. Agan, et al. "Influence of the Timing of Antiretroviral Therapy on the Potential for Normalization of Immune Status in Human Immunodeficiency Virus 1–Infected Individuals." *JAMA Internal Medicine* 175, no. 1 (2015): 88–99.

Silverman, Ed. "Orphan Drugs: 'Rare' Opportunities to Make Money," August 23, 2012.

Therapeutic Goods Administration. "Orphan drugs program." https://www.tga.gov.au/sites/default/files/consultation-orphan-drugs-program.pdf.

US Food and Drug Administration. "Developing Orphan Products: FDA and Rare Disease Day." http://www.fda.gov/ForIndustry/DevelopingProductsforRareDiseasesConditions/ucm239698.htm.

World Health Organization. "The 3 by 5 Initiative." http://www.who.int/3by5/en/.

Other Media

60 Minutes, "The Cost of Cancer Drugs." *CBSNews*, June 21, 2015: An interview with the doctors from Memorial Sloan Kettering about Zaltrap.

Jackie Judd, "Quality Care for Less Money: Can Regional Successes Go National?" *Kaiser Family Foundation* video, 1:30:28, February 15, 2012: The Kaiser Family Foundation hosted an event where a PBS documentary that explores efforts to provide low-cost, quality healthcare was shown and debated.

Shane Smith, "VICE Special Report: Countdown to Zero," *HBO*, December 1, 2015: Details current HIV/AIDS research and interviews former President George W. Bush about PEPFAR.

12 Ethics of Tiering

There may be no more powerful criticism of a healthcare idea than to accuse it of creating a two-tier system in which the well-off can avail themselves of better or more convenient care than others. This criticism seems self-evident. Indeed, the charge seems so compelling that people frequently feel as if there is no reason to give a further justification for not having a two-tier system.

What is the ethical problem of having more than one-tier of coverage?

There are at least three fundamental justifications for a one-tier system: (1) all people should be treated according to need, (2) markets are inherently unsuitable vehicles to deliver health services, and (3) higher tiers have a negative effect on the quality of care provided in the lower tiers.

On the first argument, the basic assumption is that every patient with the same disease or condition should be treated similarly. That is, every sick person should be treated, and people with the same ailment should receive the same—that is, the best—treatment regardless of who they are. Factors such as race, ethnicity, citizenship, and especially income and wealth should never determine what kind of services a sick person receives. In other words, healthcare should be distributed according to principles of strict equality. The central ethical issue revolves around the question of whether there should be inequality in access to healthcare services based on the ability to pay. Why should a rich person get access to better healthcare just because they are rich? While a rich person can get access to better food, clothing, housing, cars, entertainment, and a wide variety of other goods because of her greater income, it seems unethical to permit some people to get access to better healthcare services or live with fewer disabilities just because they have more money.

Second, markets are generally appropriate ways to distribute most goods and services, but inevitably they lead to inequalities based on ability to pay. The rich get more and higher quality goods and services than do people with lower incomes. For this reason, it is widely viewed that markets are not good ways to distribute fundamental needs—or only once those needs are satisfied past a basic threshold. Thus, everyone should get access to enough food to satisfy basic nutritional and energy requirements, regardless of income. The market is acceptable only once those basic needs are fulfilled. This is why it is viewed as unethical to distribute food through a market mechanism during a famine or widespread shortages of basic foodstuffs. This argument explains the acceptance of rationing food to people through specific and limited coupons during World Wars I and II, when there were food shortages. Inherent shortcomings of markets are also central to the ethical justification for guaranteeing lower income people basic food needs through governmental programs such as food stamps. In cases of limited food availability, either because of natural shortages or low income, income should not determine access to food, and rationing may be needed. However, beyond conditions of scarcity, a market is typically acceptable.

Like food, health is a precondition not only for life itself, but for being able to pursue any meaningful set of life goals. As such, it seems unethical to let the market distribute goods that satisfy fundamental needs—that is, those things that are necessary for life. Everyone should get access to healthcare services regardless of the ability to pay. For instance, it is widely viewed as unethical to allow the rich to buy the limited number of livers for transplantation. Livers are basic to life. Income and ability to pay should not determine who gets the livers and, therefore, who lives and who dies.

If health and healthcare are fundamental needs and should not be distributed by the market in which income determines the distribution of goods and services, it follows that there should not be a two-tier system in which ability to pay determines who gets which services.

Healthcare should not be distributed through the market; it should be distributed by medical need alone. Those who need care, services, medications, and other interventions because of their diseases and conditions should get them. Medical need, not income, should determine who gets medical care. As the health economist Alan Maynard argues (Excerpt 1):

> What principle of equity should determine access to health care? In Canada, Western Europe and Australia and increasingly in the Pacific Rim countries, the answer to this question involves repudiation of market principles of willingness and ability to pay in favor of the allocation of health care on the basis of need. . . . where need is defined as the patient's capacity to benefit from health care per unit of cost (the cost effectiveness rule).[1]

Third, in addition to these linked ethical arguments that need, not money, should be the basis for distributing healthcare goods and services, there is a powerful practical consideration that argues for a single-tier system. A system that allows the well-off to buy more healthcare will inevitably erode the tier for lower income people, making it lower both in terms of range and quality of services. Programs for the poor inevitably get underfunded and become poor programs, the argument goes.[2] As Maynard argues, a two-tier system reduces quality in the public sector as better physicians, hospitals, and other clinical services will flock to the well-off who pay more. The result is an impoverishment of the public system.[3]

Troven Brennan worries that having a luxury healthcare market for primary care—"concierge care" for the rich—will undermine access for the poor and middle class (Excerpt 2).[4] He is less worried about traditional concerns of the "physician's commitment to individual patients" and more concerned about the

---

[1] A. Maynard, "How to Defend a Public Health Care System: Lessons from Abroad," in *Access to Care, Access to Justice: The Legal Debate over Private Health Insurance in Canada*, edited by K. Roach, L. Sossin and C.M. Flood (University of Toronto Press, 2005), pp. 237–240.

[2] L. Rainwater, "Stigma in Income-Tested Programs," in *Income-Tested Transfer Programs: The Case for and Against*, edited by I. Garfinkel (Academic Press, 1982), p. 42.

[3] Maynard, "How to Defend a Public Health Care System," p. 250.

[4] T. A. Brennan, "Luxury Primary Care—Market Innovation or Threat to Access?," *New England Journal of Medicine* 346, no. 15 (2002): pp. 1165–1168.

systemic impact.[5] Brennan asks a Kantian-type question: What would happen if "all" physicians charged luxury fees? It seems disingenuous to argue that concierge or luxury care is ethical only if a few physicians do it because then it does not undermine access, but is unethical if it grows to be too much of the market. He argues that what constitutes ethical practice should not change with the situation and extent of market penetration. Since concierge medicine for the rich, if extensive, is wrong, then it should be opposed as undermining equity.

Traditionally, in Britain, two-tier medical care meant that the well-off bought private insurance for all their care bypassing the National Health Service (NHS). This manifested itself with private hospitals being cleaner and better equipped while NHS hospitals were starved for resources and became dirty, crowded, and outdated facilities.[6] But there is another way a two-tier system could impact the NHS, what is called "topping up." In this situation, people get most of their care through the NHS but can buy additional services, typically drugs, that are not covered. Thus, they don't opt out entirely to another private system; instead they top up beyond the base tier with their own money. The *Lancet* editors strongly object to topping up as it undermines solidarity and dignity by having the rich use the collective system when it suits them, but get additional personal benefits (Excerpt 3).[7] It is almost like having the state pay for part of private education.

In Canada, the Superior Court of Quebec heard a case on Quebec's prohibition of private medical insurance in 2000 and concluded (Excerpt 4):

> The evidence showed that the right to have recourse to a parallel private health care system would have repercussions on the rights of the public as a whole. We cannot act like ostriches. The result of creating a parallel private health care system would be to threaten the integrity, sound operation and viability of the public system. . . . .The only way of ensuring that all health resources will benefit all Quebecers without discrimination is to prevent a parallel system from being established.[8]

These three arguments for a one-tier system assume that all healthcare is like liver transplantation, a situation in which there is absolute scarcity and healthcare services are a matter of life and death. But a great deal of healthcare is not like that. Proponents make three points in arguing for permitting a multitiered healthcare system. First, even though John Rawls did not directly address the context of healthcare, thinkers such as Krohmal and Emanuel draw on him to argue that the principles of justice are necessary precisely because there is moderate scarcity (Excerpt 5).[9] Public spending on fundamental needs requires reasonable limits. Society cannot be required to provide its members everything they need and want. Society must provide people essential services necessary to living and pursuing a reasonable range of life goals.[10] Thus, public expenditures do not—and should not—cover every possible medical intervention.

Second, justice is concerned with an equal distribution to cover needs as well as liberties. Liberty is just as much a principle of justice as

---

[5] Brennan, "Luxury Primary Care," p. 1167.

[6] "Dirty Hospitals 'Named and Shamed'," 2001, accessed November 2, 2015, http://news.bbc.co.uk/2/hi/health/1269991.stm.

See also B. Haywood, "NHS Trust Member Condemns Dudley Hospital as Dirty and Cluttered," 2013, accessed November 2, 2015, http://www.birminghammail.co.uk/news/health/nhs-trust-member-condemns-dudley-5783638.

[7] The Lancet, "A Morally Bankrupt Government Divides the NHS," *The Lancet* 372, no. 9651 (2008): p. 1708.

[8] "Appendix A," in *Access to Care, Access to Justice: The Legal Debate over Private Health Insurance in Canada*, edited by K. Roach, L. Sossin and C.M. Flood (University of Toronto Press, 2005), p. 556.

[9] B. J. Krohmal and E. J. Emanuel, "Access and Ability to Pay: The Ethics of a Tiered Health Care System," *Archives of Internal Medicine* 167, no. 5 (2007): p. 434.

[10] Ibid., p. 434.

is the requirement that society guarantee citizens fundamental needs. Thus, beyond these essential services, people should have liberty to decide how they want to spend their money.[11,12] If some people want more healthcare, the principle of liberty means they should be free to spend their money as they want, including to spend it on additional medical services. Beyond the basic needs, people must be free to spend their own money to pursue their life goals.

Third, liberty is not unlimited. The liberty to spend private money on healthcare services has limits.[13] The well-off cannot spend their money on goods and services in ways that deprive others of access to the goods and services that satisfy fundamental needs. In this way, a multitier system is not just permitted but required to fulfill the liberty principle of justice. In more general terms, this stipulation is probably most clearly articulated in Locke's famous proviso that states people can take land as long as they leave as much and as good for others:

> Nor was this appropriation of any parcel of land, by improving it, any prejudice to any other man, since there was still enough and as good left, and more than the yet unprovided could use. So that, in effect, there was never the less left for others because of his enclosure for himself. For he that leaves as much as another can make use of does as good as take nothing at all.[14]

Similarly, the well-off can use their income to buy medical services as long as it does not compromise others receiving the healthcare services they need and to which they are entitled. This is precisely why a rich person should not be permitted to buy a liver—because, given the severe shortage, he cannot leave "as much and as good" for others who need livers. But a rich person may be permitted to buy a private hospital room, a magnetic resonance imaging (MRI) scan, brand-name drugs, and shorter waiting times for cataract surgery because these do not compromise others getting the goods and services to which they are entitled. Thus, those advocating for a multitier system argue that equality should determine the distribution of essential health services but that liberty should be allowed to determine whether people use their own money to buy services above the essential benefits, as long as they do not compromise access by all to essential health benefits.[15]

Canada is the country that enforces the single tier most actively. It has prohibited private insurance from offering to cover services that are offered by the government system, even though the very well-off can travel to the United States for treatment. The Canadian court used the Lockean argument to reject a multitier system, claiming it would compromise access to essential health services.

On the other hand, many other countries do permit a multitier system. They allow private insurance or other mechanisms for people to buy greater access to healthcare services. For instance, in the new US insurance exchanges, people can purchase insurance from one of four different "metal" tiers—bronze, silver, gold, and platinum—with the government supporting the purchase at a level equivalent to the second least expensive silver plan.[16] All metal plans must provide the same basic 10 categories of essential benefits, but the higher tiers can provide more services, a wider range of health providers, and other health benefits. Similarly, in Britain, private insurance is allowed that can replace services in the NHS, and private insurers can even buy access to beds and services in NHS hospitals.[17]

[11] Ibid., p. 435.

[12] J. Rawls, *A Theory of Justice, Revised Edition* (Cambridge: Harvard University Press, 1999).

[13] Krohmal, "Access and Ability to Pay," p. 435.

[14] J. Locke, *The Second Treatise of Government: And, A Letter Concerning Toleration* (Dover Publications, 1956), p. 15.

[15] Krohmal, "Access and Ability to Pay," p. 434.

[16] *Patient Protection and Affordable Care Act*, H.R. 3590, Section 1302.

[17] Y. Doyle and A. Bull, "Role of Private Sector in United Kingdom Healthcare System," *BMJ* 321, no. 7260 (2000): p. 563.

In Germany, well-off individuals (those making more than €52,200 annually) may opt out of the statutory social health insurance system and buy private insurance. About 11% of the country has private insurance.[18] In addition, about 9% of Germans also purchase supplemental insurance that covers healthcare goods and services not covered by the sickness funds. Thus, Germany has at least a three-tiered system.[19]

[18] S. Thomson, et al., *International Profiles of Health Care Systems, 2013* (New York: The Commonwealth Fund, 2013), p. 57.

[19] M. Tanner, "The Grass Is Not Always Greener: A Look at National Health Care Systems around the World," *Cato Policy Analysis Paper*, no. 613 (2008).

Questions for Discussion

1. Under Canadian law, private insurance companies cannot offer insurance for any medical services, such as cataract operations or hip replacements, that are provided by the provincial/territorial health insurance plans (under Canadian Medicare). What are the benefits of this law? What are the drawbacks?
2. If it has been determined that public funds should not be used to cover a bone marrow transplant, should I be allowed to buy it with my own money?
3. In Excerpt 5, Krohmal and Emanuel argue that public funds should be used to provide everyone with essential health services only—with the remainder offered in markets. Suppose you live in a society operating on this principle: what would be your biggest concern about this arrangement?
4. If you were charged with implementing a two-tier system, what ethical safeguards would you put in place?

EXCERPTS

Note: The following excerpts have generally been edited for length, and omissions are indicated with ellipses. Editing includes footnotes and endnotes, which have also been renumbered. For citation and related purposes, the full original source texts should be used.

EXCERPT 1

Abridged text from:

A. Maynard, "How to Defend a Public Health Care System: Lessons from Abroad," in *Access to Care, Access to Justice: The Legal Debate over Private Health Insurance in Canada*, edited by K. Roach, L. Sossin, and C. M. Flood (University of Toronto Press, 2005).

How to Defend a Public Health Care System: Lessons from Abroad

Alan Maynard

Introduction

. . .

What principle of equity should determine access to health care? In Canada, Western Europe and Australasia and increasingly in the Pacific Rim countries, the answer to this question involves repudiation of market principles of willingness and ability to pay in favour of the allocation of health care on the basis of need. . . .

Remember Those Equity Goals?

Health care reformers like Bismarck in Germany and Lloyd George in Britain were politicians who responded to threats similar to those now facing the architects of Canadian Medicare. The "market solution" then and now (e.g. in the US) involved both the denial of care and the bankruptcy of fellow citizens as a result of their misfortune and genetic susceptibility. Government intervention was, and is, needed to create financial protection for citizens.

. . .

The competing camps are essentially libertarian and egalitarian. For the former, the primary goal is freedom—and in health care this means freedom of choice, based on individuals' willingness and ability to pay.

Libertarians believe that individuals are the best judges of their own welfare and if this leads to unequal or no health care protection for the poor, so be it! These folk prefer under-regulated, or even better, unregulated markets as the means of delivering diversity, inequality and the protection of individual freedom.

Egalitarians place equality of opportunity above freedom and other values. They believe that all members of society have equal rights to basic goals, of which health care may be one. In societies like these in Canada, Western Europe and elsewhere, a consensus has "emerged that health care is a basic good and that in the absence of equality of opportunity, there is a moral obligation, to compensate those deprived of health care by creating public financed provision. Such intervention creates financial protection for those in need. Health care is provided **not** on the basis of willingness and ability to pay but **on the basis of need,** where need is defined as the patient's capacity to benefit from health care per unit of cost (the cost effectiveness rule).

. . .

What sort of society do Canadians, Brits and others want? Do they want to experiment with the inequality and inefficiency inherent in the diversity and (lack of) choice in the US health care system and risk the consequence that once altered any system is difficult to reverse? Or do they want to adhere to egalitarian principles and defend those principles by improving the efficiency of Medicare in Canada by mitigating its failings-, such as excessive waiting time and other inefficiencies? . . .

Improving Health Care Efficiency

. . .

Regardless of the public-private mix in the finance and provision of care and regardless of the GDP of countries, there are common failures in the provision of health care to populations. These failures in public health care systems can reinforce ideologically driven criticism. Thus waiting times in Canada, Australia and the UK generate libertarian advocacy of complementary (i.e. duplicate) private health insurance. The reluctance of public policy makers to manage their resources efficiently creates an opportunity for antipathetic ideology advocacy.

. . .

The existence of a two tier health care system creates the potential for health care activity and quality to be reduced in the public sector. In the UK the process of care in the private sector is generally regarded as superior with physicians wearing "private sector suits" and having a more bedside manner. Furthermore facilities, in terms of patients' creature comforts (e.g. TV, single room etc) are superior. With specialists "diverted" to the private sector by money, more junior practitioners may treat public patients. However whether this produces inferior outcomes is a matter of conjecture rather than something with an evidence base and again it is a product of public sector management inefficiency in not enforcing public sector employment contracts. . . .

It is important to grapple with the possibility, even the certainty that the current Canadian "crisis" over waiting times, and private insurance is an inevitable product of weak political and managerial control of a potentially fine health care system built on egalitarian principles where practice remains inefficient[1], and in so doing creates the potential for private sector development and with it the potential for damage to public sector provision.

Overview

Private health insurance based on international experience offers no remedies for the market failures outlined here and is generally designed to worsen equity. If private health insurance were to emerge in Canada, Federal and Provincial administrations would have to regulate it vigorously to avoid both "cream skimming" policies that challenge Medicare finance and equity policies and the inefficient provision of care, e.g. failure to deliver appropriate care and the propensity to deliver care of little clinical benefit to patients. Whichever ideological path is chosen, these well documented and generally ignored problems of inefficiency in the use of society's resources will have to be mitigated. Once the path of duplicated public and private health is chosen, it will be very difficult to reverse the system as the consumer and provider benefits will make electoral change costly as demonstrated by Labour's acceptance of Howard's private health insurance reforms in the last Australian election.

. . .

[1] K. Bloor, A. Maynard, and N. Freemantle, "Variation in Activity Rates of Consultant Surgeons and the Influence of Reward Structures in the English NHS," *Journal of Health Services and Research Policy* 9, no. 2 (2004): pp. 76–84.

EXCERPT 2

Abridged text from:

T. A. Brennan, "Luxury Primary Care—Market Innovation or Threat to Access?," *New England Journal of Medicine* 346, no. 15 (2002): pp. 1165–1168.

Luxury Primary Care—Market Innovation or Threat to Access?

Troven A. Brennan

Primary care practitioners in several states have recently decided to restructure their practices in a way that enables them to see a much smaller number of patients and to spend more time with the ones they do see. Patients enrolled in these practices, referred to as "luxury primary care," pay an annual fee to the practice. In return for this annual fee, they can expect certain amenities that are not currently part of primary care, such as access to their physicians 24 hours a day, 7 days a week, using cell phones or prompt paging devices.[1] When they see their primary care physicians, they can expect up to an hour-long visit. The primary care provider is no longer under pressure to see as many patients as possible each day, because the up-front fee paid by the patient changes the financial structure of the practice. Physicians can even accompany their patients on visits to specialists or to the hospital.

Many physicians are enthusiastic about this new approach because it allows them to take more time in providing care for individual patients. Many patients who dislike the rapid pace and tight schedules that have become characteristic of primary care in the United States are also attracted to this model.[2]

[1] C. Jackson, "Premium Practice: When Patients Pay Top Dollar for Exclusive Care," *American Medical News* 15 (2001).

[2] P. Belluck, "Doctors' New Practices Offer Deluxe Service for Deluxe Fee," *New York Times*, January 15, 2002.

However, some physicians have criticized this approach to primary care, pointing out that only the wealthy can afford such amenities and that physicians should not be catering to wealthy patients. They also claim that these practices are unethical, because patients who cannot afford to pay the annual fee are not allowed into the practice, and long-standing ties with such patients may be severed, disrupting the continuity of care.[3] . . .

Market Innovation

. . .

Luxury primary care is an excellent example of a market innovation that serves the interests of both consumers (patients) and suppliers (physicians). The consumers in this case are patients who wish to pay extra for certain amenities that are currently unavailable in primary care. . . .

There may be a market for practices in which physicians spend more time with patients in return for an annual fee, especially if the fee is only a supplemental payment, with the rest of the costs of health care covered by the patient's health insurance.

Most luxury primary care practices fit this model, although the details vary. The patient usually pays a set fee for entry into the practice.[4] The fee ranges from $1,000 to $20,000 annually but in most cases is at the lower end of the range. . . .

With substantial revenues from the annual fees that patients pay, physicians in luxury primary care practices can see fewer patients per day and have time for other activities, such as accompanying patients on visits to specialists. Since the average patient visits a primary care physician two to five times per year, a physician providing care for 200 to 300 patients would have a total of 1500 or fewer visits. . . .

[3] "Personal and Devoted Doctors," *Boston Globe*, January 8, 2002.

[4] Jackson, "Premium Practice."

Many providers will find this approach to primary care practice attractive. . . .

The luxury style of practice may well represent a return to what many providers consider the old days, when physicians had ample time to spend with patients and could really undertake the ethical responsibility to put the patient's welfare above everything else. In addition, the small errors that can occur with rapid-fire primary care may be reduced with luxury primary care, resulting in better care for patients.[5] Certainly, from a professional viewpoint, this new approach promises a much richer and more satisfying practice. Thus, at first blush, luxury primary care appears to be the kind of market innovation that both physicians and patients would welcome.

Although the proponents of luxury primary care acknowledge that not all patients can afford to pay for such care, they argue that there are luxuries unavailable to many people in all sectors of our economy. The analogy to education is especially telling. Many children are educated in public schools, but a substantial minority of children attend private schools that cost much more per year than a luxury primary care practice would. Neither the administrators of such schools nor the parents of the children who attend them have qualms about the fact that not all parents can afford to give their children a private education. Moreover, the teachers enjoy the same professional rewards as teachers in public schools. Like private education, luxury primary care is simply a response to a market need.

The Expectations of Insurers

. . .

Some insurers might balk at the luxury tax for primary care, for several reasons. First, they may think it is unfair for a patient who pays an insurance premium to be charged an additional premium, even if it is the patient's choice to do so. More likely, insurers may fear that patients who join luxury practices will expect not only highly personal care but also luxurious care in terms of diagnostic and therapeutic procedures. In addition, typical arrangements for ensuring that primary care providers act as gatekeepers, such as capitation mechanisms and the withholding of fees, will probably not be very effective if the primary care provider's main source of income is the luxury premium. Insurers are therefore concerned that luxury primary care will result in high rates of use of specialty services, with the patients in these practices essentially having a free ride on other patients' premiums.

Ethical Issues

. . .

There are ethical issues. The first concerns the transition to a luxury practice. Most physicians who are interested in providing luxury primary care are going to make the leap once they know that there is adequate demand for it in their own practice. That means that most practitioners will be making the move from a fully staffed, traditional primary care practice to the new practice. To do so, they must rid themselves of patients who do not wish or cannot afford to pay the luxury tax. Opponents of luxury care argue that these patients will be abandoned and that their care will suffer.

Medical ethics prohibits physicians from abandoning sick patients. This prohibition is supported by the common law, which allows patients, within the context of an established relationship with a physician, to sue the physician for inappropriately refusing to provide further care.[6] But both medical ethics and the common law allow physicians to terminate their relationships with patients. If a patient is

[5] T. Gandhi, et al., "Drug Complications in Outpatients," *Journal of General Internal Medicine* 15, no. 3 (2000): pp. 149–154.

[6] M. A. Hall, "Theory of Economic Informed Consent, A," *Georgia Law Review* 31 (1996): p. 511.

receiving treatment for an acute disorder, the physician must continue to provide care.[7] In the case of a patient with an acute problem that has been managed, however, or a patient who is relatively healthy, the relationship can be terminated by finding another physician to provide care for the patient. Therefore, as long as practitioners who make the transition to luxury care do so carefully, by winnowing down their practice and providing patients with referrals to other physicians, there should be no serious ethical or legal impediments.[8] . . .

Traditional medical ethics is rather poorly equipped to address issues related to luxury primary care. Ethical standards in medicine have focused on the physician's commitment to individual patients and have not addressed broader financial and political issues.[9] . . .

Opponents of luxury primary care argue that its effect on access is the main problem. If almost all primary care physicians charged luxury fees before providing care for patients, then access to health care would certainly be affected. Luxury primary care would have a regressive effect on the health care system, reducing access.

Advocates of luxury primary care counter that they are simply filling a small niche. They point out that at the premium level required for a true luxury practice, relatively few patients will be interested in paying for such care and that it thus does not pose a threat to health care access in general.

Since professional ethics is a matter of reasoning on the basis of principles, there is something suspect about this argument. It suggests that in the current situation—that is, with relatively little demand for luxury primary care—the practice can be endorsed by professional ethics. However, if the demand were great and access were reduced, then the practice would be considered unethical. This means that the definition of ethical practice changes with the situation—in this case, the degree of access to health care. Such situational ethics flies in the face of standard professional principles.

Luxury primary care also undermines cross-subsidized care. For the past 50 years, the American health care system has been dependent on cross-subsidies from patients with good insurance coverage to those with poor coverage or none. For example, a hospital manages to cover the costs of providing care for uninsured patients because it receives payments that exceed the costs of providing care for some well-insured patients. . . .

Indeed, such cross-subsidies can be used to justify practices that otherwise might raise serious ethical questions. For instance, some hospitals and doctors solicit wealthy patients from other countries who are willing to pay a premium for care and for deluxe hospital rooms. The key difference between this practice and luxury primary care is presumably that these hospitals and physicians also provide care to the uninsured. Physicians who provide luxury primary care have simply dropped out of the cross-subsidy system. . . .

We still might ask whether luxury primary care is more out of line with our professional commitment than are other practices we tolerate. Physicians today choose the communities and the situations in which they are going to practice. Relatively few physicians practice in impoverished inner-city or rural areas; many do not accept patients with Medicaid or those without insurance. As a result, poor people and members of minority racial or ethnic groups generally have less access to health care than other Americans. We have not, as a profession, addressed these issues in a serious fashion. Since we have accepted broad inequities in access to health care in the past, it is difficult to argue that luxury practice should be prohibited.

In this light, the development of luxury primary care might be seen as a crystallizing event. The medical community must be prepared to step forward with ideas and programs that ensure an equitable distribution of health care

---

[7] *Ricks v. Budge*, 64 P.2d 208 (Utah 1937).

[8] T. A. Brennan, "Ensuring Adequate Health Care for the Sick: The Challenge of the Acquired Immunodeficiency Syndrome as an Occupational Disease," *Duke Law Journal* 1988, no. 1 (1988): pp. 29–70.

[9] E. H. Moreim, *Holding Health Care Accountable: Law and the New Medical Marketplace* (New York: Oxford University Press, 2001).

services. No matter how innovative and attractive luxury primary care is to some patients and physicians, it poses questions about equity. We should identify ways in which luxury primary care can be regulated by the medical profession (perhaps by mandatory cross-subsidies and careful monitoring of the prevalence of such care), while also addressing other threats to access. The questions that luxury primary care poses should remind us that as physicians we have a commitment to the equitable distribution of health care and therefore a duty to address market innovations that could leave some patients without access to care.

I am indebted to Atul Gawande, Michelle Mello, David Studdert, David Fairchild, and George Thibault for their advice on earlier drafts of this article.

EXCERPT 3

Full text from:

The Lancet, "A Morally Bankrupt Government Divides the NHS," *The Lancet* 372, no. 9651 (2008): p. 1708.

A Morally Bankrupt Government Divides the NHS

The Lancet

The UK's National Health Service (NHS) is one to be proud of: free care for all at the point of delivery. But a proposal last week by the Department of Health to allow NHS patients in England who can afford to buy treatments that are not approved for NHS use to top-up their treatment heralds a truly two-tier system.

The existing system allows patients to pay for extra treatment (top-ups) but then they lose all NHS care. The new proposal, which is out for consultation until January, will allow top ups, with the rider that the extra treatment cannot be given on an NHS ward but will need to be administered in a private ward or hospital. The UK Government is clearly embarrassed, not wanting patients in adjacent NHS beds to be receiving different care.

Welfare spending (and health-service spending can be seen as part of that) affects the health of citizens. In a paper in *The Lancet* last week, the NEWS Nordic Expert Group showed that generosity in family policies is linked with lower infant mortality and that generosity in pensions is linked with lower old-age excess mortality. "Social policies are of major importance for how we can tackle the social determinants of health," the authors concluded. A Comment added: "At least in the Nordic countries, such policies have been as much about dignity and solidarity."

Dignity and solidarity are key concepts that must be applied to NHS funding. The decision to allow a two-tier NHS is undignified and divisive. The National Institute for Health and Clinical Excellence, battered this year for its decisions about high-profile drugs for renal and lung cancer, and dementia, is to review how it calculates whether a treatment is cost effective. But the funding of a national health service reaches higher, to the heart of government. This summer saw the UK Government use £400 billion of taxpayers' money to rescue ailing financial institutions. Vast sums of money can be made available when needed. The government needs to re-align its priorities, or face accusations of moral bankruptcy.

EXCERPT 4

Abridged text from:

"Appendix A," in *Access to Care, Access to Justice: The Legal Debate over Private Health Insurance in Canada*, edited by K. Roach, L. Sossin, and C. M. Flood (University of Toronto Press, 2005).

Appendix A

Chaoulli v. Quebec
Trial Judgment of February 25, 2000
Ginette Piché J. Presiding

. . .

Introduction

The present dispute concerning health and its current accessibility problems sometimes makes us forget the not too distant past, in which people who were sick did not obtain care because they simply did not have the means to do so. . . . Is it desirable to have a public health system with a parallel private health care system?

. . .

The applicants submitted to the Court a motion for a declaratory judgment asking it to rule that ss. 15 of the Health Insurance Act ("HIA") and 11 of the Hospital Insurance Act ("HIA") are unconstitutional. Those provisions prohibit insured services being paid for by private insurance when they are furnished in Quebec. . . .

The applicants asked the Court to be allowed to obtain a private insurance policy to cover the costs inherent in private health services and hospital services when the latter are furnished by physicians not participating in the Quebec public health system.

. . . Counsel for the coapplicant George Zéliotis in fact said "I am arguing for the right of more affluent people to have access to parallel health services." Why could they not purchase private insurance? Why prevent them? . . .

Were the applicants right to thus "denounce" being unable to obtain private insurance?—and what about people who suffer lengthy delays before being operated on or, for example, receiving their chemotherapy treatments? Is all this not cruel? . . .

Discussion

. . .

The Court accepts that waiting lists are too long and that even if the question is not always one of life or death all individuals are entitled to receive the care they need as promptly as possible. Yes, Quebeckers are patient and easygoing, but this does not mean that the health system should not be improved and transformed. . . .

Expert Witnesses: Their Opinions and Viewpoints

. . .

In Canada, the choice has been made to protect society against the catastrophe caused by illness by making insurance available to everyone, subsidizing those who could not pay for it and making participation compulsory for everyone. This strategic choice frees insurance from the obligation to constantly adjust the prices of its services to its claim experience. The compulsory participation of all guarantees that the effect of bad actuarial risks will be minimized in the larger number of good risks which it is possible to assemble in a society. It also permits a saving to be made on all the costs inherent in advertising and continual recruiting of participants. This in part explains the tremendous administrative effectiveness of [the Canadian] health care system, the cost of managing which is nearly four times less than in the U.S.

. . .

"For the essential portion of medically necessary services, the Quebec health care system relies on a single payer and single management in which private participants are involved. Access is not based on the ability to pay," says Dr. Howard Bergman. Opening financing up to private sources would lead to a multi-speed system depending on the type of insurance each person could afford.

. . .

In cases where there are two systems, the public one becomes a "safety net" where private hospitals transfer the worst economic risks. In Manitoba, it has been shown that health care providers who serve both private and public clientele give priority to the former, thereby lengthening the waiting period of patients in the public sector. . . .

Dr. Wright explained that:

> The principal argument for permitting a second tier private alternative system, namely that this would cause better overall access to care and relieve pressure on the public system, is not supported by any data. The information and studies compiled here suggest the opposite, namely that the major effect of allowing private alternative would be to shift energy and resources from the public system into the private system, causing deterioration of public system access. This would only be to the advantage of those who could afford to pay or to purchase additional private health care insurance.

. . .

Prof. Marmor then addressed the argument of waiting lists. Marmor explained:

> There are waiting lists in Canada. If some of those on waiting lists made private arrangements for care at their expense (but eased by insurance options), and there were no change in Medicare, everyone would be better off. Those who jumped queues would be better off, as would the health care professionals who provided their care and received income. But even those remaining on queues would benefit, since the queues would be shortened. And so, why not permit this change?

Prof. Marmor explained that it is completely mistaken to think that there would be no change in our health system if a parallel private system were allowed to develop. He explained his conclusions as follows:

> . . . waiting lists would persist in the public sector, and perhaps lengthen, as the number of patients in that system declined, since fewer hospital beds and professional staff would be serving them. (If resources were not diverted from the public system, unit costs would rise as fewer patients were treated in the same facilities, and new resources would be needed to service the private sector, increasing total Canadian spending on medical care.) Furthermore, the argument takes for granted that privately funded services can be organized as 'free-standing units.' Otherwise, such privately funded services would be unfairly subsidized by past and present public investment in research, capital improvements, and the easy availability of well-equipped modern hospitals. Thus I believe that allowing private insurance to be available as an alternative to Medicare would have profound negative impacts, on the public system rather than none as is assumed. It would not increase availability of services in the public sector or reduce waiting lists. Instead, it would divert resources from the publicly financed program to be available to private activities, and it would increase total Canadian expenditures on health. It also would give those able to secure private coverage an advantage over others.

Having a parallel insurance system would produce substantial changes and damage the health system in Canada . . .

Discussion

The Court considers that the economic barriers set up by the single payer system are closely linked to the opportunity to have access to health care. Without these rights, in view of the cost involved, access to private care is illusory. In this sense, these provisions are an obstacle to access to health services and are thus capable of infringing the life, liberty, and security of the person. . . .

Additionally, limitation of recourse to the private sector for care constitutes an infringement of the physical integrity of the person only in the event that the public system is not capable of effectively guaranteeing such access. If the public system makes the care in question available, there will not be any infringement. The Court does not believe that a constitutional right exists to choose the sources from which the medically required care will be obtained.

. . .

Principles of Fundamental Justice

. . .

The Health Insurance Act and the Hospital Insurance Act are legislation designed to create and maintain a public health system open to all residents of Quebec. They are legislation which seeks to encourage the overall health of all Quebecers without discrimination on the basis of their economic situation. In short, it is a measure by the government intended to promote the well-being of its population as a whole.

Clearly, these acts raise economic barriers against access to private care. However, these are not really measures designed to limit access to care, but measures intended to prevent the creation of a parallel private care system. Underlying these provisions is the fear that the establishing of a private care system would have the effect of diverting a substantial portion of health resources at the expense of the public sector. The Quebec government adopted these acts to guarantee that virtually all health resources existing in Quebec would be at the disposal of the Quebec population as a whole. That is clear.

The disputed provisions seek to guarantee access to health care which is equal and adequate for all Quebecers. The adoption these acts was prompted by considerations of equality and human dignity, and hence it is clear that there is no conflict with the general values expressed by the Canadian Charter or the Quebec Charter of Human Rights and Freedoms.

In closing, let us consider the question of the balance that should exist between individual rights and those of society. The Quebec public health system does not enjoy unlimited and inexhaustible resources; all the expert witnesses said so. The same might indeed be said for every health system existing in the world. In such circumstances, it is entirely justifiable for a government, having the best interests of its people at heart, to adopt a health policy solution which is designed to favour the largest possible number of people. The government limits the rights of a few to ensure that the rights of all citizens in the society will not be adversely affected.

The evidence showed that the right to have recourse to a parallel private health care system, advocated by the applicants, would have repercussions on the rights of the public as a whole. We cannot act like ostriches. The result of creating a parallel private health care system would be to threaten the integrity, sound operation and viability of the public system. . . .

The only way of ensuring that all health resources will benefit all Quebecers without discrimination is to prevent a parallel care system from being established. That is precisely what the disputed provisions in the case at bar do. . . . In the Court's opinion the infringement of the right to life, liberty and security of the person in the case at bar is not "unnecessarily broad, going beyond what is needed to accomplish the governmental objective."

Consequently, the infringement of the right to life, liberty and security of the person in the case at bar is done in accordance with the principles of fundamental justice.

. . .

FOR THESE REASONS, THE COURT:
DISMISSES the motion;
WITH costs.
GINETTE PICHÉ J.S.C.

EXCERPT 5

Abridged text from:

B. J. Krohmal and E. J. Emanuel, "Access and Ability to Pay: The Ethics of a Tiered Health Care System," *Archives of Internal Medicine* 167, no. 5 (2007): pp. 433–437.

Access and Ability to Pay: The Ethics of a Tiered Health Care System

Benjamin Krohmal and Ezekiel Emanuel

. . .

One question facing American health care reformers is whether the United States should continue to have a tiered health care system—a system that allows patients to buy access to medical services that others with the same needs cannot obtain. In America's current system, public coverage is incomplete, and the more one pays, the more options, fewer prior approvals, and faster access to care private insurance generally provides. At the other extreme, Canada favors strict equality and prohibits private payment for more, faster, or better health care options, although debate over tiered health care has intensified following a controversial 2005 Canadian Supreme Court decision that seems to be scaling back these restrictions.[1]

Single-tiered health care should be distinguished from single-payer health care. . . . The number of payers in a system refers to the number of entities that directly finance the provision of health care, whereas the number of tiers refers to the number of levels of quality, variety, or timeliness of available health care. There is no necessary connection between the number of tiers and the number of payers. For instance, the American public Social Security system has a single payer, the federal government, but there are multiple tiers of payout within the public system depending on how much an individual has paid in. . . . The question of whether there should be a single tier of health care raises substantive ethical concerns because a tiered system necessarily permits inequality in access to health care.

Many who regard America's current health care system as inadequate believe that justice requires the United States, like Canada, to have a single-tiered system that prohibits private payment for greater access to medical care. This is a mistake. . . . But a critical evaluation of the ethics suggests that far from requiring a single tier, principles of justice actually support a tiered health care system (Table [12.1]). . . .

Objections to a Tiered Health Care System

Opponents of a tiered system appeal to arguments that health care is a universally recognized need and is central to the opportunities involved in leading a normal human life.[2,3] Health is "a necessary condition for pursuing nearly all the goals around which we organize our lives."[4] Although market influences on many goods, from cars to computers, may lead to inegalitarian outcomes that are nonetheless ethical, it is claimed that inequalities are unjust when it comes to goods as fundamentally important as health care.

A second, related argument is that medical need should be the sole criterion for distributing health care. A fundamental ethical precept is treating *relevantly* similar cases alike. Students' academic records are the relevant basis for determining their grades; it would be unethical for students' grades to differ on the basis of their families' prestige or income. Similarly, it is claimed that patients' medical

---

[1] C. Krauss, "Canada's Private Clinics Surge as Public System Falters," *New York Times*, February 28, 2006.

[2] M. Walzer, *Spheres of Justice: A Defense of Pluralism and Equality* (Basic Books, 2008), ch. 3.

[3] N. Daniels, *Just Health Care* (Cambridge University Press, 1985).

[4] D. W. Brock and N. Daniels, "Ethical Foundations of the Clinton Administration's Proposed Health Care System," *Journal of the American Medical Association* 271, no. 15 (1994): p. 1191.

Table [12.1]
Arguments Against a 2-Tiered Health Care System and Responses

Objection	Description	Response
Health is too important for the market.	Unequal distributions of many goods can be ethical, but health care services are too important to be distributed unequally by the market.	The public cannot provide all patients with access to all medical services, and it would be unjust to impose equality by "leveling down," that is lowering everyone to the level society can afford.
Need is the only relevant distributive criteria.	Need is the only morally relevant basis for distributing health care. Different health care services for people with the same medical needs amounts to discrimination.	Justice is concerned with liberties in addition to needs. . . .
Health is a public good.	Because significant public funds support the health care system, the services subsidized must be equally available to all patients.	Participation in a system 45% funded with public dollars does not obligate physicians and others to provide 100% of their products and services without regard to compensation.
Tiering undermines a program.	Higher tiers of health care would undermine health care for the poor.	Undermining coverage for the disadvantaged can be avoided by meeting 5 criteria outlined for a just tiered health care system.

needs are the relevant basis for determining their access to care and that it would be unethical to provide differential access to care on the basis of patients' ability to pay.[5,6] Much like discrimination, it is argued, a tiered health care system unethically treats relevantly similar cases differently by allowing criteria other than medical need to determine access to care.

. . . The health care system is subsidized by society at every level, from research funding and public health measures to Medicare and Medicaid payments for services as well as medical education. Critics of a multi-tiered system object to making health care a public good in its creation and funding but a private market good when distributed. Because communal funds pay for the health care system, physicians must make medical services equally available to all citizens.[7]

Finally, opponents of multiple tiers emphasize a practical argument: a tiered system leads to inadequate care for the disadvantaged. It is an old adage in American politics that programs for the poor become poor programs because they lack political support.[8] Tiered systems undermine funding for adequate public coverage and produce incentive for the best practitioners to treat the richest patients.[9] . . . Opponents claim that rejecting multiple tiers is necessary to ensure that the poor and others covered by a public health care system receive adequate and dignified care.[10]

---

[5] A. J. Culyer, "Equity – Some Theory and Its Policy Implications," *Journal of Medical Ethics* 27, no. 4 (2001): pp. 275–283.

[6] B. Williams, "The Idea of Equality," in *Philosophy, Politics and Society*, edited by P. Laslett (Oxford, England: Blackwell, 1962), pp. 110–131.

[7] E-mail communication with Marcia Angell, MD, 2004

[8] R. Fein, *Medical Care, Medical Costs: The Search for a Health Insurance Policy* (Harvard University Press, 1986).

[9] A. Gutmann, "For and Against Equal Access to Health Care," *Milbank Memorial Fund Quarterly on Health and Society* 59, no. 4 (1981): pp. 542–560.

[10] S. Woolhandler, et al., "Proposal of the Physicians' Working Group for Single-Payer National Health Insurance," *Journal of the American Medical Association* 290, no. 6 (2003): pp. 798–805.

Defense of a Tiered Health Care System

Defenders of a tiered system respond that the public cannot and should not pay for everyone to have access to every benefit. The principles of justice require society to provide its members with vital goods and services essential to human flourishing. Nonetheless, Rawls reminds us that the need for distributive justice arises precisely when scarcity precludes giving everyone all that they want or need. In allocating limited funds between competing public pursuits, justice's demand that some critical services be provided is no less a requirement that other services of lesser importance or inordinate expense be forgone.[11] However, Rawls also argues that the first principle of justice is that all have the right to the greatest individual liberties compatible with the same liberties for others. Even though many worthwhile goods and services, including some health care, must go without public funding as a matter of justice, justice protects the liberty of individuals to pay for medical options that the public fails to provide.

A nation with America's enormous wealth may have a duty to provide universal health coverage, but the fiscal tribulations of Medicare and Medicaid serve as a reminder that the public budget is limited. . . . It would make no more sense for America to attempt to fund every possible medical service than it would to try to support every possible highway project, educational opportunity, or security measure.

. . .

The principles of justice require that neither the maximum amount of society's wealth be devoted to public services nor the maximum amount of that spent on public services be devoted to health care. Some health care options should not be included in public coverage because they provide insufficient benefits. At the margins, the benefits of brand name drugs, private hospital rooms, or slightly shorter waiting times for elective surgeries are not more important than the benefits of innumerable nonmedical goods—cellular phones, air travel, and single-family homes—that are properly distributed by the market. Other more beneficial medical options should be excluded from public coverage because funding them would require too great a sacrifice of other services. Just as it would be inappropriate for the state to spend scarce funds to pay for every graduate degree or for universal home security systems, the state should not spend on coverage for disproportionately expensive treatments like lung volume reduction surgery or full-mouth reconstructive surgery. With countless important services competing for scarce public funds, it is unjust to fund services simply because they are "medical," no matter how slight their benefits or how high their price. Justice is not blind to cost.

In allocating *public* funds, the state is constrained by a limited budget and required by the principles of justice to make prudent tradeoffs that reflect society's priorities. However, respect for individual liberties leads to inherently different standards for *private* spending. The right of all to the greatest individual liberty compatible with the same liberties for others is a core provision of justice and protects individuals' freedom to spend legitimately held private wealth on safe and beneficial goods or services. Indeed, one of the aims of justice is precisely to determine which goods should be publicly provided and which should be left for people to pay for in accordance with their personal values.[12] As long as the principles of justice place strict demands on state spending while protecting individual freedom of choice, there will be some medical services that should be available if and only if patients pay privately for them.

Those who object that need must be the only criterion for distributing access to care forget that justice is concerned with liberties in addition to needs. . . . A patient's need cannot be the *only* relevant criteria for distributing access to care any more than a shopper's need

[11] J. Rawls, A Theory of Justice, Revised Edition (Cambridge: Harvard University Press, 1999).

[12] Ibid.

must be the *only* relevant criteria for distributing access to groceries.

Similar considerations make it difficult to see why 45% public funding of the health care system would limit how the private 55% is distributed, let alone require that health care workers support universal access to 100% of their products and services without regard to further compensation. Health care subsidies do not require a single tier of health care any more than airline subsidies preclude the sale of first class tickets.

Perhaps the most serious objection to the claim that the principles of justice require a single-tiered health care system is its embrace of the principle that if everyone cannot have something, then nobody can. Many share the worthy goal of increasing equality by raising the level of health care available to the disadvantaged. However, there is at least the appearance of envy and resentment in preferring that some medical services be withheld from all citizens rather than benefit those who are willing and able to pay for them. Increasing equality by bringing everyone down to the level that society can afford is an example of unjust "leveling down" that makes some worse off and none better.[13] A just health care system focuses on whether all have enough access to health care, not on stopping some from getting more.

This is not to say that private payment for health care is always appropriate. When access to care is limited by scarce materials despite the commitment of public funds, as with some organs for transplantation, distribution on the basis of private payment is unethical. However, scarcity in the overall health care system is primarily the result of limited funds, not limited commodities. When fiscal scarcity limits access to a medical service, access to that service cannot simply be redistributed from those who can pay to those who cannot. Furthermore, when patients pay for pharmaceuticals or diagnostic tests, they do not meaningfully exhaust supplies; "as much and as good" is left for others. In such cases, why should we prefer that the affluent spend on foie gras, diamonds, or another sports utility vehicle than on an extra magnetic resonance imaging scan? . . .

Designing an Ethical Tiered System

If the current US health care system is unjust, it is not because it has 2 tiers but because it fails to ensure access to adequate health care for all Americans. The proper standard for evaluating the justice of a health care system is not whether everyone has access to the exact same services or whether the rich can buy more services. The primary ethical standard is whether every citizen is guaranteed, in a sustainable manner, an adequate set of benefits—a core benefits package. Universal coverage with a core benefits package is both affordable and morally imperative.[14]

With tiered health care proving to be the most just option in principle, attention should turn to the extent to which a multi-tiered health care system is compatible in practice with adequate universal coverage. . . . With proper safeguards higher tiers would avoid undermining and could even improve coverage for the disadvantaged by reducing the public burden of funding health care for the affluent.

Although a detailed reform proposal is beyond the scope of this article, a sustainable and just tiered health care system should meet 5 criteria:

1. The core benefits package should cover an adequate level of health care.
2. The core benefits package should be guaranteed to all Americans, without means testing.
3. The core benefits package should be designed to attract a sizable majority of the population to use it without supplementation to the higher tiers.
4. Payment for higher-tiered services and coverage should be made with after-tax dollars and should not provide exemption

[13] D. Parfit, "Equality and Priority," *Ratio* 10, no. 3 (1997): pp. 202–221.

[14] E. J. Emanuel and V. R. Fuchs, "Health Care Vouchers—A Proposal for Universal Coverage," *New England Journal of Medicine* 352, no. 12 (2005): pp. 1255–1260.

from tax obligations to financially support the core benefits package.

5. Easy adjustment of the core benefits package should be possible in response to changes in technology, data about efficacy, and demand for higher-tiered services.

A tiered system that meets these 5 criteria would dramatically improve health coverage in America by raising the basic tier from a safety net for the few to a solid floor for all citizens. The requisite majority of patients using unsupplemented basic tier coverage could be maintained by adjusting the core benefits package and eliminating current tax exemptions for purchasing additional health care services. With everyone covered by adequate health insurance and most patients relying on the core benefits package, treating patients with basic public coverage would no longer be a financial burden for physicians, and limiting a practice to those with higher-tier coverage would rarely be fiscally sound.

Political undermining would also be avoided by eliminating means testing. A non–means-tested universal core benefits package would benefit every citizen, and even the minority who pay for higher-tier services could pay less for supplemental coverage than they would for a full health insurance plan. Although means-tested welfare programs face an uphill battle for political support, non—means-tested Medicare and Social Security programs enjoy broad popularity despite the ability of richer beneficiaries to upgrade with Medigap insurance and private retirement savings. Eliminating means testing also circumvents the need for patients to prove that they are poor to receive benefits, and the stigma associated with public coverage would cease when the public tier is the norm.

The criteria offered require elaboration. What is an adequate core benefits package? It should begin with services that, given a fair share of society's wealth, many people would pay out of pocket to cover for themselves.[15] Such a core benefits package is likely to ensure that a relatively small proportion of Americans buy higher-tier services. Each of the top 10 rated health care systems in the United Nations' equality-oriented 2000 "World Health Report" provides excellent basic coverage to all their citizens while allowing some to purchase higher tiers of health care.[16] By following the 5 criteria given herein, there is no reason the United States could not join them.

Conclusions

What sort of replacement should we want for our troubled health care system? Many argue that justice requires prohibiting private payment for medical services to enforce a Canadian-style single-tiered health care system. This egalitarian approach, while well intentioned, fails to recognize 3 fundamental claims of justice: Public resources are limited, society cannot provide everything, and individual liberties include the freedom to pay for benefits the state does not provide. A tiered system, like English or Israeli systems, can provide broad but necessarily finite universal public coverage without trampling freedom of choice. Many questions remain for American health care reformers, but on the question of tiering, the principles of justice call for a multi-tiered health care system.

Acknowledgment: We thank John Arras, PhD, Steve Pearson, MD, Bonnie Steinbock, PhD, and Alan Wertheimer, PhD, for their critical reviews of the manuscript.

---

15 R. Dworkin, *Sovereign Virtue: The Theory and Practice of Equality* (Harvard University Press, 2002).

16 World Health Organization, *The World Health Report: Health Systems: Improving Performance* (Geneva, Switzerland: World Health Organization, 2000).

Further Resources

Relevant Organizations

Governmental

National Health Services, United Kingdom (NHS): Covers health services for all citizens, however, individuals are allowed to buy private health insurance for additional services. Additional information can be found at http://www.nhs.uk/pages/home.aspx

Quebec Health Insurance Board (RAMQ): All citizens are entitled to basic healthcare, and those involved in private prescription plan are not eligible for RAMQ's prescription plan. Additional information can be found at http://www.ramq.gouv.qc.ca/en/Pages/home.aspx

Swiss Health: Covers health services for all citizens; however, individuals are allowed to buy private health insurance for additional services. Additional information can be found at http://www.swisshealth.ch/en/

Literature

Blizzard, Rick. "The Haves and Have Notes of Healthcare," *Gallup,* August 6, 2002.

Daniels, Norman, "Justice and Access to Health Care," *The Stanford Encyclopedia of Philosophy* (Spring 2013 Edition), Edward N. Zalta (ed.), http://plato.stanford.edu/archives/spr2013/entries/justice-healthcareaccess/.

National Health Service. "Guidance on NHS Patients Who Wish to Pay for Additional Private Care." https://www.gov.uk/government/uploads/system/uploads/attachment_data/file/404423/patients-add-priv-care.pdf.

Rosemarie Day. "The Evolution of a Two-Tier Health Insurance Exchange System," *Health Affairs Blog,* August 13, 2014. https://www.healthaffairs.org/do/10.1377/hblog20140813.040707/full/.

Ruger, J. P. "Health, Capability, and Justice: Toward a New Paradigm of Health Ethics, Policy and Law." *Cornell Journal of Law and Public Policy* 15, no. 2 (Spring 2006): 403–482.

Yu, Chai Ping, David K. Whynes, and Tracey H. Sach. "Equity in Health Care Financing: The Case of Malaysia." *International Journal for Equity in Health* 7, no. 1 (2008): 1–14.

Other Media

Canada, Geoffrey. *Waiting for "Superman."* DVD. Directed by Davis Guggenheim. Burbank: Warner Bros. Entertainment Inc.: K–12 education in America is explored, comparing low-funded schools with private schools and charter schools.

Reich, Robert. *Inequality for All.* DVD. Directed by Jennifer Chaiken and Stephen M. Silverstein. New York City: RADiUS, 2014: Explores economic inequality in America and how it affects individual with low incomes, such as not having enough money to provide for their families.

13 Resource Allocation at the Bedside

Imagine you are admitted to a hospital with kidney problems. The physician describes a number of tests that will be performed, including an x-ray examination of your kidneys that involves injection of a dye into your blood to see how effectively the kidneys remove it (known as an *intravenous pyelogram*). Your physician mentions something about different contrast agents that could be used. Although you don't understand all the details, the way she talks about the options makes you think that it is OK to accept the high-osmolality agent that she seems to prefer. The test, and various other ones, goes fine. That evening at home you try to relax and surf the Internet. For some reason, the name of the contrast agent comes to your mind. You type its name in the search engine. You find out that the other options that the doctor mentioned are marginally less likely to have serious side effects but are considerably more expensive. How do you feel about your doctor?[1]

Should physicians always put their patients first? Or can there be circumstances where it is justifiable for a physician to give some priority to the larger pool of people who contributed to the funds that are used to pay for healthcare services—whether the ultimate payers are taxpayers in a publicly funded system or individuals who are members of a health insurance pool?

In rationing cases, physicians also play a role in deciding who gets the absolutely scarce healthcare resource. Yet, in policy and practice, there is typically little leeway for physician action when it comes to rationing under absolute scarcity. For example, we noted in Chapter 5 explicit criteria for listing patients on transplant waiting lists. Similarly, the American Thoracic Society's *Fair Allocation of Intensive Care Unit Resources* guidelines stipulate unambiguously that when demand exceeds supply, "medically appropriate patients should be admitted on a first-come, first-served basis . . . [as] every individual's life is equally

[1] P. A. Ubel and R. Arnold, "The Unbearable Rightness of Bedside Rationing: Physician Duties in a Climate of Cost Containment," *Archives of Internal Medicine* 155, no. 17 (1995): pp. 1837–1842.

valuable." Expressly, the guidelines note that "relative benefit, . . . relative medical need" are unfair criteria.[2] Many hospital guidelines echo this approach. But when it comes to resource allocation situations, physicians across a wide range of disciplines make countless decisions day in and day out, in which they have considerable discretion, with large and direct impacts on spending and budgets. Whose side should they be on—that of controlling cost, or doing what is best for their individual patient, regardless of total cost?

Using the analogy of a lawyer–client relationship, Levinsky argues that doctors are required to "act solely as [the] patient's advocate, against the apparent interests of society as a whole, if necessary" (Excerpt 1).[3] The patient is the only master physicians should serve. Levinsky also highlights practical problems. Individual patients are rarely identical in all their features to the statistical average of study populations. He argues that trying to connect the two spheres poses an unresolvable conundrum, leaving only arbitrary decisions:

> How is the practitioner to define "low" [value of an intervention] in everyday practice—2, 5, 10, or 20 percent likelihood of survival with a good quality of life? Even if the dividing line were defined and the requisite precision in estimating outcome could be achieved, the role of the doctor as patient advocate would be subverted by probabilistic practice.[4]

Levinsky is not blind to high cost of healthcare. His response is to focus efforts on reducing waste in the form of redundant procedures, eliminating drivers of defensive medicine, and using less expensive settings and interventions. But he does not want physicians making such resource allocation decisions when treating their patients.

Arthur Schafer's arguments against a role for physicians in resource allocation are centered around the following: (1) loss of trust, (2) discrimination, and (3) lack of training and expertise by physicians in resource allocation (Excerpt 2).[5]

First, he fears that if a patient were to discover that a physician had prescribed a suboptimal intervention on cost grounds, the trust that is essential to the doctor–patient relationship will necessarily be undermined. Second, he is concerned about arbitrary and discriminatory decisions. General bias against racial or ethnic groups, immigrants, or perhaps obese patients, alcoholics, or smokers who might be viewed as having had opportunity to avoid their health problems is prevalent in society: "it would be naïve to believe that such prejudices are not at least as prevalent among health care professionals as among the general public."[6] Thus, he worries that empowering physicians to make resource allocation decisions means that minorities, the poor, the obese, and others will not get the same services as the better-off.

Third, Schafer suggests, physicians lack the necessary will, training, time, or expertise to engage in economic evaluations of the downstream implications of different therapeutic options. In view of these constraints, he calls for more transparency in cases where priorities need to be set: "If/when [this] must occur, it is far better that [it] be done in a fair and open manner, according to publicly acceptable rules. In that way fairness prevails and is seen to prevail, and the physician's traditional role as advocate for her patients is protected."[7]

Opponents to this view often object to the courtroom analogy and adversarial construction as a mischaracterization of the professional role of physicians. Accordingly, asking which side doctors should be on—that of the individual patient before them or the more anonymous

---

[2] "Statements, Guidelines & Reports," 2015, accessed June 16, 2015, http://www.thoracic.org/statements/.

[3] N. G. Levinsky, "The Doctor's Master," *New England Journal of Medicine* 311, no. 24 (1984): p. 1573.

[4] Ibid., p. 1574.

[5] A. Schafer, "Bedside Rationing by Physicians: The Case Against," *Healthcare Papers* 2, no. 2 (2001): pp. 45–52.

[6] Ibid., p. 50.

[7] Ibid., p. 51.

community of current and future patients—is meaningless: they need to serve both. Opponents also commonly point out that doctors very routinely engage in priority-setting and find it more fruitful to acknowledge these circumstances and to identify ways in which possible drawbacks can be minimized. In this regard, disclosure and communication are central elements in Steve Pearson's proposal (Excerpt 3).[8] He suggests that instead of a Darwininan scenario in which a myriad of physician–patient dyads compete against each other for resources, a better view is what he calls *proportional advocacy*:

> patients and physicians are viewed as part of a moral community in which costs are controlled through group deliberation and decision making. [Priority-setting takes place] with the open knowledge and collaboration of their patients and the broader community.[9]

He suggests six criteria to guide proportional advocacy: (1) open communication that resource allocation is taking place, (2) communication about its justification, (3) group determination of low- and high-value services, (4) impartial application across patients and physicians, (5) reduction of physician's conflict of interest, and 6) offering opportunities for patients to appeal priority resource allocation decisions.

Ubel and Arnold discuss the frequent assertion of those opposing a role of physicians in resource allocation that explicit rules and policies are preferable options (Excerpt 4).[10] They are not opposed to rules and, indeed, see an important role for them. However, given that patients often differ significantly in their health needs and social and other relevant circumstances, they are concerned that such rules would entail considerable complexity. By contrast, physician discretion within more general guidelines can be a more effective way of fairly allocating resources.

Ubel and Arnold also emphasize that some of the concerns about the physician's role may stem from lack of clarity about the underlying reasons of decisions, concerns about who is affected by allocation decisions and what kind of services are their subject:

> The moral acceptability of bedside rationing depends crucially on which services physicians think fit to ration. For bedside rationing to be morally tolerable, physicians should base rationing decisions on medical costs and benefits, not on racial or sexual biases. In addition, they should only ration marginally beneficial services, not ones that bring significant benefits to their patients.[11]

They argue that such assessments should be centrally guided by cost-effectiveness analysis, even though they recognize CEA's methodological and value-based limitations, as outlined in Chapter 9. Physicians, they note:

> should not be expected to perform cost-effectiveness analyses at the bedside. Rather, they should become familiar enough with the concepts of cost-effectiveness so that they can more accurately identify marginally beneficial health care services.[12]

Strech and colleagues provide an empirical overview that illustrates both the urgency of clarifying physicians' role, as well as the challenges associated with calling for a more involved hands-on approach—or a more passive hands-off one (Excerpt 5).[13] They carried out a systematic review of qualitative research identifying nine studies with a total of 314

---

[8] S. D. Pearson, "Caring and Cost: The Challenge for Physician Advocacy," *Annals of Internal Medicine* 133, no. 2 (2000): pp. 148–153.

[9] Ibid., figure subtitle, p. 149.

[10] Ubel and Arnold, "The Unbearable Rightness of Bedside Rationing."

[11] Ibid., p. 1841.

[12] Ibid., p. 1842.

[13] D. Strech, M. Synofzik, and G. M. Marckmann, "How Physicians Allocate Scarce Resources at the Bedside: A Systematic Review of Qualitative Studies," *Journal of Medicine and Philosophy* 33, no. 1 (2008): pp. 80–99.

participants in six countries, mainly in primary care. They identify emerging themes in three clusters: context-, physician-, or patient-related factors; implicit and explicit strategies drawing on a range of different criteria; and consequences of resource allocation taking place in different guises in everyday practice, including impact on professionalism and emotional stress. Among their conclusions, they note that:

> the high variability of allocation criteria presented in this review calls into question the consistency of physicians' [resource allocation] decisions at the bedside . . . [which] seems to be only poorly influenced by explicit and transparent ethical criteria.[14]

Despite the importance of the issue of resource allocation at the bedside, few organizations have issued guidelines or recommendations for practicing physicians. This changed significantly in 2012, with the 6th edition of the American College of Physicians' *Ethics Manual* (Excerpt 6).[15] In line with the American Medical Association's principle that "a physician must recognize responsibility to patients first and foremost, as well as to society, to other health professionals, and to self,"[16] the *Manual* is clear that physicians have general obligations to society. These general obligations are then delineated more concretely:

> Physicians have a responsibility to practice effective and efficient health care and to use health care resources responsibly. Parsimonious care that utilizes the most efficient means to effectively diagnose a condition and treat a patient respects the need to use resources wisely.[17]

The *Manual* goes on to say that: "physicians' considered judgments should reflect the best available evidence in the biomedical literature, including data on the cost-effectiveness of different clinical approaches.[18]

It is furthermore noteworthy that, in the United States, physicians, through their specialty societies, have taken the lead in an initiative that seeks to make more progress in controlling cost by eliminating services that provide patients no added medical benefits but may add considerable cost or harm their health. Building on earlier work, the American Board of Internal Medicine Foundation invited professional societies to identify five interventions that had little to no clinical value or were predominantly harmful.[19] In the first iteration published in 2012, nine societies had joined. Each identified five commonly used tests, treatments, or services "for which the use should be re-evaluated."[20] Just a few years later, more than 70 societies have joined, identifying hundreds of practices.[21] Australia,[22] Canada,[23] Germany,[24]

---

[14] Ibid., p. 96.

[15] L. Snyder, "American College of Physicians Ethics Manual, Sixth Edition," *Annals of Internal Medicine* 156 (2012): pp. 73–104; See also E. J. Emanuel, "Review of the American College of Physicians Ethics Manual, Sixth Edition," *Annals of Internal Medicine* 156 (2012): pp. 56–57.

[16] American Medical Association, "Principles of Medical Ethics," 2001, accessed June, 2015, http://www.ama-assn.org/ama/pub/physician-resources/medical-ethics/code-medical-ethics/principles-medical-ethics.page.

[17] Snyder, "ACP Ethics Manual," p. 86.

[18] Ibid.

[19] D. Wolfson, J. Santa, and L. Slass, "Engaging Physicians and Consumers in Conversations About Treatment Overuse and Waste: A Short History of the Choosing Wisely Campaign," *Academic Medicine* 89, no. 7 (2014): pp. 990–995.

[20] C. K. Cassel and J. A. Guest, "Choosing Wisely: Helping Physicians and Patients Make Smart Decisions About Their Care," *JAMA* 307, no. 17 (2012): p. 1801.

[21] "History: Choosing Wisely," 2015, accessed June, 2015, http://www.choosingwisely.org/about-us/history/.

[22] "Choosing Wisely Australia," accessed July 29, 2015, http://www.choosingwisely.org.au/.

[23] "Choosing Wisely Canada," accessed July 29, 2015, http://www.choosingwiselycanada.org/.

[24] "Möglichkeiten Und Grenzen Einer Choosing Wisely Initiative," accessed July 29, 2015, http://www.ebm-netzwerk.de/was-wir-tun/themenportale/gemeinsam-klug-entscheiden/ziel-inhalt.

Italy,[25] the Netherlands,[26] the United Kingdom,[27] and others have launched similar efforts. Aside from having the potential to improve quality and affordability of care, the initiative can also be seen as indicative of broader cultural change regarding the professions' understanding of its role in resource allocation.

Physicians have roles in both rationing and resource allocation, although they typically have more discretion in the latter and less in the former. Choices made at higher levels (e.g., coverage decisions by health plans) have very direct consequences for particular patient groups; however, for the decision makers, the beneficiaries (and perhaps more importantly the groups losing out) are a largely invisible and anonymous group of patients. By contrast, physicians, quite literally, face the people affected by their decisions. This presence can exercise considerable pressure and lend much support to the patient advocate model, in which physicians always put their individual patients before the more amorphous interests of the collective of current and future patients in seeking to extend life and improve quality of life. But, as several of the excerpts in this chapter show, introducing the notions of high- and low-value care need not be incompatible with the professional role—in fact, recent developments in policy and practice see such conversations as an integral element of professionalism.

[25] "Slow Medicine: Fare Di Più Non Significa Fare Meglio," accessed July 29, 2015, http://www.slowmedicine.it/fare-di-piu-non-significa-fare-meglio/48-fare-di-piu-non-significa-fare-meglio/36-il-progetto.html.

[26] "Choosing Wisely Netherlands Campaign," accessed July 29, 2015, http://www.kwaliteitskoepel.nl/verstandig-kiezen/english/.

[27] "NICE 'Do Not Do' Recommendations," 2012, accessed July 29, 2015, https://www.nice.org.uk/proxy/?sourceurl=http://www.nice.org.uk/usingguidance/donotdorecommendations/index.jsp.

Questions for Discussion

1. Is it right that, in rationing situations, physicians typically have little discretion over treatment options, whereas in resource allocation they are far more free to chose among alternatives? Should the rationing context be relaxed or the resource allocation context be tightened up further?
2. Do you find Levinsky's legalistic analogy in Excerpt 1 helpful, according to which doctors are required to "act solely as [the] patient's advocate, against the apparent interests of society as a whole, if necessary"?
3. Was the American College of Physicians right to urge physicians in its *Ethics Manual* (Excerpt 6) to practice effectively and efficiently while also considering cost-effectiveness data?
4. In Excerpt 4, Ubel and Arnold argue that physicians "should only ration marginally beneficial services, not ones that bring significant benefits to their patients." Present an argument in favor and one against this position.
5. The American Board of Internal Medicine Foundation invited professional societies to identify interventions that had little to no clinical value or were predominantly harmful. Will the initiative increase or decrease trust? How can the benefits be maximized?

EXCERPTS

Note: The following excerpts have generally been edited for length, and omissions are indicated with ellipses. Editing includes footnotes and endnotes, which have also been renumbered. For citation and related purposes, the full original source texts should be used.

EXCERPT 1

Abridged text from:

N. G. Levinsky, "The Doctor's Master," *New England Journal of Medicine* 311, no. 24 (1984): pp. 1573–1575.

The Doctor's Master

N. G. Levinsky

There is increasing pressure on doctors to serve two masters. Physicians in practice are being enjoined to consider society's needs as well as each patient's needs in deciding what type and amount of medical care to deliver. Not surprisingly, many government leaders and health planners take this position. More remarkably, important elements of the medical profession are promoting this view.

I would argue the contrary, that physicians are required to do everything that they believe may benefit each patient without regard to costs or other societal considerations. In caring for an individual patient, the doctor must act solely as that patient's advocate, against the apparent interests of society as a whole, if necessary. An analogy can be drawn with the role of a lawyer defending a client against a criminal charge. The attorney is obligated to use all ethical means to defend the client, regardless of the cost of prolonged legal proceedings or even of the possibility that a guilty person may be acquitted through skillful advocacy. Similarly, in the practice of medicine, physicians are obligated to do all that they can for their patients without regard to any costs to society.

Society benefits if it expects its medical practitioners to follow this principle. As Fried[1] has eloquently argued, in any decent, advanced society there are rights in health care, in that "one is entitled to be treated decently, humanely, personally and honestly in the course of medical care. . . ." In such a just society "the physician who withholds care that it is in his power to give because he judges it is wasteful to provide it to a particular person breaks faith with his patient." A similar position has been stated by Hiatt[2]: "A physician or other provider must do all that is permitted on behalf of his patient. . . . The patient and the physician want no less, and society should settle for no less." A just society must have a group of professionals whose sole responsibility as health-care practitioners is to their patients as individuals.

The issue is not whether physicians must do everything technically possible for each patient. Rather it is that they should decide how much to do according to what they believe best for that patient, without regard for what is best for society or what it costs. I do not argue, as some have,[3] that doctors are obligated to prolong life under all circumstances or that they are required to use their expertise to confer technological immortality on dehumanized bodies. . . .

They are not entitled to discontinue treatment on the basis of other considerations, such as cost. This distinction may become blurred if physicians are pressed to balance the needs of their patients with societal needs. The practitioner may make decisions for economic reasons but rationalize them as in the best interest of the individual patient. . . .

A similar danger lurks if physicians attempt to conserve resources by using probabilities of success or failure to make decisions about the

---

[1] C. Fried, "Rights and Health Care: Beyond Equity and Efficiency," *New England Journal of Medicine* 293, no. 5 (1975): pp. 241–245.

[2] H. H. Hiatt, "Protecting the Medical Commons: Who Is Responsible?," *New England Journal of Medicine* 293, no. 5 (1975): pp. 235–241.

[3] F. H. Epstein, "The Role of the Physician in the Prolongation of Life," in *Controversy in Internal Medicine II*, edited by F. J. Ingelfinger, et al. (Philadelphia: WB Saunders, 1974).

care of individual patients. Estimates of the probable outcome of a clinical condition in a given patient are almost invariably based on "soft data": uncontrolled studies, reports of cases of dubious comparability, or the physician's anecdotal clinical experience—all further devalued by rapidly changing diagnostic and therapeutic techniques. The standard errors of such estimates are undefined but undoubtedly large. Yet leading physicians.[4,5] advise doctors to practice probabilistic medicine—i.e., to withhold expensive treatment if the probability of success is low. How is the practitioner to define "low" in everyday practice—2, 5, 10, or 20% likelihood of survival with a good quality of life? Even if the dividing line were defined and the requisite precision in estimating outcome could be achieved, the role of the doctor as patient advocate would be subverted by probabilistic practice. This point should not be blurred by using the phrase "hopelessly ill."[6] If there is no hope for a patient, then there is no problem for the doctor in discontinuing treatment. In practice, doctors can rarely be certain who is hopelessly ill. This problem is not resolved by redefining the phrase to exclude consideration of the "rare report of a patient with a similar condition who survived. . . ."[7] in deciding whether to continue aggressive treatment. Physicians cannot discharge their responsibility to their individual patients if they try to conserve societal resources by discontinuing treatment on statistical grounds.

. . .

None of the foregoing implies that in caring for individual patients doctors should disregard the escalating cost of medical care. Physicians can help control costs by choosing the most economical ways to deliver optimal care to their patients. They can use the least expensive setting, ambulatory or inpatient, in which first-class care can be given. They can eliminate redundant or useless diagnostic procedures ordered because of habit, deficient knowledge, personal financial gain, or the practice of "defensive medicine" to avoid malpractice judgments.

However, it is society, not the individual practitioner, that must make the decision to limit the availability of effective but expensive types of medical care. Heart and liver transplantation are current cases in point. These are extraordinarily expensive procedures that may prolong a life of "good quality" for some people. Society, through its elected officials, is entitled to decide that the resources required for such programs are better used for other purposes. However, a physician who thinks that his or her patient may benefit from a transplant must make that patient aware of this opinion and assist the patient in obtaining the organ.

. . .

When practicing medicine, doctors cannot serve two masters. It is to the advantage both of our society and of the individuals it comprises that physicians retain their historic single-mindedness. The doctor's master must be the patient.

[4] S. H. Wanzer, et al., "The Physician's Responsibility Toward Hopelessly Ill Patients," *New England Journal of Medicine* 310, no. 15 (1984): pp. 955–959.

[5] A. Leaf, "The Doctor's Dilemma – and Society's Too," *New England Journal of Medicine* 310, no. 11 (1984): pp. 718–721.

[6] Wanzer, "The Physician's Responsibility."

[7] Ibid.

EXCERPT 2

Abridged text from:
A. Schafer, "Bedside Rationing by Physicians: The Case Against," *Healthcare Papers* 2, no. 2 (2001): pp. 45–52.
Also available at:
A. Schafer, "Bedside Rationing by Physicians: The Case Against," Longwoods Publishing, 2001, accessed July 29, 2015, http://www.longwoods.com/content/17457.

Bedside Rationing by Physicians: The Case Against

Arthur Schafer

. . .

The argument of this paper is that even if rationing of health care resources were to prove necessary, the scheme of bedside rationing by physicians, advocated by Ubel, would be ethically unacceptable. And for several different kinds of reasons.

. . .

The Moral Weaknesses of Bedside Rationing: I) Loss of Trust

The core principle of physician ethics, incorporated in every version of physician ethics for over two thousands years affirms, in one form of words or another, that "the life and health of my patient will be my first consideration." [Declaration of Geneva] That is, a commitment to provide optimal care for one's patients constitutes the moral foundation-stone of the practice of medicine.

Now, of course, "ought implies can," as philosophers are wont to say, and if a physician lacks access to resources needed by his or her patients, then the physician is not held to be blameworthy when the care provided is sub-optimal. But were a physician deliberately to withhold optimal care from a patient, on the grounds that the physician judges it to be cost-effective for society, then the physician's obligation to her patient would be subordinated to her obligation to society. Such conduct on the part of physicians (whether undertaken to save money for society or to benefit the doctor's hospital or employer) would pose a serious risk of vitiating patient trust. That is, when patients came to realize that their doctors are no longer unqualified advocates of their best interests, they would lose trust in their doctors to an extent that would endanger the doctor-patient relationship.

Those worried about this possibility need not believe that the obligation to put the welfare of patients first must always trump a physician's obligations to society. After all, a physician's obligation to her patients is not absolute. Cases may arise in which almost everyone would concede that the physician's obligation to protect society legitimately overrides her obligation to her individual patient. For example, the protection of society against the spread of a dangerous infectious diseases could ethically oblige a physician to report a particular patient to public health authorities, in violation of the principle of doctor-patient confidentiality.

Though not absolute, the obligation of physicians to advocate for their patients and to place their patients best interests above other considerations is so fundamental to the profession of medicine that those who propose to abridge it must bear a heavy burden of proof. Consider: What would a patient be likely to think if she were to discover that her physician had prescribed for her (or for her child or parent or spouse) a pain-killing drug or a diagnostic test which was known by the physician to be sub-optimal—because the physician wanted to contain health care costs for the private insurance company, the hospital or the company by which she was employed?

There is some reason to believe that were such a practice to become widespread, as Ubel advocates it should, and were the public to become aware of it, as surely they would, there would ensue a serious erosion of trust between doctors and patients. Without a strong bond of trust, the ability of doctors to help their patients would be seriously compromised.[1] Indeed, it is difficult to think of a more serious loss to the medical profession than such an erosion of trust in the doctor's fidelity to her patients best interests. . . .

ii) arbitrary and discriminatory decisions

The likely consequences for good or ill of any health policy proposal will depend, to some considerable extent, upon the prevailing ethos and values of the society in which the proposal is embedded. North American society is marked by a worrying degree of many different kinds of social prejudice and social stigma. Blacks in the United States and First Nations people in Canada, for example, often believe, with good reason, that they are regarded by their fellow citizens as inferior, second-class, less deserving of respect and consideration when it comes to social benefits, including health care benefits. There is, as well, in North America, a widely prevalent dis-esteem for members of other minority groups, for immigrants, for elderly people, substance abusers, the mentally ill and the disabled. It would be naive to believe that such prejudices are not at least as prevalent among health care professionals as among the general public.

. . .

An illustrative example may help. Widespread use of low osmolar contrast medium for certain radiologic tests would add significant costs to the health care system, but would result in less vomiting by patients and, in rare cases, might be life-saving. Suppose that we leave to physicians at the bedside such decisions as whether to utilize low osmolar contrast medium for their patients, advising physicians to take into account the cost-effectiveness of the alternatives.

The overall costs to society of adopting the superior technology are cumulatively significant. The benefit to most patients will be slight: fewer pukes. If such decisions are left to the discretion of individual doctors, what is the likely outcome? Some doctors will conscientiously attempt to save money for the system, and will order the more expensive contrast medium only in those identifiable but rare cases in which the cheaper alternative could be dangerous to the patient. Other doctors will choose to act according to traditional medical ethics, disregard the extra costs of the low contrast medium, and order it for all their patients. Still other doctors will decide on a case-by-case basis. It would not be surprising if this latter group of doctors were to order the cheaper, but sub-optimal, medium for their poor or elderly or minority or disabled patients, while ordering the optimal medium for their wealthy, powerful, high status patients (including other doctors). Physicians who would behave in this way need not, many of them, consciously understand the discriminatory nature of their resource allocation among their patients.

This kind of bedside rationing just doesn't seem fair. . . .

iii) physicians lack the necessary will, the training, the time, or the expertise to do accurate cost-benefit calculations at the patient's bedside

A moment's reflection reveals that very few doctors have received such an education in economics as would enable them successfully to perform the micro-allocative rationing which Ubel wants us to assign to them. Moreover, the kind of cost-benefit analysis which Ubel would have them undertake for each of their treatment decisions can not be successfully carried out without a large knowledge base. Many physicians, with busy practices, can scarcely keep up with the relevant medical literature, and willy nilly receive their ongoing education from such agencies as drug company representatives—a group not known for its disinterested and benevolent advice.

Consider: in order to make sensible bedside rationing decisions, physicians would need to know both the success/failure rates of each treatment option and the comparative costs, short term and long term, direct and indirect costs, associated with each alternative. It seems likely that not one in a thousand physicians possesses such rationing knowledge and expertise or could easily acquire it.

[1] J. Katz, *The Silent World of Doctor and Patient* (Johns Hopkins University Press, 2002).

. . .

A better alternative

In the end, Ubel's argument comes down to the claim that rationing is inevitable and that, whatever the limitations of bedside rationing, there is no better alternative.

Rule-based rationing is a better alternative than bedside rationing. If/when rationing of health care resources must occur, it is far better that the rationing be done in a fair and open manner, according to publicly acceptable rules. In that way fairness prevails and is seen to prevail, and the physician's traditional role as advocate for her patients is protected. Ubel considers and rejects such a proposal, but none of his reasons for rejection strike me as persuasive.

Consider how rule-based rationing might apply to a doctor's decision to use low vs. high osmolar contrast medium. Suppose that society has decided that the expense of providing low osmolar contrast medium for every patient who could benefit would be too costly, given the minimal benefit that would be conferred. The rule, then, would be that every patient receives the cheaper contrast medium. As Ubel notes, this kind of rule will often be too simple, because there will be some patients for whom the benefits could be dramatic, for example, the small group of identifiable patients whose lives are at risk from the use of high osmolar contrast medium.

At this point, a sensible version of rule based rationing would introduce a qualification to the rule, one which permits patients whose lives would otherwise be at risk to receive the more expensive medium. Often, it will be possible explicitly to delineate the exceptions, without introducing undue complexity. But, in those cases where this would generate unwieldy complexity, the rule could specify consensus criteria to be applied in deciding which exceptions are warranted. Doctors could be allowed to apply these criteria themselves or they could be allowed, on a case-by-case basis, to seek approval from an appropriate official. Practice patterns could be audited—something which should occur in any event, as part of the move towards quality assurance and evidence-based medicine—and those with questionable patterns could be held accountable.

. . .

EXCERPT 3

Abridged text from:

S.D. Pearson, "Caring and Cost: The Challenge for Physician Advocacy," *Annals of Internal Medicine* 133, no. 2 (2000): pp. 148–153.
Also available at http://annals.org/article.aspx?articleid=713682.

Caring and Cost: The Challenge for Physician Advocacy

Steven D. Pearson

How should physicians respond to the growing tension between care and cost? One option is to reinforce the ideal of doing everything to further the best interests of the individual patient. Others, however, have argued that because health care resources are shared and limited, physicians should consciously participate in rationing by saying "no" to patients' requests for some marginally beneficial services.

But even physicians who endorse the idea of rationing wonder whether patient–physician relationships could ever survive a frank admission of rationing at the bedside. This article explores the idea that caring about costs can be brought to the bedside in a way that will sustain trust among patients and the public. By illustrating a hypothetical case and the ensuing conversation between a physician and her patient, a mode of "proportional" patient advocacy is presented in which physicians can remain forceful agents for patient good while acting within a framework that admits to the boundaries of responsible budgets for health care needs.

. . .

My experience in practice, teaching, and consulting with colleagues has led me to believe that caring about costs can be brought to the bedside in a way that will sustain the trust of patients and the public. In this article, I describe how physicians who acknowledge the need to care about costs can exercise their instinct to fight for the interests of their patients within a framework that admits to the boundaries of responsible budgets for health care needs. . . .

Traditional Patient Advocacy

In the dominant paradigm of the patient–physician relationship in the United States today, patient advocacy is encapsulated—protected, or isolated, depending on one's viewpoint—from population-based ethics, in which rationing is an ethical and practical necessity.

. . .

This kind of patient advocacy creates a significant risk for inefficient and unjust variation in care. It would hardly come as a surprise to learn that the patients who request and receive approval for marginally beneficial care are more likely to be white, affluent, and well educated. Is it fair for these patients to get marginally beneficial services when other, less advantaged patients might go without services that they need even more, just because they don't know how to ask persuasively? Resources foregone by one patient are not guaranteed to be used directly by another for greater benefit, but when physicians join with their patients to capture all the marginal care resources they can, one view is that they are not taking from administrators or insurers—they are ultimately taking from other patients.[1] . . .

An Alternative Model of Patient Advocacy

Although it may be easy intellectually to call for a "balance" between the needs of individual patients and those of other patients and other

[1] D. Eddy, "Clinical Decision Making: From Theory to Practice. Rationing Resources While Improving Quality. How to Get More for Less," *Journal of the American Medical Association* 272, no. 10 (1994): p. 817.

social priorities, practicing physicians know that this concept is difficult even to imagine when caring for a real individual patient, when pain and illness call forth the deepest human instincts to care, and to care deeply, and to care without reservation. Can these honored features of the patient–physician relationship be retained while a new model of patient advocacy that will avoid the pitfalls of Darwinian advocacy is adopted? I think it is possible, although a new model will carry its own risks. The alternative model for the patient–physician relationship is one that can be called "proportional" advocacy.[2] In this model, the key concept is that the physician and patient are linked together not as an isolated dyad but within a group in which other physicians and other patients are also drawing from a limited and shared pool of resources (bottom panel of the Figure [13.1]). The pressure to allocate and ration resources within acknowledged limits arises from within this balanced structure and is applied uniformly across physician–patient dyads that operate in open cooperation and collaboration—instead of in the competition of the Darwinian model.

Proportional advocacy requires a critical weighing of risk and benefit in every clinical decision, a process that is both logical and ethical. But this kind of balancing of multiple considerations, with ultimate integration into a coherent assessment and plan, is not foreign to physicians. Excellent physicians can make complex clinical decisions by weighing the likelihood and quality of clinical outcomes and integrating these with patient and family values. Proportional advocacy draws upon these same time-honored skills

One element of this model needs to be stressed: The individual physician is not rationing the care of his or her individual patient blindly or alone. A physician rationing care in isolation is far worse than a physician advocating for individual patients without concern for others. Physicians should ration only when they can join each other and their community in a shared quest for justice and mercy in the face of life's limits.

[2] A. R. Jonsen, *The New Medicine and the Old Ethics* (Harvard University Press, 1990).

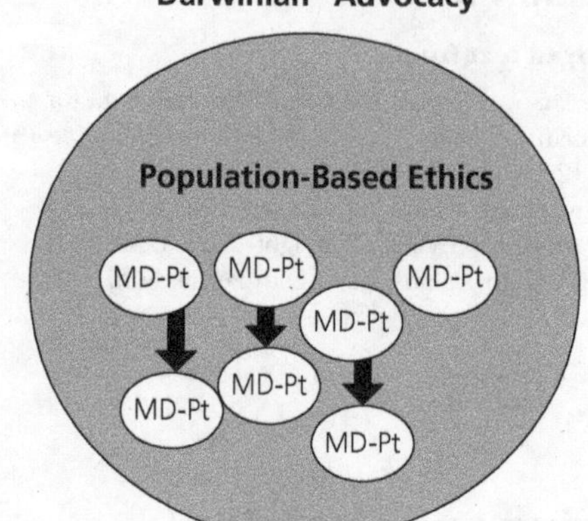

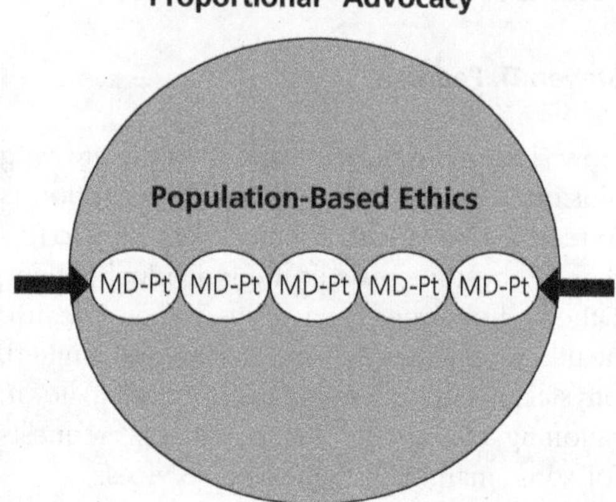

Figure [13.1] Two models of physician advocacy. *Top*: Darwinian advocacy. In this model, societal pressures to control costs are applied unevenly and even capriciously, resulting in a competitive relationship among patient–physician dyads for available resources. Some patient–physician dyads gain preferential access to services, whereas others are forced to accept less. *Bottom*: Proportional advocacy. In this model, patients and physicians are viewed as part of a moral community in which costs are controlled through group deliberation and decision-making. Physicians are called upon to ration at the bedside with the open knowledge and collaboration of their patients and the broader community.

Putting Proportional Advocacy into Action

But should proportional advocacy even be entertained as an option when for-profit health

Table [13.1]
Criteria for Ethical Proportional Advocacy

Open communication of rationing
Communication of justification of rationing
Group determination of high-value and low-value services
Impartial application: same across patients and physicians
Minimal conflict of interest for individual physicians
Recourse for challenge of any rationing decision

plans dominate the marketplace, when physicians share much of the financial risk associated with capitation while maintaining their incomes at a level significantly higher than in other countries, and when individual patients will always be vulnerable to having care withheld without their knowledge?[3,4] These are challenging questions. Yet, the advocate for proportional advocacy would argue that even if the landscape of U.S. health care were swept clean and replaced with a single-payer system, physicians would be charged with the task of prudently using the explicitly finite resources to improve health. To do that, physicians would need to discuss with patients when beneficial care did not meet the threshold for which common resources should be used to pay for it. Whether now or later, how might physicians and patients conduct these conversations? Specifically, what would patients need to hear from their physicians to believe that it was fair and reasonable for them *not* to receive coverage for a test or treatment that would be of some benefit?

My answer to this question is summarized in the Table [13.1].

Conclusion

Implicit in this discussion of proportional advocacy is the idea that rationing by physicians is best applied at the margins, where the potential or real benefit to the individual patient is small. The approach discussed above would therefore apply only to a subset of clinical scenarios. But . . . proportional advocacy need not be relegated only to situations for which the marginal benefit is easy to dismiss as vanishingly small. . . . The appropriate exercise of proportional advocacy demands constant attention to the uniqueness of individual patients, to the relative strength of the clinical evidence, and to the maturity of the collaborative decision making that has been done to justify a decision to say "no." Caution and humility are paramount. Over 25 years ago, Howard Hiatt described the need for a social compact between physicians and other groups in the society to draw the bright lines that would "protect the commons."[5] Today, that vision remains largely unfulfilled. Within our competitive and corporatized health care system, it would be a dangerous mistake for an individual physician to use proportional advocacy to justify withholding care of significant benefit. Proportional advocacy needs to remain in an incubator, but even bringing it into action sparingly, in considerations about marginally beneficial care, would be a useful first step for physicians, their patients, and a society that has been insulated from the realities of health care costs for too long.

Patients and physicians do confront choices every day that offer opportunities for the appropriate use of proportional advocacy. After a joint critical examination of the medical evidence, patients and physicians would probably find more medical care at the margin. In addition to the type of situation illustrated in the preceding section, other common

[3] S. Woolhandler and D. U. Himmelstein, "Extreme Risk: The New Corporate Proposition for Physicians," *New England Journal of Medicine* 333, no. 25 (1995): p. 1706.

[4] S. Woolhandler and D. U. Himmelstein, "When Money Is the Mission: The High Costs of Investor-Owned Care," *New England Journal of Medicine* 341, no. 6 (1999): p. 444.

[5] H. H. Hiatt, "Protecting the Medical Commons: Who Is Responsible?," *New England Journal of Medicine* 293, no. 5 (1975): pp. 235–241.

examples include decisions about maximizing patient convenience in getting a test or treatment, questions about whether to order tests meant primarily to reduce the patient's anxiety, questions about using cheaper drugs with slightly less efficacy or slightly higher risk for side effects, and questions about substituting generic or other cheaper drugs for ones the patient may already be taking.

In all of these situations, I believe physicians and patients could discuss their options using the precepts of proportional advocacy. At first, these conversations may feel awkward and create tension, and such discussions could be impeded by the pressure to spend less time with patients. Yet, as our society learns more about issues of health care rationing, I believe these conversations can be held in a way that will build trust through the honesty and forthrightness with which such "difficult" topics are addressed. Proportional advocacy offers an avowedly communitarian ethic—one that, in my experience, patients respond to positively if invited in as a partner to consider the options fairly.

Can proportional advocacy capture the ethical imagination and instincts of more practicing physicians? Can it convince patients and the public that they are valued partners in rationing decisions? I think it can. Proportional advocacy—if it can grow hand-in-hand with greater communication, collaboration, and social justice in our health care system—may offer physicians and patients a way to join together and lead the effort to find the best way to take care of all of us within a responsible budget.

EXCERPT 4

Abridged text from:

P.A. Ubel and R. Arnold, "The Unbearable Rightness of Bedside Rationing: Physician Duties in a Climate of Cost Containment," *Archives of Internal Medicine* 155, no. 17 (1995): pp. 1837–1842.

Unbearable Rightness of Bedside Rationing: Physician Duties in a Climate of Cost Containment

P. Ubel and R. Arnold

. . .

We use the term *bedside rationing* to refer to physicians' actions to withhold beneficial care from patients that the physicians were free to offer to them. As we use the term, it refers mainly to rationing that is done either without patients being aware of the rationing or, less often, with patients being aware but being given no choice. We will not concern ourselves with instances where physicians talk patients into accepting rationing.

. . .

Evaluating Cost-Control Mechanisms that Rely, at Least in Part, on Bedside Rationing

Some mechanisms control costs by strictly circumscribing physicians' actions; others control costs by setting flexible goals for physicians so they can retain control of individual clinical decisions. These mechanisms attempt to influence physicians' aggregate utilization patterns without stating when the physicians can or cannot obtain things like ankle films. For example, a system could control costs by setting global budgets or by setting spending targets for individual physicians. This system would not need to dictate clinical care to physicians. Physicians in such systems would not need to be monitored to see if they complied with elaborate practice guidelines or reimbursement rules. Rather, they could be monitored to see if they met some kind of standard for average expenditures. In meeting those standards, physicians could decide when a potential benefit was worth seeking for their patients, perhaps on occasion offering services that may not be recommended in practice guidelines and perhaps on other occasions withholding marginal benefits that they do not think justify the expense.

It is important to understand that this type of system is not necessarily devoid of rules. Utilization reviews, formulary committees, and the like may play a role in containing costs. But the rules used in this type of system will not be expected to carry the entire burden of cost containment. Instead, physicians will be allowed, perhaps even expected, to ration marginally beneficial care at the bedside. This will allow health care plans to develop rules that are more flexible and more appropriate to the complexities of clinical practice.[1,2] Consequently, the plans will be likely to result in better patient care.

The tradeoff, thus, is clear. Without bedside rationing, we can only contain costs with a complex set of rules circumscribing physicians' actions, rules that are likely to harm patients whose specific medical conditions are not adequately captured by the rules. With bedside rationing, we can contain costs with less complex rules, but we must also worry that the discretion this gives physicians will be used discriminatorily or will harm the doctor-patient relationship. What should we do?

---

[1] H. G. Welch, J. Bernat, and R. P. Mogielnicki, "Who's in Charge Here?," *Journal of General Internal Medicine* 9, no. 8 (1994): pp. 450–454.

[2] H. G. Welch, "Should the Health Care Forest Be Selectively Thinned by Physicians or Clear Cut by Payers?," *Annals of Internal Medicine* 115, no. 3 (1991): pp. 223–226.

The Short- and Medium-Run Answer

In the long run, it is not clear which of these mechanisms we should use. It is conceivable that we could devise rules and procedures that remove physicians from the need to make individualized rationing decisions, while preserving a high standard of clinical practice.[3] In this case, there would be no reason to ration at the bedside. On the other hand, it is also conceivable that no set of rules will control costs without seriously damaging the quality of patient care. Clinical medicine is a science of particulars, so even the most rigorous guidelines may not capture everything they need to. In this latter case, we will be left with a tradeoff between relying exclusively on rules to ration (while reducing the quality of patient care) or relying in part on physicians to ration (while creating the possibility that they will not do so in a fair manner).

In the short run, and probably in the medium run of the next 5 to 10 years, the moral choice is much clearer: we are in no position to eliminate bedside rationing. First, if physicians were told they could no longer ration at the bedside, the cost of health care would continue to rise even faster than it already is. While few investigators have studied the actual incidence of bedside rationing,[4] and no one that we know of has determined its economic impact, our clinical experience and our conversations with other physicians suggest that the practice is widespread. Physicians ration so often they do not even realize it. They order computed tomographic scans even though magnetic resonance imaging may yield a fraction more benefit; they prescribe Benadryl even though Seldane has fewer side effects; and they adjust the frequency of screening pap smears when the yield of more frequent screening becomes too small to be worth it. All these actions essentially save money by rationing small benefits from patients.

Second, we have not developed enough guidelines and rationing rules to effectively contain costs. Oregon has made the most serious attempt to set up an administrative rationing mechanism that will remove the need for bedside rationing. But it is too early to know whether its system will control costs. Many of the categories of covered services include generous room for physician interpretation, stating, for example, that the cost of certain cancer therapies will be reimbursed if the cancer is "treatable."[5] Physicians clinging to the traditional view of their duties could interpret this type of language in ways that will undermine Oregon's efforts to control costs.

Third, and most importantly, the ability of rules to contain costs is dependent on physicians' willingness to accept rationing. If physicians feel that their duty is to do everything within their power to benefit patients, they will find ways around all but the most stringent rules.[6] Some of us may counter that physicians who follow the spirit of the rules will not undermine their effectiveness. But the spirit of many of these rules results in rationing marginally beneficial services from patients. If that is the spirit that opponents of bedside rationing want physicians to accept, then we have a distinction without a difference, for we have accepted the notion that physicians ought to restrain their advocacy roles, if only enough to withhold marginal benefits that cost society large sums of money.

An (at Least Temporary) Ethic of Bedside Rationing

Because physicians will be required to do some amount of bedside rationing for at least

[3] D. C. Hadorn, *Basic Benefits and Clinical Guidelines* (HarperCollins Canada, 1992).

[4] B. Brody, et al., "The Impact of Economic Considerations on Clinical Decisionmaking: The Case of Thrombolytic Therapy," *Medical Care* 29, no. 9 (1991): pp. 899–910.

[5] Oregon Health Services Commission, *Prioritization of Health Services: A Report to the Governor and Legislature* (Oregon Health Services Commission, 1993).

[6] E. Morreim, "Gaming the System: Dodging the Rules, Ruling the Dodgers," *Archives of Internal Medicine* 151, no. 3 (1991): pp. 443–447.

the short and medium term, we must begin to define those factors that physicians should consider in deciding when it is appropriate to ration at the bedside.

The moral acceptability of bedside rationing depends crucially on which services physicians think fit to ration. For bedside rationing to be morally tolerable, physicians should base rationing decisions on medical costs and benefits, not on racial or sexual biases. In addition, they should only ration marginally beneficial services, not ones that bring significant benefits to their patients. We have been using the term *marginally beneficial* to describe the types of services physicians could, most plausibly, be allowed to ration. Defining this term precisely is impossible. But several concepts can help to clarify what it means in a way that can begin to settle the moral debate.

First, similar to the way we measure cost-effectiveness, physicians should think of marginally beneficial services in terms of both a numerator (costs) and a denominator (benefits). We need to know something about both before we can judge a service. Very inexpensive services, such as a screening calcium test, may offer minuscule benefits that do not justify their cost. Similarly, extremely expensive services may offer significant benefits that more than justify their cost. Oregon ignored this insight when, before developing the Medicaid plan, it decided to curtail funding for all transplants, figuring it could use the funds in more beneficial ways.[7] Its decision, ultimately repealed, concentrated only on the cost of transplantation, and thus overlooked other services which, when both cost and benefit were measured, would have proved to be a worse use of state money.

Second, the true cost-effectiveness of a health care intervention can only be determined if something is known about the costs and benefits of alternative interventions. For example, it would be wrong to determine the cost-effectiveness of a yearly pap smear by taking its costs and dividing by its benefits. This ignores the fact that most of the benefit of screening for cervical cancer can be achieved by screening every 3 years.[8] To calculate the cost-effectiveness of a yearly pap smear, one must first measure the extra cost of yearly pap smears as opposed to pap smears every 3 years and then divide this by the extra benefit brought by yearly screening. From this point of view, one would have to spend more than $1 million for every year of life gained by yearly pap smears over every 3 years.[9]

Third, the cost-effectiveness of specific therapies often varies widely depending on patient preferences.[10] For example, the cost-effectiveness of radiation therapy for prostate cancer is greater for patients who place a high value on sexual potency than for those who do not.[11] Thus, physicians need to consider patients' preferences when they are making rationing choices. This includes finding out what the patients think about various outcomes that they may experience. It also includes talking about patients' out-of-pocket costs to find out, for example, whether they are willing to pay for the small benefits that they could receive with marginally beneficial services.

While cost-effectiveness is a very helpful tool in making rationing decisions, it must be used with caution. The techniques used to measure cost and, especially, effectiveness do not necessarily reflect the relative value society places on various resources.[12] This is especially true when one is dealing with specific individuals who have potentially treatable illnesses. Society does not place a consistent value on

[7] H. G. Welch and E. B. Larson, "Dealing with Limited Resources," *New England Journal of Medicine* 319, no. 3 (1988): pp. 171–173.

[8] D. M. Eddy, "Screening for Cervical Cancer," Annals of Internal Medicine 113, no. 3 (1990): pp. 214–226.

[9] Ibid.

[10] M. F. Drummond, et al., "Selection of End Points in Economic Evaluations of Coronary Heart Disease Interventions," *Medical Decision Making* 13, no. 3 (1993): pp. 184–190.

[11] P. A. Singer, et al., "Sex or Survival: Trade-Offs Between Quality and Quantity of Life," *Journal of Clinical Oncology* 9, no. 2 (1991): pp. 328–334.

[12] D. C. Hadorn, "Setting Health Care Priorities in Oregon: Cost-Effectiveness Meets the Rule of Rescue," *Journal of the American Medical Association* 265, no. 17 (1991): pp. 2218–2225.

people's lives.[13] It is willing to spend enormous sums of money to save one child who falls into a well, yet it is unwilling to spend the same amount to save more children through prenatal care.[14] Physicians need to recognize this seeming inconsistency and factor that into their rationing decisions. Thus, physicians should be wary of withholding therapies from severely ill patients, even if cost-effectiveness studies suggest that there are better ways of spending health care dollars.

Physicians should not be expected to perform cost-effectiveness analyses at the bedside. Rather, they should become familiar enough with the concepts of cost-effectiveness so that they can more accurately identify marginally beneficial health care services. Indeed, given the necessity of bedside rationing, it is time to do more to train physicians in the economics of clinical decision making.

Conclusions

While we have only begun to discuss how and when physicians should ration at the bedside, continuing this discussion is crucial for the future of medicine. Bedside rationing is here to stay, at least for the immediate future. It creates moral problems, but these have been overstated. In addition, those mechanisms that would control costs without relying on bedside rationing raise moral problems of their own, being too primitive at present to capture the subtleties of medical practice. For at least the next 5 or 10 years, physicians will need to ration at the bedside. The medical profession needs to admit this openly, so that physicians can begin to talk openly about when they ration, and so they can learn more about when they ought to ration. Physicians are less likely to find their dual roles (as patient and societal advocates) unbearable if they can talk together about how best to balance them.

---

13 T. C. Schelling, "The Life You Save May Be Your Own," in *Problems in Public Expenditure Analysis*, edited by S. B. Chase (Washington, DC: Brookings Institution, 1968).

14 A. Gore, *Earth in the Balance: Ecology and the Human Spirit* (Plume, 1993).

EXCERPT 5

Abridged text from:

D. Strech, M. Synofzik, and G. M. Marckmann, "How Physicians Allocate Scarce Resources at the Bedside: A Systematic Review of Qualitative Studies," *Journal of Medicine and Philosophy* 33, no. 1 (2008): pp. 80–99.

How Physicians Allocate Scarce Resources at the Bedside: A Systematic Review of Qualitative Studies

Strech, Daniel, Matthis Synofzik, and Georg Marckmann

. . .

Priority setting and rationing occur at all levels in almost all health-care systems around the world. Countries with very different health-care systems and levels of health-care spending all grapple with the problem of how to reconcile a steadily increasing demand for health-care services with limited or even declining financial resources. . . . [We] need empirical information about how physicians deal with resource constraints at the bedside and about the practical challenges and opportunities in optimizing the allocation of scarce health-care resources. Quantitative and qualitative interview research with physicians on HCR provides important information about how financial constraints influence clinical decision making and the doctor-patient relationship and about the criteria that physicians use to allocate scarce resources to individual patients.

[T]here is still limited and scattered information about how physicians perceive and execute this bedside rationing (BSR) and how it can be performed in an ethically fair way. This review gives a systematic overview on physicians' perspectives on influences, strategies, and consequences of health-care rationing. Retrieved studies focused on themes that fell under three major headings: (i) conditions and influences of BSR, (ii) strategies of BSR, and (iii) consequences of BSR.

. . .

Table [13.2] summarizes the themes identified in the studies. . . .

. . .

. . .

We identified several social and psychological factors that strongly influence BSR. In particular, they are related (i) to the specific context of BSR, (ii) to the attitudes of the physician, and (iii) to the characteristics of the patient. The highly subjective nature and variability of these determinants underline the need for more explicit and consistent rationing mechanisms that clearly define which patients should get which services under certain medical conditions, for example, cost-conscious guidelines. . . . Our review shows that factors like (i) the patient's individual ability to exercise pressure, (ii) the fact whether the patient exhibits a demanding behavior, (iii) the patient's ability to articulate his/her wishes, or (iv) the physician's implicit categorization of a patient ("good performer" or "bad performer") currently might determine whether a patient gets an intervention or not. The powerful influence of individual and situational factors violates the basic ethical requirement of consistent rationing decisions.[1] Although BSR will always be influenced by case-specific factors inherent in daily medical practice, which certainly constrains the application of ethical principles and rationing standards[2], this fact does not per se eliminate the need to develop explicit and consistent rationing standards.

Our review reveals a remarkable ambivalence in physicians' attitudes toward explicit standards of care: On the one hand, several themes describe a need for relieving the burden of BSR for physicians; on the other hand, another set of themes suggests

[1] N. Daniels, "Accountability for Reasonableness," *British Medical Journal* 321 (2000): pp. 1300–1301.

[2] L. Berney, et al., "Ethical Principles and the Rationing of Health Care: A Qualitative Study in General Practice," *British Journal of General Practice* 55, no. 517 (2005): pp. 620–625.

Table [13.2]

Themes identified in the 10 references included in this review (the numbers indicate the codes used in our review to label the studies that presented quotes in relation to those themes; for further study characteristics see Table 13.1)

Conditions/factors of influence	Strategies/line of action	Consequences
Context related	Implicit	Rationing is already happening
Number of hospital beds (7)	Deferral (3, 4, 6, 8)	Rationing is already happening (1–8, 10)
Time constraints (6)	Deflection (5)	
Operating budget (7)	Delay (8)	Role conflicts
Situatedness (2, 3, 5, 6)	Early discharge (8)	Professional autonomy versus health authority guidelines (3, 6)
Availability of resources (6, 7)	Budgeting (7, 10)	
Access to relevant information (7, 10)	Remain silent (6)	Professional autonomy versus patient autonomy (3)
	Importance of intuition (2, 6)	
Influence from the pharmaceutical industry (10)	Time (6)	Patient's advocate versus society's/hospital's resources (gatekeeper) (1, 3, 5, 6, 10)
Doctor related	Negotiation (with the patient, with third parties) (3, 4, 6)	
Reluctancy to ration (1, 3, 10)	Manipulation of the system (10)	Competition for patients versus need to ration health care (3, 5)
Lack of interest (10)	Explicit	Personal interests versus patient's interests (1, 4)
Inability to maintain consistent standards of care (1–3, 6)	Need for explicit rationing (1)	
	Black list (1)	Emotional stress
Inability to change professional standards (10)	Rules/guidelines (3, 6)	Embarrassment (2, 5, 8)
Desire for satisfying patient (2, 3, 10)	Involving an interdisciplinary committee (1, 5, 7)	Frustration (6, 8)
Obligation to provide best treatment (3)	Involving politicians/government (1, 7)	
Fears regarding a shifting of costs (1, 8, 10)	Involving patients/public (1, 6, 7)	
	Criteria for prioritization	
Extremity of need/lifesaving (2, 7–9)	Effectiveness/Evidence based medicine (1, 2, 7, 9)	
Personal involvement with the patient (1, 2, 5, 6)	Cost-effectiveness (1, 2, 7–10)	
Typification and implicit categorization of patients (6)	Ability to pay co-payments (1, 3, 9)	
	Age (1, 8)	
Lack of economical competence (1, 3, 10)	Justice/fairness/equity (1, 2, 4, 5, 7)	
Patient related	Not: justice/fairness/equity (1, 3)	
Articulate patients (2, 6, 8)	Contribution to society (2, 8)	
Ability to exercise pressure (2, 3, 6, 8, 10)	Not: individual health responsibility (6, 9)	
Demanding/consumer mentality (3)		
Time-conscious patients (6) Patients preferences (2, 3)		
Personal circumstances of the patient (2, 5, 6, 10)		

physicians' inability to maintain or adapt consistent standards of care. This inability, however, apparently does not result from an inherent feature of medical practice or from irrevocable structures of our health-care systems, but rather from a personal psychological motive—the desire to satisfy the patient's preferences.

How Should We Ration?

Our review confirms that physicians see rationing as a matter of fact that is widely prevalent in everyday medical practice. This supports the view that the crucial question in the current debate is not *whether* we should ration or not, but *how* we can ration in a fair and efficient manner.[3] According to our analysis, physicians employ different *implicit* rationing strategies, such as deferral and deflection of patients. The fact that these measures are less transparent and less well controllable underlines the need for the development and implementation of *explicit* rationing mechanisms: Only if rationing is performed according to explicit, transparent, and general standards can it be performed in a (i) consistent, (ii) medically rational, and (iii) ethically fair way (since it allows an equal treatment). In fact, our analysis reveals a further argument: (iv) Explicit rationing relieves physicians from the emotional distress resulting from implicit rationing and, moreover, might put less pressure onto the physician-patient relationship.

Rationing, the Multitude of Role Conflicts and Controversial Prioritization Criteria—A Challenge for Allocation Ethics

Our results demonstrate that BSR might lead to various role conflicts for physicians. It is by now widely acknowledged that the traditional picture of a physician as acting in an encapsulated physician-patient dyad is no longer adequate, since he/she in fact maintains multiple accountabilities.[4] BSR leads to several role conflicts and ethical tensions, for example, the tension between professional autonomy and health authority guidelines or the tension between physicians' private (financial) interests and the patients' health interests. . . .

Moreover, the high variability of allocation criteria presented in this review calls into question the consistency of physicians' rationing decisions at the bedside. In contrast to the aforementioned psychological and social factors of influence, ethical criteria, however, were only rarely mentioned and their exact meaning remained opaque. In other words, BSR seems to be only poorly influenced by explicit and transparent ethical criteria. . . .

Implications for Health Policy and Health-Care Ethics

The complexity of BSR and the various context- and patient-related determinants have implications for health policy as well as for research on the ethics of rationing. Given the high variability of physicians' rationing decisions at the bedside, developing explicit and consistent rationing tools like cost-conscious guidelines should be a priority in health policy. Cost-conscious guidelines are based on the best available empirical evidence on the effectiveness and cost-effectiveness of medical interventions.[5] They allow an explicit and more systematic balancing of different allocation criteria. Instead of relying on their intuitive clinical judgment, physicians can draw on evidence-based guidance to make allocation decisions at the bedside. This can increase the transparency and consistency of BSR and

[3] P. A. Ubel, *Pricing Life: Why It's Time for Health Care Rationing* (MIT Press, 2001).

[4] S. M. Shortell, et al., "Physicians as Double Agents: Maintaining Trust in an Era of Multiple Accountabilities," *Journal of the American Medical Association* 280, no. 12 (1998): pp. 1102–1108.

[5] M. Eccles and J. Mason, "How to Develop Cost-Conscious Guidelines," *Health Technol Assess* 5, no. 16 (2001): pp. 1–69.

thereby the fairness of allocation decisions on the micro level. If the specific situation of the patient requires deviating from the recommended course of action, the physician should clearly state the underlying reasons.

The influencing factors identified in our review, however, present considerable barriers to the implementation of cost-conscious guidelines. The development and implementation of these explicit instruments for rationing decisions should, therefore, be accompanied by rigorous evaluation of their feasibility and applicability. Further quantitative and qualitative research is necessary to analyze the relative importance of the various influencing factors in different contexts of BSR.[6,7]

[6] J. J. M. van Delden, et al., "Medical Decision Making in Scarcity Situations," *Journal of Medical Ethics* 30, no. 2 (2004): pp. 207–211.

[7] S. A. Hurst, et al., "Prevalence and Determinants of Physician Bedside Rationing," *Journal of General Internal Medicine* 21, no. 11 (2006): pp. 1138–1143.

EXCERPT 6

Abridged text from:

L. Snyder, "American College of Physicians Ethics Manual, Sixth Edition," *Annals of Internal Medicine* 156 (2012): pp. 73–104.

ACP *Ethics Manual*: 6th edition: Care of Patients Near the End of Life

. . .

"Futile" Treatments

In the circumstance that no evidence shows that a specific treatment desired by the patient will provide any medical benefit, the physician is not ethically obliged to provide such treatment (although the physician should be aware of any relevant state law). The physician need not provide an effort at resuscitation that cannot conceivably restore circulation and breathing, but he or she should help the family to understand and accept this reality. The more common and much more difficult circumstance occurs when treatment offers some small prospect of benefit at a great burden of suffering (or financial cost—see "Resource Allocation" within in the Physician and Society section), but the patient or family nevertheless desires it. If the physician and patient (or appropriate surrogate) cannot agree on how to proceed, there is no easy, automatic solution. Consultation with learned colleagues or an ethics consultation may be helpful in ascertaining what interventions have a reasonable balance of burden and benefit. Timely transfer of care to another clinician who is willing to pursue the patient's preference may resolve the problem. Infrequently, resort to the courts may be necessary. Some jurisdictions have specific processes and standards for allowing these unilateral decisions.

Some institutions allow physicians to unilaterally write a DNR order over patient or family objections when the patient may survive, at most, for only a brief time in the hospital. Empathy and thoughtful exploration of options for care with patients or surrogate decision makers should make such impasses rare. Full discussion about the issue should include the indications for and outcomes of cardiopulmonary resuscitation, the physical impact on the patient, the implications for clinicians, the impact (or lack thereof) of a DNR order on other care, the legal aspects of such orders, and the physician's role as patient advocate. A physician who writes a unilateral DNR order must inform the patient or surrogate when doing so.

. . .

The Ethics of Practice

The Changing Practice Environment

. . .

Physicians have an obligation to promote their patients' welfare in an increasingly complex health care system. This entails forthrightly helping patients to understand clinical recommendations and make informed choices among all appropriate care options. It includes management of the conflicts of interest and multiple commitments that arise in any practice environment, especially in an era of cost concerns. It also includes stewardship of finite health care resources so that as many health care needs as possible can be met, whether in the physician's office, in the hospital or long-term care facility, or at home.

The patient–physician relationship and the principles that govern it should be central to the delivery of care. These principles include beneficence, honesty, confidentiality, privacy, and advocacy when patient interests may be endangered by arbitrary, unjust, or inadequately individualized programs or procedures. Health care, however, does take place in a broader context beyond the patient–physician relationship. A patient's preferences or interests may conflict with the interests or values of the physician, an institution, a payer, other members of an insurance plan who have equal claim to the same health care resources, or society.

The physician's first and primary duty is to the patient. Physicians must base their counsel on the interests of the individual patient, regardless of the insurance or medical care delivery setting. Whether financial incentives in the fee-for-service system prompt physicians to do more rather than less or capitation arrangements encourage them to do less rather than more, physicians must not allow such considerations to affect their clinical judgment or patient counseling on treatment options, including referrals.[1]

The physician's professional role is to make recommendations on the basis of the best available medical evidence and to pursue options that comport with the patient's unique health needs, values, and preferences.[2]

Physicians have a responsibility to practice effective and efficient health care and to use health care resources responsibly. Parsimonious care that utilizes the most efficient means to effectively diagnose a condition and treat a patient respects the need to use resources wisely and to help ensure that resources are equitably available. In making recommendations to patients, designing practice guidelines and formularies, and making decisions on medical benefits review boards, physicians' considered judgments should reflect the best available evidence in the biomedical literature, including data on the cost-effectiveness of different clinical approaches. When patients ask, they should be informed of the rationale that underlies the physician's recommendation.

In instances of disagreement between patient and physician for any reason, the physician is obligated to explain the basis for the disagreement, to educate the patient, and to meet the patient's needs for comfort and reassurance. Providers of health insurance are not obliged to underwrite approaches that patients may value but that are not justifiable on clinical or theoretical scientific grounds or that are relatively cost-ineffective compared with other therapies for the same condition or other therapies offered by the health plan for other conditions. However, there must be a fair appeals procedure.

The physician's duty further requires serving as the patient's agent within the health care arena, advocating through the necessary avenues to obtain treatment that is essential to the individual patient's care regardless of the barriers that may discourage the physician from doing so. Moreover, physicians should advocate just as vigorously for the needs of their most vulnerable and disadvantaged patients as for the needs of their most articulate patients.[3]

. . .

Pay-for-performance programs can help improve the quality of care, but they must be aligned with the goals of medical professionalism. The main focus of the quality movement in health care should not, however, be on "pay for" or "performance" based on limited measures. Program incentives for a few specific elements of a single disease or condition may neglect the complexity of care for the whole patient, especially patients with multiple chronic conditions. Deselection of patients and "playing to the measures" rather than focusing on the patient are also dangers. Quality programs must put the needs and interests of the patient first.[4]

Organizations that provide health insurance coverage should not restrict the information or counsel that physicians may give patients. Physicians must provide information to the patient about all appropriate care and referral options. Providers of health insurance coverage must disclose all relevant information about benefits, including any restrictions, and about financial incentives that might negatively affect patient access to care.[5]

. . .

[1] Povar, "Ethics in Practice."

[2] J. LaPuma, D. Schiedermayer and M. Seigler, "Ethical Issues in Managed Care," *Trends Health Care Law Ethics* 10 (1995): pp. 73–77.

[3] Povar, "Ethics in Practice."

[4] L. Snyder and R. L. Neubauer, "Pay-for-Performance Principles That Promote Patient-Centered Care: An Ethics Manifesto," *Annals of Internal Medicine* 147, no. 11 (2007): pp. 792–794.

[5] Povar, "Ethics in Practice."

The Physician and Society

Resource Allocation

Medical care is delivered within social and institutional systems that must take overall resources into account. Increasingly, decisions about resource allocations challenge the physician's primary role as patient advocate. This advocacy role has always had limits. For example, a physician should not lie to third-party payers for a patient in order to ensure coverage or maximize reimbursement. Moreover, a physician is not obligated to provide all treatments and diagnostics without considering their effectiveness.[6] The just allocation of resources and changing reimbursement methods present the physician with ethical problems that cannot be ignored. Two principles are agreed on:

1. As a physician performs his or her primary role as a patient's trusted advocate, he or she has a responsibility to use all health-related resources in a technically appropriate and efficient manner. He or she should plan work-ups carefully and avoid unnecessary testing, medications, surgery, and consultations.
2. Resource allocation decisions are most appropriately made at the policy level rather than entirely in the context of an individual patient–physician encounter. Ethical allocation policy is best achieved when all affected parties discuss what resources exist, to what extent they are limited, what costs attach to various benefits, and how to equitably balance all these factors.

Physicians, patient advocates, insurers, and payers should participate together in decisions at the policy level; should emphasize the value of health to society; should promote justice in the health care system; and should base allocations on medical need, efficacy, cost-effectiveness, and proper distribution of benefits and burdens in society.

[6] J. A. Tulsky and L. Snyder, "Deciding How Much Care Is Too Much," ACP Observer, 1997, www.acponline.org/journals/news/mar97/howmuch.htm.

Further Resources

Relevant Organizations

Governmental

American Board of Internal Medicine: A nonprofit organization that aims to establish uniform standards for internal medicine physicians. Additional information can be found at http://www.abim.org/about/default.aspx

American College of Physicians (ACP): A nonprofit national organization of internists that aims to enhance the quality and effectiveness of healthcare. Additional information can be found at https://www.acponline.org/

American Thoracic Society: A nonprofit organization that aims to improve health worldwide by advancing research, clinical care, and public health in respiratory disease, critical illness, and sleep disorders. Additional information can be found at http://www.thoracic.org/

Literature

Bloche, Maxwell Gregg. *The Hippocratic Myth: Why Doctors Are Under Pressure to Ration Care, Practice Politics, and Compromise Their Promise to Heal* (New York: Palgrave Macmillan, 2011).

Hurst, Samia A., Anne-Marie Slowther, Reidun Forde, Renzo Pegoraro, Stella Reiter-Theil, Arnaud Perrier, Elizabeth Garrett-Mayer, and Marion Danis. "Prevalence and Determinants of Physician Bedside Rationing: Data from Europe." *Journal of General Internal Medicine* 21, no. 11 (2006): 1138–1143.

Peter, A. Ubel. "Physicians, Thou Shalt Ration: The Necessary Role of Bedside Rationing in Controlling Healthcare Costs." *Healthcare Papers* 2, no. 2 (2002): 10–21.

Pollack, Andrew. "Cost of Treatment May Influence Doctors." *New York Times,* April 17, 2014.

Storrs, Carina, "The Doctor Will Judge You Now," *CNN,* January 19, 2016.

World Medical Association. "Declaration of Geneva." http://www.wma.net/en/30publications/10policies/g1/

Other Media

60 Minutes, "The Cost of Dying: End-Of-Life-Care." *CBSNews,* August 05, 2010: The challenges of saying no to a patient dying and the costs of this are discussed.

Bob Abernethy, "Ethics of Health Care Rationing," *PBS* video, 10:09, August 8, 2008, http://www.pbs.org/wnet/religionandethics/2008/08/08/ethics-of-health-care-rationing/16/: Staff at a hospital in Texas are interviewed about bedside rationing.

Mark Bertolini, Ralph De La Torre, Ezekiel Emanuel, and Gary Loveman, "Cost Challenges Facing the U.S. Healthcare System," *The Wall Street Journal* video, 1:00:34, September 15, 2013, http://www.wsj.com/video/cost-challenges-facing-the-us-healthcare-system/56734711-3493-47E7-ABA8-5514DB011AC0.html: Methods of containing healthcare spending are discussed, such as rationing and resource allocation by physicians.

14 Personal Responsibility for Health

Rationing and resource allocation dilemmas have in common that their impact can sometimes be lessened through changes on the demand side. If people were healthier, there would be less competition for scarce organs or limited ICU beds. Similarly, if fewer people were overweight or obese, there would be reduced need for treating (and funding) interventions for weight-related conditions such as heart disease, stroke, high blood pressure, or hip or knee replacements. In the United States, around 40% of premature mortality is attributed to behavioral patterns,[1] and it is estimated that between $300 billion and $500 billion is spent annually on preventable diseases.[2] Resources that would not be needed for these conditions could be freed for other health needs, such as pregnancy or birth-related care, accidents, many types of cancer, and a range of other conditions in which people have very limited opportunity to avoid requiring healthcare.

Countries such as Germany explicitly emphasize in health law the link between individual behavior and the efficient operation of a healthcare system. Book V of the German Social Security Code governs the provision of publicly funded healthcare. Its overarching Article 1 is entitled "Solidarity and personal responsibility" and states:

> In the spirit of a mutually supportive solidaristic community, the task of providers of statutory health insurance is to maintain, restore or improve health of the insured. The insured have co-responsibility for their health; through a health-conscious way of living, taking part in age-appropriate preventative measures [and] playing an active role in treatment and rehabilitation, they should contribute to avoiding illness and disability, and overcoming the respective

[1] S. A. Schroeder, "We Can Do Better—Improving the Health of the American People," *New England Journal of Medicine* 357, no. 12 (2007): pp. 1221–1228.

[2] PricewaterhouseCoopers' Health Research Institute, *The Price of Excess: Identifying Waste in Healthcare Spending* (2008), p. 6.

> consequences. The insurers are to assist the insured persons through the provision of information, advice and services, and should encourage a health-conscious way of living.[3]

The concept of co-responsibility implied in the German Code entails two normative assumptions. First, the community has a certain degree of responsibility for the health of each individual. In this sense, individuals are entitled to ask the community for assistance. Second, the community has certain claims against individuals. The appeal to stay healthy is made in the expectation that this will help control overall expenditure and opportunity costs and lessen resource allocation dilemmas. Not using services unnecessarily may also avoid the denial of resources to persons in need, due to absolute scarcity, thereby attenuating rationing dilemmas.[4]

The German Code's Article 2, on "necessity, efficiency, and personal responsibility" is unequivocal in stressing people's obligations in this respect:

> Services . . . are to be provided by insurers with due respect to the principle of efficiency . . . and insofar as the need for services is not attributable to the personal responsibility of the insured person. . . . Payers, providers and insured persons must seek to ensure the clinically effective and efficient utilization of services, which are only to be used insofar as necessary.[5]

The Code then embeds its concept of personal responsibility in several specific policies. For instance, there are lower dental care co-pays for patients who receive regular check-ups (annually for adults, biannually for minors). Similarly, there is the so-called healthy lifestyle bonus: insurance rebates or in-kind benefits, such as sports equipment, for participation in primary and secondary prevention check-ups or for an active gym membership. In addition, people who, over the course of a year, do not require hospitalization and do not see their primary care physician for a prescription get a bonus for having no medical claims. Financial penalties for avoidable health needs also feature in the law and include an obligation to repay part or all of the treatment cost for care that is required if an injury or a condition resulted from having engaged in criminal actions or from nontherapeutic cosmetic surgery, tattoos, or piercing.[6]

A fundamental assumption underlying the German approach is that better health will lead to lower cost to the healthcare system. This idea is most clearly reflected in the financing arrangements for the healthy lifestyle bonus program. Insurance rebates and other incentives may be funded through gain-sharing only. That means that, insofar as all those who participate in the bonus programs have lower medical claims than those who did not, the participants may receive a portion of the savings in the form of the bonus. Health plans offering this type of program must report every three years to regulatory authorities. If they cannot demonstrate lower cost for the groups participating in the incentive programs, no bonuses may be paid.[7] While it is not permissible to vary insurance premiums in publicly funded healthcare by health status, indirectly, those who make efforts to live healthily and use fewer services are able to reduce their insurance premiums through lower co-payments and bonus payments.

The German model is largely based on sharing gains resulting from savings. In the United States, by contrast, a different principle is at play. The United States permits raising costs based on health outcomes, not just participation in health programs. This can be done in two ways, which may be pursued in isolation or in combination. First, the insurance provider may impose higher insurance cost on insurance holders who do not meet

[3] H. Schmidt, "Bonuses as Incentives and Rewards for Health Responsibility: A Good Thing?," *Journal of Medicine and Philosophy* 33, no. 3 (2008): p. 200.

[4] Ibid.

[5] Ibid., pp. 200–201.

[6] Ibid.

[7] Ibid.

certain health standards. Second, providers may also shift cost among insurance holders. For example, they may offer lower premiums for those who do meet health standards and finance these discounts through surcharges for insurance holders who do not meet standards.[8] The standards are based on risk factor targets such as body mass index, blood pressure, or cholesterol thresholds: where levels are too high, insurance costs increase. Where levels are on or below target, insurance costs may be decreased. Due to the United States' fragmented healthcare system, these provisions do not apply universally, but only for group insurance (covering approximately half of the population).

The concept of *wellness incentives* implies that individuals do not always act in ways that promote their own health.[9] Similar to the German approach, rewards and penalties are deemed effective means of encouraging personal responsibility for health. However, a major difference between the US and German provisions is that both the ways and amounts used to incentivize people differ. In Germany, people who are deemed to live healthily and use services as directed receive bonuses that rarely exceed $100 annually. In the United States, people who meet health risk targets may receive lower premiums, but, more likely, those who meet targets do not face surcharges. The magnitude of these incentives can be up to 30% of the total cost of coverage (around $1,500 for single coverage) and up to 50% including the special case of tobacco use (around $2,500 for single coverage).[10]

Three ethical questions are raised by incentives in the context of resource allocation: (1) Do the different types of incentive programs work in terms of improving health? (2) Do they lead to lower cost? And (3), are there any ethical issues to be considered in designing incentive programs?

In many ways, the question of the potential of incentives to promote health is a complex and unsettled one. Several robust studies have shown great promise, but, overall, it is a field that is still in relatively nascent stages.[11] While it is difficult to generalize, incentivizing so-called simple or one-off behaviors, such as getting vaccinated, can be highly effective in terms of improving health outcomes.[12] But for "complex" behaviors, such as chronic conditions that require sustained behavior and lifestyle changes over months or years, the evidence is less clear, even if there are some robust examples.

For instance, tobacco use is harmful and highly addictive. A recent systematic review of studies that used financial incentives to help with smoking cessation[13] identified 21 randomized controlled trials (RCTs), but only two that demonstrate effectiveness beyond the period that incentives were provided.[14,15] In both studies, a bundle of incentives that were staggered over time and amounted to around $800 led to threefold higher quit rates compared to usual care that comprised informational resources and free smoking cessation aids. A review of several decades of weight-loss studies found positive effects but concluded that results varied widely and that "many important questions about the use of incentives have not yet

8 "Incentives for Nondiscriminatory Wellness Programs in Group Health Plans," *Federal Register,* 78, no. 106 (2013): pp. 33157–33192.

9 G. Loewenstein, et al., "Can Behavioural Economics Make Us Healthier?," *BMJ* 344 (2012).

10 K. Madison, H. Schmidt, and K. G. Volpp, "Smoking, Obesity, Health Insurance, and Health Incentives in the Affordable Care Act," *JAMA* 310, no. 2 (2013): pp. 143–144.

11 Loewenstein, "Can Behavioural Economics Make Us Healthier?"

12 A. Oliver and L. D. Brown, "A Consideration of User Financial Incentives to Address Health Inequalities," *J Health Polit Policy Law* 37, no. 2 (2012): pp. 201–226.

13 K. Cahill, J. Hartmann-Boyce, and R. Perera, "Incentives for Smoking Cessation," *Cochrane Database Syst Rev* 5 (2015): p. CD004307.

14 K. G. Volpp, et al., "A Randomized, Controlled Trial of Financial Incentives for Smoking Cessation," *New England Journal of Medicine* 360, no. 7 (2009): pp. 699–709.

15 S. D. Halpern, et al., "Randomized Trial of Four Financial-Incentive Programs for Smoking Cessation," *New England Journal of Medicine* 372, no. 22 (2015): pp. 2108–2117.

been clearly answered."[16] Another recent systematic review, comprising 33 studies and 63 different outcomes, concluded that the studies yielded mixed results regarding impact on health-related behaviors, substance use, and physiological markers such as blood pressures, as well as cost.[17] This review, along with further recent studies[18] and a major report to the US Congress[19] (see the short version by Mattke et al.[20]), echo the theme of limited evidence from rigorous evaluations on the effectiveness of incentives in improving health outcomes. Implementation rules by the US Government succinctly summarize the situation as follows: "insufficient broad-based evidence makes it difficult to definitely assess the impact of workplace wellness programs on health outcome and cost."[21] Nonetheless, the rules also note that "overall, employers largely report that workplace wellness programs are delivering on their intended objectives of improving health and reducing costs."[22] And indeed, an estimated 70% of all US employers providing healthcare used incentives in 2014, according to a major annual survey.[23]

Second, whether incentives reduce healthcare cost is also not straightforward. At the most general level, there is good evidence that better health increases life expectancy.[24] But it is not clear whether better health will reduce or save costs overall. Much depends on the timeframe, the health system, and which type of costs one is considering. For example, a study by Pieter van Baal and colleagues that sought to determine per capita expenditure differences between healthy people, smokers, and obese within the Dutch healthcare system found that most costs were attributable to healthy people: per capita costs from age 20 for smokers were €220,000; for obese people (BMI >30), €250,000; and for healthy people (defined as nonsmoking with a BMI 18.5–25), €281,000. The researchers found that differences were largely due to variation in life expectancy: 64.4 years for the healthy cohort, 59.9 for the obese, and 57.4 for smokers.[25] Overall, there is currently no consensus whether better health and longer life will simply delay costly care from chronic illness and make no difference to overall expenditure—as proponents of the so-called *compression thesis* would argue[26]—or increase it because there is a longer period in which a range of health services will be required, as argued by those supporting the *medicalization thesis*.[27] At the

---

16 R. W. Jeffery, "Financial Incentives and Weight Control," *Preventive Medicine* 55, no. Suppl (2012): pp. S61–S67.

17 K. C. Osilla, et al., "Systematic Review of the Impact of Worksite Wellness Programs," *The American journal of managed care* 18, no. 2 (2012): pp. e68–e81.

18 G. Gowrisankaran, et al., "A Hospital System's Wellness Program Linked to Health Plan Enrollment Cut Hospitalizations but Not Overall Costs," *Health Affairs* 32, no. 3 (2013): pp. 477–485.

19 "Report to Congress on Workplace Wellness: As Required by the Public Health Service Act, Section 2705(M)(1)," accessed June, 2015, http://aspe.hhs.gov/hsp/13/WorkplaceWellness/rpt_wellness.cfm.

20 S. Mattke, et al., *Workplace Wellness Programs Study: Final Report* (RAND, 2013).

21 "Incentives for Nondiscriminatory Wellness Programs in Group Health Plans: Final Rule," *Federal Register* 78, no. 106 (2013): p. 33169.

22 Ibid.

23 AON Hewitt, "2014 Health Care Survey," 2014, accessed June, 2015, http://www.aon.com/attachments/human-capital-consulting/2014-Aon-Health-Care-Survey.pdf.

24 K. -T. Khaw, et al., "Combined Impact of Health Behaviours and Mortality in Men and Women: The Epic-Norfolk Prospective Population Study," *PLoS Med* 5, no. 1 (2008): p. e12.

25 P. H. M. van Baal, et al., "Lifetime Medical Costs of Obesity: Prevention No Cure for Increasing Health Expenditure," *PLoS Med* 5, no. 2 (2008): p. e29.

26 L. Steinmann, H. Telser, and P. S. Zweifel, "Aging and Future Healthcare Expenditure: A Consistent Approach," *Forum for Health Economics & Policy* 10, no. 2 (2007).

27 F. Breyer, J. Costa-Font, and S. Felder, "Ageing, Health, and Health Care," *Oxford Review of Economic Policy* 26, no. 4 (2010): pp. 674–690.

See also C. Colombier and W. Weber, "Projecting Health-Care Expenditure for Switzerland: Further Evidence against the 'Red-Herring' Hypothesis," *The International Journal of Health Planning and Management* 26, no. 3 (2011): pp. 246–263.

societal level, questions about costs would also need to consider the following (among many) factors outside of the healthcare sector: behavior-associated economic benefits (such as higher tax revenues arising from purchases of tobacco or alcohol or lower state pension payments resulting from premature mortality) and costs (for example, higher rates of workplace absenteeism and lower productivity due to sickness).

The discrepancy between, on the one hand, lack of clarity about the effectiveness of incentives to improve health and reduce cost and, on the other, widespread use, can be puzzling. One possible explanation is the belief that the dictum of "an ounce of prevention saves a pound in cure" (attributed to Ben Franklin) is simply held to be self-evident. This would explain why programs are rolled out on a large scale, but only a fraction are evaluated.

Another reason may be that the option of cost-shifting can confer economic advantages to employers or health plans quite independently of the effect of reduced healthcare claims. Raising premiums on people with poor health—smokers, people with high blood pressure, or the obese—brings a net financial gain for the payer of healthcare right away.

A third explanation for the widespread use could be that the moralistic and political undercurrents of personal responsibility for health have considerable traction with payers of healthcare and are more influential in implementing policies than economic or epidemiological expectations.[28] Different and often overlapping rationales can drive incentive policies and affect their real and perceived acceptability.

The third general issue in considering the ethics of incentive programs in the context of resource allocation is how exactly programs are designed. There are numerous design elements that can be changed, giving rise to complex programs with different ethical issues. These central design elements include the following:[29]

- The *type of incentivized behavior*: Behaviors can range from "simple" to "complex," as noted earlier, and include activities that have no risks if the target behavior is achieved, such as smoking cessation, and ones where there are risks, such as overdiagnosis and overtreatment in the case of incentivized breast cancer screening.[30] The acceptability of incentives can differ across behaviors.
- The *incentivized unit*: Incentives can be offered to people individually or to groups. Group competitions for weight loss, for example, may be welcomed by some but disliked by others, especially when offered in the employment context, where there are other forms of competition.
- *The nature of the conditionality-triggering target*: One kind of target merely requires participating in an activity that is presumed to be health-conducive, such as a lecture or vaccination, which, generally, everyone is able to do. Another form is focused on accomplishing targets. These can either consist of achieving fixed threshold values, such as normal BMI, or, alternatively, and in a more person-centered way, making meaningful and measurable progress toward targets such as reducing weight by 10%. The nature of the target affects the degree of challenge and matters ethically insofar as some targets can be unreasonably ambitious.[31]
- *Currency and levels*: incentives can be financial, cash, lower or higher insurance

---

[28] K. G. Volpp and R. Galvin, "Reward-Based Incentives for Smoking Cessation: How a Carrot Became a Stick," *JAMA* 311, no. 9 (2014): pp. 909–910.

[29] H. Schmidt, "Planning, Implementing and Evaluating the Effectiveness and Ethics of Health Incentives: Key Considerations," *Eurohealth Observer* 20, no. 2 (2014): pp. 10–13.

[30] H. Schmidt, "The Ethics of Incentivizing Mammography Screening," *JAMA* 314, no. 10 (2015): pp. 995–996.

[31] H. Schmidt, D. A. Asch, and S. D. Halpern, "Fairness and Wellness Incentives: What Is the Relevance of the Process-Outcome Distinction?," *Prev Med* 55 Suppl (2012): pp. S118–S123.

premiums, or nonfinancial such as mugs, sports goods, honor badges, or wellness holidays; or take the form of access to different levels of health benefits, for example, more generous benefit packages for better health.[32] The value of incentives can range from the symbolic to the substantial and be perceived as an optional offer or coercive.

- *Mode and framing*: Incentives can be presented as rewards or "carrots" and confer a net benefit. Alternatively, the incentive could be a penalty or "stick" resulting in a net loss. Objections to rewards are generally limited to cases of what is called "cream-skimming," where, for example, people who never exercise and otherwise live unhealthily but have a healthy BMI receive a discount for a healthy body weight. One of the main concerns about penalizing "sticks" is that they may be unfair if they relate to behaviors that are beyond peoples' control in a meaningful way, as can often be the case with obesity (due to a range of powerful environmental factors).
- *Frequency and certainty*: Incentives can be offered annually, monthly, weekly, daily, or at other intervals. For example, an employer might vary insurance premiums once a year for annually measured body weight or offer incentives on a more frequent basis, for example, in line with weekly or monthly progress on a weight loss trajectory.[33] The frequency of incentives is one element of their salience and effectiveness, with direct implications for their ethics. More frequent incentives require more complex program design. Those offering them may sometimes resist elaborate designs on administrative grounds, which can undermine a program's effectiveness. However, effectiveness need not, of course, be central: Those intending to use incentives simply to shift cost—perhaps based on moralistic views about personal responsibility—will be content to use a simple design. Both frequent and infrequent incentives can also be structured as lotteries or sweepstakes. While there is less certainty of winning, rewards are typically higher, and an ethically relevant distinction of a more uncertain win is that this may prevent mercenary motives or crowding-out of motivation, which can be a concern.[34]
- *Alternative standards*: For some people, it may be impossible or unreasonably challenging to achieve the target behavior. Fairness demands that alternatives are provided in such cases.

It is clear, then, that a wide range of options exist for designing incentive programs that seek to promote personal responsibility in the context of resource allocation. Current regulations enable policy-makers to press ahead with controversial programs, with very limited opportunity for broader societal debate about the ethics of incentive programs. Feedback from employees—often fearing for the stability of their employment—is the exception, rather than the rule.[35] In view of the many drivers behind programs and the fact that normative views about personal responsibility are deeply entrenched in competing moral theories, Harald Schmidt argues that a procedural justice account is a helpful way forward (Excerpt 1).[36] He seeks to specify the relevance condition within the framework of Accountability for Reasonableness that was introduced in Chapter 9 for policies related to personal responsibility for health. He sets out a framework that suggests that, in planning,

---

[32] The Henry J. Kaiser Family Foundation, *2014 Employer Health Benefits Survey* (2014).

[33] Schmidt, "Fairness and Wellness Incentives."

[34] M. Promberger and T. M. Marteau, "When Do Financial Incentives Reduce Intrinsic Motivation? Comparing Behaviors Studied in Psychological and Economic Literatures," *Health Psychol* 32, no. 9 (2013): pp. 950–957.

[35] N. Singer, "On Campus, a Faculty Uprising over Personal Data," *New York Times*, September 14, 2013.

[36] Schmidt, "Bonuses as Incentives and Rewards."

implementing, and evaluating incentive programs, justification is owed in seven areas relating to (1) evidence, rationale, and feasibility; (2) intrusiveness; (3) attributability and opportunity of choice; (4) solidarity; (5) equity; (6) affected third parties; and (7) coherence. In a separate paper, he explores in more detail the impact incentives can have on equity. He outlines five groups of people with morally relevant differences in their motivations, behaviors, and opportunities of choice. He argues that these differences need to be considered in justifying policies, especially in programs "where the levels of incentives are substantial and already disadvantaged groups have lower chances of benefiting" (Excerpt 2).[37]

Steven Pearson and Sarah Lieber consider under what conditions it can be acceptable to impose penalties on insurance holders, such as employees of a self-insured employer (Excerpt 3).[38] They argue that rewards and penalties should not be based on outcomes, but on participation in a program. They focus on voluntariness and intentions, rather than consequences of actions, arguing that penalty programs

> should only target the voluntary action of informed employees should they choose not to take steps made available to them to try to improve their health. . . . If employees take the intended actions to improve their health, they should not be penalized, even if they do not achieve the ultimate health goal.[39]

Richard Ashcroft examines more closely the question of how incentives relate to the concept of autonomy by discussing under what circumstances programs might be coercive, constitute bribery that might unduly undermine motivation, or undermine autonomy in general (Excerpt 4).[40]

Dan Wikler argues that "personal responsibility for health might be wrong-headed, arbitrary, disingenuous, and even dangerous" and, accordingly, "deserves but a peripheral role in health policy" (Excerpt 5).[41] He outlines the philosophical debate around justice and responsibility and then raises a number of concerns around the voluntariness of actions, the possibility that deciding which behaviors people should be held responsible for can be arbitrary, difficulties with ensuring proportionality of penalties, and the importance of considering what later came to be known as the *social determinants of health*.[42]

Chronic conditions such as high blood pressure, diabetes, and cancers that are related to obesity, smoking, and other common risk factors represent an increasing proportion of the global burden of disease. Personal behavior clearly plays a role in their occurrence and treatment. More health-conducive behavior likely lessens both rationing and resource allocation dilemmas. Yet what role exactly personal behavior should play remains controversial, chiefly, because it is often unclear to what extent people can reasonably be held responsible for particular health outcomes. Despite lack of consensus in policy and practice, a wide range of policies have been put in place that appeal to personal responsibility. It is critical to review their appropriateness to determine the exact extent to which they empower patients and lead to more efficient delivery of healthcare, or, conversely, undermine autonomy and unduly penalize people for factors that are largely beyond their control.

[37] H. Schmidt, "Wellness Incentives, Equity, and the Five Groups Problem," *American Journal of Public Health* 102, no. 1 (2012): p. 53.

[38] S. D. Pearson and S. R. Lieber, "Financial Penalties for the Unhealthy? Ethical Guidelines for Holding Employees Responsible for Their Health," *Health Affairs* 28, no. 3 (2009): pp. 845–852.

[39] Ibid., p. 849.

[40] R. E. Ashcroft, "Personal Financial Incentives in Health Promotion: Where Do They Fit in an Ethic of Autonomy?," *Health Expectations* 14, no. 2 (2011): pp. 191–200.

[41] D. Wikler, "Personal and Social Responsibility for Health," in *Public Health, Ethics and Equity*, edited by S. Anand, F. Peter and A. K. Sen (Oxford University Press, 2004), pp. 109–134.

[42] M. Marmot, "Universal Health Coverage and Social Determinants of Health," *The Lancet* 382, no. 9900): pp. 1227–1228.

Questions for Discussion

1. In auto insurance, risky drivers have higher premiums. Some say that the same model should be used in health insurance. For example, they argue that obese people should pay higher premiums than people who are not overweight because they are more likely to have health problems. Do you agree?
2. To create weight control incentives, the premiums of overweight employees should be increased by how much?
3. To create weight control incentives, employees with normal BMI should receive an insurance rebate of how much?
4. Is if fair that those who meet biometric targets such as BMI thresholds or cholesterol values may receive a net reduction of up to $1,500?
5. At what point do inequalities in the capacity to use incentive programs constitute unfairness, and how should we respond in policy?

EXCERPTS

Note: The following excerpts have generally been edited for length, and omissions are indicated with ellipses. Editing includes footnotes and endnotes, which have also been renumbered. For citation and related purposes, the full original source texts should be used.

EXCERPT 1

Abridged text from:

H. Schmidt, "Bonuses as Incentives and Rewards for Health Responsibility: A Good Thing?", *Journal of Medicine and Philosophy* 33, no. 3 (2008): pp. 198–220.

Bonuses as Incentives and Rewards for Health Responsibility: A Good Thing?

Harald Schmidt

. . .

II. Solidarity and Health Responsibility—The General Legal Context

. . . I suggest that to evaluate any health responsibility–related policy, including bonus programmes, the most helpful approach is to carry out a number of "tests" that concern the impact of the respective policy on key normative and structural values and components integral to a public health-care system. These tests concern solidarity; equality and equity; intrusiveness; attributability and opportunity of choice; evidence, rationale, and feasibility; affected third parties; and coherence.

III. A Framework for Evaluating Health Responsibilities

This proposal clearly raises at least two questions: First, why the talk about tests and not ethical principles or a particular branch of moral theory? Second, why these tests, and what exactly do they involve?

At one level, deciding about an appropriate concept of health responsibility might simply be a matter of choosing the right set of principles or theoretical framework. For example, Hans Martin Sass has called for a triad of "responsibility, solidarity, and subsidiarity," viewing in particular the principle of solidarity as "deeply rooted in European culture and supported by secular . . . and Christian ethical positions" (Sass, 1995, 587). Within political philosophy, responsibility features prominently in luck egalitarianism,[1,2,3] but also in communitarian[4] and libertarian,[5] accounts. And the responsibility debate is of course also closely aligned with particular political positions. The left generally argues that the focus on the individual is misguided and that it is the environment and general living conditions that require change for people to be healthy. The right focuses more strongly on individual behavior and notions of desert, coupling entitlements to health and other social care more closely to responsibilities.[6]

---

[1] J. E. Roemer, *Egalitarian Perspectives* (Cambridge: Cambridge University Press, 1994).

[2] R. J. Arneson, "Equality and Equal Opportunity for Welfare," in *Equality: Selected Readings*, edited by L. P. Pojmanand and R. Westmoreland (New York: Oxford University Press, 1997), pp. 229–241.

[3] R. Dworkin, *Sovereign Virtue: The Theory and Practice of Equality* (Harvard University Press, 2002).

[4] D. Callahan, *False Hopes: Overcoming the Obstacles to a Sustainable, Affordable Medicine* (Rutgers University Press, 1999).

[5] H. T. Engelhardt, "Human Well-Being and Medicine: Some Basic Value-Judgments in the Medical Sciences," in *Biomedical Ethics*, edited by T. A. Mappes and J. S. Zempaty (New York: McGraw-Hill, 1981), pp. 213–222.

[6] H. Schmidt, "Health Responsibility, the Left, and the Right," Hastings Center Bioethics Forum, 2007, http://www.bioethicsforum.org/personal-responsibility-health-care-Medicaid-Membership-Agreement.asp.

So in one sense, the question of health responsibilities might simply be a matter of choosing "the right" normative framework. However, there are two principal problems with this approach. First, in value pluralistic societies, agreement about what constitutes the right framework remains generally elusive. Second, even if we suppose that we are able to find a country in which all residents (or just citizens) can agree on a single monolithic theory or accept a set of principles such as Sass' triad, such value systems are typically of a very general nature and may not tell us more geometrico how to decide particular cases, or, in the present context, judge concrete policies. The approach proposed here, focusing on addressing questions around health responsibility with a number of tests, by contrast, has several advantages, and can be used in three different ways.

First, the tests specify clearly the areas in which justification is required. In one sense, they might be understood to be complementary to the aforementioned normative frameworks, within which subsequent justification in each particular area may be provided. On this view, the tests may be seen as a necessary, although not sufficient, condition of relating abstract theory to specific policy proposals and making sense of the meaning of health responsibility.

Alternatively, the "fact of pluralism," characterizing modern liberal societies, might be taken more seriously, and the focus on particular normative frameworks for justification may be relegated to the background. Accordingly, setting out a range of tests can be useful, if not constitutive, in a more policy-orientated approach that focuses on "accountability for reasonableness," as set out by Norman Daniels and James Sabin.[7] Here, the idea that a universally accepted notion of personal responsibility can be realized in pluralistic societies is abandoned, but the argument might be made that as long as policies fulfill four conditions (relating to publicity, relevance, revision and appeals, and regulation) and as long as explicit justification in each of the areas specified by the tests is provided, reasonable policy has been secured.[8]

Lastly, the fact of pluralism and the normative value of justification may be acknowledged by using the tests within a contractualist framework, as presented, for example, by contemporary proponents such as Thomas Scanlon. Although, for space and other reasons, I shall not pursue this general project here, I contend that this is in fact the most promising strategy, not least because of Scanlon's discussion around responsibility. I will return to his useful distinction between responsibility as attributability and substantive responsibility below, and I will assume in the following that it makes sense to use the tests sketched out here in a project that focuses on identifying those principles or policies that, provided people have certain choices, "no-one could reasonably reject."[9] The corollary is that such norms have particular robustness and in fact special moral value. However, even if the reader is not inclined to make this leap at this stage, it will become clear that the proposed framework is well suited to interrogate the German policy on health-care bonuses as set out in SGB V and provide helpful illumination of significant ethical tensions.

The seven tests proposed here are not intended as an exhaustive list. However, they are informed by an analysis of the kinds of issues raised by legal and policy provisions found in major patient charters and similar documents[10,11,12] and by the range of arguments

[7] N. Daniels, "Accountability for Reasonableness," *British Medical Journal* 321 (2000): pp. 1300–1301.

[8] H. Schmidt, "Just Health Responsibility," *Journal of Medical Ethics* 35, no. 1 (2009): p. 21.

[9] T. Scanlon, *What We Owe to Each Other* (Belknap Press, 2000), p. 153.

[10] D. C. English, "Moral Obligations of Patients: A Clinical View," *Journal of Medicine and Philosophy* 30, no. 2 (2005): pp. 139–152.

[11] A. S. Iltis and L. M. Rasmussen, "Patient Ethics and Responsibilities," *Journal of Medicine and Philosophy* 30, no. 2 (2005): pp. 131–137.

[12] H. Schmidt, "Patients' Characters and Health Responsibilities," *British Medical Journal* 335, no. 7631 (2007): pp. 1187–1189.

typically set forth by proponents and opponents of health responsibility.[13,14,15,16,17,18]

Solidarity Test

Health as a good is special in at least two ways: first, in a very obvious sense, good health matters in our lives in experiential, if not existential terms. Second, health has a clear impact on one's civic and economic livelihood and the options one can make use of in a society based on fair equality of opportunity.[19] On an individual basis, regaining health in the case of sickness can be extremely costly, if not impossible to afford. Admittedly, countries that have made social health insurance mandatory have taken away a degree of liberty in relation to whether or not people should protect themselves against the consequences of poor health. But nonetheless, it is plausible to describe those brought together in social health insurance systems as being in a solidaristic relationship with others, which has the aim of providing mutual protection against the negative implication of diseases. . . .

The general concept of solidarity is highly complex. In addition to the two notions introduced here, recent work examining its motivation, function, and role in different European health-care systems has analyzed it among other things, as attitudes of individuals or descriptions of communal arrangements, and has explored notions of fellowship, compassion, charity, altruism, universal or group-specific brotherhood, friendship, interest coalitions, civic duties, or mutual recognition and interdependency of individuals.[20]

Although there are hence a range of different candidates that might explain why solidarity should matter, it is clear that a functional baseline description of solidarity in public health-care systems would be focused around the notion of achieving collectively a degree of security that could not generally be achieved individually. In this sense, solidarity has also been characterized as "the 'beating heart' of a social health insurance approach."[21,22,23] It is equally clear, then, that any evaluation of appeals to health responsibilities, whether in the form of bonus systems or policies that have a more negative character, needs to consider whether they are likely to enhance this central concept or will be to its detriment.

Equity and Equality Test

Broadly speaking, inequalities relate to the uneven distribution of goods (or access to them), and such distributions are inequitable

[13] D. Wikler, "Persuasion and Coercion for Health: Ethical Issues in Government Efforts to Change Life-Styles," *Millbank Memorial Fund Quarterly/Health and Society* 56, no. 3 (1978): pp. 303–338.

[14] D. Wikler, "Personal and Social Responsibility for Health," in *Public Health, Ethics and Equity,* edited by S. Anand, F. Peter, and A. K. Sen (Oxford University Press, 2004), pp. 109–134.

[15] A. W. Cappelen and O. F. Norheim, "Responsibility in Health Care: A Liberal Egalitarian Approach," *Journal of Medical Ethics* 31, no. 8 (2005): pp. 476–480.

[16] E. Feiring, "Lifestyle, Responsibility and Justice," *Journal of Medical Ethics* 34, no. 1 (2008): pp. 33–36.

[17] C. C. Gauthier, "The Virtue of Moral Responsibility and the Obligations of Patients," *Journal of Medicine and Philosophy* 30, no. 2 (2005): pp. 153–166.

[18] M. Kelley, "Limits on Patient Responsibility," *Journal of Medicine and Philosophy* 30, no. 2 (2005): pp. 189–206.

[19] N. Daniels, *Just Health: Meeting Health Needs Fairly* (Cambridge University Press, 2007).

[20] R. Houtepen and R. Meulen, "New Types of Solidarity in the European Welfare State," *Health Care Analysis* 8, no. 4 (2000): pp. 329–340.

[21] R. Saltman, "The Historical and Social Base of Social Health Insurance Systems," in *Social Health Insurance Systems in Western Europe,* edited by R. Saltman, R. Busse, and J. Figueras (Maidenhead, UK: Open University Press, 2004).

[22] R. Houtepen and R. Meulen, "The Expectation(s) of Solidarity: Matters of Justice, Responsibility and Identity in the Reconstruction of the Health Care System," *Health Care Analysis* 8, no. 4 (2000): pp. 355–376.

[23] H. Schmidt, "Germany Institutes Incentives for Cancer Patients," Hastings Center Bioethics Forum, 2008, http://www.bioethicsforum.org/health-responsibility-Germany.asp.

when they are unfair or unjust. In one sense, one could assume that assessing a policy in terms of its impact on solidarity is the same as assessing it in terms of its impact on equality and equity. However, this is not necessarily the case, as there can be arrangements that satisfy a particular concept of solidarity, although they may not treat everyone equally and/or equitably. For example, although a system might be described as solidaristic in view of the mechanisms of financing and access to health services, other organizational arrangements or societal factors may mean that some groups of people benefit more than others. Given that the reduction of inequalities in health and social status through largely prioritarian strategies is an explicit goal of all liberal European states, it is therefore useful to assess whether particular responsibilities are likely to contribute to reducing inequalities or not.

Intrusiveness Test

Promoting personal responsibility is often seen as synonymous with imposing highly intrusive and paternalistic measures. However, this is far from necessary, and the means available include mere provision of information or nondirective education, targeted and directive education and persuasion; the use of financial and other incentives and disincentives, possibly targeted at different populations (taxes, different levels of insurance contribution or copayments, bonuses, etc.); restricting access to particular interventions; and ultimately infringing civil liberties (such as mandatory isolation of people with highly infectious diseases who refuse to accept the responsibility not to harm others).[24]

Minimizing intrusion is not only of relevance in terms of respect for autonomy but also with regard to the acceptability and sustainability of a program seeking to promote responsibility. The intrusiveness test therefore concerns the extent of interference and in a wider assessment whether a particular measure is likely to be the least intrusive, but most effective of a set of available options.

Attributability and Opportunities of Choice Test

One of the most controversial issues in the debate about health responsibilities concerns the question of how to consider, in praising or blaming, or making decisions about access to health care, the extent to which people's behavior contributed to a good or bad health outcome. Controversy surrounds, in particular, the discussion around negative health outcomes and their association with blame and reduced access to health care.

For some, the question of holding people responsible or imposing sanctions is the same as assessing the extent to which an action is attributable. . . . However, attributability can admit of degrees, and the question might then turn on what degree or threshold of attributability should be sufficient. This is particularly relevant in considering responsibility in the health-care context. For, clearly, disease development is affected by a highly complex range of factors that include genetic predispositions, biological processes, and environmental conditions, in addition to behavior. It would amount to a Kafkaesque situation to say someone has only themselves to blame for a health outcome and has lost all claims to assistance if the actual causal factors were in fact fully, or to a significant extent, outside of that person's control. One option, therefore, is to abandon any talk about apportioning responsibility for bad health outcomes.

Another is to analyze more closely the kinds of responsibilities involved. Scanlon distinguishes two principal types. Responsibility as attributability concerns our assessments relating to praise and blame and rests on whether a given action is attributable in the sense that the choices were guided by the attitudes of the person who is judged.[25] Hence, we might acknowledge that in the case of some people, their behavior played a certain causal role in contributing to a disease but not feel it appropriate to blame them for it. There may be others, however, where we might want

[24] Nuffield Council on Bioethics, *Public Health: Ethical Issues* (London: 2007).

[25] Scanlon, *What We Owe to Each Other*, p. 290.

to do so, provided their behavior was guided by their attitudes. And equally we might praise people in cases where their attitudes led to behavior that produced a good health state. However, adapting Scanlon's model, none of these assessments determine what people are owed. Such obligations rest on substantive responsibility, which can be independent of the choices a person has made. On this view, what a person is owed is determined primarily, if not exclusively, by the opportunities a person had for making the right choices: "what matters is the value of the opportunity to choose that the person is presented with. If a person has been placed in a sufficiently good position, this can make it the case that he or she has no valid complaint about what results, whether or not it is produced by his or her active choice."[26] In deciding what kind of opportunities need to be provided in this respect, Scanlon suggests that we should be guided by reasons "that people in general have reason to value," as "the justifiability of a moral principle must rest on [generic reasons]" people have in a given situation and not on their particular values and attitudes.[27]

For the evaluation of particular polices, it then follows that a close assessment is required of the kinds of opportunities that they create and how they relate to the general opportunities that people have in their lives. People's claims against the solidaristic community may only be lessened if the policies have provided them with option sets that allow people motivated by generic reasons to prevent harm. In a positive sense, substantive responsibility may justify offering rewards for positive behavior. And independently of the question of substantive responsibility, the notion of attributive responsibility may still allow us to praise or blame people's behavior, or to appeal to them to change their behavior where we judge they should behave differently and it is in their power to do so. But the latter judgments are distinct from decisions about what people are owed.

[26] Ibid., p. 258.

[27] Ibid., pp. 263, 205.

Evidence and Rationale, Feasibility Test

In view of possible opportunity costs, personal responsibility can be emphasized on the grounds of fairness toward others in the solidaristic community. Or it may be based on a more general appeal to efficient use of health-care resources. In any case, evidence is required that a particular policy and means used to enforce it will actually help realize the justificatory reasons. Being explicit about evidence and underlying rationales is crucial in justifying and securing support for particular health responsibility policies, and to avoid "legal moralism," where particular behaviors are rewarded or penalized simply because those setting policy have a like or dislike for them.[28] An assessment of the rationale may also help us to understand better the primary beneficiaries of particular polices, who may not always be individual people, or the solidaristic community, but perhaps (also) insurance providers or government departments receiving taxes.

In considering different policy options, an assessment is furthermore required of the administrative and general organizational effort necessary to set out health responsibilities, and, where deemed appropriate, to enforce them. It may be that although some types of responsibility can be clearly specified, and are reasonable, their enforcement would simply be disproportionate in terms of cost or effort.

Affected Third Parties Test

The implementation of responsibilities set out in law or policy also needs to consider the effect on third parties. Doctors may (or may not) wish to appeal to patients' responsibilities to change their behavior. However, depending on the type of responsibility, doctors may also be required to pass on information to sickness funds or similar agencies about whether or not people comply with particular obligations. This may affect the doctor-patient relationship, as it may give an unwelcome policing function to

[28] Wikler, "Persuasion and Coercion for Health," pp. 316, 332.

health-care professionals or may have a negative impact on people's willingness to come into contact with health services. The implications of particular responsibilities for the various agents involved and the relationships between them, therefore, also require close scrutiny.

Coherence Test

Justice, in one meaning, demands treating similar cases similarly. Particular forms of health responsibility therefore need to be compared to other health responsibilities and to obligations in social policy more widely.

A comparison to other areas of social policy may furthermore be interesting since many of the hard questions in apportioning responsibility also arise in other contexts, such as criminal, tort, and liability law. For example, in the United Kingdom and Germany, contributory negligence (Eigenverschulden) commonly leads to reductions in personal injury claims brought by victims of traffic accidents who failed to wear a seat belt (if wearing the seatbelt would have prevented or significantly limited the harm caused). Of course, such comparisons do not mean that identical standards need to be implemented in the health context—there may be morally relevant differences. But ultimately, a coherent use of responsibility would be the ideal outcome, whether this means similar or distinct policies. . . .

EXCERPT 2

Abridged text from:

H. Schmidt, "Wellness Incentives, Equity, and the Five Groups Problem," *American Journal of Public Health* 102, no. 1 (2012): pp. 49–54.

Wellness Incentives, Equity, and the Five Groups Problem

Harald Schmidt

Incentives aimed at individuals increasingly play a role in the organization of health care systems.[1,2] Wellness incentives are intended to encourage uptake of prevention and health promotion programs. A recent survey also found that 56% of large US employers see wellness programs as 1 of the top 3 strategies for curbing cost.[3] Savings may result, for example, from reduced health care expenditure owing to a healthier workforce or from incentives structured in a way that shifts health care cost from employers to employees. The goals of health promotion and cost containment may come into conflict, and the fairness of wellness programs depends significantly on their implementation. Various ethical issues may arise, but a central concern is equity, because ideally, all who are offered incentive programs should enjoy equal opportunity to access them, especially when associated benefits are substantial. . . .

The 5 Groups Problem

To understand these issues, it is useful to consider the responses of 5 types of people to incentive programs that are offered universally to all enrollees of a health plan:

1. the "lucky ones,"
2. the "yes-I-can" group,
3. the "I'll-do-it-tomorrow" group,
4. the "unlucky ones," and
5. the "leave-me-alone" group.

Depending on the exact characteristics of particular programs, the impact on these groups varies, of course. Nonetheless, this somewhat abstract model may bring clarity to the ongoing debate about the acceptability of different incentive programs, whether they focus on process or outcomes. The framework illuminates significant differences across groups of enrollees in the extent that programs succeed in promoting behavior change. It also shows that people differ in their ability to make use of incentive programs. The 5 groups problem therefore concerns this question: At what point do disparities in the capacity to use incentive programs constitute unfairness, and how should policymakers respond? . . .

Characteristics of the 5 Groups

The lucky ones. Almost any incentive program will cover people who qualify for associated reimbursements without any form of behavior change. By habit, some people simply enjoy eating healthily and exercising regularly and do so quite effortlessly. Their behavior is hence compatible with the wellness program spirit, even if the incentive benefit–for example, a process-based reimbursement for going to the gym regularly or an outcome-based incentive for meeting certain BMI thresholds or for not smoking–does not lead to behavior change and, strictly speaking, does not function as an

---

[1] K. G. Volpp, A. B. Troxel, and M. V. Pauly, "A Randomized Controlled Trial of Financial Incentives for Smoking Cessation," *New England Journal of Medicine* 360, no. 7 (2009): p. 699.

[2] K. Baicker, D. Cutler, and Z. Song, "Workplace Wellness Programs Can Generate Savings," *Health Affairs (Millwood)* 29, no. 2 (2010): p. 304.

[3] *Survey: Large Employers' 2011 Health Plan Design Changes* (National Business Group on Health, 2010).

incentive. Others whose actions may remain unaffected are people whose dispositions are not as well aligned. For example, some people may eat in the most unhealthy ways and never exercise and still have favorable BMI values. Despite the dissonance between their motivations and a wellness program's spirit, they may reap the same benefits as their health-conscious counterparts, without any change in behavior or motivation (to some extent, such behavior is related to the concept of free riding in the economic literature).[4]

The yes-I-can group. Another group of people would not normally have performed the benefit-qualifying behavior, but the incentive may be a welcome occasion–though perhaps not the sole reason–for trying to overcome inertia or lack of determination. The incentive's nudge, coupled with their underlying motivation, provides an effective basis for action. For most in this group, incentives are likely to feel like a deserved reward. The benefit may help initiate behavior change in the first place, or sustain it, where intrinsic motivation is not yet sufficiently developed.

Alignment of motivation and action cannot be taken for granted: behavior change may also occur more grudgingly, for example, where people care less about the supposed health benefit but participate mainly because they feel bribed by the level of the incentive. The yes-I-can group may therefore have subgroups: happy and grumpy. Conceptually and in practical terms, the yes-I-can group is also known as the group of responders in the literature, yet it cannot be assumed that all–or even the majority–of those offered incentive programs are, in fact, responders. Furthermore, it is plausible to assume that responders' attitudes differ by the mode of incentive: some may find a soft process incentive most attractive and feel overly pressured by a hard outcome incentive that requires, for example, meeting BMI targets. Others may respond better to a more robust challenge that requires meeting hard thresholds. Such variation needs to be considered in designing an effective and acceptable intervention.

The I'll-do-it-tomorrow group. Some people share the desire for behavior change with the yes-I-can group but, for a range of reasons, may not act on it. They may feel unable to try, or when they try they often fail. The reasons may stem from their everyday circumstances, such as poor availability of affordable and healthy food or insufficient time to prepare it. They may lack access and time for physical exercise in a safe environment. They may face above-average levels of professional or personal stress and resort to coping mechanisms such as smoking. Such factors can render outcome incentive programs, such as quitting smoking or achieving specific BMI values, significantly more challenging. Upbringing may also play a role: some participants likely received more encouragement than others to be self-motivated and self-efficacious. Therefore, even process incentives such as lower health care costs in return for gym attendance may be taken up more readily by some than by others. For many in this group, incentives may be extremely tempting, yet the amounts at stake can be as far out of reach as the branches of the fruit-laden trees were for the mythical Tantalus.

The unlucky ones. For biological, medical, or other reasons that are completely external to their volition, some people face such strong constraints that, whatever they might do, they are simply unable to meet the criteria associated with specific outcome or process incentives such as BMI targets or gym participation. For example, some people with genetic mutations will always be obese, regardless of how much they exercise or control their energy intake. As with the I'll-do-it-tomorrow group, incentives that are simply out of reach will make little sense for the unlucky ones.

---

[4] R. Cornes and T. Sandler, *The Theory of Externalities, Public Goods, and Club Goods* (Cambridge: Cambridge University Press, 1996).

The leave-me-alone group. Some people might qualify for wellness incentives but voluntarily decide not to use them. They may already meet targets or could do so easily or could effortlessly participate in incentivized activities, but still resist. They may feel patronized or "nannied" by wellness programs; they may also believe that incentives introduce an inappropriate element of competition in health plans that they think ought to be based on a principle of mutuality and fair risk sharing. Or, on quite practical grounds, they might judge the effort required to register for programs to be too burdensome.

Fairness Issues

It is clear, then, that universally offered wellness incentive programs can give rise to several equity problems:

- Some people may receive benefits, even if their motivation and behavior run counter to the spirit of wellness programs.
- Behavior change is not always required, and some people may receive benefits for default behavior–whether this is the result of deliberate previous choice or unreflective habit.
- Some people face constraints attributable to weakness of the will, poorly developed self-efficacy, or strong medical or societal constraints. Meeting targets or participating in health promotion activities requires a much greater effort of them than of others. Still, when they fail to begin or complete an incentive program, they must forgo the benefit in the same way as those who had sufficient opportunity of choice, but who voluntarily chose not to take part.

Clearly, the extent to which inequalities in incentive use occur in practice and the extent to which we might find them unfair depend critically on the way incentive programs are implemented. Many more people will typically be able to use process than outcome incentives. Therefore, an employer who uses process incentives only is more likely to enable all to secure associated monetary benefits.

One of the most important equity questions is how easy it is for employees with different backgrounds and abilities to avail themselves of the opportunities created by incentive programs. In addition, consideration should be given to the level of benefits. Disparities can become more inequitable if benefits (which, often, may only be open to some) are substantial. The recent health reforms significantly increased the reward levels for outcome incentives. This change, and the interest of employers in using incentives for cost shifting and cost reduction, may result in a scenario where only a relatively small number of people among the lucky ones and the yes-I-can group benefit from large incentives, with others, particularly the I'll-do-it-tomorrow group, at a disadvantage.

Policy Options

The relevance of this analysis clearly needs to be ascertained in empirical studies of specific programs, and in light of the scarcity of such work to date, my framework is intended to help guide such research. Several policy options (which may change in the wake of empirical analysis) may be considered to respond to the 5 groups problem: (1) continue to offer incentives universally, (2) offer them universally but with modifications, (3) offer targeted rather than universal programs, or (4) abandon incentive programs altogether (Table [14.1]). . . .

. . .

Table [14.1]
Implications of Policy Responses to the 5 Groups Problem in Wellness Incentive Programs

Policy Options	Groups[a] Lucky Ones	Yes-I-Can	I'll-Do-It-Tomorrow	Unlucky Ones	Leave-Me-Alone	Analysis
Offer universally	Benefit	Benefit	Don't benefit	Don't benefit	Don't benefit	Unlucky ones lose out. I'll-do-it-tomorrow group, treated identical to leave-me-alone group. Some lucky ones reap benefits even if they do not change behavior or comply with spirit of policy.
Offer universally, modified	Benefit	Benefit	May benefit	May benefit	Don't benefit	Create alternative standards for unlucky ones and I'll-do-it-tomorrow group; this can improve fairness but faces practical and arbitrariness challenges. Shift from offering alternative standards in response mode to proactive mode to reduce negative aspects of petitioning. Shift focus from outcome to process incentives.
Targeted, not universal	Don't benefit	Benefit	Benefit	May benefit	Don't benefit	No incentives for lucky ones because they do not require further encouragement. Potential for curbing cost, if focus is on improving health status of worst off. Minimizes potential for exacerbating existing disparities in health and wealth. Reverses financing of benefits where benefits result from cost shifting; instead of the poorer and unhealthy financing the benefits of the better off and more healthy, controversially, the opposite happens.
Abandon	Don't benefit	Don't benefit	Don't benefit	Don't benefit	Don't benefit	No unfairness from different use of incentives, but also no potential to use incentives as complement to action at the level of social determinants of health for health promotion. Strongest case if it can be shown that other measures to improve population health are equally or more effective.

[a]Lucky ones qualify for incentives without behavior change; yes-I-can only qualify if they succeed in changing behavior, which may be more likely because of the incentive; I'll-do-it-tomorrow only qualify if they change behavior but perceive obstacles to change; unlucky ones are practically impossible to qualify; leave-me-alone could qualify in principle, but refuse to do so.

EXCERPT 3

Full text from:

S. D. Pearson and S. R. Lieber, "Financial Penalties for the Unhealthy? Ethical Guidelines for Holding Employees Responsible for Their Health," *Health Affairs* 28, no. 3 (2009): pp. 845–852.

Financial Penalties for the Unhealthy?: Ethical Guidelines for Holding Employees Responsible for Their Health

S. D. Pearson and S. R. Lieber

As health care costs continue to rise, an increasing number of self-insured employers are using financial rewards or penalties to promote healthy behavior and control costs. These incentive programs have triggered a backlash from those concerned that holding employees responsible for their health, particularly through the use of penalties, violates individual liberties and discriminates against the unhealthy. This paper offers an ethical analysis of employee health incentive programs and presents an argument for a set of conditions under which penalties can be used in an ethical and responsible way to contain health care costs and encourage healthy behavior among employees.

Penalty programs must offer employees fair and equal opportunities to improve their health.

Rising health care costs and increasing rates of chronic illness threaten the future of the U.S. health care system.[1] Purchasers and health plans have responded with a variety of strategies to try to contain costs while maintaining or improving quality. Employee health education and wellness programs, disease management, pay-for-performance (P4P), public reporting of quality performance, tiered formularies, tiered physician networks—all of these strategies have been tried, but none has been able to tame the rise in chronic disease rates or overall health care costs.

Recently, a growing number of self-insured employers have devised new strategies, using financial incentives to promote healthy behavior and thereby reduce preventable health care costs.[2] Major corporations, including Dell, Scott's Miracle-Gro, Meritain Health's Weyco Inc., and Clarian Health are directly rewarding or penalizing employees for changing unhealthy behavior such as smoking and, in some cases, for achieving targets on "biometric" outcomes such as weight, blood pressure, and cholesterol level.[3] Nearly half of employers surveyed in 2007 by Hewitt Associates reported that they now offer employees incentives to participate in health promotion services; just over two-thirds planned to use more-aggressive wellness and disease management programs by the end of 2008.[4]

The federal Health Insurance Portability and Accountability Act (HIPAA) sets boundaries on the use of financial incentives for behavior change or biometric outcomes by requiring all workers covered under a particular employer-sponsored health plan to pay the same premiums regardless of their health status. In July 2008, however, federal agencies finalized rules granting some exceptions from HIPAA to certain wellness programs. According

---

[1] R. DeVol and A. Bedroussian, "An Unhealthy America: The Economic Burden of Chronic Disease," 2007, accessed February 18, 2009, http://www.milkeninstitute.org/pdf/chronic_disease_report.pdf.

[2] K. Jochelson, "Paying the Patient: Improving Health Using Financial Incentives," 2007, accessed February 17, 2009, http://www.kingsfund.org.uk/publications/other_work_by_our_staff/paying_the.html.

[3] B. Baker, "Now, the Stick: Workers Pay for Poor Health Habits," *Washington Post*, November 13, 2007.

[4] Business Wire, "Hewitt Study Shows Companies Plan to Invest More in the Health of Their Employees," 2007, accessed February 19, 2009, http://www.redorbit.com/news/health/907738/hewitt_study_shows_companies_plan_to_invest_more_in_the/index.html.). A case study of one company, Clarian Health, is available online at http://content.healthaffairs.org/cgi/content/full/28/3/845/DC1.

to these rules, employers can offer rewards or penalties of as much as 20% of the total cost of covering an employee.[5] In December 2007 the U.S. Department of Labor issued guidelines that narrow the definition of types of supplemental coverage through which employers can provide such incentives, but interest in these programs remains high: companies such as BeniComp Group and Vital Measures, a unit of United-Health Group, help design and manage incentive programs for a growing clientele of both small and large employers.[6]

Early reports and anecdotal information suggest that direct financial incentives can effectively motivate employees to change their health behavior, but employers are facing a backlash from organized unions and others who contend that workplace incentive programs, particularly penalty programs, are unethical.[7] Employers that use penalty programs have said that they are acting in the best interest of both individual employees and the collective workforce, which has a shared interest in keeping health care premiums in check. To some employees and workers' rights protection groups, however, penalty programs are a thinly veiled, discriminatory attempt to make sicker employees shoulder increased health care costs.[8]

Given the growing interest in using direct reward and penalty programs, and the starkly competing views of whether they are fair and ethical, all such programs should be subject to careful ethical analysis. Consideration must be given to determining whether it is possible to strike a proper balance between holding employees responsible for their health and providing a fair system of health insurance that protects individual liberties.

This paper analyzes the arguments for and against employee health incentive programs, with a focus on penalty programs. Positive incentive programs (rewards) raise many of the same ethical concerns, but penalties heighten the potential for coercion and inequity. Nonetheless, penalty programs seem poised to play a larger role if early anecdotal reports of their success are confirmed more broadly. The goal should be to establish an ethical balance between holding employees responsible and protecting their liberties.

Ethical Foundation for Penalty Programs

Economic harms

Before exploring in detail how to achieve an ethical balance, we first consider the underlying justification for penalty programs. Employers have an ethical duty to provide responsible stewardship for the health care programs they administer that pool limited resources to help cover health care costs. The primary principle supporting employers' use of penalty programs is that employees should be held responsible if, through their voluntary actions, they harm fellow employees. Given that costs are shared, an unhealthy employee will drive up costs for others who are contributing to the collective pool. The impact of unhealthy behavior and its

---

5 "Nondiscrimination and Wellness Programs in Health Coverage in the Group Market," *Federal Register* 71, no. 239 (2006): pp. 75014–75055.

6 V. Knight, "Wellness Programs May Face Legal Tests: Plans That Penalize Unhealthy Workers Could Get Tighter Rules," *Wall Street Journal*, January 16, 2008.

7 R. Ozminkowski et al., "Long-Term Impact of Johnson and Johnson's Health and Wellness Program on Health Care Utilization and Expenditures," *Journal of Occupational and Environmental Medicine* 44, no. 1 (2002): pp. 21–29; E. Finkelstein et al., "A Pilot Study Testing the Effect of Different Levels of Financial Incentives on Weight Loss among Overweight Employees," *Journal of Occupational and Environmental Medicine* 49, no. 9 (2007): pp. 981–989; Associated Press, "Employees Starting to Pay for Poor Health: Are You Obese or Have High Blood Pressure? Your Insurance May Go Up," 2007, accessed January 20, 2008, http://www.msnbc.msn.com/id/20625381.

8 Baker, "Now, the Stick"; and AP, "Employees Starting to Pay for Poor Health."

attendant outcomes is significant: health care costs for "moderately" obese workers are about 21% higher than they are for workers of normal weight, costing employers an additional $670 per employee each year. Similarly, health care costs are 75% higher for "severely" obese workers (an additional $2,441 annually per employee).[9] Such costs burden fellow employees by leading to lower wages and higher premiums for group insurance coverage.

"Benign paternalism" versus coercion

Another argument advanced to justify penalty programs is that, ultimately, their goal is to motivate behavior change that benefits the individual as well as the group. By itself, this "benign paternalism" is a weak justification, easily counterbalanced by the specter of coercion. The primary justification for penalty programs must rest on the economic harms imposed on others when employees engage in unhealthy behavior. Considerations of the key concepts underlying when and how it is ethical to hold employees responsible for these harms form the core of the criteria that we propose for ethical penalty programs (Figure [14.1]).

Responsibility for Unhealthy Behavior

Penalty programs should hold employees responsible for behavior that leads to poor health and increased health care costs only if employees voluntarily refuse to take action to change their behavior.

Key elements of voluntary action

First, employees must be informed. Employers must assure that employees are fully aware of the medical—and economic—reasons why they should change their unhealthy behavior. Second, there must be clearly defined steps that employees can take to try to change their behavior. And third, employers must provide or assure that all employees have equal and unencumbered access to the programs, medications, or other interventions that can help change such behavior. Income, job duties, or other barriers beyond employees' control must not be allowed to become a barrier to the tools to support behavior change.

Beyond a person's control

Although some behavior that increases health risks may be under a person's full control, the ability to change behavior is often diminished in several ways. Many biological, psychological, and sociological factors undermine a person's control over his or her behavior; people are frequently restricted in their ability to change their behavior because of "encumbrances on the will," which "preclude or impede authentic, reasoned choice."[10]

Consider the example of smoking, one of the most common targets of penalty programs. For smoking to be an ethically acceptable target of a penalty program, the act of quitting smoking would have to be voluntary. But the effects of nicotine addiction undermine a person's ability to follow through on a choice to quit. The act of continued smoking is thus not fully voluntary, and therefore smoking itself is not behavior for which a smoker should be held fully responsible.

A result of choice

In contrast, choices made concerning whether or not to attempt to quit smoking are far more voluntary for most people. If an employee is made aware that entering a smoking cessation program could help him quit smoking, the employee can voluntarily choose to enter—or not to enter—the program. Should he

[9] D. M. Huse, "Obesity in the Workforce: Health Effects and Healthcare Costs," 2007, accessed February 13, 2008, http://employer.thomsonhealthcare.com/uploadedFiles/Cost_of_Obesity_in_the%20Workplace.pdf.

[10] D. Wikler, "Who Should Be Blamed for Being Sick?", *Health Education Quarterly* 14, no. 1 (1987): pp. 11–25.

Selecting Targets for Penalties	
Criteria	**Examples/Methods**
Measured targets are failures to take voluntary actions to improve health behavior: Information on unhealthy behavior is shared with employees Employees are informed what actions to take to improve health Actions are voluntary; ability to take action not undermined by biological, psychological, and sociological factors	Example: Even though informed of the health benefits of these actions and free to adopt them, employees: Do not take cholesterol-lowering medication Do not attend diet counseling sessions Do not get cancer screening Do not enroll in smoking cessation programs Example: Programs targeting smoking should not penalize employees for the presence of nicotine in the body: instead, employees should be penalized for not entering a smoking cessation program
Biometric outcomes are not the measured target for penalties	Example: Employees should not be penalized for high cholesterol levels, because some are genetically predisposed to high cholesterol
No discrimination: Behavior selected leads to poor health outcomes and increased health care costs Selection not based on stigmatization of the behavior or of individuals prone to the behavior	Transparency: selection process and justification for selection made public Evidence-based: behavior selection supported by robust empirical data
Accommodation for fundamental behavior	Examples: sexual activity, child bearing, outdoor sports, and recreation
Administration of penalties	
Fair and equal opportunities to change behavior: Programs provide necessary tools to take voluntary actions to change unhealthy behavior All employees have equal access to services for behavior change and improved health	Health education Examples: nutrition counseling, prevention and health management information sessions Health promotion tools Examples: weight-loss programs, on-site gym facilities, health clinics, health coaches, pharmacies, smoking cessation programs
Opt-out appeals process Exemptions permitted on medical or personal grounds	Example: an employee with severe osteoarthritis is exempted from participation in exercise classes
Fair notice Employees have reasonable time to take actions to improve their health	Example: employees are given six months to reflect, quit smoking on their own, or prepare to be penalized on not entering a smoking cessation program if they are still smoking
Fair magnitude of penalty Fair limits set so that penalty acts as incentive to change behavior, not to recoup health care costs	Lowest monetary value needed to motivate change in behavior Penalty amounts scaled to personal salary
Privacy protection	Careful adherence to HIPAA confidentiality rules

HIPAA, Health Insurance Portability and Accountability Act.

Figure [14.1] Criteria for ethical penalty programs encouraging employee behavior change.

voluntarily decide to forgo this option, his failure to act justifies holding him responsible for not taking the necessary steps toward improved health. Thus, although the ultimate goal is to motivate employees to change their unhealthy behavior such as smoking, the actual measure by which employees are judged should only be the failure to take voluntary actions to change behavior and improve health. Health programs should not penalize employees for the mere presence of nicotine in the body. Rather, it would be reasonable to penalize an employee for not enrolling in a smoking cessation program so long as that employee has an informed and unencumbered choice to take this step toward improving his or her health.

Responsibility for Biometric Health Measures

An obvious corollary to the argument above is that an important distinction needs to be made between holding employees responsible for behavior and holding them responsible for biometric health outcomes such as obesity, hypertension, or high cholesterol levels. People do not voluntarily choose their health outcomes—poor personal health is not a simple product of informed voluntary choices. Biological, environmental, and socioeconomic factors greatly affect health, regardless of how a person behaves.

The obesity example

Here obesity provides a valuable example. The causes of obesity are a complex web of factors and may include detrimental workplace design and other workplace policies over which employees have no control at all. Employees cannot exercise a truly voluntary choice not to be obese. On a practical level, workplace health programs might need to use certain biometric measures such as weight, blood pressure, and cholesterol to assess problematic areas in an employee's health. But penalty programs should not assign financial penalties using these measures themselves as targets. Rather, as in the case of smoking, penalty programs should only target the voluntary action of informed employees should they choose not to take steps made available to them to try to improve their health. For obesity, penalty programs might target participation in nutritional counseling offered in the workplace; for hypertension, the target might be attendance at regular monitoring sessions; and for high cholesterol, the penalty target might be adherence to prescribed medication. If employees take the intended actions to improve their health, they should not be penalized, even if they do not achieve the ultimate health goal.

The case of medication adherence

Penalties for medication adherence conflict with competent patients' general right to decline any treatment, and therefore they must be framed cautiously and narrowly. Penalty programs should only consider as potential targets treatments prescribed by an independent physician who has judged, in discussion with the employee, that the medication is likely to confer a positive net health benefit on the employee. If this condition can be met, then it is reasonable to consider adherence to the prescription as a voluntary action for which an employee can be held responsible.

Discrimination

A separate ethical concern for penalty programs lies in the risk that types of behavior will be selected as targets because of discrimination. The evidence linking behavior with poor health and increased costs must be evaluated in an even-handed way; penalty programs should not be based on moral judgments made by employers in a discriminatory and stigmatizing manner.

The risk is that penalty programs will find it easiest to focus on behavior and outcomes that are generally viewed as "socially unacceptable" within a workplace community or society at large. As one commentator has written, "Not all choices leading to illness are counted alike. Those that are targeted tend to be sins—sloth, gluttony, lust, to use their old-fashioned names—or to be behavior, such as drug addiction, of the marginalized."[11] It is hard not to notice that all of the early penalty programs target employees who are obese and employees who smoke. Were other potentially costly types of behavior considered in the selection process? Is it for evidence, practicality, or other reasons that penalties were not focused on excessive alcohol intake, failure to get cancer screening, engagement in risky outdoor sports, or other potentially unhealthy types of behavior that might have imposed unfair financial burdens on the workforce?

To avoid discriminating and stigmatizing practices, a transparent and evidence-based process should guide the selection of targets for any penalty program. The components of a fair, evidence-based process to select targets for penalties mirrors those described as the basis for legitimate efforts to set limits fairly in all health care systems.[12] Thus, a central component of penalty programs must be that decisions regarding which types of behavior receive penalties are made with the participation of employees and use publicly accessible, evidence-based reasons as justification.

Accommodation for Fundamental Behaviors

Another ethical criterion for penalty programs is the exclusion of penalties for "unhealthy" types of behavior that society acknowledges to be fundamental elements of personal freedom and identity. Holding employees responsible for the costs of any behavior that increases health care costs would undermine the liberty of choosing for oneself how to live one's life.[13]

For example, penalties should not be considered for behavior such as sexual activity, bearing children, and most recreational activities and sports. Although these types of behavior may entail increased health risks and costs, they are widely accepted in our society as critical components of self-expression, free choice, and personal identity. Admittedly, it is a matter of judgment whether some activities that increase risks and costs, such as "extreme" sports, are worthy of accommodation on this basis. Do these activities constitute essential elements of personal expression, or are they merely risky, superficial enjoyments that merit consideration as the target of penalties? The answer lies in value judgments that may vary legitimately among the employees and cultures of different organizations. Thus, as with avoidance of discrimination in target selection, an ethical penalty program must ground its decisions to exempt certain types of behavior in a fair, participatory, and transparent decision-making process.

Fair Administration of Penalty Programs

A partnership between employer and employees

Given that the core ethical justification for penalty programs is that employees should be held responsible for voluntary actions that cause harm to others, the voices of employees should help guide the key decisions about how to implement any penalty program. A positive example exists in the employee smoking cessation program created in 2008 by the insurer

[11] D. Wikler, "Personal and Social Responsibility for Health," in *Public Health, Ethics and Equity*, edited by S. Anand, F. Peter, and A. K. Sen (Oxford University Press, 2004), pp. 109–134.

[12] N. Daniels and J. Sabin, "The Ethics of Accountability in Managed Care Reform," *Health Affairs* 17, no. 5 (1998): pp. 50–64.

[13] S. Shiffrin, "Egalitarianism, Choice-Sensitivity, and Accommodation," in *Reason and Value: Themes from the Work of Joseph Raz*, edited by R. Wallace et al. (Oxford: Oxford University Press, 2004).

Humana.[14] The program description states that it is being designed by a project team of employees including a mix of tobacco nonusers, former tobacco users, and current tobacco users. Whether through mechanisms like this or through working with representative groups such as employee unions, employers must reach out to engage employees in a partnership to guide the administration of an ethical penalty program.

Access to health promotion tools

As described above, employers considering a penalty program must also recognize their responsibility to provide health promotion tools that can give every employee a fully voluntary choice to attempt to modify unhealthy behavior. Even small businesses with limited resources can offer cost-effective tools to employees to improve their health. In the areas of smoking and obesity, these tools might include health coaching, online support tools, time during working hours to exercise, and reduced copays for certain medications and health services. Other innovative strategies to give all employees the means to improve health include weight-loss competitions, organized corporate races, and outdoor activities.[15]

Opt-out processes

Another important element of fair administration of penalty programs is the establishment of an opt-out process for employees who have legitimate medical or personal reasons that make it impossible for them to participate in the health-promoting behavior that is targeted by ethical penalty programs. For example, an employee with severe arthritis might not be able to take part in exercise classes meant to reduce obesity; similarly, an employee might have contraindications to taking cholesterol-lowering medications.

An opt-out requirement is in keeping with new nondiscrimination provisions in HIPAA. According to these federal regulations, incentive programs should have a "reasonable alternative standard" that exempts employees from penalties when it is unreasonably difficult or medically inadvisable to meet certain health benchmarks.[16] Under these regulations, employees can justify their appeals with the testimony of a medical professional and must be offered an alternative target for a health behavior change or biometric outcome. One way to implement this kind of process would be to establish a review committee of managers, employees, and medical professionals.

It is important to note that HIPAA's current provisions for a reasonable alternative standard seem only to apply to "wellness programs" that presumably use "rewards." Federal regulations in the future should specify more clearly that these requirements apply to penalty programs as well.

Fair notice

Employees should be given enough lead time both before and after the implementation of a penalty program so that they have a reasonable chance to plan how they will approach the challenge of changing their health behavior. For example, smokers might be given six months' notice that there would be a penalty program instituted that targets documented smoking cessation or attendance at smoking cessation classes. Then, once implemented, the program would give smokers six months to either quit on their own or enter a cessation program. To determine what would constitute a fair amount of time to change a specific type of behavior, health programs should look to empirical data and personal accounts from employees for evidence on how long it generally takes to change certain behavior and the factors that influence this length of time.

---

[14] Gregory Matthews, Consumer Innovations, Humana, personal communication, 18 July 2008.

[15] S. Okie, "The Employer as Health Coach," *New England Journal of Medicine* 357, no. 15 (2007): pp. 1465–1469.

[16] "Nondiscrimination and Wellness Programs in Health Coverage."

Fair magnitude of penalty

Penalty programs must ensure that the magnitude of penalties is fairly selected. The goal of penalties should not be to recoup costs attributed to unhealthy behavior. The economic harm that penalty programs might cause individual employees may strike low-income workers particularly severely; penalties should serve only as incentives to encourage changes in behavior, not as tools to drive at-risk employees out of their health insurance. The ethical balance sought for penalty programs therefore requires that penalties be scaled only to motivate employees to adopt healthier behavior.

The magnitude of penalties necessary to motivate behavior change will always be difficult to estimate, but there should be a transparent and collaborative process for setting the amount. Existing HIPAA regulations set reward cutoffs at 20% of the cost of health care coverage without giving any rationale for this limit.[17] Using any single flat rate for penalties might disproportionately burden low-income employees while providing less of an incentive for highly compensated employees to change health behavior. Thus, if it is administratively possible, motivational penalties should be scaled in some way to an employee's personal salary or wages and seek to use the lowest magnitude that will provide a reasonable incentive to change behavior.

Privacy protection

In accordance with current HIPAA policies, medical data or information that is used to assign penalties to employees must be kept confidential. Health records and information should be accessible to only third-party health plan administrators or other outside vendors authorized by the employee. After collecting and storing employee health information, these outside organizations can only use de-identified data to determine risk factors within a work-force and subsequently design health interventions.[18] Employers in penalty programs will not be able to access this information or discriminate against employees based on their health records.

Despite many threats to its future, employer-based health insurance is still the dominant form of health care coverage in America. As health care costs continue to rise and employers adopt new strategies to contain costs, clear ethical guidelines need to be established to ensure that when employers use financial incentives, there is an appropriate balance between holding employees responsible for increased health care costs and protecting individual liberties.

The workplace offers a unique environment in which employees can be encouraged to improve their health and provided the appropriate medical attention and services to help them change unhealthy behavior. In society at large, it is difficult to hold people responsible for being unhealthy, especially given that there is no universal health care system in place and people do not have fair and equal opportunities to improve health. In the workplace, however, it is possible to identify a shared interest among employees in healthy behavior and restraint on health care costs. The workplace offers an excellent access point for the delivery of health promotion and behavior-change tools, which can empower those who are at risk and enable them to change their health for the better. Therefore, unless a deus ex machina appears on the horizon, it is likely that financial incentive programs for health in the work-place will gain increasing attention. Penalty programs may have an important role within this movement, but they should only be considered after broad reflection by employers and employees on the important criteria that must be met if these programs are to be used in an ethical way.

[17] Ibid.

[18] Okie, "The Employer as Health Coach."

EXCERPT 4

Abridged text from:

R. E. Ashcroft, "Personal Financial Incentives in Health Promotion: Where Do They Fit in an Ethic of Autonomy?", *Health Expectations* 14, no. 2 (2011): pp. 191–200.

Personal Financial Incentives in Health Promotion: Where Do They Fit in an Ethic of Autonomy

Richard E. Ashcroft

. . . One type of intervention to support personal behaviour change which has received considerable attention is the use of personal financial incentives. Money incentives—as well shall see—are intended to reinforce the desirability or feasibility of behaviour changes which a patient may wish to perform but for one reason or another fails to do in the absence of an incentive. They bring long term goals into the short term decision horizon, for instance.[1] In this paper I will give a preliminary account of the moral issues which arise in the use of such incentives in health promotion, paying particular attention to considerations of personal decision-making autonomy. It is not my intention here to give conclusive arguments about the merits and disadvantages of this type of intervention, or specific instances of it, but rather to give an overview of the types of arguments which arise.

A Case Study

Consider a 14-year-old young woman, Holly, who has been offered Chlamydia screening, and has either declined it or failed to attend her appointment. The local healthcare provider (in England, the Primary Care Trust), noting low rates of uptake of the programme in this age group, has established a scheme whereby if young adults between the ages of 12 and 18 come for screening, they will be given a £10 mobile telephone credit. Learning of this scheme, Holly presents herself for screening. There are three broad concerns here: coercion, bribery, and undermining her autonomy.

Coercion

The ethical arguments here are diverse. A first argument, often mentioned in media debates about this type of incentive scheme, is that it involves coercion. The reasoning is that Holly has changed her behaviour in response to the offer. But for the offer, she would—it is assumed—not have come for screening. It is further assumed that her non-attendance reflects a considered choice on Holly's part, and that therefore she has good reasons not to attend. The offer of a financial incentive has overborne her considered choice, essentially making her do something that all other things considered she does not wish to do. . . .

The coercion theory is very difficult to make out, purely on the basis of making sense of an individual's response to an incentive. It may be that some version of the coercion theory can be sustained, under specific conditions. One way it may work is that if the subject is offered a significant amount of money, conditional on completing a particular series of actions, then what is most salient to them is not the value of the actions in themselves, but the fear of loss of the reward. Behavioural economists point to well documented phenomena of fear of anticipated regret.[2] Coercion typically works by forcing an agent to do something through

[1] J. L. Grand, "The Giants of Excess: A Challenge to the Nation's Health," *Journal of the Royal Statistical Society: Series A* 171, no. 4 (2008): pp. 843–856.

[2] C. Starmer, "Preference Reversals," in *Behavioural and Experimental Economics*, edited by S. N. Durlauf and L. E. Blume (London: Palgrave Macmillan, 2010), pp. 206–211.

fear of the consequences of not doing it. To force you to do something, I must arrange that the costs to you of not doing so are both large and frightening to you. And I must arrange that your welfare is dependent on my will, so that you have an interest in keeping me happy, on pain of your feared loss. So, in the incentive situation, if the structure of my offer of money is such that you come to consider the money as "already" yours, then my proposal not to pay you unless you do as I ask is framed as a loss. And if the loss is big enough, you may feel coerced to comply. The scale of the loss here is to some extent subjective: one element of some acts of coercion is that they work by taking advantage of pre-existing needs, so that offers of even small amounts of money might coerce somebody in poverty. This would be explicable in two, possibly interacting, ways: first, the degree of desperation induced by severe poverty might make even a small incentive much-needed; and second, the utility of a small amount of additional money can be predicted to be much greater than the utility of the same amount of money to someone much better off, due to the well-attested phenomenon of the diminishing marginal utility of money.[3,4] These questions are ripe for empirical investigation since much of our ethical argument here depends on the specific features of the psychological mechanisms in play, and since much of our policy choice will turn on how and when these mechanisms work as well as when interventions based on them are morally justified

Bribery

Suppose Holly does not feel coerced, and no impartial observer would consider her choice to be coerced. Another moral difficulty with her decision to take part in screening may then arise. This is the claim that she has been bribed to take part. There are two different moral concerns here. One is that she has been paid to do something which she should have been doing anyway. This is the type of bribery that concerns us in connection with paying bribes to public officials merely to do their jobs in a timely and professional way. The other is that she has been paid to do something which she should *not* have been doing anyway. This is the type of bribery that concerns us in connection with paying bribes to public officials to secure (unfairly) a benefit to the payer of the bribe. . . .

This concern can also be analysed further. First, there is the concern that payment may weaken internal motivation, and second, that it may undermine prosocial behaviours.[5] The weakening of internal motivation concern is that we may shift people from doing things because they are the right thing to do, or because it is in their own best interests, to doing things in order to get external rewards. If I do something for the money, the thought goes, I am orientating my practical reason toward the reward, and overlooking the reasons which properly *ought* to motivate me (my health or the public good, for instance).[6] I may even come to *expect* reward, so that I am less likely to act on intrinsic motivations than I was before. Indeed, this attitude might come to infect my decision-making outside the context of this particular incentive scheme, and become a more general feature of my expectations and motivations. This takes us to the second concern, that I may be more likely to act in ways which benefit others only where there is some tangible benefit in there for me. This has sometimes been

[3] B. Stevenson and J. Wolfers, "Economic Growth and Subjective Well-Being: Reassessing the Easterlin Paradox," *Brookings Papers on Economic Activity* (2008): pp. 1–102.

[4] P. Dasgupta, *An Inquiry into the Sources of Well-Being and Destitution* (Oxford: Oxford University Press, 1993).

[5] R. M. Ryan and E. L. Deci, "Self-Regulation and the Problem of Human Autonomy: Does Psychology Need Choice, Self-Determination, and Will?," *Journal of Personality* 74, no. 6 (2006): pp. 1557–1586.

[6] C. M. Korsgaard, *Self-Constitution: Agency, Identity, and Integrity* (Oxford: Oxford University Press, 2009).

argued in the context of payments to research subjects in social survey research; if no payment is offered at all, then a certain response rate might be typical across society at large, but if some payment is offered, not only may response rates in surveys which do pay *fall* (if people think the payment is insufficient), they may fall further in surveys which do not pay, as there is an expectation that researchers should pay and that payment signals that the research is "really" just in the interest of the researcher and not in the general public interest. This concern is sometimes studied by economists under the label "motivation crowding out."[7]

How are we to evaluate these arguments? The first observation, again, is that largely they depend on testable empirical hypotheses, and there is an extensive literature in psychology and behavioural economics on just these hypotheses in other contexts.[8] Secondly, as with the coercion objection, the bribery objections—they are really as I have shown here a family of objections rather than just one—may prove too much. There are many activities where payment is necessary and expected, and where the remunerated behaviour is in the interest of the agent or the public, but we do not label the payment bribery and evaluate its moral status as such. Philosophy lecturers typically expect to be paid for their work, for instance, even if they would philosophise without payment and even if doing philosophy is in the public interest. To make sense of the bribery claim we need a much finer grained and contextually sensitive account of the moral wrong the bribery claims are trying to identify. . . .

Undermining Autonomy

The purported moral wrongs in coercion and in bribery are in a sense external threats to autonomy. They rest on the assumption that the agent is autonomous, and address her as such. Holly, it is assumed, knows that she should go to be screened, but cannot be bothered, and has to be bribed to do what she should. Or, she is a fine upstanding woman, who rejects the offer because she has firm moral objections to it. But the offer of money corrupts her resolve, either through need of the inducement, or fear of the loss, or some other reason to do with being distracted by a powerful extrinsic motivation.

Some criticisms of inducements see them as undermining autonomy itself. On the above account, Holly's autonomy is not undermined, so much as suborned. But if she were to feel that actually she was not the author of her choice to be screened in any meaningful way, or that her status as a person was in doubt or under threat, we might want to say that her autonomy *as such* was undermined. Noting that in Holly's case, given the nature of the intervention and the types of incentive used, this is unlikely, let us turn to cases where autonomy is already fragile: mental illness and drug dependency.

Notice first that there are forms of coercion which are so extreme as to involve "breaking the will" of the agent. Torture is a typical example.[9,10] So far as I am aware no critic of incentives in health promotion alleges that incentives break the will of agents, and arguably even very large sums of money would not do so in the way that physical pain or intense and acute psychic distress do. What very large incentives might do is induce someone to do something which radically disrupts the narrative unity of their personhood.

[7] B. S. Frey and F. Oberholzer-Gee, "The Cost of Price Incentives: An Empirical Analysis of Motivation Crowding-Out," *The American Economic Review* (1997): pp. 746–755.

[8] J. Andreoni, W. T. Harbaugh and L. Vesterlund, "Altruism in Experiments," in *Behavioural and Experimental Economics*, edited by S. N. Durlauf and L. E. Blume (London: Palgrave Macmillan, 2010), pp. 6–13.

[9] E. Scarry, *The Body in Pain: The Making and Unmaking of the World* (Oxford University Press, 1985).

[10] S. J. Brison, *Aftermath: Violence and the Remaking of a Self* (Princeton University Press, 2011).

The standard example here is the "indecent proposal," where someone may be induced to betray some important personal or normative commitment under the lure of large financial gain.[11] There are two elements to the concern here: one is with personal integrity itself, and the other is with the behavioural change induced. In the health context, it is hard to imagine a personal behavioural change which would involve a radically disruptive change in someone's self-image, in ways which neither the person evaluating the decision prospectively nor the person looking back on the decision would endorse as being "their own decision." Decisions to break an addiction may well involve a breach in the narrative unity of the self—I might well see "me as an addict" and "me clean" as truly different people. But this could be something I profoundly wish after the change, and profoundly endorse beforehand.[12,13] The most likely case involves inducing someone to take long term antipsychotic medication in a context where all things considered they dislike the side effects of the medication and see their unmedicated self as their true, authentic self.[14] This is indeed a troubling problem in the ethics of psychiatry. But it should be stressed that the moral status of inducement here does not depend on this dilemma. The dilemma exists whether or not the inducement is offered, and insofar as we dislike an inducement in this context, it is arguably because it is an inducement to do something we dislike, or judge to be wrong, rather than because of anything inherently wrong in the inducement itself.[15] . . .

How may inducements undermine the quality of the decision? Recall the concern about extrinsic motivation. That was introduced as a concern about undermining people's ability to do the right thing for the right moral reason. However, it may be that it applies here too, in a different way. If the moral justification of the treatment rests on the deliberative endorsement of the treatment (assume here that we are discussing long term treatment of the mentally ill in the community, rather than crisis treatment of someone acutely mentally ill), then what may be from a legal point of view a valid, capacitous consent may fail to be a morally valid consent. If it matters that the patient is doing it in full knowledge of the risks and implications of accepting treatment (and of the alternatives and their consequences), then a decision which is actually made with one eye on the money may not meet this test. In some cases this is clear: a patient who *really* does not want the treatment, but desperately needs the money, and consents specifically in order to get the money is perhaps better described as being coerced, as above. But consider the more subtle case of the patient who, perhaps distracted by the money, fails to deliberate carefully enough and consents in a spirit of "oh, all right then." Has he been nudged in an insidious way? Has the focus on the *mechanisms of his personality* come to treat his *person* as merely phenomenal, in such a way that his moral autonomy has been undermined?[16]

Much of the discussion of incentives in the policy literature builds on the work popularised in Sunstein and Thaler's "Nudge" . . . that involve building on evidence from psychology and behavioural economics about the ways in which my decision-making may be erratic, irrational or self-subverting. These experimentally-inspired (and sometimes experimentally evaluated) interventions aim both to understand how we manage to make choices which are incoherent with our stated preferences or the values of our best selves, and to restructure the conditions under which we make choices

---

[11] H. Lindemann Nelson, *Damaged Identities, Narrative Repair* (Ithaca, NY: Cornell University Press, 2001).

[12] J. Elster, *Strong Feelings: Emotion, Addiction, and Human Behavior* (MIT Press, 2000).

[13] G. Ainslie, *Breakdown of Will* (Cambridge University Press, 2001).

[14] G. Szmukler and P. S. Appelbaum, "Treatment Pressures, Leverage, Coercion, and Compulsion in Mental Health Care," *Journal of Mental Health* 17, no. 3 (2008): pp. 233–244.

[15] D. Claassen, "Financial Incentives for Antipsychotic Depot Medication: Ethical Issues," *Journal of Medical Ethics* 33, no. 4 (2007): pp. 189–193.

[16] Korsgaard, *Self-Constitution: Agency, Identity, and Integrity.*

so that they are not subverted in the same way. However, it is arguable that the strategy is troubling. Typically, these interventions do not work by *unbiassing* our decisions and choice frameworks. Instead, they work by *using* the same biases to produce choices which fit with our stated preferences or values of our best selves. So the idea is not actually to improve the quality of our decision-making, but to trick ourselves.

This may not matter. Although "Ulysses contracts," for instance, are controversial, this is not because of how they work in the present, by making us pre-commit to a certain course of action and making us stick to it. The idea of a Ulysses contract draws on the classical myth of Odysseus/Ulysses, who wished to hear the song of the Sirens without risking being lured to his death. He instructed his sailors to tie him to the mast, and not to untie him until they had passed the Sirens, whatever he might say thereafter, and no matter how forcefully he insisted.[17,18] In psychiatry and dementia care, a Ulysses contract is a form of advance decision whereby the patient, while competent, binds himself to a certain treatment plan even if, later, he says (competently or otherwise) that he wishes to be released from it. It is because they bind future selves to the wishes of present selves in ways which the future selves may not truly endorse. A person can rationally sign a Ulysses contract, endorsing both the course of action committed to, and the mechanism of enforcement. They are vulnerable to the charges that people may change their minds and that they are incentive to changes in external circumstance. Now consider the incentive scheme which seeks to nudge us into giving up smoking by offering us small short term rewards, and thus overcoming the weak influence long run future health states have over the present desire to smoke. If I consent both to the incentive scheme's structure, and to the plan to give up smoking, and to the psychological mechanism, then I have consented in full to intervention. But it is likely that absent a good explanation, I do not grasp the way in which the scheme works. And my consent may indeed by framed by factors other than deliberative endorsement of the smoking cessation intervention. It may be that my apparently autonomous decision-making is being tweaked by this psychological sleight of hand.

In a healthcare ethics arena in which we place enormous moral and epistemological emphasis on autonomous choice, the idea that we "cheat" autonomy in this way is controversial. There are a number of possible responses here. First, it is clear that autonomous choice, given the pervasiveness of cognitive biases, is empirically, if not normatively, much more complex and perhaps compromised than we ordinarily allow.

Second, it is also true that many actors in the health field are making a lot of use of these cognitive biases in ways we often overlook or are unaware of—notably the behaviour of the food, tobacco and other industries and companies. In light of the pervasiveness of cognitive biases, we should of course highlight the way that corporate actors intervene in ways which trade on these biases. But this will not eradicate those biases. Indeed, most likely nothing can. Given that, making good and morally careful use of them is sound policy. Moreover, if it can be done in a way which commands reflective deliberative endorsement by citizens and patients, then arguably it is morally justified, provided it is fair, effective and efficient. . . .

[17] J. Elster, *Ulysses and the Sirens: Studies in Rationality and Irrationality* (Cambridge University Press, 1979).

[18] I. Gremmen, "Ulysses Arrangements in Psychiatry: From Normative Ethics to Empirical Research, and Back," in *Empirical Ethics in Psychiatry*, edited by G. Widdershoven, et al. (Oxford: Oxford University Press, 2008), pp. 171–185.

EXCERPT 5

Abridged text from:

D. Wikler, "Personal and Social Responsibility for Health," in *Public Health, Ethics and Equity*, edited by S. Anand, F. Peter, and A. K. Sen (Oxford University Press, 2004), pp. 109–134.

6.4. A Role for Personal Responsibility for Health?

The notion that people should bear responsibility for the consequences of their voluntary choices makes up part of the bedrock of our moral and political culture. It is, in John Roemer's words, "the cost of freedom," the dues we pay when we assert our right to self-determination as free adult citizens. The same freedom that permits us to act on our personal tastes and preferences, pursuant to our individual goals, plans, and values, reduces the scope of excuses for these choices should they turn out badly. Just as we expect to be left alone to decide which risks to take, others expect to hold us accountable for the consequences. If the condition of evading or denying responsibility for the consequences of our choices were the denial of the freedom to choose, the price would often be too high.

In the field of health, personal responsibility can be life-giving. Because health and longevity depend so much on whether a person adopts healthy living habits, encouraging people to take good care of themselves is a key to a population free of avoidable infirmity and premature mortality. The first steps toward adoption of healthier living habits are understanding the causal links between behaviour and health, and accepting and acting upon the notion that to this large extent, we can control our state of health in the future.

Despite these considerations, I will argue that personal responsibility for health deserves but a peripheral role in health policy. This conclusion should be reached, in my view, whether or not we think that personal responsibility should be central to our thinking about distributive justice generally. I will begin with a brief account of arguments against emphasising personal responsibility in the theory of justice, for if we reject the broader view we have little reason to support it in the special case of health. On the chance that these arguments are not convincing, I proceed to offer reasons to reject any attempt to move from the general thesis to its application to health. I close with a word on how a very limited, but constructive, role for personal responsibility might be envisioned within health policy.

6.4.1. Justice and responsibility

A full assessment of the debate over the role of personal responsibility in the general theory of justice is not possible within the confines of the present chapter. But it is worth noting some of the grounds on which such objections might be made. As Elizabeth Anderson points out in her paper, "What is the point of equality," some implications of luck egalitarianism are highly counterintuitive, and an important source of these problems is the view's preoccupation with individual choice. The fundamental idea, that bad (brute) luck deserves compensation but that the consequences of voluntary trades, gambles, risks, and tradeoffs do not, seems to yield appropriate concern on neither point. For example, such a regime would in effect punish many people who seem to have done no wrong, such as those who voluntarily refrain from work in order to care for dependents, or people who suffer when prudent risks go bad. These people will lose out in a luck egalitarian society because their deprivation stemmed from their free choices. On the other hand, luck egalitarianism might call for compensation to a person with better than average income who, through no fault of his own, had developed inalterable tastes for champagne and caviar. Anderson notes that while luck egalitarianism might seem at first sight to offer the best of capitalism and socialism by encouraging personal responsibility under the protection of a safety net against bad luck, it is also vulnerable to the charge that it combines some of the worst features of the two systems. In seeking to remove every difference in involuntary advantage, it is a

Utopian project to "correct" for cosmic injustice, differences in prospects which are the fault of no person or society. At the same time, it assigns responsibility, and withholds assistance, regardless of need, whenever people make choices, standing in stern judgement of what, in actual human beings, is often a halting and uncertain effort to secure well-being. Its echo of the Elizabethan poor laws is a case in point; and the medical implications are another.

Given that most, if not all, of the philosophers contributing to the luck egalitarian literature hail from the left side of the political spectrum (in some cases, far from the centre), it is startling when the views they express on some issues exceed in their judgemental rigour positions which are prevalent even on the right. In this regard, the luck egalitarian position does not close the gap Scheffler alleged to exist between theorists of justice and contemporary popular political morality; it opens a new gap to the opposite side.

Again, the medical examples are the clearest example. The record shows that proposals to assign personal responsibility for health along the lines discussed in this essay have been relatively rare in any political milieu. Though proposals to this effect have appeared occasionally in the literature of medicine and bioethics, no significant figures in health policy or politics have taken up John Knowles's theme. Physicians, who in the United States lean toward the right, tend to be even more emphatic on the requirement that patients be cared for without regard to fault. The near-unanimity of liver transplant surgeons on the need to avoid "moralizing" about the responsibility of alcoholics is particularly noteworthy, in light of the absolute need to establish priorities among patients whose lives hang in the balance.

It is true that some respondents in focus groups studied by health economists indicated that rationing should take into account the contribution of the individual to his or her own plight. But in nearly every case, those who voiced this sentiment were in the minority. Moreover, several investigators noted that support for assigning lower priority to individuals at fault waned during deliberation.[1,2,3] And the proposition has been rejected outright by some deliberative bodies seeking to establish basic principles for prioritisation.[4]

Even the minority view on personal responsibility for health which appears to tally with the luck egalitarian verdicts may, in the view of one group of researchers, stem from quite different premises. Ubel et al.[5] sought to distinguish between three grounds for assigning lower priority to patients whose behaviour may have contributed to their susceptibility to illness or injury. These respondents declined to change their priorities when told that the capacity for treatment, that is, likelihood of recovery with a given amount of resources, was the same for both sets of patients. But they were unmoved also when told that, after all, the patients' behaviour had not in fact been a contributing factor in their ill health. The reason that these respondents favoured lower priority for treatment for the likes of alcoholics and addicts was that they did not think that the lives of people of this sort were as worthy of care. This position, of course, is antithetical to the egalitarian emphasis of the luck egalitarian viewpoint which, superficially, leads to similar conclusions on personal responsibility for health.

The lack of correspondence between the luck egalitarian view and conventional morality need not be understood as any kind of rebuttal

[1] E. Nord, et al., "Maximizing Health Benefits Vs Egalitarianism: An Australian Survey of Health Issues," *Social Science and Medicine* 41, no. 10 (1995): pp. 1429–1437.

[2] P. Dolan, R. Cookson, and B. Ferguson, "Effect of Discussion and Deliberation on the Public's Views of Priority Setting in Health Care: Focus Group Study," *British Medical Journal* 318 (1999): pp. 916–919.

[3] E. Nord and J. Richardson, Cost-Value Analysis in Health Care (Cambridge: Cambridge University Press, 1999).

[4] Ibid.

[5] P. A. Ubel, J. Baron, and D. A. Asch, "Social Acceptability, Personal Responsibility, and Prognosis in Public Judgments and Transplant Allocation," *Bioethics* 13, no. 1 (1999): pp. 57–68.

of the former; ordinary thinking about these moral issues might be wrong. But in this case the charge against Rawls and other liberals, that their views are seriously out of step with mainstream opinion, does not recommend luck egalitarianism as an alternative.

In the view of luck egalitarianism, informed and voluntary choices establish a moral fact, that of individual responsibility, from which important consequences flow. The more plausible alternative is of course that the more fundamental consideration is that of need. And it is the need of patients, without regard to responsibility, that is counted as the only relevant consideration in conventional medical ethics, and apparently in the mind of most members of the public as well.

A theory of justice which does not give a central role to personal responsibility need not dismiss the moral significance of choice entirely. It can be given due emphasis on instrumental grounds. Where people, or whole societies, might be harmed by relieving people of responsibility for the consequences of their choices, this accountability can be imposed. But where the consequences of doing so would, on the whole, be adverse, there would remain no reason to do so. J. S. Mill[6] as noted by Richard Arneson (himself a luck egalitarian), urged that assistance be given to the impoverished up to the point at which further aid becomes harmful.[7] The point applies still more forcefully to health, since it is very unlikely that the threat of forfeiture of health care can serve as a deterrent to risk taking, and in particular that the harm that would be averted would be greater than that inflicted in denying care to the sick and injured.

6.4.2. The context of personal responsibility for health

These brief remarks do not tell against luck egalitarianism, or indeed against any theory of justice which has the consequence that individual responsibility for health should be assigned a central role in health policy decisions. This must be determined on the merits of these theories as general theories of justice. Though the medical examples are instructive, they appear in this literature only as illustrations; the tail does not wag the dog. This task cannot be undertaken here, but there are further considerations that tell against any attempt to put personal responsibility closer to the centre of the health policy stage, however well-founded the theory of justice which recommends doing so. These considerations are a mixture of practical and philosophical concerns.

Which actions are voluntary?

A moral viewpoint that puts great store on individual choice and responsibility must offer a criterion for determining which choices incur these obligations. The web of complications that stand in the way is, as we know from criminal law, extremely broad. But in criminal law we have at least a set of precedents and statutory specifications that guide us. In the case of personal responsibility for health, we have only the intuitions of one observer, set against that of another.

Moreover, actions only rarely have all the attributes—informed, voluntary, uncoerced, spontaneous, deliberated, etc.—that, in the ideal case, are preconditions for full personal responsibility. This is a particular problem in the case of lifestyles, which are matters of habit ingrained over many years and may have been learned from the individual's principal role models. The most dangerous elements of lifestyle, such as smoking or alcohol abuse, involve addiction, and the status of the smoker's decision to light up the next cigarette is anything but clear. One way around this problem is to assign personal responsibility on the basis of the initial decision to smoke, or the rational deliberation of the then-unaddicted individual to accept risk to health as the price of anticipated pleasure. This is the same strategy used by prosecutors of witchcraft in colonial Salem, Massachusetts, where both statute and common law viewed the acts of witchcraft as those of the inhabiting spirits and punished the witch

---

6 J. S. Mill, *Principles of Political Economy* (Toronto: University of Toronto Press, 1965), p. 961.

7 R. Arneson, "Egalitarianism and the Undeserving Poor," *Journal of Political Philosophy* 5, no. 4 (1997): pp. 327–350.

for having permitted the devil to assume her shape, or by having communed with the devil by commissioning him to do acts of mischief. As with the magistrates in Salem, it is no easy matter to establish when and where this originating sin occurs, or to link the severity of the sentence to the degree of wrongful risk that we might imagine has been assumed.

At the most fundamental level, this requirement takes us directly to the ancient question of freedom of the will. Any policy debate which awaits resolution of these uncertainties is a long way from closure. John Roemer, a luck egalitarian theorist, has taken up the challenge and offers, in the abstract, a method. Once again, a health example—responsibility for the consequences of smoking—is chosen as a focus for discussion.

Roemer's elegant proposal[8],[9] imagines that among factors leading to the act of smoking we can sort those over which the individual has control from those over which this is lacking. The circumstances of one's birth; one's gender; and perhaps one's social class, for example, may not be matters of one's choosing. But all of these seem to influence a person's pattern of tobacco use. Roemer recognises that different societies will identify the locus of control differently: the factors counted in one culture as beyond individual control may be regarded otherwise elsewhere. Roemer suggests that each society list the factors it wishes to recognise as beyond control, which in turn will delimit a "type"—for example, female schoolteachers, or male steelworkers. These "types," subject to different factors beyond individual control, will display different ranges of behaviour; for example, the steelworkers might smoke more than the schoolteachers. But, in Roemer's view, their degree of responsibility is not proportionate. Instead, Roemer suggests that the median individual in each type (as measured, for example, in the number of cigarettes smoked per day) should be assigned null responsibility, with accounting in a positive or negative direction proceeding from this midpoint. Roemer does not propose any particular list of such factors, and indeed is not committed to the premise that this question admits of anything other than a conventional answer. Still, in Roemer's view, the proposal will ensure that, in every society, responsibility will be assigned in proportion to the degree of personal control, as understood by that society. In Roemer's words, this is "A pragmatic theory of responsibility for the egalitarian planner".

It is as a pragmatic theory for planning purposes, however, that the first questions arise. For the debate within societies, including Roemer's, over how much control individuals have over their behaviour, much of the controversy is precisely over which factors should be on this list. The prospect that different societies will construct their lists in different ways, however responsive to cultural differences, itself advertises the likelihood that all these lists will reflect not metaphysical bedrock—that is, whether the individual really does have control, or lacks it—but rather the consensus of opinion. A dissident who rejects this consensus will thus have no reason to change his or her views. Finally, it is not clear how finely these "types" will be differentiated. Each individual's path to tobacco or obesity is distinct, channelled or inhibited by influences, opportunities, inclinations, and preferences unique to that person. Male steelworkers, even if they tend to smoke more than female schoolteachers, are an otherwise heterogeneous lot. If we classify like with exactly like, the groups will be too small and too homogeneous to admit of enough deviation from the median to generate Roemer's interesting result. The question of what counts as "a factor," that is, how precisely to account for a particular individual's behaviour, takes us directly back to the controversy, which the proposal was designed to resolve, over the possibility and scope of free choice given the apparent determinants in one's internal and external environments. Arneson, a luck egalitarian, moderates the policy impact of this approach in pointing out that responsibility and desert are proportional not only to the consequences of one's actions but also

[8] J. E. Roemer, "A Pragmatic Theory of Responsibility for the Egalitarian Planner," *Philosophy & Public Affairs* (1993): pp. 146–166.

[9] J. Roemer, "Equality and Responsibility," *Boston Review* 20, no. 2 (1995): pp. 3–7.

to the difficulty one faced in attempting to be prudent. Pill and Stott[10],[11] found that working class respondents trusted health information if obtained from someone they knew, but seldom otherwise; individuals vary, to some extent as a matter of chance, in the sources of information offered to them. These variations at the individual level are unlikely to be measurable at the societal level. And even when they are, we may not agree on their significance. Studies of the origins of class differences in health-related behaviour, for example, demonstrate that unhealthy habits of living are strongly predicted by poverty in childhood and throughout the lifespan.[12] Some people transcend these origins and life prudently; there is at least as much disagreement over the freedom of the others to do likewise as on any other issue in this complex debate.

Adverse effects of assigning responsibility

On a less metaphysical plane, an important consideration weighing against emphasis on personal responsibility for health is the potential harm that the enterprise might inflict upon the enterprise of health care, and on social policy on health affairs. One plausible ground for the resistance of physicians to basing treatment decisions on assessments of personal responsibility is the prospect that the very useful and virtuous first instinct of the doctor or nurse, that of sympathy and care for the suffering patient, might be attenuated—put on an unstable hold, as it were, until the verdict of fault comes in. All of us gain if and when doctors think of patients as patients (a point which tells also against financial screening of patients at the hospital door). The same point can be made for societies as a whole: it is not salutary for people to become used to withholding sympathy for sick fellow-citizens unless and until it is established that those who are sick could not have stayed healthy by acting more prudently.

Arbitrariness of fault-finding

The empirical findings of Ubel et al., mentioned above, point to a further reason for concern with the notion of assessing personal responsibility for health. Ubel's sample, it will be recalled, included people whose concern was less with the contribution to illness made by voluntary choice than with distaste for the kinds of people who were thought to make these choices. An examination of the small literature, beginning with Knowles, that has proposed a greater role for personal responsibility reveals that not all choices leading to illness are counted alike. Those that are targeted tend to be sins—sloth, gluttony, lust, to use their old-fashioned names—or to be behaviour, such as drug addiction, of the marginalised. We could, but do not, augment this list by adding other kinds of choices, also having a pronounced effect on health—of which we tend to approve. For example, the decision to have children, now that this involves a definite intention for many people, risks the health of the mother. A decision to postpone childbearing until advanced education has been completed markedly increases the risks for cervical and breast cancer. Daredevilry in sports and adventure risks life and limb, but the survivors are treated as heroes. If the moral principle underlying a move to give greater prominence to personal responsibility for health is that those who generate costs should pay for them, we should not expect that the only ones made to shoulder the costs are those who behave in ways that offend their neighbours. The point is not that a society must either demand compensation for all avoidable costs or else demand none. But the coincidence of two lists, that of lifestyles deemed burdensomely expensive and that of lifestyles deemed sinful, or of people deemed

[10] R. Pill and N. Stott, "Concepts of Illness Causation and Responsibility: Some Preliminary Data from a Sample of Working Class Mothers," *Social Science and Medicine* 16 (1982): pp. 43–52.

[11] R. Pill and N. Stott, "Choice or Chance: Further Evidence on Ideas of Illness and Responsibility for Health," *Social Science and Medicine* 20, no. 10 (1985): pp. 981–991.

[12] J. W. Lynch, G. A. Kaplan, and J. T. Salonen, "Why Do Poor People Behave Poorly? Variation in Adult Health Behaviors and Characteristics by Stages of the Socioeconomic Lifecourse," *Social Science and Medicine* 44, no. 6 (1997): pp. 809–819.

unworthy, suggests a different agenda from the stated one.

A sense of disproportion

Finally, a policy in which individuals are made to shoulder the burden caused by adverse consequences of choices they have made must make "the punishment fit the crime": the burden reimposed on the risk-taker should be proportional to the burden imposed by the risk taking. But there is no metric to permit this. One problem is that similar behaviour in different people, and in different circumstances, represents quite different levels of risk (Japanese men, for example, are less likely to contract lung cancer from smoking than American men). Moreover, some habits which are unhealthy, even lethal for some are actually health-giving to others; alcohol is the outstanding example. And some habits, because they are taxed, may present a net economic gain to their societies. When cigarette taxes are high, for example, the added medical costs generated by the use of tobacco are more than offset by the payment of taxes and the elimination of pensions when smokers die. Those who have taken care of themselves, in that kind of regime, are the real threat to their neighbours' well-being.

Exaggeration of interpersonal differences

When critics of the emerging literature on the influence of social status on health attempt to explain away the evident health impact of social inequality, the thrust of their commentary is to shift responsibility away from social institutions and social structure and onto individuals. But to make this plausible, a series of exaggerations are required. First, almost all of the measured differences in health status between social groups is attributed to behaviour. Second, almost all of that behaviour is characterised as purely voluntary. But neither claim is supportable. Though it is certainly true that working class adults in the United Kingdom and United States smoke more and weigh more than their well-to-do fellow citizens, on average, these differences account for only part of the difference in health. One widely cited study which examined the leading risk behaviours put the figure at 15% (Lantz et al. 1998).[13] Though others give higher estimates (and there is not agreement on what these figures mean), no investigators explain virtually all health differences associated with social status to differing lifestyles. Moreover, where these behavioural differences do exist, the extent to which these can reasonably be viewed as free, informed, and voluntary choices is partial at best. Even assuming that some of the behavioural differences reflect different values, goals, or attitudes toward time, the remainder is occasion enough for concern over the fairness of the distribution of health.

In this light, proposals to attach importance in health policy to imprudent health-related behaviour involve a great deal of hand-waving. A sense of proportion is elusive. This should not be surprising. The administration of the criminal law, in which degree of responsibility must be determined as closely as possible, requires the elaborate and expense apparatus of the courts, attorneys, and lengthy trials. There is nothing comparable in the medical world, and there is no common law built of precedents, penalties attached to particular kinds of acts over many years, adopted in the interest of a smoothly functioning society. Nor is there likely to be, nor would it be desirable if there were to be.

Taken together, these considerations suggest that health policies that would give personal responsibility for health a central role face severe objections. The theory of justice which seems most supportive of this policy is questionable on its own terms, and in any case does not lend this support without a number of dubious accompanying assumptions. These reservations are joined by a number of objections of a more practical nature which suggest that a commitment to assessing personal responsibility for health might be wrong-headed, arbitrary, disingenuous, and even dangerous.

---

[13] P. M. Lantz, et al., "Socioeconomic Factors, Health Behaviors, and Mortality: Results from a Nationally Representative Prospective Study of US Adults," *Journal of the American Medical Association* 279 (1998): pp. 1703–1708.

This account should not, however, end on that note. For a number of reasons, it is both practical and desirable that personal responsibility play a role (though not a central role) in public health and clinical medicine in the future.

One reason that personal responsibility for health should not be wholly ignored is the inherent desirability of free choice, and assumption of responsibility, for personal development and for the management of one's life course. Interpersonal variation in goals, preferences, and tastes—beyond the reckoning of the most omniscient managers—requires individual liberty so that circumstances can be tailored to the individual. Assumption of risk by the individual enables society to condone this freedom. This shouldering of the risk has numerous further benefits for the individual as well (though these can be overshadowed by seriously adverse consequences). . . .

Further Resources

Nongovernmental

Kaiser Family Foundation (KFF): Publishes an annual survey on employer health benefits, including data on different types of wellness incentives. Additional information can be found at http://kff.org/health-costs/report/2015-employer-health-benefits-survey/

Health Research & Educational Trust (HRET): Publishes an annual survey on employer health benefits, including data on different types of wellness incentives. Additional information can be found at http://www.hret.org/

Literature

Forde, Ian, and Rosalind Raine. "Placing the Individual within a Social Determinants Approach to Health Inequity." *The Lancet* 372, no. 9650: 1694–1696.

Horwitz, Jill R., Brenna D. Kelly, and John E. DiNardo. "Wellness Incentives in the Workplace: Cost Savings through Cost Shifting to Unhealthy Workers." *Health Affairs* 32, no. 3 (March 1, 2013): 468–476.

Sen, Aditi P., Taylor B. Sewell, E. Brooks Riley, Beth Stearman, Scarlett L. Bellamy, Michelle F. Hu, Yuanyuan Tao, et al. "Financial Incentives for Home-Based Health Monitoring: A Randomized Controlled Trial." *Journal of General Internal Medicine* 29, no. 5 (2014): 770–777.

Other Media

Dan Chaykin, "To Win, We Have to Lose—The Weight of the Nation," *HBO* video, 2012. http://theweightofthenation.hbo.com/watch/main-films/Consequences: Examines how America's weight problem affects all individuals, and the potential contribution wellness programs might make.

"Debating 'No Smoker' Hiring Policies." Narrated by Tracey Matisak. *WHYY*, April 5, 2013. http://whyy.org/cms/radiotimes/2013/04/05/debating-no-smoker-hiring-policies/: A debate over the ethics, benefits, and flaws of "no smoker" hiring policies.

"The Bottom Line," *PBS* video, 11:46, http://www.pbs.org/now/shows/health-care-reform/ : Discusses employer-provided healthcare and wellness incentives

15 Global Health Priorities

When it comes to funding global health, the world faces some stark choices. In 2000, the United Nations adopted eight Millennium Development Goals (MDGs) that included three fundamental health targets: (1) combatting HIV/AIDS, malaria, and tuberculosis (TB); (2) reducing child mortality by two-thirds between 1990 and 2015; and (3) improving maternal health and reducing maternal deaths.[1] To succeed the MDGs, the UN adopted in 2015 the significantly expanded Sustainable Development Goals (SDGs) that comprised 17 individual goals. Goal 3 focused specifically on health and set out 13 targets (see Box 15.1). In moving forward, it pays to look back: making progress toward the SDGs health goal benefits considerably from learning priority-setting lessons emerging from striving to achieve the MDGs.

Concomitantly, various official bodies, such as the World Health Organization (WHO) Commission on Microeconomics and Health and the Lancet Commission, have determined the minimal healthcare needs to achieve these types of health goals. These healthcare services typically include antiretroviral treatments for HIV/AIDS, a set of childhood vaccinations, and primary care. There have been estimates made about the amount of money needed to provide these basic healthcare services. In 2001, the WHO Commission on Macroeconomics and Health estimated this type of package costs about $34 per person per year.[2] More recently, the Lancet Commission estimated incremental costs of $26 per person per year in 2015.[3]

The problem is, however, that funding is not matching the need for financial support. The decade immediately after 2000 saw a significant increase in total global health assistance from annually just under $12 billion in 2000 to $35.9

---

[1] United Nations, *The Millennium Development Goals Report: 2015* (New York: 2015).

[2] Commission on Macroeconomics and Health, *Macroeconomics and Health: Investing in Health for Economic Development* (Geneva: World Health Organization, 2001), p. 11.

[3] D. T. Jamison, et al., "Global Health 2035: A World Converging within a Generation," *The Lancet* 382 (2013): pp. 1898–1955.

Box 15.1 *Goal Three of the UN's Sustainable Development Goals*

Goal 3. Ensure healthy lives and promote well-being for all at all ages.

3.1: By 2030, reduce the global maternal mortality ratio to less than 70 per 100,000 live births
3.2: By 2030, end preventable deaths of newborns and under-five children
3.3: By 2030, end the epidemics of AIDS, tuberculosis, malaria, and neglected tropical diseases and combat hepatitis, water-borne diseases, and other communicable diseases
3.4: By 2030, reduce by one-third premature mortality from noncommunicable diseases (NCDs) through prevention and treatment, and promote mental health and well-being
3.5: Strengthen prevention and treatment of substance abuse, including narcotic drug abuse and harmful use of alcohol
3.6: By 2020, halve global deaths and injuries from road traffic accidents
3.7: By 2030, ensure universal access to sexual and reproductive health care services, including for family planning, information and education, and the integration of reproductive health into national strategies and programmes
3.8: Achieve universal health coverage (UHC), including financial risk protection; access to quality essential health care services; and access to safe, effective, quality, and affordable essential medicines and vaccines for all
3.9: By 2030, substantially reduce the number of deaths and illnesses from hazardous chemicals and air, water, and soil pollution and contamination
3.a: Strengthen implementation of the Framework Convention on Tobacco Control in all countries as appropriate
3.b: Support research and development of vaccines and medicines for the communicable and noncommunicable diseases that primarily affect developing countries, provide access to affordable essential medicines and vaccines, in accordance with the Doha Declaration which affirms the right of developing countries to use to the full the provisions in the TRIPS agreement regarding flexibilities to protect public health and, in particular, provide access to medicines for all
3.c: Increase substantially health financing and the recruitment, development, and training and retention of the health workforce in developing countries, especially in LDCs and SIDS
3.d: Strengthen the capacity of all countries, particularly developing countries, for early warning, risk reduction, and management of national and global health risks

Source: United Nations, *Zero Draft of the Outcome Document*, p. 11.

billion in 2014.[4] While many factors contributed to this increased funding, the leading factor was an increase in US funding and especially the President's Emergency Plan for AIDS Relief (PEPFAR).[5] US aid increased from $2.7 billion in 2000 to $13.0 billion in 2011 before declining to $12.4 billion in 2014.[6,7] However, since about 2010, funding has slowed and even decreased from 2013 to 2014. In 2013, all the donor countries, foundations, and nongovernmental aid organizations combined contributed about $36.5 billion for global health assistance. More importantly, this amount has remained relatively flat for the past 4 years.[8] Many experts believe global health assistance is unlikely to increase significantly.[9] There may be temporary rises because of emergency situations such as the 2014 Ebola epidemic in West Africa (to which the US appropriated $5.4 billion in a spending bill at the year's end).[10] But it appears that the initial increase in global health aid has

[4] Institute for Health Metrics and Evaluation, *Financing Global Health 2014: Shifts in Funding as the MDG Era Closes* (Seattle, WA: IHME, 2015), p. 9, 21.

[5] Ibid., p. 22.

[6] Ibid., pp. 96–97.

[7] The Henry J. Kaiser Family Foundation, *Fact Sheet: The US President's Emergency Plan for AIDS Relief (PEPFAR)* (2014).

[8] Institute for Health Metrics and Evaluation, *Financing Global Health 2014*, pp. 9, 96–97.

[9] Ibid., p. 13.

[10] A. Parker and J. Weisman, "Congressional Leaders Reach Deal on Spending," *New York Times*, December 9, 2014.

come to an end, and, as the Institute for Health Metrics and Evaluation suggests, austerity has become the new normal.[11]

One consequence of the gap between the needs and available funding has been that the world has made less progress than envisaged with meeting the targets set out under the MDGs. For instance, while under-five mortality has dropped by almost 50%, from 90 deaths per 1,000 live births in 1990 to 43 in 2015, it is still far from the target of a two-thirds reduction.[12]

The needs are huge, and the funding is limited. Not all health needs can be met. This raises the fundamental question: What should be the priorities for global health assistance? Another way of framing the issue is to ask where should the next dollar, euro, pound, yen, or kroner in health assistance go? Should it fund additional antiretroviral treatment for HIV/AIDS? Should it fund more bed nets or antimalarial drugs? Should it fund the distribution of more advanced equipment to rapidly diagnose TB? What about expanding childhood vaccinations for pneumococcal pneumonia and rotavirus? Or what about expanding treatment for intestinal parasites? Should more health aid instead go to fund training of midwives for safe childbirth? Should priority be placed on the construction of additional clinics? Programs for community healthcare workers? The pessimistic way of putting the issue is this: If global health assistance actually declines, the question then becomes, "From what kind of programs should health assistance be cut?"

So, where *should* the next dollar, euro, pound, yen, or kroner in global health assistance go? Since countries differ considerably in the funding they make available (Table 15.1), should there be more effective supranational governance structures that promote proportionate efforts by all countries with sufficiently strong economies?

In making such resource allocation decisions, it is important to have some facts on global health. According to the WHO, in

Table 15.1
2014 Development Assistance for Health (DAH) by Country[13]

Country	Total 2014 DAH (in millions USD)
United States	12,385.93
United Kingdom	3,789.27
Germany	1,284.94
Canada	1,150.10
Japan	1,071.22
France	1,027.72
Australia	964.30
Norway	845.14
Netherlands	675.41
Sweden	313.73
South Korea	272.22
Belgium	206.04
Denmark	192.68
Switzerland	130.88
Spain	129.11
Austria	121.96
Italy	110.49
Ireland	93.08
Luxembourg	51.46
New Zealand	35.41
Finland	35.13
Portugal	7.93
Greece	0.28

low-income countries, the leading cause of death is lower respiratory infections—essentially pneumonia—followed by HIV/AIDS, diarrhea, and cardiovascular diseases including stroke and heart attacks (Figure 15.1). The ordering is similar for disability-adjusted life years (DALYs), where lower respiratory infections cause the most loss of DALYs, followed by HIV/AIDS and diarrhea (Table 15.2). Similarly, evaluations of current global funding allocations show that approximately 30.3% went to HIV/AIDS in 2014[14] (Figure 15.2).

[11] Institute for Health Metrics and Evaluation, *Financing Global Health 2013: Transition in an Age of Austerity* (Seattle, WA: IHME, 2014).

[12] United Nations, *The Millennium Development Goals Report: 2015*, p. 32.

[13] Institute for Health Metrics and Evaluation, *Financing Global Health 2014*, pp. 96–97, Table B2.

[14] Ibid., pp. 116–117.

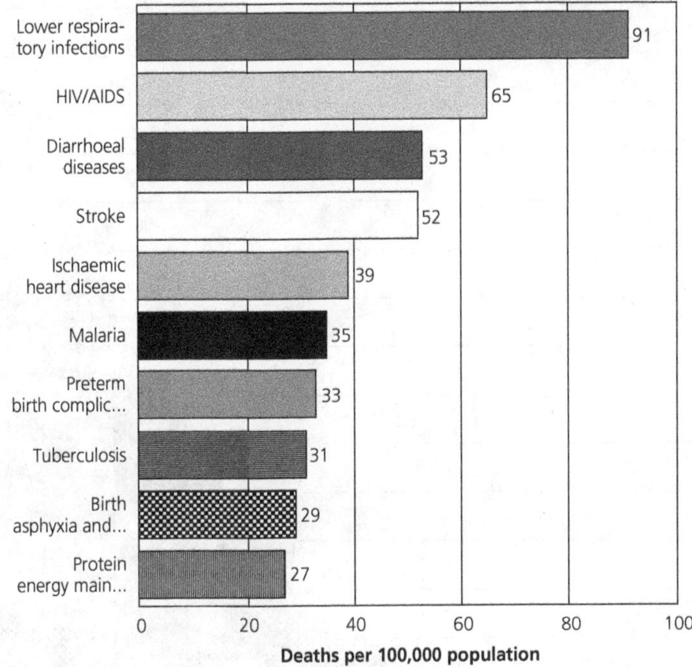

Figure 15.1 The top 10 causes of death in low-income countries, 2012.

World Health Organization, "The Top 10 Causes of Death: 2012," 2014, accessed October 31, 2015, http://www.who.int/mediacentre/factsheets/fs310/en/index1.html.

Table 15.2
Top 10 Leading Causes of DALYs in Low-Income Countries, 2012[15]

Cause	DALYs (000s)	% DALYs	DALYs per 100,000 population
All Causes	507,628	100.0	59979
Lower respiratory infections	46,610	9.2	5507
HIV/AIDS	34,610	6.8	4089
Diarrheal diseases	33,538	6.6	3963
Malaria	26,359	5.2	3114
Preterm birth complications	26,026	5.1	3075
Birth asphyxia and birth trauma	23,863	4.7	2820
Protein-energy malnutrition	13,956	2.8	1649
Tuberculosis	13,068	2.6	1544
Neonatal sepsis and infections	12,694	2.5	1500
Meningitis	11,445	2.3	1352

[15] World Health Organization, "Estimates for 2000–2012: Disease Burden," 2015, accessed November 2, 2015, http://www.who.int/healthinfo/global_burden_disease/estimates/en/index2.html.

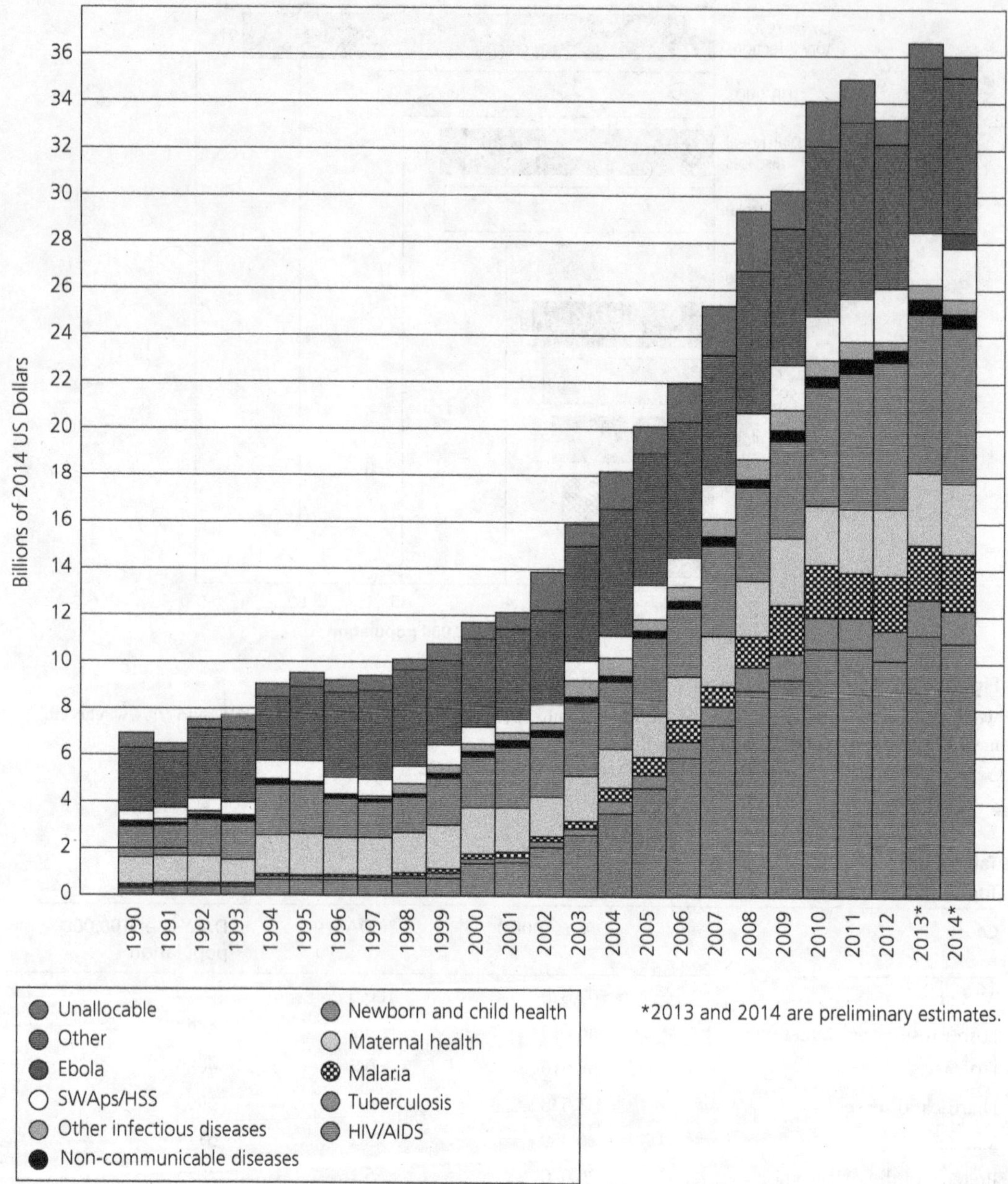

Figure 15.2 DAH by health focus area, 1990–2014.

Institute for Health Metrics and Evaluation, *Financing Global Health 2013*, p. 23, figure 6.

Johri and colleagues review four dominant philosophical theories of justice to elucidate their views of global health assistance (Excerpt 1).[16]

[16] M. Johri, et al., "Global Health and National Borders: The Ethics of Foreign Aid in a Time of Financial Crisis," *Globalization and Health* 8, no. 1 (2012): pp. 1–10.

There are significant differences between these theories. For instance, Singer is a consequentialist who believes national borders have no moral significance and calls upon all individuals to contribute to the healthcare of the less fortunate as long as the gain from that contribution will outweigh the loss caused by the contribution.

Pogge argues that the world order is rigged in favor of well-off countries, which are major contributors to worldwide poverty and ill health. Consequently, these wealthy countries have a duty not to harm people in developing countries, and this entails both changing the world order and aiding disadvantaged populations. His emphasis is on ensuring provision of essential medicines that he believes is obstructed by various international agreements that prioritize patent rights and other advantages for developed countries.

Shue recognizes the importance of ensuring all people have the security and subsistence that are preconditions for the exercise of all other rights and freedoms within national boundaries. The responsibility for providing security and subsistence normally falls to national governments. However, where national governments fail, other countries have a duty to ensure these responsibilities for security and subsistence are fulfilled. In this way, national governments of well-off countries have a duty to ensure that poor people have a basic minimum of security and subsistence to exercise their rights and freedoms.

Finally, Rawls—while not focusing on health specifically but instead on development efforts more broadly—provides a more complex argument. He recognizes that there are what he calls "burdened societies," those that are so deprived they cannot form just political institutions.[17] Well-ordered countries have duties to assist burdened societies to achieve a minimal level of development that allows them to be just. After that minimal level of assistance, any additional aid arises not out of an obligation but out of charity.

Johri and colleagues contend there is sufficient overlap among these four theories to justify a duty to provide global health assistance: "responsibilities to provide international assistance are significant for all four theories."[18] And "interventions for health enjoyed consistent prominence," reflecting the importance of health to living a fulfilling life.[19] But they do not go into detail about what kinds and how much of global health assistance would take priority.

[17] Ibid., p. 7.

[18] Ibid., p. 8.

[19] Ibid., p. 1.

Eeva Ollila tries to address this question directly (Excerpt 2).[20] She argues that the way global health assistance is prioritized reflects less the health needs of developing countries and more the fears and interests of developed aid donors:

> The lists of the current global health priorities can be seen as reflecting health related problems in the developing countries that are perceived to threaten the vital interests of industrialized countries.[21]

Concretely, this means an emphasis on infectious diseases and the use of technology to tackle these problems. Ollila objects to this prioritization on two grounds. First, noncommunicable diseases account for the "majority of ill-health in developing countries, and their importance is increasing rapidly." They are not receiving sufficient funding. Second, funding flows to "selected interventions," especially "the use of new technologies," rather than funding sustainable healthcare infrastructure is a mistake.[22]

The Commission on Smart Global Health Policy established by the US Center for Strategic and International Studies (CSIS), an influential independent think-tank, offers its own prioritization of US health assistance (Excerpt 3).[23] The priority-setting criteria are encapsulated in five points. First, the Commission urges maintaining funding for PEPFAR and especially HIV/AIDS treatment. Second, it recommends doubling funding for interventions aimed at women and children, especially those seeking to reduce infant deaths in the first month of life and those expanding vaccination efforts and access to family planning methods. Third, the Commission recommends long-range investments on preparedness to fight health hazards. The fourth recommendation is to create

[20] E. Ollila, "Global Health Priorities—Priorities of the Wealthy?", Globalization and Health 1, no. 6 (2005).

[21] Ibid.

[22] Ibid.

[23] W. J. Fallon and H. D. Gayle, Report of the CSIS Commission on Smart Global Health Policy: A Healthier, Safer, and More Prosperous World (Washington, DC: CSIS, 2010), pp. 8–13.

long-term predictability in global health assistance with, for example, a 15-year strategy that links funding to achieving performance targets. Finally, the Commission recommends focusing attention on multilateral organizations that can pool resources rather than do everything alone. Overall, the Commission recommends aiming toward $25 billion in US global health assistance by 2025 to support these five priorities,[24] representing more than a doubling of current assistance levels.[25]

Denny and Emanuel argue that increasing HIV/AIDS funding through PEPFAR or the Global Fund to Fight AIDS, Tuberculosis, and Malaria is not the best use of additional global health assistance dollars (Excerpt 4).[26] They argue that the focus on HIV/AIDS "fails to address many of the developing world's most serious health threats."[27] Instead, they argue that global health assistance should follow three fundamental principles: (1) save the most lives, (2) save young lives in particular, and (3) use "finite resources most effectively"; that is, allocate resources to the most cost-effective interventions.[28] Concretely, this means maintaining funding for HIV/AIDS but increasing funding for the health needs of mothers and children, specifically preventing and treating diarrhea, respiratory infections, TB, malaria, vaccine-preventable diseases, neonatal conditions, and maternal problems during delivery, such as infections and hemorrhage. Within these areas, funding should "emphasize cost-effective" interventions such as community-based care for neonatal pneumonia or insecticide-treated bed nets in malaria-infested areas.[29]

Onarheim and colleagues examine the health impact of increasing coverage for 14 interventions targeting child mortality in order to provide data on health impacts for policymakers who must choose where to spend global health assistance (Excerpt 5).[30] The interventions they evaluate range from institutional child delivery to oral rehydration for diarrhea to antimalarial drugs to pneumococcal vaccines to measles vaccines to improved water supplies. Somewhat surprisingly, the analysis shows that:

> If the policy makers opt for a few very effective interventions at a high coverage rate, [the package should include five interventions:] institutional delivery, oral rehydration solutions, case management of pneumonia, breastfeeding, and case management of severe neonatal infection.[31]

The authors show that institutional delivery saves five times more lives than insecticide-treated bed nets to prevent malaria.

In September 2015, the UN agreed upon SDGs that aim to set out "integrated, indivisible . . . global priorities for sustainable development."[32] Expanding the MDGs initial eight goals to 17, Goal 3 concerns health and urges states to "ensure healthy lives and promote well-being for all at all ages" by working toward 13 targets including, in Section 3.4, reducing by 2030 "by one-third pre-mature mortality from non-communicable diseases" (see also Box 15.1).[33] Imagine you are thrust into the role of a global health policy-maker and must allocate an additional $100 million in health aid. Where does it go? What are your priorities?

---

[24] Ibid., p. 32.

[25] Institute for Health Metrics and Evaluation, *Financing Global Health 2014*, pp. 96–97.

[26] C. C. Denny and E. J. Emanuel, "US Health Aids Beyond PEPFAR: The Mother & Child Campaign," *JAMA* 300, no. 17 (2008): pp. 2048–2051.

[27] Ibid., p. 2048.

[28] Ibid., p. 2049.

[29] Ibid.

[30] K. H. Onarheim, et al., "Prioritizing Child Heath Interventions in Ethiopia: Modeling Impact on Child Mortality, Life Expectancy and Inequality in Age at Death," *PLoS ONE* 7, no. 8 (2012).

[31] Ibid., pp. 4–5.

[32] United Nations, *Zero Draft of the Outcome Document for the UN Summit to Adopt the Post-2015 Development Agenda* (2015), p. 43.

[33] Ibid., pp. 9, 11.

Questions for Discussion

1. According to the WHHHO, there is roughly a $35 billion/year gap between the funds needed to meet all of the UN's health-related MDGs and the total aid funds available. If the global community increased aid by 0.05%, the gap would be closed. But the gap won't be closed. Or will it? What do you perceive as the primary obstacles to increasing funding, and how might they be overcome?
2. Which of the four theories of global health assistance that Johri and colleagues identify (Excerpt 1) do you find most persuasive?
3. In what way are noncommunicable diseases especially relevant in setting priorities for global health?
4. Denny and Emanuel argue in Excerpt 4 that global health assistance should follow three fundamental principles: (1) save the most lives, (2) save young lives in particular, and (3) allocate resources to the most cost-effective interventions. What challenges might this approach face?

EXCERPTS

Note: The following excerpts have generally been edited for length, and omissions are indicated with ellipses. Editing includes footnotes and endnotes, which have also been renumbered. For citation and related purposes, the full original source texts should be used.

EXCERPT 1

Abridged text from:

M. Johri, et al., "Global Health and National Borders: The Ethics of Foreign Aid in a Time of Financial Crisis," *Globalization and Health* 8, no. 1 (2012): pp. 1–10.

Global Health and National Borders: The Ethics of Foreign Aid in a Time of Financial Crisis

Mira Johri, Ryoa Chung, Angus Dawson, and Ted Schrecker

. . .

Background

In keeping with the vision of "a more peaceful, prosperous and just world" enshrined in the United Nations Millennium Development Goals (MDGs),[1] initiatives to improve global health and human development have proliferated over the last decade.[2,3,4,5] Although developing countries play the leading role, the success of these strategies depends critically on the participation of the citizens and governments of the donor nations (principally, the state members of the Group of Eight Countries (G8) and the European Union) through financial assistance and supportive policies. International development assistance for health (DAH) has enjoyed a special priority among donors in recent years.[6] Resources quadrupled from $5.6 billion in 1990 to $21.8 billion in 2007, and the rate of growth accelerated sharply after 2002.[7]

The future of global health financing is much more uncertain. The global financial crisis that began in 2008 has placed aid budgets under pressure.[8] Although DAH continued to expand between 2007 and 2010, the rate of growth slowed dramatically.[9] Competition among global health priorities may also have intensified. In 2010, world leaders endorsed an ambitious new scheme to reach the MDGs by the 2015 target date through a focus on the health of the most vulnerable women and children.[10] Yet, funding for international assistance for HIV and AIDS

[1] United Nations General Assembly, "United Nations Millennium Declaration," 2000.

[2] Commission on Macroeconomics and Health, *Macroeconomics and Health: Investing in Health for Economic Development* (Geneva: World Health Organization, 2001).

[3] WHO Commission on Social Determinants of Health, *Closing the Gap in a Generation: Health Equity through Action on the Social Determinants of Health: Commission on Social Determinants of Health Final Report* (World Health Organization, 2008).

[4] GAVI Alliance, http://www.gavialliance.org/

[5] The Global Fund to Fight AIDS, Tuberculosis and Malaria, http://www.theglobalfund.org/en/

[6] N. Ravishankar, et al., "Financing of Global Health: Tracking Development Assistance for Health from 1990 to 2007," Lancet 373, no. 9681 (2009): pp. 2113–2124.

[7] Ibid.

[8] D. W. Te Velde, "The Global Financial Crisis and Developing Countries," *ODI Background Note.* (London: Overseas Development Institute, 2008).

[9] C. J. Murray, et al., "Development Assistance for Health: Trends and Prospects," *Lancet* 378, no. 9785 (2011): pp. 8–10.

[10] United Nations, *Global Strategy for Women's and Children's Health* (Geneva: UN, 2010), p. 20.

provided by donor governments declined by 10% over the 2009–2010 period, marking the first time year-to-year support for HIV and AIDS has fallen in more than a decade.[11]

It is too early to know what the 2011 Eurozone crisis will mean for global health funding; however, a slowdown in global growth[12] and fiscal austerity in Europe and elsewhere will almost certainly put additional downward pressure on meeting aid targets.[13,14,15] The United States Congress is now considering the first significant cuts in overseas aid in nearly two decades, on the order of $12 billion, or 20% of the President's request for 2012.[16,17]

The competition between national priorities and foreign aid commitments raises important ethical questions. For some, the motivation to support global health is based on a principle of universal solidarity among human beings.[18] However, for many, national borders delimit the prime locus of moral responsibility. The duty to alleviate suffering abroad is seen as discretionary, and distinctly secondary to domestic concerns. Two arguments dovetail to support this latter perspective. A realist conception of international relations suggests that the proper role of every national government is to represent and advance the interests of its own nation. Similarly, many ethicists hold that we have more important moral duties towards co-nationals, with whom we share a common past, the benefits and burdens of social cooperation, and a common destiny.[19] The view that "charity begins at home" may seem particularly salient in the current context of financial uncertainty and the prospect of a global economic recession.

To ensure that global health priorities receive adequate and stable funding it will be essential not only to demonstrate the effectiveness of interventions and programmes[20], but also to clarify the reasons for our commitment to this goal. . . .

Results

We reviewed four theories representing consequentialist (Singer), relational (Pogge), human rights (Shue), and social contract (Rawls) approaches. . . .

Four theories of justice

. . . Table [15.3] provides an overview of the four theories, Table [15.4] presents common objections to each view, and Table [15.5] offers examples of the types of policies that could be supported by each approach.[21]

. . .

---

[11] Kaiser Family Foundation and the Joint United Nations Programme on HIV/AIDS (UNAIDS), *Financing the Response to Aids in Low- and Middle-Income Countries: International Assistance from the G8, European Commission and Other Donor Governments in 2010.* (Geneva: KFF/UNAIDS, 2010).

[12] International Monetary Fund, *World Economic Outlook (WEO): Slowing Growth, Rising Risks* (Washington: International Monetary Fund, 2011).

[13] I. Massa, J. Keane, and J. Kennan, *The Euro Zone Crisis: Risks for Developing Countries* (London: Overseas Development Institute, 2011), p. 7.

[14] D. Saunders, "Foreign Aid Taking a Back Seat to Euro Crisis at G20," *The Globe and Mail*, November 3, 2011.

[15] L. Bryant, "G20 Summit Gives Less Aid to Poor Countries," *Voice of America*, November 4, 2011.

[16] S. L. Myers, "Foreign Aid Set to Take a Hit in US Budget Crisis," *New York Times*, October 4, 2011.

[17] D. Gartner, *Congress and Foreign Aid* (Brookings Institution, 2011).

[18] WHO Commission on Social Determinants of Health, *Closing the Gap*.

[19] Miller D., *On Nationality* (Clarendon, 1995).

[20] Murray, "Development Assistance for Health."

[21] Department of Health, "Health Is Global: Proposals for a UK Government-Wide Strategy. A Report from the UK's Chief Medical Adviser Sir Liam Donaldson," 2007.

Table [15.3]
Importance of the Health of the Global Poor[a] on Four Accounts of Justice

	Singer	Pogge	Shue	Rawls
Addressed to whom?	Individual moral agents	Individuals & national governments	Individuals & national governments	National governments & their peoples
National borders important?	No	Possibly	Yes	Yes
Key concepts	Individuals have an obligation to prevent the occurrence of something significantly bad if they can do so at acceptable cost to themselves.	We have a duty not to cause severe harm for minor gain. This obligation remains equally valid if an agent is responsible for causing harm in a jurisdiction outside his or her national borders, and is independent of whether we should privilege obligations to compatriots.	Two basic rights—subsistence and security–constitute preconditions for the enjoyment and exercise of all other rights and freedoms. Liberal democratic states have a duty to adopt foreign policies consistent with these fundamental human rights.	Under an idealised form of social contract, representatives of free and equal societies would adopt 8 principles of governance that enable an ideal global community to live together over time in peace, harmony and mutual respect.
Is health of the global poor important?	Yes	Yes, under certain conditions	Yes, to a limited extent	Yes, if useful to achieve just political arrangements
Why?	The global rich can ameliorate the suffering of the global poor with little sacrifice to themselves.	The international community is in some instances causally implicated in the genesis and perpetuation of severe poverty and ill health worldwide.	In instances where national governments fail to protect basic rights, others have a duty to guarantee their fulfilment. The right to subsistence guarantees every person worldwide a decent chance at a long and healthy life.	The 8 principles include a duty to "assist other peoples living under unfavourable conditions that prevent their having a just or decent political and social regime." Empirical evidence shows that population health contributes to just political arrangements.
What kind of obligation?[b]	Justice	Justice	Justice	Justice or charity[c]

What is the extent of the obligation?	Until suffering has been eliminated	Until causal responsibility for harm has been corrected and adequately compensated[d]	Until a basic minimum has been provided	Until the international community has enabled burdened societies to develop just political arrangements
Which health-related strategies should be privileged?	Poverty alleviation & action on other determinants of health	Examination of national policy coherence to avoid causing or contributing to harms abroad;	Examination of national policy coherence to avoid depriving or contributing to deprivation abroad;	Those that strengthen basic institutions to a minimally decent threshold, enabling further social development.
	Provision of health care	Analysis of the effects of global institutions Institutional reforms to promote satisfaction of human rights[e]	Provision of aid to ensure subsistence rights[f], including guarantees related to the social determinants of health and minimal preventive health care.	Candidate strategies could (1) promote equality of opportunity (especially in education and training), e.g. through child health; (2) offer additional synergies for development, e.g. by focussing on the rights and fundamental interests of women.

[a] The World Bank defines poverty as "pronounced deprivation in well-being" comprising multiple dimensions such as low incomes and the inability to acquire the basic goods and services necessary for survival with dignity, low levels of health and education, poor access to clean water and sanitation, inadequate physical security, lack of voice, and insufficient capacity and opportunity to better one's life. The global poor are poor in an absolute sense.[i]

[b] Each theory takes a position on the question of whether duties towards the health of those outside our borders are matters of "justice" or "charity." Duties of justice are precise, owed to specifiable others, and can in principle be legally enforced, whereas duties of charity admit of discretion in relation to their nature, timing, and choice of beneficiary. Charitable duties are adopted through conscious choice and are not legally enforceable.

[c] For Rawls, the duty to assist is a duty of justice under the principles of the Law of Peoples. Beyond the threshold of minimal decency, the duty to assist becomes charity.

[d] According to Pogge, degree of responsibility is proportional to benefits reaped and is discharged when proportional compensation is made.[ii]

[e] For Pogge, a guarantee of human rights aims to confer on all human beings worldwide "secure access" to "minimally adequate shares" of basic freedoms of participation, of food, drink, clothing, shelter, education and health care.[iii]

[f] For Shue, minimal economic security, or subsistence, entails "unpolluted air, unpolluted water, adequate food, adequate clothing, adequate shelter, and minimal preventive public health care.[iv]

[i] J. Haughton and S. R. Khandker, *Handbook on Poverty and Inequality* (Washington, D.C.: The World Bank, 2009).

[ii] T. Pogge, "Severe Poverty as a Violation of Negative Duties," *Ethics & International Affairs* 19, no. 01 (2005): pp. 55–83.

[iii] T. W. Pogge, *World Poverty and Human Rights* (Cambridge: Polity Press, 2002).

[iv] H. Shue, *Basic Rights: Subsistence, Affluence, and US Foreign Policy* (Princeton University Press, 1996).

Table [15.4]
Common Criticisms of the Four Theories[a]

	Criticisms	Rejoinders
Singer[b]	Moral priorities should focus on local need, for reasons similar to those raised in relation to national borders.	Singer allows that psychologically it might make a difference whether an individual is in severe need in front of one's eyes or in a far-away country, but that it makes no moral difference.
	Singer demands too much of individuals as there will always be further work to do to relieve suffering somewhere in the world. All of one's time could be spent relieving suffering, potentially endangering one's own well-being.	This is unlikely to pose a problem in practice. Singer's recent work aims to define attainable standards for living an ethical life in a world that contains great affluence and extreme poverty.[c]
	Any obligation to respond to the challenges of global health should be understood as one of charity rather than justice.	For Singer, the severity of the suffering involved means that talk of charity is inappropriate. Provision of toys to children may be a fit subject for "charity," but not meeting essential health needs.
Pogge	Does Pogge's analysis of harm cohere with ordinary usage? Does it satisfy the description of a negative duty (i.e. an injunction to refrain from doing something, in this case, causing harm)?	Harm is always properly judged in relation to a subjunctive standard (i.e., the possibility of an alternative institutional order in which fewer serious harms are committed).
	Is Pogge's empirical description of the global order accurate? Local factors such as poor governance or corruption are important in explaining the poverty of developing countries.	Pogge emphasises that local and global factors often interact in complex ways, and that local factors may often have current or past non-local causes.[d] While it may often be sufficient to point either to local causes or to global causes to explain the persistence a phenomenon such as severe poverty or poor health status, this recognition cannot diminish the share of moral responsibility attributable to either set of factors.[e]
Shue	Shue's concept of subsistence rights is indeterminate and may open the door to unduly extensive obligations	The concept of subsistence rights is not designed to foster global economic equality and is sufficiently clear to guide foreign policy.

Rawls	Individuals may be poorly served by a theory addressed primarily to peoples. One's nation of birth is a matter of luck rather than choice, and is hence morally arbitrary. It should not influence life chances unduly. In addition, citizens may not be well represented by their head of state. We have stronger duties towards individuals than Rawls's theory suggests.	If we address our theory to individuals rather than peoples, we risk undue interference in the domestic affairs of independent peoples and exceed the proper scope of justice.
	Is the thesis of explanatory nationalism, which holds that the key ingredient in how a country fares is its own political culture and traditions, correct?	Depends on one's interpretation of empirical evidence.

[a] These are criticisms commonly raised in the philosophical literature and by no means represent an exhaustive list. Rejoinders presented are consistent with the authors' standpoint.

[b] A general criticism of all consequentialist approaches would be that factors other than consequences are relevant to determining moral duties. Singer, like other consequentialists, would disagree.

[c] Singer, *The Life You Can Save*.

[d] T. W. Pogge, "Responsibilities for Poverty-Related Ill Health," *Ethics & International Affairs* 16, no. 02 (2002): pp. 71–79.

[e] Pogge, *World Poverty and Human Rights*.

Table [15.5]
Examples of Policies that Cohere with Each of the Four Accounts of Justice[a,b]

Policies	Singer	Pogge	Shue	Rawls
Reform of international arrangements governing medical research and development[c]		X	X	X
Sustainable domestic policies for high-income countries in relation to human resources for health[d]		X	X	
Proportional compensation for the health effects of environmental pollution & climate change		X	X	X
Ensuring transparency and coherence in the effects of foreign and domestic policies on health worldwide		X	X	
Reducing inequalities in health between countries through foreign and domestic policies				
Reducing agricultural trade subsidies & other protectionist practices		X	X	X
Regulatory measures to contain speculation in financial and commodity markets		X		
Meeting financial commitments to global development initiatives, such as 0.7% GDP	X	X	X	
Support for the health-related MDGs	X	X	X	X
Support for the Global Fund to Fight AIDS, Tuberculosis and Malaria (GFATM)	X	X	X	X
Support for the Global Alliance for Vaccines and Immunisation (GAVI)	X	X	X	X
Support for the UN Global Strategy for Women's and Children's Health	X	X	X	X

[a] Several of these policies were drawn from the UK "Health is global" report.[i]
[b] An "X" indicates that the policy would be supported. Detailed reasons are provided in the Additional file 2. Absence of an "X" means either that the answer is indeterminate (the theory is silent on these points) or negative.
[c] Examples include the trade-related aspects of intellectual property rights (TRIPS) agreement, and so-called "TRIPS plus" bilateral agreements.
[d] Specifically, ceasing to underfund medical training at the domestic level and to import qualified professionals from the developing world.
[i] Department of Health, "Health Is Global."

Peter Singer and the requirements to aid others in need

. . .

Consequentialists believe that consideration of outcomes forms the relevant basis for deciding which policies and practices are morally correct. Some versions may specify a single good, such as pleasure or the avoidance of pain,[22] while others promote the satisfaction of preferences,[23] or an objective list of several goods to be promoted equally. Most forms of consequentialism focus on maximising beneficial outcomes, but this is not always the case.

. . . Every human being has the capacity for suffering and enjoyment or happiness, and is thus deserving of equal consideration.[24] Contrasting the estimated 8.8 million child deaths worldwide in 2008 due to preventable, poverty-related causes[25] with the relative comfort in which almost 1 billion people live, Singer maintains that the global rich have an obligation to alleviate the suffering of the

22 J. Bentham, *The Principles of Morals and Legislation* (Clarendon Press, 1879).

23 P. Singer, Practical Ethics (Cambridge University Press, 1979).

24 Ibid.

25 R. E. Black, et al., "Global, Regional, and National Causes of Child Mortality in 2008: A Systematic Analysis," *Lancet* 375, no. 9730 (2010): pp. 1969–1987.

global poor. He argues that, if we can prevent something importantly bad without sacrificing anything of comparable significance, we ought to do so. As the morbidity and premature death linked to extreme poverty is deeply bad and a significant proportion can be prevented without undue sacrifice, this ought to be done.[26]

. . . The consequentialist moral point of view is inherently radically impartial, surmounting specific attachments to individuals, communities and countries.

Thomas Pogge on global institutions and the duty not to harm

. . .

. . . First, the governments of wealthy nations "enjoy a crushing advantage in terms of bargaining power and expertise;" and second, international negotiations are based on an adversarial system in which country level representatives seek to advance the best interests of their nation. Systematic consideration of the needs of the global poor is not a part of the mandate of any of the powerful parties to the negotiation. The cumulative results are a grossly unfair global order in which benefits flow predominantly to the affluent.[27]

. . . First, decisions taken by global institutions, state actors or corporations may cause or aggravate problems in securing critical determinants of health. Negative consequences disproportionately impact the global poor, while the benefits of development have fallen mainly to the affluent. Second, decisions have at times impeded the ability of developing country governments to provide health care to their own citizens, for example through structural adjustment or trade policies. For Pogge, a particularly important issue concerns essential medicines.[28] He believes that the global medical innovation system embodied in the World Trade Organization (WTO)'s Trade Related Intellectual Property Rights (TRIPS) agreement is unjust. An independent commission confirmed that the benefits of the current system flow disproportionately towards rich countries.[29]

Pogge invokes a central element of Western morality: it is wrong severely to harm innocent people for minor gains. The duty not to harm (a so-called negative duty, as distinct from positive duties like those to render assistance) is considered a strict obligation applicable equally to fellow citizens and foreigners. If Pogge is correct about the harm caused by our global institutions, this implies that we have an immediate duty of justice to those harmed regardless of where they live.[30]

There has been much debate about Pogge's proposal and the correct baseline for determining harm. Taking a "state of nature" perspective one might perhaps argue that, in the absence of something like the current global order, the global poor would have been no worse off.

This objection misconstrues Pogge's claim. Pogge proposes that we appeal to human rights as a minimum standard for judging the adequacy of institutions. Inspired by the 1948 Universal Declaration of Human Rights which states: "Everyone is entitled to a social and international order in which the rights and freedoms set forth in this Declaration can be fully realized,"[31] he argues that any justifiable international order must be designed insofar as reasonably possible to guarantee human rights including basic freedoms of participation, subsistence, education and health care. Pogge argues that the attribution of harm implicitly involves a "subjunctive" (as opposed to an historical) comparison, and that the correct subjunctive comparison would be the possibility of a feasible alternative institutional order in

[26] P. Singer, *The Life You Can Save: How to Do Your Part to End World Poverty* (Random House Publishing Group, 2010).

[27] A. Sen, "Why Health Equity?," *Health Economics* 11, no. 8 (2002): pp. 659–666.

[28] T. W. Pogge, "Human Rights and Global Health: A Research Program," *Metaphilosophy* 36, no. 1–2 (2005): pp. 182–209.

[29] World Health Organization, *Public Health-Innovation and Intellectual Property Rights: Report of the Commission on Intellectual Property Rights, Innovation and Public Health* (World Health Organization, 2006).

[30] Pogge, "World Poverty and Human Rights."

[31] United Nations General Assembly, *The Universal Declaration of Human Rights* (Geneva: World Health Organization, 1948).

which fewer human rights deficits would be produced.[32,33,34]

In sum, for Pogge, a set of global institutional arrangements is unjust if it foreseeably perpetuates large-scale human rights deficits that could reasonably be avoided through feasible institutional modifications. He amasses empirical evidence to demonstrate that the citizens of wealthy nations via their elected governments contribute to the perpetuation of global poverty and ill health. If Pogge's analysis is correct, we have a strict obligation of justice, grounded in the duty not to cause harm, to change our institutions and take concrete compensatory actions.[35]

Henry Shue on "basic rights"

Oxford University's Henry Shue focusses on the role of human rights, especially economic rights, in international affairs. Discussions of human rights in the West have generally distinguished "civil and political" from "social, economic and cultural" rights and given priority to the former. Shue argues that the most fundamental core of the economic rights, which he calls "subsistence rights," ought also to receive priority.[36]

Shue maintains that there are basic rights to security and subsistence. His defence of subsistence as a basic right has three main components.

(1) Some charge that the right to subsistence is a "positive right" and thus inherently of lower priority. According to a commonly held liberal view, positive rights entail correlative duties to act, whereas negative rights entail duties merely not to violate and not to interfere with other's fundamental freedoms. For example, the (negative) right to physical security can be understood as a right held by all implying a universal injunction to refrain from threatening the physical integrity of others. On this view, negative rights represent obligations for which one has a right to compel performance and impose sanctions for non-performance. Positive rights are more indeterminate; moreover, failure to comply confers no legal sanction. Shue counters this charge noting that all rights are in fact mixed and require both negative and positive actions to secure their enjoyment. For instance, the right to physical security implies not only that all citizens within a state refrain from assaulting one another, but also that the government undertake substantive steps to sustain a coercive system of justice and a police force.

(2) The right to physical integrity is often argued to have special priority in that no one can fully enjoy any right if her physical integrity is threatened. Shue makes a parallel case for subsistence rights. He argues that the rights to physical integrity and subsistence collectively provide the material preconditions necessary to the enjoyment of all other rights, such as the right to property, the right to equal political participation, and the right to freedom of association.

(3) To complement the idea of basic rights, Shue offers a theory of related duties. Essentially, "basic rights are everyone's minimum reasonable demands upon the rest of humanity"; they call for three kinds of duties incumbent upon individuals and societies. These are: 1) the duty to avoid depriving; 2) the duty to protect from deprivation; and 3) the duty to aid the deprived.

What does Shue's thesis about "basic rights" imply about transnational duties towards health? His response is somewhat ambivalent and falls short of asserting universal duties towards all those deprived of their basic rights. A particularly important challenge comes from an interlocutor who accepts the notion of universal subsistence rights, but argues that responsibility

[32] Pogge, "Severe Poverty as a Violation of Negative Duties."

[33] Pogge, "World Poverty and Human Rights."

[34] Pogge, "Responsibilities for Poverty-Related Ill Health."

[35] Pogge, "World Poverty and Human Rights."

[36] Shue, *Basic Rights*.

for their fulfilment rests with the nation of the bearer of the duty.[37] For Shue, duties beyond borders figure principally as "a back-up arrangement for the failure of so-called national governments" and come into play "where the state with the primary duty to protect rights fails for lack of will or lack of capacity to fulfill its duty."[38] In essence, to the extent that liberal democracies accept that basic rights are fundamental to domestic justice, Shue argues that a principle of consistency requires that they also respect and promote basic rights through foreign policy in countries where appropriate institutional provisions are absent or incomplete. Therefore, even if national boundaries legitimately delimit political communities whose members share strong ties and obligations, states espousing liberal democratic values have a duty to adopt foreign policies consistent with basic rights.

The right to subsistence aims to guarantee every human being worldwide a decent chance at living a long and healthy life, and includes protection from extreme poverty and guarantees related to the social determinants of health, as well as elementary health care.[39]

John Rawls and the duty of assistance

Perhaps the most influential analyst of international responsibilities from a liberal perspective, the late Harvard philosopher John Rawls addressed the question of how reasonable citizens and peoples might live together peacefully in a just world. His work is animated by the belief that the greatest evils of human history—including war, persecution, starvation and poverty—are the consequence of political injustice, and the removal of such injustice the key to their resolution.[40] For Rawls, the fundamental subjects of international law are political societies or "peoples," collective entities with specific concepts of right and justice whose territory is bounded by borders. The diversity of values and cultures among peoples is the result of legitimate free exercise of human reason, and tolerance requires that we refrain from imposition of a supposedly universal conception of human rights and liberal democracy at the international level.

Rawls's description of a just international community is based on his description of justice at the national level.[41] Speaking of modern constitutional democracies, Rawls argues that a just state must structure economic opportunities and social conditions so as to guarantee "fair equality of opportunity" in terms of life chances of the members of different sectors of society. Within a framework of guaranteed rights and liberties, Rawls proposes that social and economic inequalities be permitted only to the extent that they are of greatest benefit to the least advantaged. He argues that these principles of social cooperation reflect the notion of "reciprocity," or what it would be reasonable for free and equal persons ignorant of their specific future roles to accept in an ideal form of social contract.[42]

At the international level Rawls envisages a similar hypothetical social contract. The representatives of peoples come together in a context of reciprocity, characterised by symmetry, freedom and equality of the parties. In a situation that masks specific knowledge of features such as country size, wealth and history, Rawls claims that the representatives would define eight principles of mutual governance, including a duty to "assist other peoples living under unfavourable conditions that prevent their having a just or decent political and social regime."[43]

The duty to aid burdened societies

Rawls distinguishes duties and norms of conduct governing the relationship of "well-ordered peoples" (generally, liberal democracies) to two types of societies: "outlaw states" that refuse to comply with international law, and—the focus

---

[37] Ibid.

[38] Ibid.

[39] Ibid.

[40] J. Rawls, *The Law of Peoples* (Harvard University Press, 1999).

[41] J. Rawls, *A Theory of Justice, Revised Edition* (Cambridge: Harvard University Press, 1999).

[42] M. Marmot, "Health in an Unequal World," *The Lancet* 368, no. 9552 (2006): pp. 2081–2094.

[43] Rawls, *The Law of Peoples*.

of our interest—"burdened societies." Rawls defines burdened societies as those that suffer from unfavourable circumstances that preclude them from developing just political institutions. Moreover, he maintains that the key element in how a country fares overall is its own political culture and traditions, rather than poor luck in its share of natural resources or external factors related to interactions between states.[44] This thesis, known as "explanatory nationalism," is highly contested. In keeping with this view, Rawls limits universally valid human rights to political rights.

Although his eight rules of governance do not include a principle of distributive justice, Rawls holds that well-ordered societies have an important duty to assist burdened societies. He offers three points of guidance. First, mechanisms for assistance should be chosen so as to effect a change in the political culture and institutions of the burdened society. Rawls argues that economic transfers may not be most appropriate for realising this goal.[45] Among recommended courses of action, Rawls stresses the importance of policies and interventions that emphasise human rights, particularly those that further the rights and fundamental interests of women.[46] Second, while recognising that poverty and a lack of material resources may impact on a country's ability to develop and maintain positive political institutions, the aim of the duty of assistance is not to compensate for material lacks, to equalise levels of wealth across societies, or to permit continuous economic growth. Third, the objective of assistance is to enable burdened societies to achieve just political arrangements. When this is achieved further assistance is not required, even if the society remains relatively poor.[47]

Health & the duty of assistance

The aim of Rawls' duty of assistance is to enable burdened societies to achieve just political arrangements. As this duty is framed in political terms it entails no obvious health-related obligations. Candidate strategies must be justified by demonstrating their contribution to just political arrangements. We argue that supporters of a rawlsian position should privilege health-related interventions, as empirical evidence shows that interventions to improve global health make an essential contribution to achieving just political arrangements. We offer two complementary reasons.

Unhealthy societies cannot be politically just. Rawls describes several criteria that must be satisfied in order for a society to be just. At the domestic level, a just society must satisfy Rawls's principle of equality of opportunity.[48] Yet, there is extensive empirical evidence that health problems are disproportionately concentrated in disadvantaged population sub-groups, reflecting and exacerbating social and economic differences between the members of a society.[49] Everywhere the burden of disease is high, the chance to survive to adulthood, when the rights and privileges of democratic citizenship can be exercised, differs sharply across social groups. Deeply unhealthy societies therefore cannot guarantee that those with similar abilities, skills and initiative have similar life chances, regardless of starting point.

Out of respect for national sovereignty, Rawls offers a less stringent version of the equality of opportunity principle for state members of the just international community. The international version stipulates that all states must, at a minimum, maintain equality of opportunity in education and training.[50] However, child survival, school performance and life prospects are importantly affected by preventable and treatable health conditions, and negative effects are concentrated among vulnerable population sub-groups.[51] Where the burden of disease is high, the principle of equality of opportunity in education and training cannot be met.

---

44 Ibid.

45 Ibid.

46 Ibid.

47 Ibid.

48 Rawls, *A Theory of Justice*.

49 Marmot, "Health in an Unequal World."

50 Rawls, *The Law of Peoples*.

51 WHO Commission on Social Determinants of Health, *Closing the Gap*.

Rawls also views basic economic entitlements as essential to just political arrangements.[52] A high burden of disease contributes to the entrenchment of poverty and threatens subsistence rights, with greatest impact upon the vulnerable and powerless.[53,54] For this ensemble of reasons, societies with a high burden of disease necessarily fail to meet criteria for just political arrangements.

Health interventions are a particularly effective way to promote just political arrangements. Conversely, for many otherwise vibrantly democratic developing nations, failure to achieve a reasonable standard of population health is a major impediment to achieving just political arrangements. Where the burden of disease is still high, improvements in population health would speed the process of transition to just societies by making it possible for individuals to enjoy real exercise of their rights, liberties and opportunities and to avoid destitution. Such policies would disproportionately promote the well-being and empowerment of women and children. Health interventions are also potentially very effective in stimulating sustainable economic growth and alleviating poverty.[55]

Discussion

The moral significance of national borders is perhaps the central question facing contemporary theories of justice. Noting that one's country of birth is a matter of moral luck, cosmopolitan philosophers[56,57] argue that the deep inequalities that characterise our globe are injustices that ought to be corrected by the international community. Their nationalist counterparts[58,59] argue that the concept of justice does not properly apply in the international context. These philosophers highlight the absence of legitimate institutions of common governance at the global level and the importance of preserving national autonomy.

We have reviewed four theories taking different positions in this debate and highlighted the reasons that each might give to support initiatives to improve the health of the worst off worldwide [Table [15.3]]. The four theories offer distinct rationales for intervention and suggest different limits on responsibilities, with cosmopolitan theories (Singer, Pogge) generally upholding more widespread and urgent responsibilities for health beyond borders than their nationalist counterparts (Shue, Rawls), who seek to qualify the scope of such duties. Notwithstanding, some important commonalities emerge.

First, whether conceived as obligations of justice or charity, responsibilities to provide international assistance are significant for all four theories (Table [15.3]). Even those theorists who see national borders as highly morally salient recognise the importance of some supranational obligations, in contradiction to the popular presumption that domestic concerns always have priority. In other words, there are limits to the scope of acceptable national autonomy.

Second, among the range of potential aid foci, interventions for health enjoy consistent prominence (Table [15.3]). This reflects the inherent importance of health to individuals and its contribution to leading a dignified and fulfilling life [36], as well as the intimate link between health and development.[60] The importance of global health is explicit for Singer, Pogge and Shue, while for Rawls it follows from the effectiveness of health interventions in strengthening equality of opportunity and thereby, just political arrangements.

[52] Rawls, *The Law of Peoples*.

[53] Marmot, "Health in an Unequal World."

[54] D. McIntyre, et al., "What Are the Economic Consequences for Households of Illness and of Paying for Health Care in Low- and Middle-Income Country Contexts?," *Social Science and Medicine* 62, no. 4 (2006): pp. 858–865.

[55] Commission on Macroeconomics and Health, *Macroeconomics and Health*.

[56] Pogge, *World Poverty and Human Rights*.

[57] Singer, *The Life You Can Save*.

[58] Shue, *Basic Rights*.

[59] Rawls, *The Law of Peoples*.

[60] Commission on Macroeconomics and Health, *Macroeconomics and Health*.

Third, despite significant theoretical disagreements (Tables [15.3], [15.4]), many of the most important current initiatives to promote global health can be supported by all four views (Table [15.5]). An "overlapping consensus"[61] at the level of policy can thus be upheld from a variety of moral perspectives and by way of diverging views about the importance of national borders.

Our analysis has two important limitations. First, as this argument was developed through a review of the work of four contemporary philosophers, our conclusions reflect the frameworks selected for inclusion and the specific interpretations given these theories. Our selection of theories was careful and purposive, and we believe that they do represent the most important viewpoints in contemporary discussions of justice. Moreover, although limitations of space prevent us from undertaking a demonstration, we believe that the overwhelming majority of contemporary theories of justice could support a similar justification for action on global health. While we acknowledge the existence of viewpoints that might not support our conclusions, we wish to underscore the remarkable degree of support for current global health interventions among prominent competing frameworks.

Second, given the inherently controversial nature of ethical choices, a separate challenge relates to the value of pursuing a normative approach. One might ask, would it not be preferable to base the argument on pragmatic reasons for action such as enlightened self-interest, or protection of common interests? Pragmatic reasons offer extremely important sources of motivation in many instances. However, our self-interest is not always served by doing what is right. The current global situation has clear winners and losers. To the extent that the contemporary state of global health reflects "a toxic combination of poor social policies and programmes, unfair economic arrangements, and bad politics,"[62] the remedy cannot come from the powerless.

The MDGs represent a landmark pledge of solidarity on the part of the international community towards the global poor. As the target date for their fulfilment approaches, recent crises related to instability in financial markets and in food and commodity prices, as well as environmental change, threaten to undermine hard-won gains in health and prosperity while jeopardising future availability of overseas development assistance (ODA). ODA is only one of many policy channels affecting global health and development [38]; however, it plays a crucial role.[63] Choices made by the citizens and governments of the wealthy nations in the next short while will be particularly decisive. The overlapping normative consensus we have identified in favour of action on global health is undoubtedly fragile; yet, it resonates with the broad based public support enjoyed by key global health initiatives. We are hopeful that an informed dialogue on ethics can enable individuals and governments to find a more reasoned basis for their views. The most effective resource of the global poor may be a transformation of moral vision on the part of the powerful.[64]

Abbreviations

AIDS: Acquired Immune Deficiency Syndrome; DAH: International Development Assistance for Health; G8: Group of Eight Countries; HIV: Human Immunodeficiency Virus; MDGs: Millennium Development Goals; ODA: Overseas Development Assistance; TRIPS: Trade Related Intellectual Property Rights; WTO: World Trade Organization.

[61] J. Rawls, *Political Liberalism* (Columbia University Press, 2005).

[62] T. Addison, C. Arndt, and F. Tarp, "The Triple Crisis and the Global Aid Architecture," *African Development Review* 23, no. 4 (2011): pp. 461–478.

[63] Ibid.

[64] Pogge, *World Poverty and Human Rights.*

Competing interests

The authors declare that they have no competing interests, financial or otherwise, in completion of this work. MJ collaborates on a pro bono basis with the World Health Organization (WHO), the GAVI Alliance, and the Global Fund to Fight AIDS, Tuberculosis and Malaria (GFATM), and has received research funding from GFATM and WHO unrelated to this project. RC has no relationships to disclose. On a pro bono basis, AJD has collaborated with WHO in the past, and is a current member of the Research Ethics Board of Médecins Sans Frontières (MSF) and the Public and Political Support Working Group for the Decade of Vaccines Collaboration. He has received research support from the Bill and Melinda Gates Foundation unrelated to this project. TS coordinated the Globalization Knowledge Network of the WHO Commission on Social Determinants Of Health (CSDH) with funding from the International Affairs Directorate, Health Canada. The authors assume sole responsibility for the opinions expressed in this work.

Authors' contributions

MJ conceived the study and drafted the manuscript. RC and AJD contributed to conception and design of the study, drafting of the manuscript, and critical revision of the manuscript for important intellectual content. TS contributed to conception and design of the study and revision of the manuscript for important intellectual content. All authors have approved the final version.

Acknowledgments

Salary support for MJ was provided by the Canadian Institutes of Health Research (CIHR) in the form of a New Investigator Award. Partial support for TS's work on this paper was provided via CIHR research Grant No. 79153. The study sponsor played no role in study design, interpretation of data, writing of the report, or in the decision to submit the paper for publication. The authors would like to thank participants and fellow panellists at the session on "Global Health Equity" at the 2009 Canadian Conference on International Health (CCIH), and the workshop on "Health and Justice" at the 2011 International Studies Association (ISA) Annual Convention "Global Governance: Political Authority In Transition." The paper has benefitted greatly from the comments of Daniel Wikler, Alan Whiteside, and three outstanding anonymous reviewers.

EXCERPT 2

Abridged text from:

E. Ollila, "Global Health Priorities—Priorities of the Wealthy?," *Globalization and Health* 1, no. 6 (2005).

Global Health Priorities: Priorities of the Wealthy?

Eeva Ollila

. . .

Global Health Policy Actors

The major actors in global health policy are changing. New actors are entering and old ones are losing power; the overall change has seen a shift from global nation-based health-policy-making structures towards more diversity that puts emphasis on private sector actors. In the 1980s and 1990s there was a shift in global health policy making from the UN agencies towards financial institutions. This shift has meant increasing attention being given to involving private actors in health policy[1,2,3,4] . . . This development was partly due to the declining levels of development assistance of the OECD (Organisation for Economic Co-operation and Development) countries to the UN. . . .

In the UN forums, civil society has become recognized as an important body of actors in global policy-making. . . . Recently the public health NGOs have been important, for example, in shaping pharmaceutical policies and emphasising the needs and rights of HIV-infected people. . . .

Development aid to health has continued to grow substantially since 1992 despite the fall in total official development assistance (ODA) since that time. The USA provides about one third of the total bilateral aid to health. . . . The multilateral agencies provide one third of the total official development assistance to health.[5] As a new funding source, the Global Health programme of the Bill and Melinda Gates Foundation (BMGF) has become not only significant in size, but also in setting health policy. . . .

During the past decade, the USA has been active in lifting global health issues in new forums, such as the G8. The USA was also instrumental in the creation of the GFATM, towards which the EU, for instance, was initially more critical. . . .

Global Health Priorities

. . .

Millennium Development Goals (MDGs)[6] are a product of consultations between international agencies, but were also adopted by the United Nations (UN) General Assembly in September 2001 as part of the road map for implementing the substantially broader Millennium Declaration, which it had adopted in September 2000.[7]

---

[1] M. Koivusalo and E. Ollila, *Making a Healthy World: Agencies, Actors, and Policies in International Health* (London: Zek Books, 1997).

[2] E. Ollila, "Restructuring Global Health Policy Making: The Role of Global Public-Private Partnerships," in *Commercialization of Health Care: Global and Local Dynamics and Policy Responses*, edited by M. Mcintosh and M. Koivusalo (Palgrave Macmillan, 2005).

[3] M. Koivusalo, "The Impact on WTO Trade Agreements on Health and Development Policies," in *Global Social Governance. Themes and Prospects*, edited by B. Deacon, et al. (Helsinki: Ministry of Foreign Affairs of Finland, 2003).

[4] J. Lethbridge, "International Finance Corporate (IFC) Health Care Policy Briefing," *Global Social Policy* 2, no. 3 (2002): pp. 349–353.

[5] OECD, "Recent Trends in Official Development Assistance to Health," 2000, http://www.oecd.org/dataoecd/22/31/25503059.pdf.

[6] United Nations, "Road Map Towards the Implementation of the United Nations Millennium Declaration. Report of the Secretary-General," 2001.

[7] United Nations General Assembly, "United Nations Millennium Declaration. Resolution," 2000.

The MDGs have eight goals, three of which are health-focussed, namely those on child mortality, maternal health, and HIV/AIDS, malaria and other diseases.

The UN-led Millennium Project, directed by the economist Jeffrey Sachs, has the objective of ensuring that all developing countries meet the MDGs. The whole UN system has since been requested to adapt to addressing the MDGs, and to report to the Secretary General on their achievements in that direction. For health policies, this has meant, for example, pressures from some of the member states, such as the UK, for the WHO to refocus its work on the MDGs, most notably to the goal concerning HIV/AIDS, malaria and tuberculosis, while its wider mandate as the normative health organisation that sets norms and standards and promotes the building up a wider health systems would not be so emphasised.[8] The MDGs have become an important tool to steer both the UN system towards a narrower agenda with more emphasis on selected interventions and country presences. . . .

Development aid for health is also largely steered towards tackling communicable infectious.[9] USAID has financed population programmes, including family planning, for three decades, while its emphasis on health issues is more recent. In 2002, the USAID population, health, and nutrition funding covered HIV/AIDS, family planning/reproductive health, child survival/maternal health, and infectious diseases.[10] The BMGF has provided strategic funding for the founding of new structures for global health policy making—such as GAVI and GAIN. . . Its Global Health programme focuses on infectious disease prevention, vaccine research and development, and reproductive and child health, with emphasis on the development and implementation of technologies, though recurrent costs or chronic conditions are not financed[11]. . . .

According to global mortality and burden-of-disease calculations, the above-set priorities indeed represent the majority of deaths and ill-health in sub-Saharan Africa,[12] but do not represent the majority of ill-health in any other region. They cover less that a third of the global ill-health.[13,14] Today, non-communicable diseases are a cause of the majority of ill-health in developing countries, and their importance is increasing rapidly. They affect all socioeconomic groups and in many cases the risks are biggest in the poorest sections of the populations.[15]

. . .

The lists of the current global health priorities can be seen as reflecting health-related problems in the developing countries that are perceived to threaten the vital interests of industrialised countries. Linking national interests to development aid is by no means new. In the 1970s, such concerns were central in, for example, the argumentation for population programme implementation.[16,17] Nevertheless, it is noteworthy that since the mid-1990s the arguments for a greater US engagement in global health have been expressed increasingly

[8] R. Horton, "WHO's Mandate: A Damaging Reinterpretation Is Taking Place," *Lancet* 360, no. 9338 (2002): pp. 960–961.

[9] D. Yach, et al., "The Global Burden of Chronic Diseases: Overcoming Impediments to Prevention and Control," *Journal of the American Medical Association* 291, no. 21 (2004): pp. 2616–2622.

[10] USAID, "Total Population, Health and Nutrition Funding," 2002, http://www.usaid.gov/our_work/global_health/home/Funding/index.html.

[11] Bill and Melinda Gates Foundation, "Global Health Programme Fact Sheet," http://www.gatesfoundation.org/GlobalHealth/RelatedInfo/GlobalHealthFactSheet-021201.htm.

[12] World Health Organization, *World Health Report 2002. Reducing Risks, Promoting Healthy Life* (Geneva: WHO, 2002).

[13] Commission on Macroeconomics and Health, "Macroeconomics and Health: Investing in Health for Economic Development," 2001.

[14] WHO, *World Health Report 2002.*

[15] Yach, "The Global Burden of Chronic Diseases."

[16] S. Grimes, "From Population Control to "Reproductive Rights": Ideological Influences in Population Policy," *Third World Quarterly* 19, no. 3 (1998): pp. 375–393.

[17] National Security Council, "National Security Memorandum 200," 1974.

in terms of national interests or enlightened self-interest.[18,19]

The joint strategic plan of the US Department of State and the US Agency for International Development (USAID) for the fiscal years 2004–2009 states that US foreign policy and development policy are fully aligned to advance the National Security Strategy. The strategy sets out its mission as being to create a more secure, democratic and prosperous world for the benefit of the American people and the international community. The purpose of the Strategy is to help American business succeed in foreign markets and help developing countries create conditions for investment and trade.[20] . . .

Approaches for Improved Global Health

Health policy-making has become increasingly fragmented and verticalized, with the increasing emphases on selected interventions, the increasing number of partnerships and especially because of the founding of new entities for various health issues. Little emphasis has been put on comprehensive infrastructure building. These trends are in contrast to the stated aims of integrating health policy making with the broader development agenda or with comprehensive health sector planning.

An emphasis on innovations and innovative approaches encourages the use of new technologies and the building of new structures. Problems of unsustainability and inequity have arisen with the high levels of funding required, an emphasis on fast results, and the construction of new structures both at global and national levels[21,22,23,24]. . . .

The inclusion of business as an integral part of public policy making may weaken the vital role of the public sector in norm and standard setting and monitoring, as the public sector has been made an equal partner with business, sharing a common purpose and tasks. The WHO collaboration with business has caused harm to the credibility of the WHO's normative functions.[25,26,27,28,29] The legally independent global PPPs are structured so that public bodies with normative functions hold seats in the policy-making bodies together with business representatives both at global and national levels. This "forced marriage" within the legally independent PPPs may harm not only the credibility of the normative functions of the regulators, but also the normative functions as such. . . .

---

[18] I. Kickbusch, "Influence and Opportunity: Reflections on the US Role in Global Public Health," *Health Affairs (Millwood)* 21, no. 6 (2002): pp. 131–141.

[19] M. Koivusalo and E. Ollila, "Digest," *Global Social Policy* 1 (2001).

[20] US Department of State and US Agency for International Development, "Security, Democracy, Prosperity. Strategic Plan Fiscal Years 2004–2009," 2003, http://www.state.gov/m/rm/rls/dosstrat/2004/.

[21] Ollila, "Restructuring Global Health Policy Making."

[22] A. Hardon, "Immunization for All? A Critical Look at the First GAVI Partners Meeting," *HAI-Lights* 6, no. 1 (2000).

[23] G. Yamey, "Faltering Steps Towards Partnerships," *British Medical Journal* 325, no. 7374 (2002): pp. 1236–1240.

[24] P. Poore, "The Global Fund to Fight Aids, Tuberculosis and Malaria (GFATM)," *Health Policy Planning* 19 (2004): pp. 52–53.

[25] J. Richter, *Public-Private Partnerships and International Health Policy-Making. How Can Public Interests Be Safeguarded?* (Helsinki: Ministry of Foreign Affairs of Finland, 2004).

[26] A. Chetley, *A Healthy Business?: World Health and the Pharmaceutical Industry* (Zed Books, 1990).

[27] A. Hardon, "Consumers Versus Producers: Power Play Behind the Scenes," in *Drugs Policy in Developing Countries*, edited by N. Kanji, et al. (London and New Jersey: Zed Books, 1992).

[28] C. Kopp, "WHO Industry Partnership on the Hot Seat," *British Medical Journal* 321 (2000): p. 958.

[29] L. Hayes, "Industry's Growing Influence at the WHO," 2001, http://www.globalpolicy.org/reform/2001/0223who.htm.

Conclusion

While globalisation increases the risk that infectious diseases travel from South to North, it has also increased the risk that major risk factors for non-communicable diseases travel from North to South. Currently, global public health policies are concentrated on selected conditions around infectious diseases and on the technological solutions for them. Addressing infectious diseases in the South is important. However, other health matters are increasingly being left for private actors to deal with. Addressing the most important risk factors of non-communicable diseases, namely tobacco, alcohol and unhealthy foods, would benefit from normative actions, including restrictions on trade and marketing.[30] Simultaneously, global health policy making is increasingly aligned with industrial and trade policies, and is being done hand in hand with business, thus weakening the firewalls necessary for effective regulation and normative actions both at global and national levels.

Acknowledgments

I would like to thank Mark Phillips for editing the language, as well as the editors and the anonymous reviewers for their comments on the earlier draft.

---

[30] Yach, "The Global Burden of Chronic Diseases."

EXCERPT 3

Abridged text from:

W. J. Fallon and H. D. Gayle, *Report of the CSIS Commission on Smart Global Health Policy: A Healthier, Safer, and More Prosperous World* (Washington, DC: CSIS, 2010).

Report of CSIS Commission on Smart Global Health Policy

CSIS Commission

Synopsis

"We have before us the chance to accelerate our recent historic successes in advancing global health. If Americans seize this moment, take the long strategic view, make the commitment—with our friends and allies—the lives of millions will be lifted in the coming decades. The world will be safer and healthier. Our nation will have shown its best."

—Helene D. Gayle

As the United States applies smart power to advance US interests around the world, it is time to leverage the essential role that US global health policy can play.

Americans have long understood that promoting global health advances our basic humanitarian values in saving and enhancing lives. In recent years, support for global health has also proven its broader value in bolstering US national security and building constructive new partnerships.

A smart, strategic, long-term global health policy will advance America's core interests, building on remarkable recent successes, making better use of the influence and special capabilities of the United States, motivating others to do more, and creating lasting collaborations that could save and lift the lives of millions worldwide. . . .

And it will enhance America's influence, credibility, and reservoir of global goodwill.

The CSIS Commission on Smart Global Health Policy calls on Washington policymakers to embrace a five-point agenda for global health—a mutually reinforcing set of goals to achieve US ambitions and partner country needs.

1. Maintain the commitment to the fight against HIV/AIDS, malaria, and tuberculosis

It is critical that the United States keep its HIV/AIDS, malaria, and tuberculosis programs on a consistent trajectory, even in the face of a grave fiscal situation and competition from other worthy priorities. Today, more than 2.4 million persons living with HIV are directly supported by the United States with life-extending antiretroviral treatment (ART). Many others are ready to begin treatment. If we continue investing steadily in these programs, the Obama administration can realize its goal of funding antiretroviral treatment for more than 4 million people over the next five years; and our AIDS and malaria platforms can expand successfully into other health areas, in partnership with able international alliances like the Global Fund to Fight AIDS, Tuberculosis and Malaria.

It won't be easy. Over the past year, the pace of growth in treatment has slowed. Budgets have tightened. Concerns have mounted over the long-term costof treatment, especially if resistance develops to current medications. In this difficult climate, tensions have risen among global health advocates. But compassionate, realistic, patient US leadership can transcend fragmentation, ameliorate conflict across health constituencies, and ensure that immediate budgetary woes do not derail our efforts. We can leverage our existing disease-focused investments to create lasting health systems, with long-term solutions based on steady growth that reduce mortality and illness, and build partner country capacities.

2. Prioritize women and children in US global health efforts

The United States should move swiftly and resolutely to bring about major gains in maternal and child health, through proven models of care prior to, during, and after birth, and through expanded access to contraceptives and immunizations. A doubling of US effort—to $2 billion per year—will catalyze inspiring results. Direct US investments are best focused on a few core countries in Africa and South Asia where there is clear need, the United States can make a distinctive contribution, partner governments are willingly engaged, and there is a genuine prospect of concrete health gains and increasing country capacities. . . .

Closing gaps in the critical services and protections provided to mothers and children is a smart, concrete, and effective means to strengthen health systems and lower maternal and child mortality and illness. Affordable tools exist to reduce infant deaths in the first month of life; expanded immunizations can improve child survival; and expanded access to contraceptives can bolster women's health.

US leadership in collaboration with others will lift the lives of the next generation of girls and women, strengthen families and communities, and enhance economic development worldwide. It will also accelerate progress toward the major Millennium Development Goal (MDG) of improving maternal mortality, where efforts during the past two decades have yielded scant gains.

. . .

3. Strengthen prevention and capabilities to manage health emergencies

. . .

Meeting emerging threats requires long-range collaborative investments: building preparedness among partner countries to prevent, detect, and respond to the full range of health hazards, including infectious diseases; and creating reliable opportunities for poor countries to access affordable vaccines and medications that will be crucial in combating pandemics. . . .

4. Ensure the United States has the capacity to match our global health ambitions

In an era where much more is possible in global health, and much more is at stake, the US government needs greater predictability, order, evaluation, leadership, partnerships, and dialogue with the American people.

An essential step is to forge a global health strategy, organized around a forward-looking commitmentof about 15 years, careful planning, and long-term funding tied to performance targets. Such an approach could preserve our gains and provide the long-term predictability and time to achieve substantial progress in reaching our core goals: improving maternal and child health, access to contraceptives, preparedness capacities, control of infectious diseases, and means to address chronic disorders. Strengthening skilled workforces and infrastructure around these objectives typically requires 15 to 25 years. . . .

In the face of our current fiscal constraints, we will need to stay on course to fulfill the president's Global Health Initiative (FY2009–FY2014). Over the longer period, 2010 to 2025, a reasonable growth target is for US annual commitments to global health to be in the range of $25 billion (inflation adjusted) by 2025.

There is much to be gained if the administration and Congress both alter their practices to allow for multiyear budgeting of long-term global health programs, as well as for support of innovative financing methods. . . .

5. Make smart investments in multilateral institutions

The Commission recommends that the United States bolster its collaboration with partner institutions capable of achieving significant health outcomes: the World Health Organization (WHO); the World Bank; the GAVI Alliance; the Global Fund to Fight AIDS, Tuberculosis and Malaria; and traditional UN agencies such as UNICEF. The United States will continue to put a strong focus on its direct investments, since such a bilateral approach affords greater control and accountability and strengthens bilateral partnerships and goodwill, but multilateral approaches offer a vital and necessary complement. By pooling resources and efforts with others, the United States is better able to build health systems, extend the reach of vaccine and infectious disease programs beyond US partner countries, devise alliances to meet trans-sovereign challenges, and mobilize resources and leadership among our partners. . . . We need to look realistically beyond 2015 to the considerable additional work that will likely be required over the following decade to consolidate and sustain MDG progress.

Enhanced US leadership and engagement multilaterally will be crucial in three areas: finance, coordination, and strategic problem solving.

Finance: . . . The Commission recommends that the United States increase the share of global health resources dedicated to multilateral organizations from 15 to at least 20%. . . . The United States should press the World Bank to significantly step up its role in building health systems. . . .

Coordination: . . . There is a counterproductive proliferation of uncoordinated donor demands for data. This obstacle to efficiency, in part exacerbated by US programs, results in duplicated effort and wasted resources. TheUnited States could work more closely with other governments, donors, and organizations in support of strengthened national health plans aiming for greater efficiency and streamlined efforts.

. . .

If we pursue these steps, we can accomplish great things in the next 15 years

We can cut the rate of new HIV infections by two-thirds, end the threat of drug-resistant tuberculosis, and eliminate malaria deaths.

We can significantly expand access to contraceptives, which will substantially improve the health of mothers and their families.

We can reduce by three-quarters the 500,000 mothers who die each year in pregnancy; save over 2.6 million newborn babies from perishing in their first month of life; and significantly reduce the more than 2 million deaths of children under five years of age caused each year by vaccine-preventable diseases.

Using existing medicines, we can control or eliminate many neglected diseases that affect billions of people in the developing world.

We can help build the basic means to detect and respond to emerging health hazards and build a better system for ensuring access to essential vaccines and medications when severe pandemics strike.

And with US assistance, developing and middle-income countries alike can greatly reduce the premature death and illness associated with diabetes, cardiovascular disease, tobacco use, and traffic accidents.

Put simply, we can give global public health an excellent prognosis for lasting progress.

. . .

EXCERPT 4

Abridged text from:

C. C. Denny and E. J. Emanuel, "US Health Aids Beyond Pepfar: The Mother & Child Campaign," *JAMA* 300, no. 17 (2008): pp. 2048–2051.

US Health Aids Beyond PEPFAR: The Mother & Child Campaign

Colleen C. Denny and Ezekiel J. Emanuel

One of the George W. Bush Administration's biggest successes has been the President's Emergency Plan for AIDS Relief (PEPFAR).[1] Even the president's critics acknowledge the important benefits PEPFAR has produced, both for those countries most seriously affected by human immunodeficiency virus (HIV)/AIDS and for the United States' moral legitimacy and diplomatic reputation. It was accordingly unsurprising that the president used his final State of the Union address to call for a doubling of PEPFAR's funds. . . .

Yet doubling or tripling PEPFAR's funding is not the best use of international health funding. In focusing so heavily on HIV/AIDS treatments, the United States misses huge opportunities. By extending funds to simple but more deadly diseases, such as respiratory and diarrheal illnesses, the US government could save more lives—especially young lives—at substantially lower cost. Rather than inflating PEPFAR funding, the newly pledged billions could launch a new proposal program called the Mother & Child Campaign.

PEPFAR's Purview

In 2003, Congress appropriated PEPFAR $15 billion over 5 years to combat HIV/AIDS in developing regions. By September 2007, the program had prevented mother-to-child transmission for 10 million pregnancies, supported outreach activities aimed at preventing transmission to 61.5 million people, and provided antiretroviral treatment (ART) to 1.45 million individuals.[2] United States citizens generally strongly support PEPFAR, partly because of the devastating effects of HIV/AIDS—the disease claims 1.9 million lives annually in lower-income countries—but also because HIV/AIDS is one of the few major health problems the United States shares with the developing world, and because it primarily affects adults, who have greater economic and political power.[3]

Yet despite being "the largest commitment ever by a single nation toward an international health initiative,"[4] PEPFAR fails to address many of the developing world's most serious health threats. In lower-income countries, mundane but deadly diseases cause more harm than HIV/AIDS. Respiratory infections alone claim 2.86 million lives each year.[5] Another 2.2 million die annually from diarrheal diseases,[6] and 1.24 million and 1.6 million die from malaria[3] and tuberculosis,[7] respectively. Even though a few smaller government-sponsored initiatives do target some of these illnesses, such efforts pale in comparison with the sheer funding and attention that PEPFAR provides for HIV/AIDS.

[1] Office of US Global AIDS Coordinator, "The United States President's Emergency Plan for Aids Relief," 2008, http://www.pepfar.gov/.

[2] Ibid.

[3] UN AIDS, "Global Summary of the Aids Epidemic," 2007, http://data.unaids.org/pub/EPISlides/2007/071118_epicore2007_slides_en.pdf.

[4] Office of US Global AIDS Coordinator, "The United States President's Emergency Plan for Aids Relief."

[5] World Health Organization, "The Top 10 Causes of Death: 2007," 2008, http://www.who.int/mediacentre/factsheets/fs310/en/index.html.

[6] World Health Organization, "Water-Related Diseases," 2015, http://www.who.int/water_sanitation_health/diseases/diarrhoea/en/.

[7] World Health Organization, "Tuberculosis: Fact Sheet 104," 2015, http://www.who.int/mediacentre/factsheets/fs104/en/index.html.

Principles for International Health Aid

International aid is inherently limited; it is impossible to address all health problems in developing countries simultaneously. Consequently, it is extremely important to consider how this finite aid is distributed. The allocation of international health aid should be guided by 3 fundamental principles: (1) to save the most lives; (2) to save young lives in particular; and (3) to do so using finite resources most effectively.

Saving the most lives has intuitive appeal: There are clear ethical obligations to help others, especially to avoid death, and it is imperative to meet that obligation for as many individuals as possible.[8] This requires paying particular attention to the health problems inflicting the greatest burden on the greatest number of individuals.[6]

The focus on saving children reflects the particular need and condition of this population. Young children in developing regions have a proportionally greater disease burden than any other age group: 1 in 6 children born in sub-Saharan Africa dies before age 5 years.[9] Furthermore, while every premature death is distressing, death in childhood is particularly tragic, as children lose more future years and stages of life than adults. Additionally, the effort required to prevent these deaths is small: of the 10 million annual deaths that occur among young children, 70% are attributed to easily avoidable causes such as pneumonia, diarrhea, malaria, and neonatal complications.[10] Thus, children in developing regions likely represent the population most deserving of aid: a greater percentage die, losing more potential life, from causes that could be easily averted.

Because resources devoted to international health aid are inherently limited, seemingly economic considerations about cost-effectiveness actually reflect fundamental ethical principles. The more cost-effectively resources are used, the more lives can be saved.

Assessing PEPFAR

PEPFAR's strategy falls short of these 3 principles. Although annual mortality from HIV/AIDS is staggering, more lives could be saved by combating simple illnesses such as respiratory disease and diarrhea. PEPFAR also fails to focus on children: as Jones et al note, "levels of attention and effort directed at preventing the small proportion of child deaths due to AIDS with a new, complex, and expensive intervention seem . . . to be outstripping the efforts to save millions of children every year."[11]

Even though some HIV/AIDS-related interventions, such as condom distribution, are indeed cost-effective, other PEPFAR-funded interventions prove significantly less so. ART, for example, has a cost-effectiveness ratio between \$350 to \$2010 per disability-adjusted life-year (DALY) averted.[12,13] Increasing US spending on such interventions means that health needs unrelated to HIV/AIDS will remain unmet.

The Mother & Child Campaign

What is the alternative? . . .

The Mother & Child Campaign would focus on the health needs of those hit hardest by simple but deadly diseases: young children

---

[8] P. Singer, "Famine, Affluence, and Morality," *Philosophy & Public Affairs* (1972): pp. 229–243.

[9] United Nations International Children's Emergency Fund, "Millennium Development Goals: Reduce Child Mortality," 2015, http://www.unicef.org/mdg/childmortality.html.

[10] Ibid.

[11] G. Jones, et al., "How Many Child Deaths Can We Prevent This Year?," *Lancet* 362, no. 9377 (2003): pp. 65–71.

[12] A. Creese, et al., "Cost-Effectiveness of HIV/AIDS Interventions in Africa: A Systematic Review of the Evidence," *Lancet* 359, no. 9318 (2002): pp. 1635–1643.

[13] D. R. Hogan, et al., "Cost Effectiveness Analysis of Strategies to Combat HIV/AIDS in Developing Countries," *British Medical Journal* 331, no. 7530 (2005): pp. 1431–1437.

Table [15.6]
Treatment Options and Cost-effectiveness in Lower-income Regions

Annual Deaths in Lower-Income Regions	Sample Interventions	Cost-effectiveness Ratio, $/DALY[a]	Cost per Intervention, $	DALYs Averted for 1 Year of PEPFAR-Level Funding ($3 Billion), in Millions
HIV/AIDS				
1.9 Million total (280 000 in children <15 y)	Condom promotion and distribution	1 (for sex workers) through 99 (medium-risk women)	11–17 per infection prevented	15–3 Billion
	Prevention of mother-to-child transmission	1–34	20–47 per infection prevented	250–600
	Voluntary counseling and testing	18–22, 82	393–1315 per infection prevented	36.6–167
	First-line ART	350–2010	28038–185396 per infection averted	1.5–8.5
Respiratory illness				
2.86 Million total (2 million in children <5 y)	Community-based case management for neonatal pneumonia	1		3 Billion
	Treatment of nonsevere pneumonia at the facility level	24–50	2 per treatment episode	125
	Case management of pneumonia	62–87	3–6 per treatment episode	34–48
Diarrheal disease				
2.2 Million total (1.9 million in children <5 y)	Oral rehydration therapy	24–139	0.50–6 per treatment for a child	125
	Water supply and sanitation: hygiene education, program design, and regulation added to existing infrastructure	20 (1.67–140)	NA	150
Malaria				
1.24 Million total (848,000 in children <5 y)	Case management with artemisinin-based combination therapy	12	NA	250
	Indoor residual spraying of long-lasting insecticides	9–41	NA	250–333
	Insecticide-treated bed nets	11–41	5 per insecticide-treated bed net	176–273
Vaccine-preventable disease				
2.1 Million total (1.4 million in children <5 y)	Traditional immunization program (diphtheria, pertussis, polio, tetanus, and measles)	7	14 per fully immunized child	429
Tuberculosis				
1.1 Million (100 000 child deaths)	DOTS treatment of new smear-positive cases only	6–8	443–590 per treatment	500
	DOTS therapy plus therapy for resistant cases	11–15	465–460 per treatment	200–273
Maternal conditions and neonatal complications[b]				
529 000 Maternal and 4 million neonatal deaths	Community newborn care package	9	NA	333
	Antenatal tetanus toxoid immunizations	12	NA	250
	Iron and folic acid nutritional supplementation	13	NA	231
	WHO mother-and-baby package[c]	77–151	NA	20–39
	Routine maternity care[d]	86–125	NA	24–35

ART, antiretroviral therapy; *DALY*, disability-adjusted life-years; *DOTS*, directly observed treatment, short-course; *HIV*, human immunodeficiency virus; *NA*, not found or available; *PEPFAR*, President's Emergency Plan for AIDS Relief; *WHO*, World Health Organization.

[a]Data in this column were calculated using information from references 9-15.

[b]Primarily neonatal sepsis/pneumonia, preterm delivery, and asphyxia at birth.

[c]WHO mother-and-baby package with magnesium sulfate and active management of labor.

[d]Ninety percent coverage of prenatal care, normal delivery with skilled attendance, postnatal care, and treatment of sexually transmitted infections, syphilis, anemia, eclampsia, obstructed labor, postpartum hemorrhage, and sepsis.

and their mothers. Accordingly, the campaign would support efforts to prevent and treat diarrheal disease, respiratory infections, tuberculosis, malaria, vaccine-preventable diseases, neonatal conditions, and obstetric and maternal health problems.

Funding distribution would emphasize cost-effectiveness. For example, rather than financing treatments of neonatal jaundice ($652 per DALY averted), the program would first provide community-based care for neonatal pneumonia ($1 per DALY averted), nutritional supplements for anemic pregnant women ($13 per DALY averted), and insecticide-treated bed nets in areas of endemic malaria ($11-$41 per DALY averted) (Table [15.6]). Even anticipating start-up costs, these lifesaving interventions would prove considerably more cost-effective than some currently funded interventions. Emerging cost-efficiency data would be incorporated into future Mother & Child Campaign funding decisions, continuously refining the program to maximize benefit.

To appreciate the potential health effects, compare the available treatment options under the 2 programs. In 2007, $1.34 billion, nearly 50% of PEPFAR's annual budget, was spent supporting ART treatment for 1.45 million individuals.[1] For this same amount, the Mother & Child Campaign could vaccinate more than 44 million children against diphtheria, pertussis, polio, tetanus, and measles, and provide 134 million insecticide-treated bed nets to prevent malaria.[14,15] . . .

The Mother & Child Campaign also more fully meets the 3 evaluative principles. Addressing maternal and pediatric health works to save as many lives as possible by targeting 2 populations enduring much preventable morbidity and mortality; like young children, women of childbearing age in developing regions have a particularly great burden of disease.[16] The campaign also promotes children's health, both directly and by aiding mothers: motherless children are 10 times more likely to die within 2 years of their mother's death.[17] Moreover, the Mother & Child Campaign overtly considers cost-effectiveness in distributing finite resources.

It would be unethical and impractical to abandon or decrease programs developed under PEPFAR given fiduciary relationships, the threat of drug-resistant HIV/AIDS, and the devastation the disease wreaks on societal infrastructure. But the choices are not "double or nothing." Government pledges to vastly increase PEPFAR funding create new options for international health aid. By allotting these newly pledged billions to the Mother & Child Campaign, the United States could continue PEPFAR programs at their current high level while using the newly committed funding to launch a more cost-effective program targeting basic health problems. This would respect the continuing need for HIV/AIDS work while acting upon the moral, economic, and practical advantages of devoting funding to diseases afflicting mothers and children in the developing world.

. . .

[14] World Health Organization, "Choosing Interventions That Are Cost-Effective (WHO-Choice)," 2008, http://www.who.int/choice/results/en.

[15] D. T. Jamison, et al., *Disease Control Priorities in Developing Countries* (World Bank Publications, 2006).

[16] Ibid.

[17] World Health Organization, "Why Do So Many Women Still Die in Pregnancy or Childbirth?", 2014, http://www.who.int/features/qa/12/en/index.html.

EXCERPT 5

Abridged text from:

K. H. Onarheim, et al., "Prioritizing Child Health Interventions in Ethiopia: Modeling Impact on Child Mortality, Life Expectancy and Inequality in Age at Death," *PLoS ONE* 7, no. 8 (2012).

Prioritizing Child Health Interventions in Ethiopia: Modeling Impact on Child Mortality, Life Expectancy and Inequality in Age at Death

Kristine Husøy Onarheim, Solomon Tessema, Kjell Arne Johansson, Kristiane Tislevoll Eide, Ole Frithjof Norheim, and Ingrid Miljeteig

. . .

Introduction

The fourth Millennium Development Goal (MDG 4) calls for a two-thirds reduction in deaths of children younger than five years between 1990 and 2015. Fortunately, the under-5 mortality rate (U5MR) is declining in all regions, but many countries are still far from achieving the goal.[1,2] In Ethiopia, the second most populated country in Africa, the decline in child mortality after 1990 has been steeper than in several other sub-Saharan African countries.[3] Rajaratnam et al. estimated a decrease in U5MR in Ethiopia from 201.9 per 1000 live births in 1990 to 101.0 per 1000 live births in 2010[4]. . . . (See Table [15.7].)

Table [15.7]
Sociodemographic Characteristics for Ethiopia (1, 5–9)

Population Indicators	
Total population (000)	82825
Population aged under 15	44%
Life expectancy at birth (years)	59.3
Health indicators	
Total Fertility Rate	3.9
Maternal Mortality Ratio (per 100,000 live births)	590
Neonatal Mortality Rate (per 1000 live births)	35
Infant Mortality Rate (per 1000 live births)	68.5
Under-5 Mortality Rate (per 1000 live births)	101
One year olds fully immunized against measles	75%
Stunting in children under 5 years of age	47%
HIV prevalence rate	2.1%
Physician per 10,000 population	0.2
Development indicators	
Adult literacy rate (>15 years)	29.8%
Gross Domestic Product per capita (PPP $)	934
People living below 1,25 $ a day	39%
Human development index	0.363
Multidimensional Poverty Index	0.562
Income Gini coefficient	29.8
Health expenditure as % of GDP	4.3%
Per capita total expenditure on health (PPP $)	37

doi:10.1371/journal.pone.0041521.t001

[1] J. K. Rajaratnam, et al., "Neonatal, Postneonatal, Childhood, and Under-5 Mortality for 187 Countries, 1970–2010: A Systematic Analysis of Progress Towards Millennium Development Goal 4," *Lancet* 375, no. 9730 (2010): pp. 1988–2008.

[2] Z. A. Bhutta, et al., "Countdown to 2015 Decade Report (2000–10): Taking Stock of Maternal, Newborn, and Child Survival," *Lancet* 375, no. 9730 (2010): pp. 2032–2044.

[3] S. Accorsi, et al., "Countdown to 2015: Comparing Progress Towards the Achievement of the Health Millennium Development Goals in Ethiopia and Other Sub-Saharan African Countries," *Transactions of the Royal Society, Tropical Medicine and Hygiene* 104, no. 5 (2010): pp. 336–342.

[4] Rajaratnam, "Neonatal, Postneonatal, Childhood, and Under-5."

But the gap between those in need of care and those who in reality have access to care is large.[5,6,7] When the burden of disease is high and there are limited resources to invest in health care, decision makers face difficult dilemmas on where to invest their resources. To make these assessments, decision makers need valid and relevant information concerning the different alternatives and their distributive consequences as well as opportunity costs.[8,9]

However, we lack information on which services will promote rapid health gains and which services to prioritize in a specific country. As of today, models on possible impacts and costs of introducing new interventions and scale-up of interventions exist for larger WHO regions.[10,11,12,13,14,15] Contextualized models applying best local evidence give information that is more relevant for decision makers at the country level. Marginal Budgeting for Bottlenecks (MBB) and the Lives Saved Tool (LiST) are new analytic epidemiological tools for policy makers and researchers to evaluate the possible health impacts of scaling-up interventions.[16,17] . . .

This study aims to estimate the potential health impact of increasing coverage of 14 selected health care interventions targeting child mortality in Ethiopia. We also explore the impact on life expectancy and inequality in the age of death (measured by $\text{Gini}_{\text{health}}$).

. . .

[5] Bhutta, "Countdown to 2015 Decade Report."

[6] Central Statistical Authority, *Ethiopia Demographic and Health Survey 2005*, (Addis Ababa: Central Statistical Authority, 2006).

[7] M. V. Kinney, et al., "Sub-Saharan Africa's Mothers, Newborns, and Children: Where and Why Do They Die?," *PLoS Medicine* 7, no. 6 (2010).

[8] O. F. Norheim, "Healthcare Rationing: Are Additional Criteria Needed for Assessing Evidence Based Clinical Practice Guidelines?," *British Medical Journal* 319, no. 7222 (1999): pp. 1426–1429.

[9] R. Baltussen, O. F. Norheim, and M. Johri, "Fairness in Service Choice: An Important yet Underdeveloped Path to Universal Coverage," *Tropical Medicine and International Health* 16, no. 7 (2011): pp. 838–839.

[10] I. K. Friberg, et al., "Sub-Saharan Africa's Mothers, Newborns, and Children: How Many Lives Could Be Saved with Targeted Health Interventions?," *PLoS Medicine* 7, no. 6 (2010).

[11] G. L. Darmstadt, et al., "Saving Newborn Lives in Asia and Africa: Cost and Impact of Phased Scale-up of Interventions within the Continuum of Care," *Health Policy Planning* 23, no. 2 (2008): pp. 101–117.

[12] T. T. Edejer, et al., "Cost Effectiveness Analysis of Strategies for Child Health in Developing Countries," *British Medical Journal* 331, no. 7526 (2005): p. 1177.

[13] T. Adam, et al., "Cost Effectiveness Analysis of Strategies for Maternal and Neonatal Health in Developing Countries," *British Medical Journal* 331, no. 7525 (2005): p. 1107.

[14] D. T. Jamison, et al., *Disease Control Priorities in Developing Countries* (World Bank Publications, 2006).

[15] D. Chisholm, et al., "What Are the Priorities for Prevention and Control of Non-Communicable Diseases and Injuries in Sub-Saharan Africa and South East Asia?," *British Medical Jouranl* 344 (2012): p. e586.

[16] R. Knippenberg, A. Soucat, and W. Vanlerberghe, "Marginal Budgeting for Bottlenecks: A Tool for Performance Based Planning of Health and Nutrition Services for Achieving Millennium Development Goals," World Bank, UNICEF, WHO (2003).

[17] R. Steinglass, et al., "Development and Use of the Lives Saved Tool (List): A Model to Estimate the Impact of Scaling up Proven Interventions on Maternal, Neonatal and Child Mortality," *International Journal of Epidemiology* 40, no. 2 (2011): pp. 519–520.

Results

Increasing coverage of the 14 interventions to target levels in the Ethiopian HSDP IV could avert 114,600 child deaths by 2015 (Table [15.8]).

By increasing coverage to 90% of all 14 interventions, an additional 102,600 deaths could be averted (217,200 deaths averted in total). The five most effective interventions are: 1) institutional delivery, 2) oral rehydration solutions (ORS), 3) case management of pneumonia, 4) breastfeeding and 5) case management of severe neonatal infections. Together, these interventions account for 57.8% and 65.7% of the deaths averted in Scenario 1 (SC1) and Scenario 2 (SC2), respectively. . . .

Compared to the current U5MR, the reduction is then 32.6%, 58.7% and 44.4%. Ethiopia can therefore reach MDG 4 within a period of 5 years. . . .

Life expectancy at birth increases to 62.5 (+2.6), 64.2 (+4.3) and 63.4 (+3.5) by increasing coverage of interventions according to SC1, SC2 and SC3, respectively. This corresponds to a 4.4%, 7.2% and 5.9% increase in life expectancy at birth. Without scale-up of interventions, $\text{Gini}_{\text{health}}$ in Ethiopia is estimated to be 0.24 in 2015. Scaling-up to SC1, SC2 and SC3 levels would lead to a reduction in inequality in age at death ($\text{Gini}_{\text{health}}$) at 0.21 (20.03), 0.18 (20.06) and 0.19 (20.05). . . .

Discussion

. . . Scaling-up selected child health interventions can have great impact on mortality, life expectancy and inequality in age at death. . . . The MDG 4 target of an U5MR of 68 per 1000 live births is achievable. Our estimates provide support for giving priority to child health interventions in Ethiopia also in a broader perspective. . . . It is also important to note that prioritizing child health will have great impacts towards a more equal distribution of health in the population. . . .

Which Interventions to Prioritize?

Given budget constraints, policy makers in Ethiopia must deal with the tragic trade-off: should they opt for a package of a few very effective interventions at a high coverage rate, a large package at a medium coverage rate, or a mix of these packages? . . .

If the policy makers opt for a few very effective interventions at a high coverage rate, our results indicate that a package of institutional delivery, oral rehydration solution (ORS), case management of pneumonia, breastfeeding and case management of severe neonatal infection could have considerable impact on child survival. . . . A high-impact intervention such as institutional delivery will save five times more lives than insecticide-treated materials or indoor residual spraying intervention, but will also require more investment in terms of resources and funding than typical "quick-fix" solutions. Although policymakers might prioritize more comprehensive interventions when aiming at averting most deaths, other factors like lack of health workers, people's preferences or donor-driven priorities might force decision makers to compromise their overall strategy.

. . .

Extending the Results: Adding Life Expectancy and Ginihealth

Within the literature of disease control priorities, much attention has been given to lives saved and mortality reductions, as well as cost-effectiveness of interventions.[18] There has been less discussion of reducing inequality in age at death.[19] . . . We believe it is relevant to look at overall health outcomes in addition to child mortality rates alone.

. . . Our analysis shows that if fewer children (and their mothers) die prematurely, life expectancy would increase substantially. Further, our analysis shows that an investment in child

[18] Jamison, *Disease Control Priorities.*

[19] D. W. Brock and D. Wikler, "Ethical Issues in Resource Allocation, Research, and New Product Development," in *Disease Control Priorities in Developing Countries, 2nd Edition*, edited by D. Jamison, et al. (Washington, DC: Oxford University Press and The World Bank, 2006), pp. 259–270.

Table [15.8]
Estimated Deaths Averted from Scaling-Up Health in Ethiopia from 2011 to 2015

Intervention	Current coverage (2011)	Scenario 1	Deaths averted Scenario 1	Scenario 2	Deaths averted Scenario 2	Scenario 3	Deaths Averted Scenario 3
Institutional delivery	15.7%	65.0%	26700	90.0%	45900	90.0%	45900
Labor and delivery management[a]	3.1%	45.5%	11800	90.0%	21500	90.0%	21500
Oral rehydration Solution	37.0%	65.0%	26700	90.0%	42600	90.0%	52800
Case management of pneumonia	0.0%	17.0%	4200	90.0%	20800	90.0%	27000
Breastfeeding	49.0%	57.0%	2800	90.0%	17600	90.0%	18500
Case management of severe neonatal infection	25.0%	42.0%	5800	90.0%	15700	90.0%	20200
Antimalarials	8.0%	54.0%	8900	90.0%	12600	8.0%	0
Pneumococcal vaccine	0.0%	90.0%	12600	90.0%	12500	0.0%	0
Zinc for treatment	0.0%	62.0%	9900	90.0%	12000	0.0%	0
Insecticide treated materials or indoor residual spraying	42.0%	65.0%	4200	90.0%	8900	42.0%	0
Preventive postnatal care	5.0%	25.0%	2300	90.0%	8700	5.0%	0
Kangaroo mother care	6.3%	45.5%	4800	90.0%	8200	6.3%	0
Prevention of Mother-to-Child Transmission of HIV (PMTCT)	8.0%	76.0%	5700	90.0%	7200	8.0%	0
Improved water source	65.2%	98.3%	5800	90.0%	4400	90.0%	0
Measles vaccine	77.0%	90.0%	100	90.0%	100	77.0%	0
Total			**114600**		**217200**		**164400**

.... We model scale-up in three scenarios. Current coverage data (2011) are from HSDP IV and the Ethiopian Demographic and Health Survey (2005). The definitions of the interventions can be accessed through Appendix S1 and details about scenarios 1, 2 and 3 can be found in Figure 1.

[a]Labor and delivery management is a subcomponent of the institutional delivery intervention. doi:10.1371/journal.pone.0041521.t002

health will reduce inequality in age at death by up to 25.8% (SC 2). By studying $Gini_{health}$, we get information about the impacts on the overall distribution of health within the population. Our empirical analysis suggests that an improvement in child health would both increase life expectancy and reduce inequality in age at death, as there are many potential life-years lost when large parts of the population die prematurely. . . .

Acknowledgments

We thank the Ethiopian Ministry of Health for sharing information and plans. We thank Ingrid Friberg at Johns Hopkins Bloomberg School of Public Health and John Stover at Futures Institute for technical assistance and feedback on the LiST analysis. We thank the Global Health research group at the University of Bergen for valuable feedback.

Author Contributions

Conceived and designed the experiments: KHO, OFN, IM. Performed the experiments: KHO, ST. Analyzed the data: KHO, ST, IM, OFN. Wrote the paper: KHO, ST, KAJ, KTE, OFN, IM.

Further Resources

Relevant Organizations

Governmental

The US President's Emergency Plan for Aids Relief: Initiative to help save the lives of those suffering from HIV/AIDS around the world. Additional information can be found at http://www.pepfar.gov/

The World Bank: The World Bank is an international financial institution that provides financial and technical assistance to developing countries around the world. Additional information can be found at http://www.worldbank.org/

United Nations (UN): An international organization made up of 193 member states; it takes action or make recommendations on many topics, such as health emergencies. Additional information can be found at www.un.org

World Health Organization (WHO): The WHO is a UN specialized agency concentrating on health by providing technical cooperation and carrying out programs to control and eradicate disease. Additional information can be found at http://www.who.int/en/

World Trade Organization (WTO): Organizes agreements between its member governments in regard to goods, services, and intellectual property. Additional information can be found at https://www.wto.org/

Nongovernmental

Bill & Melinda Gates Foundation: The Gates Foundation is a nonprofit organization that works with partner organizations to tackle issues such as global health. Additional information can be found at http://www.gatesfoundation.org/

Center for Strategic & International Studies: A nonprofit organization focused on defense and security, regional stability, and transnational challenges ranging from energy and climate to global development and economic integration. Additional information can be found at http://csis.org/

GAVI: An nonprofit international organization that aims to bring together public and private sectors with the shared goal of creating equal access to new and underused vaccines for children living in the world's poorest countries. Additional information can be found at http://www.gavi.org/

Partners in Health (PIH): A nonprofit organization that aims to build health systems in poor countries by training local workers, in addition to building medical schools and residency programs. Additional information can be found at http://www.pih.org/

Literature

Chisholm, Dan, Kim Sweeny, Peter Sheehan, Bruce Rasmussen, Filip Smit, Pim Cuijpers, and Shekhar Saxena. "Scaling-up Treatment of Depression and Anxiety: A Global Return on Investment Analysis." *The Lancet Psychiatry* 3, no. 5: 415–424.

Daar, Abdallah S., Peter A. Singer, Deepa Leah Persad, Stig K. Pramming, David R. Matthews, Robert Beaglehole, Alan Bernstein, et al. "Grand Challenges in Chronic Non-Communicable Diseases." *Nature* 450, no. 7169 (11/22/print 2007): 494–496.

Dugger, Celia W. "As Donors Focus on AIDS, Child Illnesses Languish," *New York Times,* October 29, 2009.

Kaiser Family Foundation. "The US Global Health Budget: Analysis of the Fiscal Year 2017 Budget Request." http://kff.org/global-health-policy/issue-brief/the-u-s-global-health-budget-analysis-of-the-fiscal-year-2017-budget-request/.

Other Media

Bilheimer, Robert. *A Closer Walk.* DVD. Directed by Robert Billheimer. Bloomfied: Worldwide Documentaries, Inc., 2003: Explores the spectrum of the global AIDS experience, interviewing individuals who have been infected, doctors and nurses helping them, government leaders, and also NGO officials.

"Fiscal Transfers for Better Health—Podcast with Amanda Glassman and Anit Mukherjee."

Narrated by Rajesh Mirchandani. Center for Global Development, December 17, 2015. http://www.cgdev.org/blog/fiscal-transfers-better-health-podcast-amanda-glassman-and-anit-mukherjee: A conversation about global health and how focusing on health budgets in developing countries can improve health.

Paul Farmer, "I Believe in Health Care as a Human Right," *TED* video, 3:27, http://ed.ted.com/on/rqg025vx: Discussed is the death of individuals from lack of basic resources such as water and vaccines.

"United in the Fight Against NCDs," *World Health Organization* video, 6:17, 2011, http://www.euro.who.int/en/health-topics/noncommunicable-diseases/ncd-background-information/who-video-unite-in-the-fight-against-ncds: Features material from countries in each WHO region discussing the importance of investing in noncommunicable diseases.

Index

Note: Tables, figures, and boxes are indicated by an italic *t*, *f*, or *b* following the page number.